Colorectal Cancer - Surgery, Diagnostics and Treatment

http://dx.doi.org/10.5772/50593

Edited by Jim S Khan

Contributors

Nikola Kolev, Krassimir Ivanov, Valentin Ignatov, Anton Tonev, Shteryu Shterev, Tanya Kirilova, Tsvetelina Teneva, Elitsa Encheva, Robert Partyka, Georgi Ivanov, Alexander Zlatarov, Georgi Todorov, Vasil Bojkov, Ivan Shterev, C. Alberto Blanco Álvarez, Raúl Sanchez-Jiménez, Emilia Balboa, Francisco Barros Angueira, Angel Carracedo, Teodoro Palomares, Ana Alonso-Varona, Ignacio García-Alonso, Vicente Portugal, Jonathan Blackburn, Mario Sansone, Roberta Fusco, Mario Petrillo, Antonio Avallone, Paolo Delrio, Fabiana Tatangelo, Antonella Petrillo, Martina Perse, Syed Abul Hassan Naqvi, Syeda Farah Nazir, Hitoshi Okamura, Andra-Iulia Suceveanu, Laura Mazilu, Adrian-Paul Suceveanu, Zoran Krivokapic, Goran Zoran Stanojevic, Garrett, Fabio Cianchi, Fabio Staderini, Benedetta Badii, Syed Mudassar Andrabi, Jim S Khan

Published by InTech

Janeza Trdine 9, 51000 Rijeka, Croatia

Notice

Publishing Process Manager Sandra Bakic

Technical Editor InTech DTP team

Cover InTech Design team

Additional hard copies can be obtained from orders@intechopen.com

Colorectal Cancer - Surgery, Diagnostics and Treatment, Edited by Jim S Khan

p. cm.

ISBN 978-953-51-1231-0

For EU product safety concerns:
IN TECH d.o.o., Prolaz Marije Krucifikse Kozulić 3, 51000 Rijeka, Croatia,
info@intechopen.com or visit our website at intechopen.com.

Meet the editor

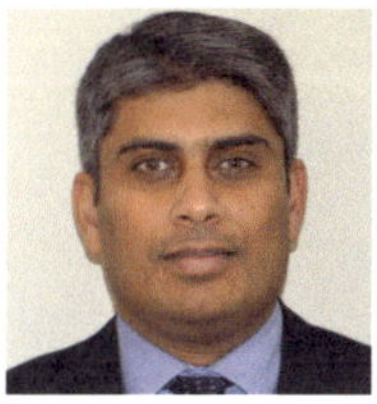

Jim Khan is a specialist colorectal surgeon with a comprehensive training in general, colorectal, laparoscopic and robotic surgery. After graduation in 1996, he specialised in general surgery and became a fellow of the Royal College of Physicians & Surgeons Glasgow. He completed his specialist registrar training in colorectal surgery in Wessex. He learned complex pelvic and rectal cancer surgery while working with Professor Heald at Basingstoke. His specialist colorectal training included the UK National Laparoscopic Fellowship at Colchester, where he received training from Prof Roger Motson in advanced laparoscopic pelvic surgery. Later on he was awarded a travelling clinical fellowship at Mayo Clinic Rochester (US). He has vast experience of laparoscopic surgery and his main practice is application of laparoscopic and robotic surgery for treating colorectal cancer and inflammatory bowel disease. He, in collaboration with Prof Amjad Parvaiz, has published and presented widely on this subject. At Portsmouth he is actively involved in medical education and clinical training. He trains on a variety of courses both nationally and internationally including basic surgical skills, laparoscopic skills, ATLS, TEMS, Laparoscopic colorectal surgery and coloproctology courses. He has been a national trainer for consultants' training in laparoscopic colorectal surgery (LapCo)—a programme run by the Department of Health for promotion of training in key-hole bowel cancer surgery.

Contents

Preface

Colorectal cancer is one of the commonest cancers affecting both men and women in the western world. Surgery has been the mainstay of treatment with 5 years survival rates between 80-90% for stage I and II and dropping to 40% for advanced disease. The last decade has seen significant developments in the diagnosis and management of colorectal cancer. Better survival and improved patient outcomes have been reported across the globe due to advances in technology, better diagnostics and improvements in adjuvant therapy.

It's extremely important for any clinician dealing with colorectal cancer patients to stay up to date with their knowledge of the disease, its behavior, management options and response to therapy. This book provides state of the art papers on some very important topics in the field of management of colorectal cancer. The chapter on screening critically analyses the different screening tests and also gives a comprehensive review of different screening modalities used in different countries. An update on MRI, PET and Ultrasound imaging for colorectal cancer is provided. Advances in surgical technology including laparoscopic surgery, single port surgery and robotic surgery are discussed in detail and the data from published literature & authors experiences are presented in a simple and comprehensible way for the readers. Section on adjuvant therapy covers the role of chemotherapy and radiotherapy very well, with particular emphasis on newer biological agents and targeted therapy. Genomics in colorectal cancer have been the focus of some significant research and this area has been covered very well by expert authors sharing their experience and providing useful insights into the topic.

This book will be an interesting read for any clinician dealing with colorectal cancer in their practice. This will also prove a useful update manual for any trainees in colorectal surgery, gastroenterology and radiology. I am grateful to all the authors for sharing their experience and valuable work and also would like to thank Sandra Bakic for her unreserved support in editing this work. Last but not least I am very grateful to my wife, Sadaf for providing me with the inspiration and help all the way along, enabling me to complete this task.

Jim Khan
Consultant Colorectal & Minimal Access Surgeon
Portsmouth Hospitals NHS Trust
Portsmouth, UK

Section 1

Screening

Chapter 1

Screening for Colorectal Cancer

Syed Naqvi and Syeda Farah Nazir

Additional information is available at the end of the chapter

http://dx.doi.org/10.5772/57506

1. Introduction

It has become an acknowledged fact that Colorectal Cancer (CRC) is a worldwide problem, with an annual incidence of approximately 1 million cases and an annual mortality of more than 500,000. Furthermore, the absolute number of cases will increase over the next two decades as a result of the aging and expansion of populations in both the developed and developing countries.

Apparently, CRC is the second most common cause of cancer related mortality among men and women in the world; so, most CRCs arise from sporadic adenomas, and a few from genetic polyposis syndromes or inflammatory bowel disease (IBD). The term "polyp" refers to a discrete mass that protrudes into the intestinal lumen. Therefore, the reported prevalence of adenomatous polyps, on the basis of screening colonoscopy data, is in the range of 18–36%.

The fact is that the risk for CRC varies from country to country and even within countries; the risk also varies among individual people based on diet, lifestyle, and hereditary factors. The most common neoplastic outcome of colorectal cancer screening is the adenoma. After having removed, patients need to be placed in a follow-up surveillance programme, very much similar to the patients with identified and treated cancer.

In the western world, we are very much aware that colorectal cancer has become an important health problem as each year, over 380,000 persons are diagnosed with colorectal cancer; bout half of these, patients die of the disease making colorectal cancer the second leading cause of cancer deaths in Europe. An estimated figure reveals that almost one million people suffering from colorectal cancer are going through cost – intensive treatments putting a huge burden on the healthcare system.

Screening is defined as population based testing in an asymptomatic individual to identify particular disease. The aim of screening is to lower the burden of cancer in the population by discovering latent disease in its early stages and treating it more effectively than diagnosed later when symptoms have appeared. As such, screening is a commendable method to reduce the burden of the disease. However, population screening targets a predominantly healthy population, and should therefore only be conducted after a careful consideration of both harms and benefits.

In 1968 the World Health Organization [1] (WHO) defined the first set of principles of population screening (Wilson &Junger 1968). These principles are still valid today.

The desirable features for community screening program for any disease are:

1. The disease should be an important health problem
2. Natural history of the disease must be known
3. The disease should be detectable at an early stage
4. Benefits of early detection should be there
5. Simple test should be available at early stage
6. The test should have high sensitivity and specificity and should be safe, effective, acceptable, inexpensive, and repeatable after an interval
7. Services should be in place to treat the early disease
8. Benefits of decrease mortality and morbidity should be there

Recommendation for action- general:

- Develop and disseminate structured educational programme for members of the public, providers, health-care systems, and policy-makers/political leaders. Effective educational programmes should be directed to each of the important participants in an acceptable manner.
- Develop evidence-based standards for quality throughout the screening process.
- Develop and disseminate inexpensive, easy-to-use clinical management systems.
- Advocate screening through national and local venues.
- Promote colorectal cancer screening as a part of comprehensive clinical preventive care.

Recommendation for action –Programme design:

Planning the screening programme:

- A target population should identify-asymptomatic men and women, age, risk factors (e.g., familial)
- The decision to implement colorectal cancer screening should be based on the relative burden of the colorectal cancer in the population to be screened.
- The screening strategy (test, interval, age range) should be based on medical evidence (guidelines), availability of resources, level of risk, and cultural acceptance by population.

http://dx.doi.org/10.5772/57506

- Support by influential professional and patient advocacy groups and from the media is essential.
- Evaluate the feasibility of the proposed programme. Address the development and allocation of the resources (financial, personnel, facilities).
- Evaluate the specific cultural and language needs of the population.

Implementation of screening programme:

- Identify the target unit for implementation, and ensure communication (training and education) with providers (general practitioners and others) and the target population.
- Develop and disseminate guidelines on screening, diagnosis, treatment, and surveillance in a patient friendly and culture sensitive manner.
- Develop methods for initial patient enrollment and follow-up.

Monitoring the Screening program:

- Careful, timely monitoring of following rates: screening uptake, re-screening, and follow-up of the positive test.
- Compliance with surveillance recommendations.
- Measurement of the programme quality should be in place, and evaluated regularly.
- Outcomes, including detection rates, cancer stage distribution, adenoma detection, complications, and finally, the effect on the population incidence and mortality.

2. Colorectal cancer risk assessment tools and referral system in different countries in the world

It is believed that colorectal cancer risk varies regionally according to geographical distribution of the population. As we will see in following sections, colorectal screening is yet to be implemented fully in general population of developed countries of the world. So in different regions, colorectal cancer risk assessment tools has been introduced to identify the high risk patients needs to be screened in general population of the society. Usually these risk assessment tools are for GPs and primary care units to identify the high risk patients to be screened.

2.1. Hamilton risk assessment tool for colorectal cancer

The risk assessment tool was based on work done by Professor Willie Hamilton in the CAPER studies (Cancer Prediction in Exeter), a series of case control studies which identified symptoms of common cancers that were presented to primary care and quantified the risk of cancer associated with them. The tool acts as reminder to GPs to consider the likelihood of an individual patient aged 40 or over having lung or bowel cancer given the symptom or combination of symptoms they present with. It is presented as three tables (colorectal cancer, lung cancer for non smokers and lung cancer for smokers) containing the risk values for each symptom in isolation or combination and is available as mouse mat or a desk easel so as to be easy to hand.

The parameter used in Hamilton risk assessment tool are: constipation, diarrhoea, rectal bleeding, loss of weight, abdominal pain, abdominal tenderness, abnormal rectal examination and haemoglobin <10g/dl.

2.2. USA National Cancer Institute (NCI USA TOOL)

A recent online tool for calculating colorectal cancer risk in men and women age 50 or older was launched, based on a new risk assessment model developed by researchers at the National Cancer Institute (NCI), part of the National Institute of Health. This new tool may help health care providers and their patients in making informed choices about when and how to screen for colorectal cancers and can be used in designing colorectal cancer screening and prevention trials.

So, by using easily obtainable information (e.g., personal and family medical history, lifestyle behaviours, and age), the tool provides an estimate of an individual`s risk of developing colorectal cancer over certain time periods (within five years, ten years, and over the course of lifetime). This risk-assessment model is first to provide an absolute risk estimate for colorectal cancer (i.e., the probability of developing colorectal cancer over a given period of time) for general non –Hispanic white population age 50 or older in United States.

In order to develop the risk assessment model, the researcher used data from two large- based case control studies. Several factors that have been previously associated with colorectal risk were shown to be predicted of a colorectal cancer diagnosis in those two studies including age; family history of colorectal cancer; consumption of vegetables; body mass index; cigarette smoking; use of aspirin or other non-steroidal anti inflammatory drugs; physical activity; use of hormone replacement therapy; previous history of sigmoidoscopy and/or colonoscopy; and history of polyps. Estimates of relative risk (comparisons of risk in one group to another) from the case-control studies were combined with population based data on colorectal cancer incidence from NCI`sSEER (Surveillance, Epidemiology and End Results) cancer registries to make the model broadly applicable in United States. [2]

"This colorectal cancer risk model should provide physicians and their patients a new tool to help in making informed decisions about cancer screening and other cancer prevention strategies. It may also assist policy makers in evaluating the usefulness of current and future population colorectal cancer screening approaches" said Andrew Freedman,Ph.D., lead author of the paper that describes the development of the risk-assessment model.

It has been observed that the majority of participants in the two case-control studies used to develop the model were non-Hispanic whites aged 50 or older, the researchers were unable to estimate relative risks for other age and racial/ethnic groups. However, there are plans to expand the tool to include these populations in the future. In addition, the tool is not applicable to individuals with certain gastrointestinal disorders (such as ulcerative colitis or Crohn`s disease), certain inherited genetic conditions, such as familial adenomatous polyposis or hereditary nonpolyposis colorectal cancers) or a personal history of colorectal cancer. These conditions are known to carry a high risk of colorectal cancer.

2.3. Asia-Pacific Colorectal Screening (APCS) score

From a development set of 860 asymptomatic subjects undergoing screening colonoscopy, multiple logistic regression was applied to identify significant risk factors advanced colorectal neoplasia defined as invasive carcinoma or advance adenoma. Odd Ratios for significant risk factors were utilised to develop risk score ranging from 0 to 7 (Asia- pacific Colorectal Screening (APCS score). Three tiers of risk were arbitrarily defined:0-1 `average risk` (AR); 2-3 `moderate risk` (MR); 4-7 `high risk` (HR). In this study performance of the APCS score in predicting risk of advanced neoplasia was evaluated

3. Current tests for colorectal screening and emerging screening tools

The following screening methods are currently used globally:

Guaiac-Based faecal occult bleeding test (gFOBT) is at present the most frequently used method in screening programme throughout the world. It detects the peroxidase reaction of Hemoglobin, which causes the detection paper impregnated with guaiac resin to turn blue. As it can react with animal haemoglobin, dietetic restrictions are necessary to exclude the false- positive results. A number of studies showed limited sensitivity of this test for both, advanced adenomas (11%) and carcinomas (13%). With gFOBT, a decrease in mortality for colorectal cancer by 15 to 33% has been proved.

Immunological faecal occult bleeding test (iFOBT) reacts exclusively to human haemoglobin, so no dietetic restrictions are seen as necessary.Taking and assessing the stool samples are easier than the case with gFOBTs, which may explain a higher participation in the target population. A wide range of qualitative and quantitative tests are available, with varying levels of sensitivity and specificity. The advantage of quantitative tests is the possibility to set cut-off limits; the most frequently used values are 75 or 10 ng/ml. The disadvantage of iFOBT is its cost. It is, no doubt, an expensive test as compared to gFOBT. But, presently, the price is approaching that of gFOBT for qualitative tests. As this test has higher sensitivity and specificity as compared to gFOBT, iFOBT is being increasingly used in screening programmes.

New screening methods include tests which examine the stool for the presence of abnormal DNA. Generally, these tests have higher sensitivity but lower specificity than gFOBT. They are expensive tests and a major obstacle in their implementation is their price. [3]

Flexible sigmoidoscopy is an endoscopic examination with maximum reach to splenic flexure. On the basis of emerging evidence---this is a promising screening test. A number of studies are under progress to accumulate enough evidence for usage of flexible sigmoidoscopy as a screening test based on WHO guidelines. Recommended interval varies from 3 to 5 years. A recent pilot study carried out in Darby UK* [36]. In the UK flexible sigmoidoscopy trial, 90% of all CRC detected at screening was found in the distal colon. According to one report by Sophie White et al from university of Sheffield, more than 60% adenomas are detected in left side of colon at screening age of the population and more than 70% CRC detected by flexible sigmoidoscopy at the screening age of the population.

Colonoscopy is another screening tool used in diagnostic and therapeutic endoscopic procedure which also detects lesion in proximal colon. It is more sensitive in detecting both adenomas and carcinomas. This is an established screening procedure for synchronous and metachronous tumours and surveillance of polyposis and non polyposis hereditary colorectal cancers. This is also a primary surveillance tool for multiple polyps according to guidelines. The risk of serious adverse events is higher than any other screening test with one in five hundred colonic perforation rate in expert hands. In spite of being gold standard, colonoscopy will not establish itself as an ideal population screening test due to its cost and adverse events and a lack of wide spread skills available.

Computed tomographic colonography (virtual colonoscopy) can detect lesions in the colon and rectum by reconstructing two-and three-dimentional images. To date, there is no evidence of reduction in incidence and mortality of colorectal cancer by this method in comparison with other screening tools. In cases, where caecum is not reached during colonoscopy due to patient related factors, CT colonography is the preferable screening tool to complete the examination. According to current NICE guidelines, the evidence of meta-analysis of data of 14 studies with a total of 1324 patients concluded that for CT colonography, the pooled per-patient sensitivity for polyps 10mm or larger was 88%, for polyps 6-9mm it was 84% and for polyps 5mm or smaller it was 65%. The pooled per-polyp sensitivity for polyps 10mm or larger was 81%, for polyps 6-9mm it was 62% and for polyp 5mm or smaller it was 43%. The overall specificity for the detection of polyps 10mm or larger was 95%. No significant complications were reported in the studies

Double contrast barium enema shows entire colon and rectum, although with significantly lower sensitivity and specificity than colonoscopy. The percentage of undetected carcinomas is upto 22%. This test is no longer widespread and in clinical practice due to its low sensitivity and specificity and availability of other better screening tools. Despite the fact, it still has a role in the areas in the world where colonoscopy and flexible sigmoidoscopy resources are severely limited.

It is quite obvious that Colorectal Screening is a complex process which in order to function requires the coexistence of number of factors such as a functioning invitation-reminder system, media campaigns targeted at the general public, the development of recommendations for general practitioners, patients compliance, sufficient funding, stratification of risks, and last but not least the election of the most suitable screening test. Among all available screening tests, only Fecal Occult Blood Test meets the WHO criteria.

http://dx.doi.org/10.5772/57506

4. Current global colorectal cancer screening pathways

4.1. Europe

Until 2007 Colorectal Cancer Screening was running or being established in 19 of 27 European countries [4] The target group contains approximately 136 million individuals suitable for colorectal screening (aged 50 to 74 years). Of this number, 43% individual come from 12 countries where colorectal population screening is performed or being prepared on either national or regional level; 34% come from the five countries where national population screening has been implemented (Finland, France, Italy, Poland and United Kingdom).

In 2007,gFOBT (which in 2003 was the only test recommended by the council of the European union) was used as the only screening method in twelve countries (Bulgaria, Czech republic, Finland, France, Hungary, Latvia, Portgal, Romania, Slovena, Spain, Sweedon, and United Kingdom). Colonoscopy was the only screening method used in Poland. In six countries, two types of the tests were used: i FOBT and flexible sigmoidoscopy in Italy, and g FOBT and colonoscopy in Austria, Cyprus, Germany, Greece, and Slovak republic. In the remaining 8 states, (Belgium, Denmark, Estonia, Ireland, Lithuania, Luxembourg, Malta, and the Netherlands), colorectal cancer screening has not been implemented yet. The age limit for target population varies across EU countries.

After 2007 Report, EU countries progressed toward the implementation of population screening programme. Recently, new EU guidelines for screening of colorectal cancers have been introduced.

In United Kingdom, a screening programme was announced in 2004 and initiated in 2006, with prospects of national coverage in 2009. It has been designed in two stages: with gFOBT tests at two yearly intervals with colonoscopy for positive tests. In 2007, the compliance was 52%. The program is carried out through regional centres falling under one of the five national hubs. The role of general practitioners is less significant here. [5]

The NHS Bowel Cancer Screening has achieved nation-wide coverage by 2010. The programme hubs operate a national call and recall system to send out FOBT kits, analyse samples and dispatch results. Consequently, each hub is responsible for coordinating the programme in their area and works up-to 20 local screening centres. The screening centres provide endoscopy services and specialist screening nurse clinics for people receiving abnormal results. Screening centres are also responsible for referring those requiring treatment to local hospital multidisciplinary team (MDT).

In Ireland, colorectal screening programme was launched in 2009 after National Screening Board Report which was published in December 2008 [6] A summary of the screening programme highlights:

- An immunochemical faecal occult blood test (iFOBT) is the primary screening tool for population-based colorectal screening programme.
- A target population for screening of all men and women aged 55 and 74 years with a screening interval of two years.

- Colonoscopy to be offered to those individuals who test positive with iFOBT

In France, Screening program was initiated in 2003, based on gFOBT tests at 2 years intervals with colonoscopy for positive result [7]. The role of general practitioners as coordinators is of crucial importance. The major advantage of French program is its good organization, with a call-recall system comprising central management at national level and individual steps taken by centres in individual departments. Asymptomatic individuals aged from 50-70yrs are mailed gFOBT tests, with the reminder at three monthly intervals for nonparticipants. Compliance in referred districts achieved 42%, and overall positive test rate was 2.7%. The screening programme has been generalised to the whole French territory since 2008.

In Italy, a nation-wide campaign was initiated in 2005; the implementation was entrusted entirely to 21 regional centres, including choice of the testing method. In Piedmont region, flexible sigmoidoscopy is the method of choice, in other regions iFOBT, with colonoscopy for positive tests. [8]

In Spain, the main obstacle to its implementation was the highly heterogeneous healthcare system, in terms of organization and insurance coverage in individual self governing units. That is why they are behind in implementation of screening program as compared to the UK, Germany, France, Italy and Finland.

In Finland, a structured screening programme was initiated in 2004. The target population, aged from 60 to 69 years (106000 individuals), was randomised into two groups. Individuals in the screening group were mailed a gFOBT test at intervals of 2 years. The finish program shows a high level compliance of the target population (70.8%), particularly for females [9]

Poland is the only state at the moment using colonoscopy as the only screening method, without the alternative of of FOBTs. An opportunistic screening programme was initiated in 2000, and by 2005, this had grown to 57 centres across Poland. The program is financed by ministry of health, independent of the overall healthcare system. The target population (Asymptomatic individuals aged 55-66 years) is recruited through general practitioners. High emphasis is placed on the quality control of the colonoscopies, with complications reported for 0.1% of the procedures, and no patient mortality. The advantage of the programme is through monitoring and evaluation, including monitoring of interval cancers. [10]

Germany was the first country to introduce a population screening program (in 1976) based on annual gFOBT for individuals more than 44 year of age. Since 2002, it has been offering participants a choice between colonoscopy at 55 year of age and FOBT at annual intervals between 50 and 55 year of age. After 55 year of age, examinations are carried out at 2 year, if the test results are positive colonoscopy is indicated. Those who undergo a screening colonoscopy with no neoplasia detected at initial examination are recommended re-examination at 10 years time if the first colonoscopy was carried out before they were 65. The positive feature of screening and data gathering is the emphasis on staging the disease at the time of its diagnosis. [11]

In the Czech Republic, CRC screening has many years of tradition. The country was the second in the world to start screening nation-wide, in 2000. In the initial years, gFOBT was offered to asymptomatic individuals more than 50 years of age by their general practitioners at preventative medical checks, followed by colonoscopies if tests were positive. Now both gFOBT and iFOBT are being offered. The implementation of the newly designed programme is supported by intense media campaign. [12,13]

Recently, the following EU guidelines for Colorectal Screening are published:

4.2. Australia

According to a recent survey, one in 12 Australians are likely to develop the colorectal cancers in their lifetime. [14] In Australia, CRC is second most common cause of cancer-related mortality. [15] survival from colorectal cancer is stage-dependent, yet fewer than 40% of individuals are diagnosed at a localised stage. [16]

In Australia, clinical practice guidelines for the prevention, early detection and management of colorectal cancer (the national guidelines) recommend that asymptomatic people classified as "at or slightly above risk" receive FOBT screening biennially, commencing at 50 years of age, with sigmoidoscopy (preferable flexible) consider every 5 yrs. [17]. Colonoscopy screening is endorsed only for asymptomatic people who are considered to be at "moderately increased risk" or "potentially high risk"due to risk features including personal or family history of CRC, adenoma and chronic ulcerative colitis. The recently re-funded National Bowel Cancer Screening Programme (NBCSP) offers one-off Immunochemical FOBT screening to people turning 50, 55 or 65 years of age.

Implementation of biennial CRC screening in Australia for all those aged 50-74 years could prevent up to 500 deaths per year, [18] with cost effectiveness comparable to breast and cervical cancer screening Programs. [19]

4.3. United States

In USA, men and women who are 50 to 75 year old should be screened for colorectal cancer in one of the following three ways; [20]

- A high-sensitivity faecal occult blood test (FOBT) every year.
- Sigmoidoscopy every five years and a high-sensitivity FOBT every three years.
- A colonoscopy every10 year.

Colorectal screening rates rose for both men and women. The rate for women increased slightly faster, so that the rates for men and women were about the same in 2010 [58.5% for men and 50.8%for women.The colorectal cancer screening was 58.6%, below the target of 70.5%.

4.4. Asia

In Asia colorectal screening percentage is at its lowest level and research revealed that colorectal cancer burden rapidly increasing in Asian countries [21]. A study to evaluate the cost-effectiveness of FOBT, flexible sigmoidoscopy and colonoscopy in Asian countries indicated that FOBT is cost-effective compared to flexible sigmoidoscopy or colonoscopy for colorectal screening in average risk population. [22]

The Increasing rate of colorectal cancer in Asia means that we need to take action immediately to prevent colorectal cancer and to diagnose the disease at early stages. The cost-effectiveness of screening programmes must be assessed in each individual country and research should be done to elucidate the epidemiology, genetic and environmental factors in development of colorectal cancer. [21]

5. Management of screening detected polyps

It is now widely accepted that the majority of colonic cancers arise from pre-existing adenomatous polyps (adenoma-carcinoma sequence).The supporting evidence being as follows: [23]

1. The prevalence of adenomas correlates well with that of carcinomas, average age of adenoma patients being around 5 years younger than patients with carcinomas.
2. Adenomatous tissue often accompanies cancer, and it is unusual to find small cancers with no contagious adenomatous tissue.
3. Sporadic adenomas are identical histologically to the adenomas of familial adenomatous polyposis (FAP), and this condition is unequivocal premalignant.
4. Large adenomas are more likely to display cellular atypia and genetic abnormalities than small lesions.
5. Distribution of adenomas throughout the colon is similar to that of carcinomas.
6. Adenomas are found up to one-third of all surgical specimens resected for colorectal cancers
7. The incidence of colorectal cancer has been shown to fall with long-term screening programme involving colonoscopy and polypectomy.

The patients who have undergone colonoscopy and had adenomas removed are at increased risk of developing colorectal cancer (CRC) in future, and therefore might benefit from colonoscopic surveillance. [24]

Surveillance Guidelines about colorectal adenomas are established by British Society of Gastroentrology. According to these guidelines surveillance of the colorectal adenomas depends upon ; number of polys, size of polyps and grade of dysplasia present in histology. Risk of colorectal cancer and adenomas with advanced pathology (>1cm or severely dysplastic) is greater. Risk can be stratified according to the findings at baseline and refined at each subsequent surveillance examination.

A Summary of surveillance guidelines [25] is:

- Low risk Patients with only 1-2 small <1cm) adenomas. No follow up or five yearly until one negative examination.

- Intermediate risk; Patients with 3-4 small adenomas or at least one >1cm.Three yearly colonoscopy until two consecutive negative examinations.
- High risk; Patients with >5 adenomas or > 3 adenomas at least one of which >1cm. An extra examination should be undertaken at 12 months before returning to three yearly surveillance.

The cut off age for stopping surveillance is usually 75 years but should also depends upon patients wishes and comorbidity.

Patients with incomplete examinations due to failed colonoscopies, for whatever reasons, should undergo repeat colonoscopy or alternative complete colonic examination (ct colonography). These guidelines are based on accurate detection of adenomas; otherwise risk status will be under estimated.

Large sessile adenomas removed piecemeal should be re-examined every three months. Small areas of residual polyp can be retreated endoscopically, for further check for complete eradications in three months. If extensive residual polyp is seen, open surgical resection needs to be considered. If there is complete healing of polypectomy site, then there should be sigmoidoscopy or colonoscopy at one year before returning to three yearly Surveillance. India ink tattooing aids recognition of the polypectomy site at follow up.

Stopping Surveillance.

The cut-off age for stopping surveillance is usually quoted as 75 years as the remaining life expectancy is likely to be less than the average time required for new adenomas to become malignant. After this age, it is unlikely that the benefits of surveillance will outweigh the potential risk of the procedure. However, this should not preclude further surveillance in a fit and motivated person who has a tendency to produce multiple or advanced adenomas at follow up.

The risk and benefit of adenoma surveillance needs to be balanced at all ages, particularly in patients who have significant co morbidity.

The decision to undertake each colonoscopy examination at follow up should depend not only on the number and type of adenomas, but also on the patient's age and wishes, and the presence of significant co morbidity. The Patient status should be established prior to attendance for each examination possibly by questionnaires.

6. Importance of audit in screening and screening relating colonoscopies

In any screening programme, as with any other medical service programme, adequate steps must be taken to ensure that the original objectives are being met and that methodology meets appropriate standard. The importance of maintaining the quality of screening programmes should never be under estimated. Evaluation, audit and quality control should be an integral part of any screening programme to ensure that it is achieving what it meant to be.

Colonoscopy is gold standard in important ultimate diagnostic tool in population screening programmes. Skilful colonoscopy with more then 95% caecal intubation rate is requirement for effective colorectal screening.

In the UK, before rolling out of the National Bowel Cancer Screening Programme, a large-scale study of colonoscopy practice was carried out. [26] The study demonstrated disappointing results with poor caecal intubation rates (76.95) and higher than expected complication rates. Since then there has been significant investment in endoscopic training, a quality assurance framework for endoscopic units has been implemented and National Bowel Screening Programme (NBSP) has been rolled out.

A nationwide audit of colonoscopy practice was conducted over a 2-weeks periods from 28 February 2011 until 11 March 2011. [27]. The study was performed prospectively, with the data entry occurring electronically through the purpose built website. All units performing >100 colonoscopies annually on NHS patients were included. Data on 20085 colonoscopies and 2681 colonoscopists were collected from 301units. Results showed 95.8% adjusted caecal intubation, 32.1% polyp detection rate, 92.3% resected polyps were retrieved and 90.2% o procedures achieved acceptable level of comfort. A total of 8 perforations and 52 significant haemorrhages were reported. Eight patients underwent surgery as a consequence of a complication.

The audit confirms that there has been significant improvement in performance of colonoscopy in UK since the last study reported 7 Years ago (caecal intubation rate 76.9%) and the performance is above the required national standard. But there is continuous need for assessment and audit of screening tools to keep the required national standard.

7. Colonoscopy capacity, training and accreditation

Most colon cancers are assumed to have adenomatous polyp phase. Therefore, colonoscopic detection and polypectomy provides the opportunity for cancer prevention [25]. So, colonoscopy is gold standard in high risk patients and patients with FOBT positive in population screening program. As we have discussed in previous sections, effective colorectal screening depends on available colonoscopy expertise in different part of the world

The aim of colonoscopy is to visualize whole of the colonic mucosa in order to identify pathology. A systemic review [28] of back-to-back studies has shown polyp miss rate at colonoscopy of 22% even in expert hands, especially polyps less than 1cm. Available data about polyp miss rates have shown a variation in performance between endoscopists, but this can be wider in very expert endoscopists. This shows that there is link between individual technical skill and polyps detection rate [29]. The single most important factor in the technique is withdrawal time after caecal intubation. The current recommendation is that colonoscopists should spend 6-10 minutes during withdrawal inspecting the colonic mucosa [30].

Skills in colonoscopy technique and coecal intubation rates are directly proportional to adenoma detection rate. In a standard endoscopy unit, single adenoma detection rate should not be less than 20%. Inadequate skills in colonoscopy can also lead to higher percentage of the procedure related complications.

In 2004, the largest prospective study of colonoscopic practice in UK revealed poor outcome in terms of completion and perforation rate, as well as deficiencies in all aspect of training. The guidelines on training have been published both in UK and the USA. [30-31]

Colonoscopy training and its accreditation is a challenging task. Structured colonoscopy training is lacking in most of the countries. The NHS Bowel Cancer Screening Programme (NHS BCSP) commenced in July 2006 and recruited expert colonoscopists to carry out colonoscopies in the programme. Owing to the known variability in colonoscopy skills, strict criteria have been developed for the accreditation of screening endoscopists to minimize the risk of the complications and inaccurate and incomplete examinations.

The Joint Advisory Group of GI Endoscopy (JAG) was established under the Academy of Medical Royal Colleges and now has a number of colleges and societies with an interest in endoscopy as members who are responsible for agreeing and setting policy and strategy and advising its constituent bodies and organizations (such as GMC and NHS)on standard and in endoscopy. The Jag office manages the administrative functions of the screening Assessor Accreditation System process on behalf of the NHS BCSP which is a web-based application process.

There are several advantages of this accreditation process, to both the unit and the individual endoscopists involved. Accreditation is an essential part of preparation for the implementation of local screening programme in UK. It also provides opportunities to demonstrate high level colonoscopic skills and improve the local endoscopy service. In addition it helps clinicians who wish to teach colonoscopy locally or on courses. The accreditation process leads to the Joint Advisory Group on GI Endoscopy (JAG) certificate of competency to perform screening derived colonoscopy.

8. Hereditary risk cancer and colorectal cancer screening protocol

Inherited bowel cancer comprises of 5% of the total colorectal cancers. Based on risk of Inherited bowel cancer population can be divided into three groups: Low risk group, Moderate risk group and High risk group based on family history. Approach for screening surveillance is different in three groups:

8.1. Low risk group

It includes the individuals with:

1. No personal history of bowel cancer: no confirmed family history of bowel cancer; or
2. No first degree relative (i.e. parent sibling or child) with bowel cancer; or
3. One first degree relative with bowel cancer at or above the age of 40 years.

In this group, the risk of bowel cancer may be twice the average risk [31] and there is no evidence to support invasive surveillance in his group [24]. These individuals should be explained that they are atonly marginally increased risk of developing colorectal cancer, and that this risk is not sufficient to outweigh the disadvantages of colonoscopy. They should be educated regarding symptoms of colorectal cancer, and importance of reporting if further members of the family develop cancers. And they should be encouraged to take part in the population screening for colorectal cancer.

8.2. Moderate risk group

Individuals are included in this category if there is:

1. One first-degree relative with colorectal cancer below the age of 45 without any feature of high risk group.

2. Two first-degree relatives with bowel cancer diagnosed at any age without any of the feature of high risk group.

In this group there is three to six fold relative risk of colorectal cancer. [31]. There is only marginal benefit from invasive surveillance (colonoscopy). Current recommendations are that individuals should be offered colonoscopy at 35-40 year of age (or at presentation if they are older), and again at the age of 55 years. [24]. Coecal intubation is mandatory, as neoplasms in individuals with a strong family history are often proximal; if the caecum is not reached, virtual colonoscopy should be performed.

8.3. High risk group

In this group, hereditary non-polyposis colorectal cancer (HNPCC) and various polyposis syndromes are included. Criteria for inclusion in this group includes:

1. Family member of familial adenomatous polyposis (FAP) or other polyposis syndrome; or

2. Member of family with known lynch syndrome; or

3. Pedigree suggestive of autosomal dominantly inherited colorectal (or other lynch syndrome associated) cancers.

In this group the individuals have one upto a 1 in 2 chance of inheriting a lifetime risk and more than 50 % chances of developing colorectal cancers. They must be referred to a clinical genetics service.

According to World Gastroenterology Organisation, the low risk group and population without obvious inherited colorectal cancer history are labelled as average risk population, while moderate rick and high risk groups are considered as one group with increased risk of colorectal cancer. Global screening guidelines cascades are established in 2007 based on these risk groups.

http://dx.doi.org/10.5772/57506

8.4. Lynch syndrome or Hereditary Non Polyposis Colorectal Cancers (HNPCC)

Lynch syndrome is inherited as an autosomal dominant fashion. It comprises of 2% of the colorectal cancers and is commonest of inherited bowel cancers. It is associated with endometrial carcinoma (30-70%), gastric carcinoma (5-10%), ovarian carcinoma in females (5-10%), urothelial carcinoma (5%) and others (small bowel pancreas and brain)< %5

Predictive genetic testing should be offered. These individuals should have first colonoscopy at the age of 25 years or five years before earliest colonoscopy in the family and gastroscopy at the age of 50 or five years before earliest gastric cancer in family. [24]. Colonoscopy and gastroscopy should be done two yearly.

Screening for extracoloic cancers in Lynch syndrome is available. There is little evidence of benefit. Recommendation varies from centre to centre, but surveillance is advised if there is family history of particular cancer. Recommended options for extracolonic surveillance [32] are;

- Annual transvaginal ultrasound, colour flow Doppler imaging and endometrial sampling.
- Annual CA125 level and clinical examination (pelvic and abdominal).
- Upper gastrointestinal endoscopy every two years.
- Annual urinalysis /cytology.
- Annual abdominal ultrasound of renal tracts, pelvis, and pancreas.
- Annual liver function tests,CA19-9,CEA

Familial adenomatous polyposis (FAP)

It is less common than Lynch syndrome. In FAP risk of colorectal cancer is 100%.

FAP is characterised by:

- Hundred of colorectal adenomatous polyps at a young age (second or third decade of life);
- Duodenal adenomatous polyps;
- extra-intestinal manifestation;
- Mutation in the APC gene at chromosome5q

If family mutation is known, at risk family member should be offered predictive genetic testing in their early teens. If this is not possible, then clinical surveillance is required. Usually, polys develop in teenage. Colonoscopy should only be performed in symptomatic children before teenage years. Otherwise annual flexible sigmoidoscopy starting at 13-15 years of age is recommended. If no polyps are detected, 5 yearly colonoscopy at the age of 20 years with annual flexible sigmoidoscopy in the intervening years. [24]. Flexible sigmoidoscopy should be performed carefully to avoid false negative results. Chromo-endoscopy is an option in doubtful cases.

9. Future research for improvement of screening programme

Although most of the screening programme based on research has shown improved survival in patients whose tumours are detected by screening, all population screening studies are prone to biases.

Selection bias arises from the tendency of people who accept screening to be particularly health conscious and therefore atypical of population as a whole.

Length bias indicates the tendency for screening to detect a disproportionate number of cancers which are slow growing, which thereby has good prognosis.

Lead-time bias results from the time between the date detection of cancer by screening and date when it would have been diagnosed had the subject not been screened. As survival is measured from time of diagnosis, screening advances the date at which diagnosis is made, thus lengthening the survival time without necessarily altering the date of death.

Because of these biases effectiveness of any screening can be assessed only by well designed randomized trials comparing disease –specific mortality in a population offered screening with that in an identical population not offered screening.

Initially three large randomized trials, using FOBT (Minnesota, Nottingham, in Funen Denmark) [33,34,35] showed reduction in mortality. These trials provided solid ground to initiate colorectal screening programme in western countries and US.

Randomized controlled trials are expensive and difficult to manage and may be ethically questionable in situations where control group is denied treatment for the condition in question. Despite this, UK National Screening Committee will only recommend the introduction of any new programme after assessing the findings of a properly conducted randomized controlled trial. The committee also keeps all screening programmes under regular review to ensure that they continue to perform in the way intended and continue to be effective.

9.1. Bowel cancer screening programme research committee

The research committee considers the feasibility and scientific value of research projects that arises from the screening programme in UK. It encourages collaboration between researchers and tries to prevent duplication.

The committee, chaired by Professor John Scholefield, meets quarterly and has considered over 60 research applications. The area of research considered by the committee included uptake/ acceptability of screening test, epidemiology/histopathology and screening technologies. Here we will mention some important research project in relation with screening.

9.2. False positive research study

A research project to investigate the causes of false positive results on Foecal Occult Blood (FOB) testing is now under way. The five year project, funded by cancer research UK is a collaboration between university of Oxford and newly formed NHS cancer screening programmes` Research unit, which is based in the university` cancer epidemiology unit.

The pilot studies started early in 2008 and the study will eventually involve over 200,000 screening programme participants, including about 2,500people with a positive FOB test result who are categorized as normal following a colonoscopy.

9.3. UK flexible sigmoidoscopy screening trial

This trial looked at bowel cancer incidence and mortality reduction 11 years after a single screening examination with flexible sigmoidoscopy [36]

It examined the efficacy and duration of effect of ;

- A once only flexible sigmoidoscopy screen between ages 55 and 64 years.
- Removal of small polyps (<10m) during screening
- Colonoscopy only for high risk adenomas.

170,000 people were entered into the trial. Cumulative incidence, including prevalent cancers detected at screening, was reduced by 50% for the cancers in the rectum and sigmoid colon, and 33 percent for bowel cancer overall. Bowel cancer mortality was reduced by 43 percent.

The trial concluded that flexible sigmoidoscopy screening-with removal of small polyps at the examination is safe and, when offered only once between the ages 55 and 64, confers a substantial and long lasting benefit.

9.4. HTA: Frequency of follow-up for patients with intermediate grade colorectal adenomas

Beginning in September 2006, this study examined the effort of extending intervals between follow-up colonoscopies in people found to have intermediate adenomas, as defined by the British Society of Gastroentrology guidelines. It is using data from hospitals ad from bowel cancer screening initiatives to identify groups of patients with intermediate adenomas. The risk of cancer and severe adenomas will be assessed according to the interval between examinations and the number, size and features of adenomas detected.

Firstly, the study will identify whether all patients with intermediate adenomas require surveillance; secondly, whether the intervals are of the appropriate length; thirdly, it should also demonstrate how many follow-up examinations are needed. Finally, it will determine whether informing patients they need to have colonoscopy distresses them or whether they feel reassured as a result. A health economist will analyze the cost to individual patients and to the NHS and compare these with any potential benefit.

9.5. NHS bowel cancer screening programme evaluation group

The NHS Bowel Cancer Screening Programme Evaluation Group reviews and develops criteria used for evaluation and monitoring the progress of the Bowel Cancer Screening Programme.

It Includes representatives from all the professional groups in the programme as from the Cancer Screening Evaluation Unit, the Health and Social Care Information Centre and Bowel Screening Wales.

10. Current screening percentage of at risk world population and future of colorectal screening

World Gastroenterology Organization (WGO), in affiliation with International Digetive Cancer Alliance (IDCA), launched guidelines for international colorectal screening programmes after indicating the low percentage of screening programme in place in different coutries of the world. In these guidelines, they emphasise the need of some kind of screening programme in place based on locally available screening facilities

As mentioned earlier, the risk for colorectal cancers varies from country to country and even within countries. The risk also varies among individual people based on diet, lifestyle, and hereditary factors. Colorectal cancer screening is particularly challenging, as reflected in current low screening rates in most countries where there is high risk for colorectal cancer. Colorectal cancer screening is complex as there are multiple options, it requires considerable patient effort (Fecal Occult Blood Slides, Colonoscopy Preparation etc.), and it requires sedation and health-care partner for some tests (colonoscopy). [37]

It is an acknowledged fact that the lowest screening percentage of on risk population for colorectal cancer is in Asia and Africa. In most Asian and African countries, National Health Care systems and Health Insurance cover only a minority of people. So, access to healthcare facilities is limited in many rural areas and communities of low socio-economic status. In Asian countries, there is little health authority support for colorectal cancer screening and very low public awareness for this emerging epidemic in Asia. [38]

For the screening programme to be successful, multiple steps need to be taken correctly, beginning from awareness and recommendation from the primary-care physician, patient acceptance, financial coverage, risk stratification, screening test, timely diagnosis, timely treatment and appropriate follow-up. If any one of these steps is left faulty or not of high quality, the screening programme will certainly fail. (WGO)

10.1. International colorectal screening cascade

According to WGO guidelines, colorectal screening cascade consist of set of recommendations based on availability of resources in different countries of the world beginning with 1 (highest resources available) and ending with 6 (minimal resources available. [37]

10.1.1. Cascade Level 1

This is a set of recommendations for countries where high level of resources (Financial, professional, facilities) available.

http://dx.doi.org/10.5772/57506

For average- risk 10 yearly colonoscopies starting at 50 years.

For increased- risk patients more frequently two yearly or five yearly colonoscopies starting at 40 yrs of age.

10.1.2. Cascade Level 2

Recommendations are same as cascade level 1 but they apply when colonoscopy resources are more limited.

For average- risk once in life time colonoscopy at the age of 50.

For increased risk recommendations are same as cascade1.

10.1.3. Cascade Level 3

Recommendation are same as cascade level 1 but apply when colonoscopy resources are more limited but flexible sigmoidoscopy resources are available.

For average- risk flexible colonoscopy 5 yearly starting from 50 years of age with diagnostic workup with full colonoscopy in case of positive flexible sigmoidoscopy.

Recommendations for increased- risk are same as level 1 cascade.

10.1.4. Cascade Level 4

Recommendations are same as level 3 but they apply when flexible sigmoidoscopy and colonoscopy resources are more limited.

For average-risk screening flexible sigmoidoscopy once in life time at the age of 50 years. Diagnostic colonoscopy workup for positive flexible sigmoidoscopy or neoplasia depending on availability of resources.

Recommendations for increased risk are same as level 1 cascade.

10.1.5. Cascade level 5

Recommendations are same as resource level 4 but they apply when diagnostic colonoscopy is severely limited.

For average- risk population flexible sigmoidoscopy is recommended once in a life time at the age of 50 years. Diagnostic colonoscopy only when advanced neoplasia is detected.

Recommendations for screening increased-risk patients depend on colonoscopy resources available.

10.1.6. Cascade Level 6

Recommendations are same as for level 1 but they apply when flexible sigmoidoscopy and colonoscopy resources are severely limited.

For average -risk population, Faecal Occult Blood Testing (FOBT) should be done every year starting at the age of 50 years. The type of test used depends upon colonoscopy resources available and dietary habits of the population. The diagnostic work-up can be done either with colonoscopy, if available or barium enema, if colonoscopy is not readily available.

Therefore, recommendations for increased risk individuals are to identify them separately for special screening (level 1) and the decision depends on available colonoscopy resources. If not available, these people can be screened with average-risk individuals.

These guidelines are established considering a lack of resources in poor socioeconomically countries and can provide a base for the structured global screening programme. We hope the world will take measures to implement population screening programmes to save mankind from the cruel hands of colorectal cancer.

Author details

Syed Naqvi* and Syeda Farah Nazir

FRCS Colorectal surgery, RCSI, Dublin, Ireland

References

[1] Wilson JMG, JungerG (1968). Priciples and practice of Screeningfor Disease. Geneva: World Health Organization.

[2] Freedman AN, Slattery ML, BallardBarbash R, Willis G, Cann BJ, Pee D, Gail MH, and Pfeiffer RM. A Colorectal Cancer Risk Prediction Tool for White Men and Women Without Known Susceptibility. JCO. Online December 29, 2008.

[3] Ahlquist DA, Sargent Dj, Loprinzi cL et al. Stool DNA and occult blood testing for screen detection of colorectal neoplasia. Ann Intern Med.2008:149:441450,W81

[4] Von Karsa L, Anttila A, Ronco G et al. Cancer screening in European Union. Report on the implementation of the council recommendation on cancer screening. First report ISBN 9789279089343.European communities (publ.) Printed in Luxembourg by services of European commission.Lyon:IARC Press; 2008.

[5] West NJ, Boustiere C, Fischbach W, Parente F, Leicester RJ. Colorectal cancer screening in Europe, differences in approach; similar barriers to overcome. \int J Colorectal Dis.2009; 24:731740.

[6] National Cancer Screening Services, recommendation for colorectal screening programme in Ireland. 3, December 2008

[7] Goulard H, BoussacZarebska M,AncellePark R, Bloch J. French colorectal cancer screening pilot programme. : results of first rounds.J MED Screen. 2008;15:143148.

[8] Zorzi M, Falcini F, Fedato C, Grazini G et al. Screening for colorectal cancer in Italy.: 2006 survey.Epidemiol prev.2008;32:5568.

[9] Malila N, Oivanen T, Malminiemi O, Hakama M. Test, episode, and programme sensitivities of screening for colorectal cancers as a public health policies in Finland. Experimental design.BMJ. 2008;337:a2261

[10] Regula J, Rupinski M, Kraszewska E, Polkowski M, et al colonoscopy in colorectal-cancer screening for detection of advanced neoplasia. N Eng J Med. 2006;355:18631872.

[11] Pox C, Schmiegel W, Classen M. Current status of screening colonoscopy in Europe and in united states. Endoscopy.2007;39:168173

[12] Fric P, Zavoral M, Dvorakova H, Zoubek, et al. An adapted programme of colorectal cancer screening – 7 years experianceand cost benefit analysis. Hepatogastroentrology. 1994:41:413416

[13] Zavoral M, Zavada Filip, Salek C, Czech society of gastroenterology: colorectal cancer screening in Czech republic. Endoscopy. 2006;38:7480

[14] Australian institute of health and welfare. Australian cancer incidence and mortality (ACIM) books. Bowel Cancer for Australia Canberra:AIHW, 2011. http://www.aihw.gov.au/acimbooks

[15] Australian institute of health and welfare. Cancer in Australia 2010:An Overview.Canberra :AIHW,2010 (AIHWCat No.CAN 56. Cancer Series No. 60. http://www.aihw.gov.au/publicationdetail/?id=6442472459

[16] National Cancer Institute.Surveilance epidemiology and end results. SEER Stat Fact Sheets: colon and rectum. (http://seer.cancer.gov/statfacts/html/colorec.html.

[17] Australian Cancer Network Colorectal Guidelines revision Comittee. Guidelines for prevention, early detection and management of colorectal cancer. Sydney: The cancer council Australia and Australian Cancer Network.,2005. http://www.nhmrc.gov.au/filesnhmrc/publications/attachments/cp106 0 pdf

[18] Pignone MP, Flitcroft KL, Howard K et al. Costs and cost effectiveness of full implementation of biennial foecal occult blood test screening program for bowel cancer in Australia. Med J Aust 2011;194:180185.

[19] Anderson R, Haas M, Shanahan M. Cost –effectiveness of cervical screening in Australia:what is the inpact of screening in different intervels or over a different age range.Aust N ZJ Public Health 2008:32: 4352.

[20] .Centre for Disease Control and Prevention (CDC). Cancer screening –United states. 2010 MMWR2012;61 (3):4145

[21] .M Amin P, increased burden of colorectal cancer in asia.World J Gasrointest Oncol 2012 April15;4 (4):6870.

[22] .Tsoi KK, Ng SS, Leung MC, Sung JJ. Cost–effectiveness analysis on screening for colorectal neoplasm and management of colorectal cancer in Asia. Aliment pharmacol ther 2008;28:353363

[23] Leslie A, Carey FA, Pratt NR et al. Colorectal adenomacarcinoma sequence. Br J Surgery2002;89:84560

[24] Dunlop MG. Guidance on large bowel surveillance for people with two first degree relatives with colorectal cancer under 45 years. Gut 2002;51 (SupplV):1720

[25] W S Atkin, B P Sounders. Surveillance guidelines after removal of colorectal adenomatous polyp. Gut2002;51:v6v9doi:10.1136/gut.51.suppl_5.v6

[26] Bowels CJ, Leicester R, Romaya C, et al. Prospective study of colonoscopic practice in the UK today:are we adequately prepared for national colorectal cancer screening tomorrow.

[27] OC007 The national colonoscopy audit : a nationwide assessment of the quality and safety of colonoscopy in the UK. Gut2012;61: A3doi:10.1136 / gutjnl2012

[28] Van Rijn JC,reitsma JB, Stoker J et al. Polyp miss rate determined tandem colonoscopy: a systemic review.Am J Gastroenterol 2006;101 (2):34350

[29] Rex DK, Cutler CS, Lemal GTet al. Colonoscopic miss rate of adenoma determined by backtoback colonoscopies.Gastroentrology 1997 ;112 (1):248

[30] Bond J, Winawer S et al. Quality in the technical performance colonoscopy and continuous quality improvement process for colonoscopy. Recommendations of US MultiSociety Task Force on colorectal cancer.Am J Gastroenteral 2002;97 (6):1296308

[31] Houlston RS, Murday V,Harocopos C et al. Screening and genetic counselling for relatives of patients with colorectal cancer in a family cancer clinic.Br Med J 1990:301:3668

[32] Vasen HFA, Moselein G, Alonso A et al.Guidelines for clinical management of Lynch Syndrome (Hereditary Non Polyposis Colorectal Cancers). J Med Genet 2007;44:35362

[33] Mandel JS, Church TR, Ederer F et al. Colorectal cancer mortality: effectiveness of biennial screening for fecal occult blood. J Natl Cancer cancer inst199;91:4347

[34] Hardcastle JD, Robinson MHE,Moss SM et al. randomized controlled trial of fecal occult blood screening for colorectal cancer. Lancet 1996;348;14727

[35] Kronborg O, Fenegar C Olsen J et al. Rndomised study of screening for colorectal cancer with fecal occult blood test at Funen in Denmark. Lancet 1996.;348:146771.

[36] Prof Wendy S Atkin, Rob E, Ines K H, et al.Onceonly flexible sigmoidoscopy screening in prevention of colorectal cancer: a multicentricrandomised control trial.Lancet, Volume 375, issue 9726,pages 16241633 8 May 2010.

[37] World gastroenterology organization (WGO)/International Digestive Cancer Alliance. Practice guidelines for colorectal cancer screening ; 2007.

[38] Sung J. Colorectal Cancer Screening: Its time for action in Asia. Cancer Detect Prev 2007;31:12

Section 2

Diagnostics

Chapter 2

Diagnostic Modalities in Colorectal Cancer –Endoscopy, Ct and Pet Scanning, Magnetic Resonance Imaging (Mri), Endoluminal Ultrasound and Intraoperative Ultrasound

Valentin Ignatov, Nikola Kolev, Anton Tonev, Shteryu Shterev, Elitsa Encheva, Tanya Kirilova, Tsvetelina Teneva and Krassimir Ivanov

Additional information is available at the end of the chapter

http://dx.doi.org/10.5772/57508

1. Introduction

Colorectal cancer (CRC) is the third most diagnosed cancer in men, next to prostate and lung cancer. In women it is the second most diagnosed cancer, next to breast cancer. In a time of limited resources in health care, there has been considerable debate which imaging modality offers the best non-invasive examination of colorectal cancer, offering both detection and characterization. The use of multiple diagnostic modalities is both costly and time-consuming. Clinical evidence amassed over the last several decades indicates that routine colorectal cancer (CRC) screening, compared to no screening, detects CRC at an earlier stage, reduces the incidence of CRC or the progression early CRC through polypectomy, and reduces CRC mortality.

2. Endoscopy

The first complete examination of the colon using a flexible fiber optic endoscope is reported by Wolff and Shinya in 1971 [42]. Nowadays colonoscopy is the gold standard for evaluation of the entire colonic mucosa with therapeutic capability of resecting detected malignancies.

In the last years the colonoscopy is the modality of choice to detect and correct the adenomatous polyps and colorectal cancer. The diagnosis CRC can be confirmed after biopsy in a known malignant pathology and by obtaining more tissue sampling and/or a second opinion from a consulting pathologist in none diagnostic, highly suspected colon lesion. Besides the role as a diagnostic tool in CRC, colonoscopy identifies subsequent lesions at the time of surgery, which is called preoperative endoscopic marking. It is performed through metallic clip placement and endoscopic tattooing.

The colonoscopic equipment consists of camera and four-way tip controls [43]. The camera can produce images of high-definition quality. The four way tip controls include (1) examination of a found patch to confirm an abnormal growth; (2) insufflating air to dilate the lumen for mucosal inspection and relieving air after examination, (3) irrigating a suspected region; (4) suctioning to avoid missing lesions under fluid, and (5) inserting biopsy devices.

The patient must undergo bowel preparation - taking clear liquid diet and ingesting laxative solutions for colon cleansing the day before examination. Sedation is needed to relieve the discomfort during the procedure, but it increases the costs. The complication of sedation are different cardiac disturbances such as hypotension, arrhythmias,oxygen desaturation, and others. The preparation with purgatives may cause abdominal discomfort, nausea, and other symptoms. The colonoscopy continues from 30 minutes to an hour. The risk during colonoscopy consists in colonic perforation in 0,1 % of cases. Colonoscopy fails to visualize the entire colon in 10–15% and it may miss up to 10–20% of polyps fewer than 10 mm.

Colonoscopy is golden standard for diagnosing of CRC but there are more symptoms which could be evaluated and appreciated by endoscopic examination, for example- abdominal pain, unexplained gastrointestinal bleeding, diarrhea of unexplained origin, chronic inflammatory bowel disease, etc. It is also the most common interventional modality for polypectomy, hemostasis, balloon dilation, foreign body removal, palliative treatment of neoplasms, etc. Colonoscopy could be the best screening option for all none specific underdiagnosed gastrointestinal symptoms.

Colonoscopy removes all detected polyps, regardless of histology type- adenomatous or hyperplastic. Not all of them must undergo resection. The polyps vary in size and polyps under 5 mm are not detected endoscopic. For detection of polyps smaller than 5 mm the virtual colonospcopy is the alternative to the conventional colonoscopy.

3. Virtual colonoscopy

Virtual Colonoscopy uses computed tomography (CT) imaging virtual- reality technology for the purpose of screening the entire colon which is reconstructed from abdominal CT images.

The technique starts after cleansing of the colon with oral laxatives with inflation of air or CO2 introduced through rectal tube [71]. Then abdominal CT images are taken during a single breath holding with sub mm resolution in axial and transverse directions. The volume model of the colon is constructed from the spiral CT images. Image segmentation is necessary for the reconstruction of an accurate colon model [72]. Computer graphics navigate inside the 3D colon model, the navigation is called fly through model. For validating the detection in the 3D colon model, interpretation of the 2D image slices at transverse, sagital and coronal directions is often included in the procedure.

The virtual colonoscopy achieves higher sensitivity and specificity rates compared to conventional colonoscopy for detecting polyps, which are 8 mm and larger by the same bowel preparation, and for polyps larger than 10 mm they have a comparable performance. CTC can be a potential screening tool to supplement OC for colorectal cancer. CTC is refused to be included in Medicare coverage because of its radiation risk- in about 50 mAs or 2 rads. Reducing the radiation could be achieved by decreasing of the mAs level optimization of kVp value, X-ray flux beam collimation, filtering, etc. The low-mAs strategy will lead to higher noise in the acquired data which results in steak artifacts. The significant amount of X-ray radiation exposure and the data noise cannot be disregarded and allowed to the CTC to be a preferred screening modality.

An alternative method to minimize the radiation is to use magnetic resonance imaging (MRI), i.e., MR colonography (MRC). However, this MRC has several limitation compared to CTC-high costs, sensitiveness to motion and other artifacts, and has lower spatial resolution. Modern CT can reach sub-millimeter spatial resolution and acquire a volumetric image of the abdomen, detecting polyps which are smaller than 5mm.

There are other reasons responsibe for missing small polyps.

The main reason is due to the partial colon cleansing and air/CO2 inflation and this will not generate a good interface between the colon wall and the lumen. Others include loss of image information in post-imaging processing, different anatomical characteristics in the bowel mucosa, residual fluid or stool covering the polyps. The solution could be virtual or electronic colon cleansing (ECC) - special type of software programming for virtually cleansing of the colon. It consists of three main components - (1) fecal tagging, (2) image segmentation for classifying the tagged image voxels, and (3) post-segmentation operation for cleansing the colon. ECC works virtually on the residual faecal materials with or without adequate bowel preparation with purgatives (the so called cathartic-free CTC). The ECC must handle with the partial volume (PV) effect and with the non-uniformly altered image intensity distribution. Partial volume (PV) effect is the interface between the colon wall and the fecal materials with heterogeneously enhanced image intensities. The PV effect blurs the interface over several image voxels, causing the loss of details about the interface what results in the misdetection of small polyps. A dual energy scans of a modern CT device or a dual X-ray source scanner is a new challenging imagining modality. Two volumetric images can be acquired simultaneously at two energy levels. It is expected that the polyps would have different image contrasts in the two scans and if the contrasts are insufficient for segmenting the image voxels, oral contrast media may be utilized to increase the density of the polyps. The ECC role in this dual energy strategy is to segment the colonic materials from multi-spectral CT images. After ECC-cleansing the colon lumen could be easily inspected for abnormalities and polyps along the long colon during the fly-through navigation.

Variation among readers with different experience has been noticed. Computer-aided detection (CAD) can minimize the variation among readers' assessments. CAD system's disadvantages are many false positives (FPs), such as partial bowel cleansing, image noise, motion artifacts, colon fold structures, etc. High sensitivity CAD with minimal number of FPs and development of various texture features and virtual biopsy features remains an innovative research goal.

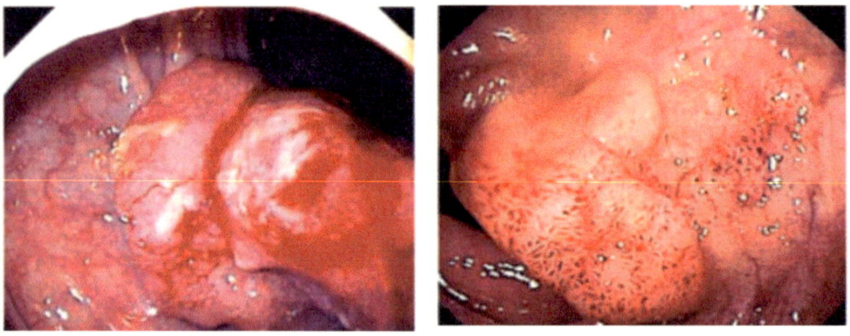

Figure 1. Endoscopic view of corectal tumor – conventional endoscopy

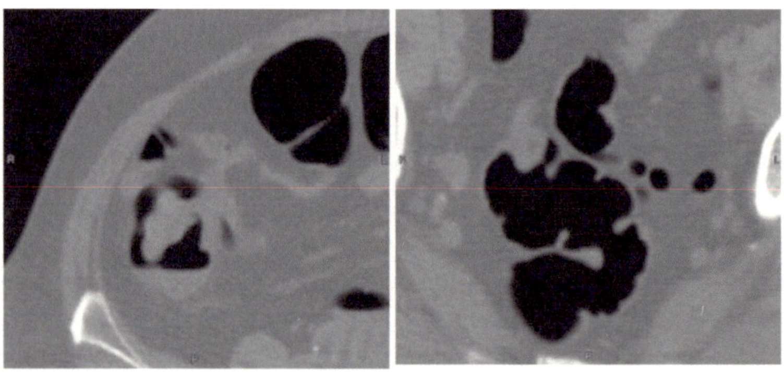

Figure 2. Virtual colonoscopy – a view of pediculaneted polypus and a small carcinoma - CT images.

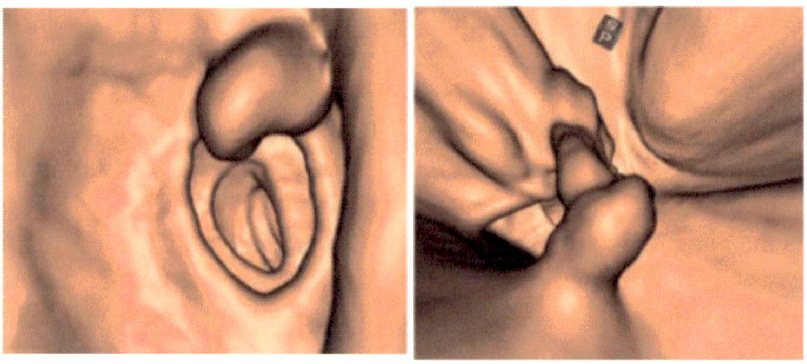

Figure 3. Virtual colonoscopy – a view of pediculaneted polypus and a small carcinoma - a 3-D reconstruction after software rendering.

4. Imaging diagnostics in rectal cancer

Staging of rectal cancer is of great importance before the surgical treatment, because staging predicts the management, prognosis, recurrence and/or metastatic disease risk (13). Staging is divided into local and distant staging. Local staging points at wall invasion, resection margin involvement and the nodal status for metastasis and distant staging refers to presence or absence of metastatic disease. Rectal examination using proctoscopy may be considered as an important tool for newly diagnosed rectal cancers. Proctoscopy may determine better visualization, localization and fixity of the tumor, including taking biopsy, which may affects positively the staging of the rectal cancer.

Nowadays several imaging modalities or combination of these are available for evaluating preoperative staging of colorectal cancer- computed tomography (CT), magnetic resonance imaging (MRI), and/or endorectal ultrasonography (EUS). EUS and MRI of the pelvis are used to appreciate the local dissemination while CT defines systemic dissemination. PET is indicated when there is clinical, biochemical or radiological suspicion of local recurrence or systemic disease. Functional imaging such as diffusion weighted MRI imaging (DWI) and CT/PET are used to distinguish fibrosis from tumor [33].

The T staging accuracy in more advanced cancer is achieved by using MR imaging modality because MRI can distinguish between mesorectum and mesorectal fascia. The N staging accuracy is also provided by MRI particularly using superparamagnetic iron oxide particles.

4.1. Endorectal ultrasound

The advancing of imaging technologies has made endoscopic ultrasound a modality of choice in gastrointestinal diseases, regarding diagnosis, staging and prognosis stratification. These novel techniques assign excellent to rectal tumors.

Endorectal ultrasound (EUS) is useful in evaluating early rectal cancers (T1 and T2 lesions) and post transanal surgery. EUS can visualize the rectal wall without distinguishing of mesorectal fascia, peritumor inflammation, or faeces collections. The accuracy of the T stage evaluation varies from 60%-90% [45].

In comparison to MRI EUS was found to be highly accurate in early lesions (for T1 and T2 the accuracy can reach to 100%), as well as for nodal metastases. For evaluation of metastatic disease neither MRI nor EUS enable reliable diagnosis.

Besides the misleading lymph node assessment, EUS has its disadvantages in detecting T3 lesions (advanced, stenotic, bulky lesions) or tumors after neoadjuvant therapy, and the technique is operator dependent.

Hypoechoic appearance, size > 5 mm, round shape, peritumoral location are characteristics suggestive of malignant involvement of lymph nodes [45,46,51-53]. EUS-guided fine-needle aspiration can be carried out from the lesion or suspiciously looking lymph nodes.

An newer technique is the three-dimensional ERUS (3D-ERUS). It consists of transverse, coronal and sagittal scan and has been found to be more reliable in staging colon cancer to two-dimensional EUS and CT. The accuracy of 3D-ERUS for assessing the depth of cancer infiltration and for nodal involvement is with 10% more than the other imaging modalities. 3D images have proved a better visualization of the mesorectal margins. With 3D-ERUS the surgeon can perform endoscopic mucosal resections of early tumors. A reliable predictor for response after chemoradiation therapy are the accurate volumetric measurements achieved by 3D-ERUS. Using Doppler signal enhancers tumor perfusion can be determine, coming to better results in neoadjuvant therapy and antiangiogenesis treatment.

3D-ERUS, elastography, and contrast enhancement might bring additional information, increasing diagnostic accuracy of ERUS and amplifying its roles in the complex management in rectal cancer.

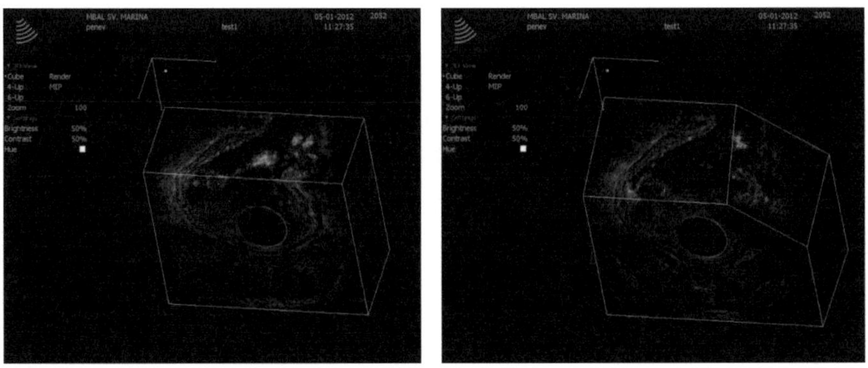

Figure 4. Endorectal ultrasonography – a view of T-3 carcinoma - 3-D reconstruction after real-time software rendering.

T and LN staging

In colon cancer patients it is essential to correctly determine the TNM stage. The modalities of choice are CT, MRI and, as mentioned above, the novel technique ERUS.

ERUS shows high sensitivity and specificity in T-staging and is prior to CT and MRI for staging superficial rectal tumors, with accuracy in evaluating rectal wall invasion to 97% [23,24]. For T1, T2, T3 and T4 staging accuracy of ERUS is more than 80%. One common finding is a lower accuracy for T2 tumors, because the impossibility in distinguishing those tumors that have deep invasion into the muscularis propria from those with microscopic invasion into the perirectal fat.

Transanal endoscopic microsurgery (TEM) and endoscopic submucosal dissections are novel important strategies which directs the mode of surgery because of the ability to visualize the submucosa. This can lead to down- or upstaging of the detected rectal cancer. Besides ERUS can detect recurrence at the anastomosis site and to differentiate between postoperative scars and local recurrences. Unfortunately assessment for nodal metastases is less accurate than that for tumor depth and reaches 75%. For rectal cancer in particular, over half of the metastatic nodes are less than 5 mm and are located within 3 cm of the primary tumor [31]. Metastatic disease was shown to predict local recurrence.

The sensitivity of ERUS in detecting LN metastasis ranges from 50% to 83%, because small lymph node (less than 5mm) is not observed with ERUS and it has limited field of view. Factors for malignancy in lymph node besides node size, echogenicity, shape, border, include: hypoechogenicity, short axis ≥ 5 mm, long axis length greater than 9 mm.

Detecting of iliac adenopathy is crucial because it goes after total mesorectal excision. This is possible through flexible not rigid probes. In general, ERUS is better at detecting lymph nodes in the distal and middle thirds of the rectum [21,33]. The reactive swollen lymph nodes, small blood vessels, urethra, and seminal vesicle often are mistaken for malignant lymph nodes and these results in over staging of the disease. On the other hand, the major reason for nodal status under staging is misdetecting of very small involved nodes (less than 2 mm) and nodes outside the perirectal tissue [21,33].

Preoperative chemoradiation is a limiting factor affecting accurate staging of rectal cancer. There are associated reactive and inflammatory changes in the rectum wall after radiotherapy. However, radiotherapy affects the wall thickness but does not change the five-layered image.

The 3D reconstruction allows improved T and N staging through direct visualization of subtle protrusions of tumors infiltrating into adjacent tissues and organs.

Limitations of ERUS are several. Firstly it is operator's experience dependent; it varies after partial excision or neoadjuvant chemoradiation. It has poor patient acceptability and it has limited depth of penetration; Another disadvantages are those that it cannot be performed in obstructive tumors [16,21]; it is unable to visualize tumors located higher with a rigid probe. It is insufficient in detecting lymph nodes outside the range of the transducer, or visualize mesorectal fascia because of its limited field of view. In addition, accuracy is affected by villous or pedunculated tumors, inflammation, hemorrhage [22,31].

MRI

MRI obtain image identification of the distance of the CRM to the tumor, the relation to pelvic floor and anal sphincter complex, differentiation between mucinous and none mucinous neoplasia. T staging accuracy of MRI is 52% when compared to histology, because of the interface between muscularis propria, perirectal fat and mesorectal fascia. MRI cannot distinguish between T1 and T2 lesions, as well as between T2 and T3 cancer.

T staging

The depth of invasion through the muscle wall is one important element seen on MRI that can help guide clinical decision making for patients with rectal cancer. Not only does the incidence of nodal involvement increase with increasing tumor penetration [19,20], but clinical studies have shown that patients with stage ◎ (T1-2 N0) rectal cancer do not benefit from neoadjuvant radiotherapy [21] and may be amenable to a less than radical surgical treatment [22]. Patients with clinically staged T3-4 tumors typically require preoperative CRT since it reduces the rates of local recurrence more effectively than either postoperative CRT or preopera-

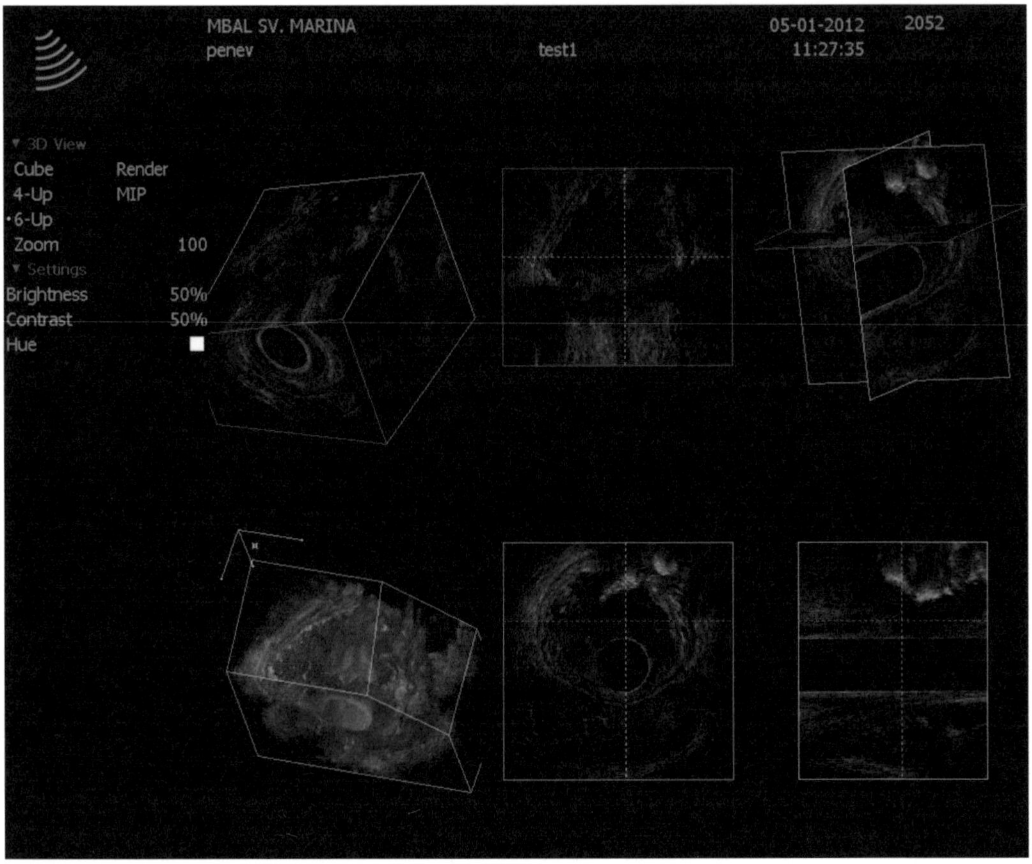

Figure 5. Endorectal ultrasonography – a real time 3-D reconstruction with different options for endorectal evaluation of the tumor process.

tive radiotherapy alone [23-25]. However, some problems remain with T stage determination on MR imaging. Overall, the agreement between MRI and histology for T staging has ranged from 66%-94% [18,26-28]. One of the main problems of T staging on MRI is the distinction between T2 and T3 tumors. In fact, investigators have shown that the negative predictive value for invasion beyond the muscularis propria varied from 93% (expert reading) to 76% (general radiologist reading) [26]. This difficulty is attributed to the presence of desmoplastic reactions around the tumor. This reaction makes it difficult to distinguish between spiculation in the perirectal fat caused by fibrosis alone from that caused by fibrous tissue that contains tumor cells [26]. In contrast, MRI has been shown to be more accurate in imaging the more advanced tumors (T4) [27,29]. According to a metaanalysis, MRI for T4 lesions has a specificity of 96% [30].

CRM

The CRM (lateral, radial) is defined as the surgical cut surface of the connective tissues (i.e. lymphovascular, fatty and neural tissue) that circumferentially encase the rectum. It equates to the mesorectal fascia that forms the plane of dissection in rectal cancer surgery. It is assessed by marking the outer surface (i.e. the CRM) with ink, taking serial cuts through the specimen and examining the macroscopic and microscopic relations between the tumor and the inked margin. The CRM gives significant information not only about the quality of the performed operation but also prognosis of the disease. Indeed, in a recent study based on the data from a randomized clinical trial, Nagtegaal *et al* [31] demonstrated in a multivariate model that the CRM is more important than the T stage for the prognosis of rectal cancer. The definition of a positive CRM remains a matter of debate. A review of the literature in 2006 showed that the majority of studies that dealt with CRM status used the ≤ 1 mm definition for positive CRM (91.1%; 7373 of 8094 patients) [32].

Six distinct types of CRM involvement have been described; direct tumor spread which occurs in 18% to 29% of cases; discontinuous tumor spread in 14% to 67% of cases; lymph node metastases in 12% to 14% of cases; venous invasion in 14% to 57% of cases; lymphatic invasion in 9% of cases; and perineural tumor spread in 7% to 14% of cases [32]. In approximately 30% of patients, there is more than one type of margin involvement. In contrast to direct tumor spread, the involvement of the CRM by lymph node metastases is not associated with local recurrence [32]. MRI is highly accurate and reliable for prediction of the CRM [33,34]. In their most recent study of 98 rectal cancer patients, Brown *et al* [27] reported a 92% agreement between MRI images and histologic findings for prediction of CRM involvement. In another study assessing the tumor relationship to the mesorectal fascia, two observers independently scored the tumor stage and the distance to the mesorectal fascia on MRI and compared these observations with the final histological findings [26]. For twelve tumors with involved mesorectal fascia, and thus, a CRM of 0 mm, the accuracy in predicting the CRM was 100% for both readers. In 29 patients with a wide CRM (10 mm), the accuracy for predicting the negative margin was 97% (27 of 28) for one reader and 93% (26 of 28) for the other [26]. It is relevant to point out that 5 mm of mesorectal tissue surrounding the lateral tumor edge on MRI was shown to equal a CRM of 2 mm in the surgical specimen [26]. In the report by Nagtegaal *et al* [35], a linear regression curve showed that the crucial distance of at least 2 mm could be predicted with 97% confidence when the distance on MRI is at least 6 mm. Therefore, the safe rule to predict CRM involvement on MRI is considered to be an MRI measurement minus 4 mm due to shrinkage of the specimen with fixation [6]. Of note, the CRM becomes more difficult to identify in low, anterior tumors and in patients with a limited amount of perirectal fat [36]. In a recent study by Frasson *et al* [37], the 5-year local recurrence rates for patients with a preoperative CRM of < 2 mm on MRI or EUS who did not receive preoperative chemoradiation was 19.4% compared to 5.4% for patients with a non-threatened margin. It is important to realize that a short course of preoperative radiotherapy has limited ability to control positive CRM. An analysis of more than 17 500 pathologic specimens by Nagtegaal *et al* [32] revealed that the chance of local recurrence was higher for patients with a positive CRM after neoadjuvant treatment (both radiotherapy and radiochemotherapy) than those with a positive CRM following immediate surgery (Hazard ratio 6.3 *vs* 2.0, respectively). Similar results have been reported following postoperative treatment [38]. In the MRC CR-07 trial, patients with positive radial margins who were selected to receive postoperative chemoradiation had a 21% local recurrence rate [39]. Thus, in cases where the tumors are close (< 2 mm) or through the mesorectal margin on preoperative MRI, a more aggressive treatment regimen is required with neoadjuvant CRT or an upfront regimen of chemotherapy before chemoradiation prior to operation. In contrast, patients with a free margin > 2 mm from mesorectal fascia may undergo surgery [total mesorectal excision (TME)] alone, avoiding preoperative chemoradiation. Interestingly, MRI-based therapy for CRM positive tumors was able to reduce the frequency of neoadjuvant therapy for rectal carcinoma by 35% without the risk of worsening the oncological results [40]. However, omitting preoperative chemoradiation for all CRM-negative tumors on MRI needs to be further investigated in prospective clinical trials before it is adopted as standard therapy.

N staging

The presence of involved lymph nodes is an indicator for the likelihood of systemic disease and local recurrence [41]. Therefore node-positive disease is generally an indication for preoperative chemoradiation. However, radiological evaluation of lymph node metastatic involvement remains a challenge. Results of anatomic studies show that over half of the metastatic nodes from rectal cancer are within 3 cm of the primary tumor and are smaller than 5 mm in size [42]. With a standard TME, the perirectal nodes are removed with the primary tumor, but the internal iliac and obturator nodes are left in place. Moriya *et al* [43] reported that as many as 28% of lymph node-positive distal rectal cancers have involvement of lateral nodes and in 6% of cases, these were the only nodes involved. This means that in 6% of patients, the disease was incorrectly staged postoperatively as node-negative at TME. For pre-operative lymph node imaging, MRI at present is only moderately accurate, although this could change with advances in new MR techniques. Currently, the reported accuracy rate of MRI for nodal staging ranges from 71% to 91% [42]. On MRI, lymph nodes typically have lower signal intensity than the perirectal fat but higher signal intensity than arteries and veins. In patients with mucinous carcinoma, metastatic lymph nodes are visualized as hyperintense nodules alone or as hyperintense areas within hypointense nodules. A node is considered enlarged if the major axis length is more than 5 mm (mesorectal), 7 mm (internal iliac), 10 mm (external iliac), or 9 mm (common iliac) [44]. However, the morphological features or signal intensity of the nodes on MRI may more accurately determine metastatic involvement rather than measurement of size. Brown *et al* [45] demonstrated that an irregular border or mixed signal intensity of lymph nodes on MRI improved the specificity of predicting nodal status from 68% (based on size alone) to 97%. One of the more promising advances of MRI may be the use of new lymphographic agents that help assess tumor spread to lymph nodes. In a recent study, gadofosveset-enhanced MRI improved the specificity of nodal staging from 82% achieved with standard MRI to 97% [46]. Fusion of diffusion-weighted MR with T2-weighted images improves identification of pelvic lymph nodes compared with T2-weighted images alone. Using fusion images, 29% additional nodes were detected compared with T2-weighted images alone [47]. The improved nodal identification may aid in treatment planning.

For the vast majority of rectal carcinomas, MRI is currently the most accurate modality on which to base treatment decisions for patients with rectal cancer. Traditionally, the decision to apply preoperative treatment for rectal cancer patients has been based on the T- and N-stage. Lately, other MRI findings such as the radial distance of the tumor to the CRM and extramural vascular invasion score have been identified as important risk factors for local failure and survival. Every center that treats patients with rectal cancer should develop a multidisciplinary team featuring a description of the MRI findings and their implementation in the treatment strategy with the aim of increasing resectability, reducing the local recurrence and treatment morbidity, and improving the quality of life.

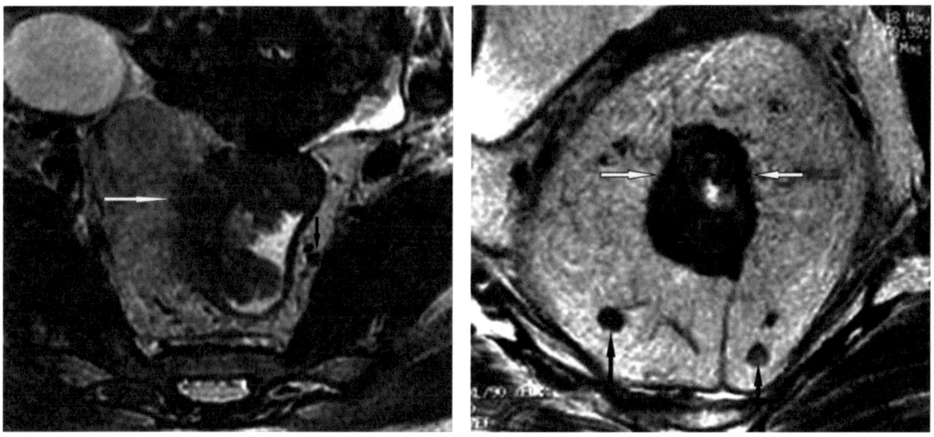

Figure 6. MRI – a view of T-3 carcinoma - 3-D reconstruction after real-time software rendering.

CT, MRI and intraoperative ultrasound for evaluation of the systematic progression in colorectal cancer

The morbidity rate for patients with cancer depends on the early detection of liver metastases. The presence of liver metastases makes of the primary tumour non-resectable for oncologic reasons, except for tumour palliative treatment (for example resection for obstruction of the gastrointestinal tract). For a few malignancies, as in colorectal carcinoma, resection of liver metastases has been shown to improve the survival of the patients. The hepatic metastases are divided into synchronous (i.e. occurring at the time of diagnosis of the primary tumour) and metachronous (occurring after diagnosis of the primary tumour). The surgical resection of the metastases depends on the division, number, size, regional distribution and all clinical parameters of the patient, which makes resectable only 30% of all colorectal patients with metastases. The 5-year survival rate of these patients is more than 30% in comparison to a survival of less than 5% of patients with liver metastases not amenable to liver surgery [1–4].

The goal of imaging modalities is to assess the presence or absence of liver metastases in surgical candidates. Different studies indicate ferumoxide-enhanced magnetic resonance (MR) imaging as more sensitive and specific than contrast-enhanced computed tomography (CT) in detection of hepatic metastases. The different MR pulse sequences and MR contrast media agents makes MRI the modality of choice for non-invasive lesion characterization.

Preoperative assessment of surgical candidates

Preoperative assessment of metastatic liver involvement should be performed for all surgery candidates. This preoperative staging is conceivable by contrast-enhanced CT and/or MRI in

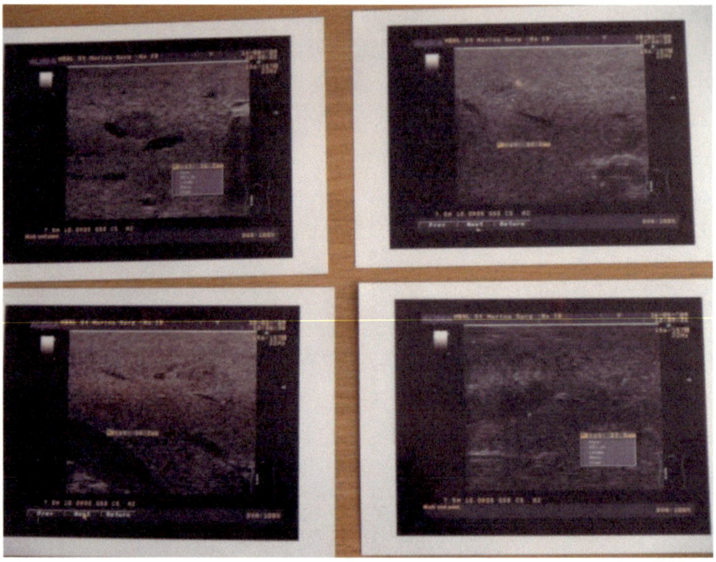

Figure 7. Intraoperative ultrasound of the liver

most oncologic centers. All imaging modalities present different false-positive or false-negative diagnoses- for helical CT- in 42%, intraoperative US- in 22.8%, mangafodipir-enhanced MRI- in 10%, ferumoxide-enhanced MRI technique is accurate as CT during arterioportography (CTAP)- in 19%. Another study found that FDG-PET CT is the most sensitive method for detection of metastases. There is no firm statement which is the best imaging modality, further more the choice depends on local equipment, availability, and operator expertise. MDCT is preferred as a screening method for hepatic lesions because of its ability to reduce respiration-related artifacts, to shorten scan time, to perform multiphase scanning. The disadvantage is the high radiation exposure.

Clinical Role of Intraoperative US

Intraoperative US provide more diagnostic and staging information to the surgeon during hepatic resection. Intraoperative US supplies 35% more information about the lesion type, localization and expansion to adjacent tissues, relation to vascular structures, providing more specificity in the evaluation of liver lesions. In addition intraoperative US represent 25% more lesions than did preoperative US, CT, or angiography. This results in correction in disease staging, which affects the surgical management and postoperative treatment. The intraoperative US has a positive effect on patient care, surgical planning, and clinical outcome.

Magnetic resonance imaging

The standard phased array MRI produces good quality images with good contrast resolution and a relatively large field of view, so it is the modality of choice for preoperative staging of rectal primary tumor. MRI is reliable for assessment of the tumor and its locoregional extension, for identifying recurrence and for planning radiation therapy. The disadvantage of MRI is impossibility in evaluation nodal metastases.

http://dx.doi.org/10.5772/57508

Deciding in management of rectal cancer is the differentiation of the mesorectal fascia-circumstance, which is possible using phased-array coils (confirmed from the multicentre European MERCURY study)(21,23).

MRI may not be the examination of choice for every patient. Patients with contraindications to MRI (e.g. implantable pacemakers), or unable to tolerate MRI (e.g. due to claustrophobia) would preferably undergo preoperative imaging with CT. Motion related imaging artifacts that can severely dampen the diagnostic quality of MRI will occur in patients who are unable to breath hold for longer than 20 seconds.

FDG PET in the Initial Staging of CRC

FDG PET is not a routine investigation for primary cancer due to its limited spatial resolution. PET cannot define the T-category of the primary tumor, but PET is superior to other imaging modalities in detecting of lymph node and distant metastases- an important prognostic factor. After PET-CT investigation the patient could be upstaged in 17% because of identifying unsuspected systemic and lymph node metastases. But the specificity of PET in nodal staging does not be higher than multi-detector CT scan (MDCT).

The principle of positron emission tomography (PET) (and Fluoro-deoxy-glucose (FDG) used as tracer or enhancer) is based on the differential metabolic profile of tumors - higher metabolic activity, change in the tumor biology. FDG/PET is mainly useful in the assessment of local recurrence and metastases. Besides in neoplastic cells FDG accumulates in areas of inflammation, infection, in organs of increased metabolic activity such as brain, myocardium, liver or kidneys leading to false positive results. Interpretation of PET without anatomic correlation is difficult which results in necessity of fusing PET with CT images- PET-CT fusion scans are invented. This offers a detailed anatomical and functional imaging. The combination provides additional value to localize the hot spots. The false positive rates are due to other diseases and physiological processes. PET scans improve the management plan for rectal cancer. The addition of FDG-PET changes patient management in up to 30% of patients with potentially resectable liver metastases, mainly by detecting previously unknown extrahepatic disease. Furthermore, FDG-PET is useful in the follow-up of patients who underwent surgical procedures of the liver, since it is sensitive in detecting residual or relapse malignancy in scarred liver tissue following both resection and local ablative techniques. For follow-up during systemic therapy, early FDG-PET appears predictive for response to therapy. FDG-PET, computerized tomography and magnetic resonance imaging are complementary techniques in staging and restaging patients with advanced colorectal cancer. A combination of FDG-PET and CT scanning characteristics seems promising, and integrated PET/ CT is becoming more widely available, although the exact clinical value and efficacy is not yet fully established. In addition, assessment of these modalities in joint reading sessions with radiologist, nuclear medicine physician, medical and surgical oncologists significantly impacts upon patient management. This review evaluates the potential of FDG-PET and combined PET/CT in patients with colorectal liver metastases and discusses potential future possibilities.

Suggested investigations for tumor staging of rectal cancer

CT scanning is still the current standard for distant staging, but not to stage the local neoplasm. The combination of CT and PET offers both anatomical and functional imaging, so it is sufficient for recurrent rectal cancers. MRI and EUS should be considered as the initial modalities to stage the local tumor. For T1-T2 lesions EUS is more appropriate, whereas MRI is used in advanced rectal cancer. MRI has been shown to be highly accurate in predicting a clear circumferential resection margin in patients undergoing TME.

Suggested investigation for nodal staging of rectal cancer

Significant malignant lymph nodes (more than 1cm in diameter), in conjunction with size, shape and morphology, are identified through MRI, CT and EUS studies. The enlarged lymph node can be as a result of the inflammatory process but normal size nodes can have micrometastases. Moreover the halves of nodes less than 5 mm are proved to be malignant. One novel technique involves use of a contrast media containing superparamagnetic iron oxide particles SPIO which accumulates in normal lymph nodes, but not in malignant nodes due to poor uptake. Then, using T2 weighted imaging, these nodes can be identified. Initial studies are promising but further research is needed [35].

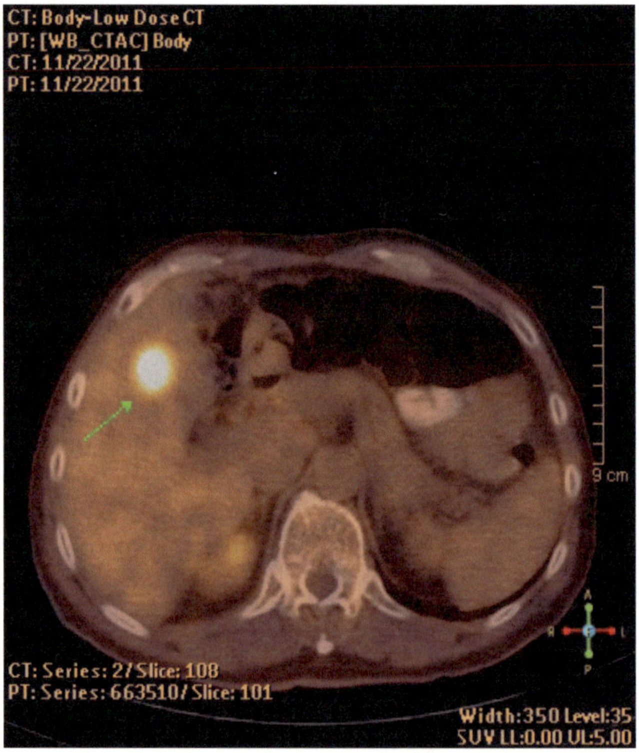

Figure 8. Positron emission tomography of the liver – an observation of metastasis from colorectal origin

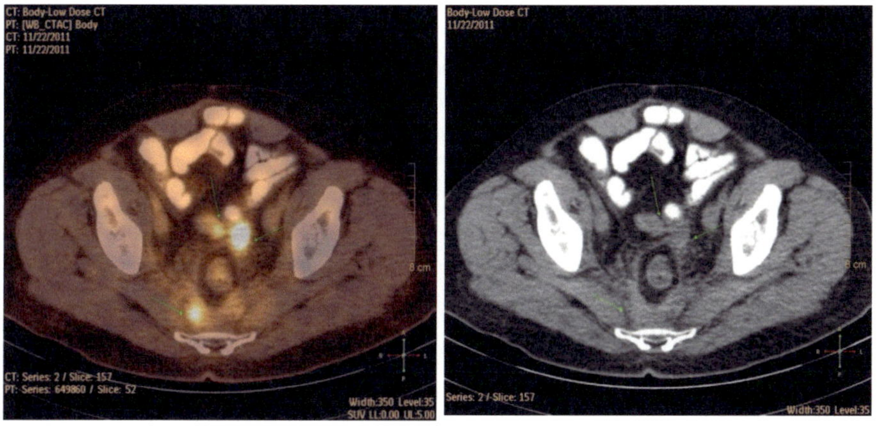

Figure 9. Positron emission tomography of the body – an observation of perirectal lymphadenopathy

5. Conclusion

Optical colonoscopy (OC) and virtual colonoscopy (VC) (i.e. CT colonoscopy and MR colonoscopy) are constantly developing and adapting to the new clinical needs. The optical colonoscopy has the advantage of being both diagnostic and therapeutic procedure for patients with positive findings on screening tests. The virtual colonoscopy is much less invasive method and can be used for mass screening because of the high prevalence of the colorectal cancer. As a screening test the VC has advantages over OC and other options such as FOBT, FIT, stool DNA testing, and DCBE. These methods can make a good combination of VC screening with OC follow-up on the positive findings. The current imaging modalities for VC are CT and MRI and in the future other modalities might be available.

The imaging standard for accurate diagnostics for colorectal cancer includes ultrasound (US), CT and MRI. The nuclear medicine has its role in finding extra-regional localization of the main disease by FDG-PET and FDG-PET/CT. The protocol for liver metastases includes CT as a first choice, which is followed by US. Lung-metastases are evaluated by X-ray or chest CT. The extrahepatic metastases are assessed by CT. The present guidelines could be adjusted by conducting comparative studies on different strategies for colon and rectal cancer, such as CT liver/abdomen vs. MRI liver/abdomen for liver and extrahepatic metastases, X-ray chest and CT chest for lung metastases.

The screening of asymptomatic patients is justified due to the high prevalence of colon carcinoma and the mortality can be effectively reduced by removing adenomatous polyps. Although effective, this method consumes large resources if applied to the whole target population. The currently available screening options have limitations. The VC has the option to identify patients with adenomatous polyps. The combination of VC screening and OC follow-up might prove as a cost-effective measure against colorectal cancer.

The challenges of VC are the associated radiation and the differentiation of the colonic materials from the colon wall. The MRI-based VC has no radiation and has better potential in differentiation of colonic materials from the colonic wall, but it has lower spatial resolution and is prone to motion artifacts. CT and MRI VC require sophisticated software processing to construct the colon model and real-time fly-through inside the lumen. More sophisticated image processing is important for the differentiation of adenomatous from hyperplastic ones. The extraction of the colon wall can be performed by the new method of electronic colon cleansing and analysis of texture features from image intensity of the wall. These processing methods are step toward computer-aided detection and diagnosis. Despite recent advances in chemotherapeutic agents, the prognosis for metastatic colon cancer remains poor. Over the past two decades, hepatic metastasectomy has emerged as a promising technique for improving survival in patients with metastatic colon cancer and in some cases providing long-term cure. To maximize safety and efficacy of metastasectomy, appropriate pre-operative imaging is needed. Advancements in computed tomography (CT), magnetic resonance imaging (MRI) and positron emission tomography (PET) have led to improved detection of occult lesions and better definition of surgical anatomy. While CT, PET and MRI have a comparable sensitivity for detection of large liver metastases, MRI excels at detection of subcentimeter liver metastases compared to CT and FDG-PET, especially with the combination of diffusion weighted imaging (DWI) and hepatocyte-specific contrast agents. CT may be useful as a screening modality or in preoperative planning such as volumetric estimation of the remnant liver size or in defining preoperative arterial anatomy for hepatic artery infusion pump placement. While technologic advancements have led to unprecedented image quality and clarity, this does not replace the need for a dedicated, competent radiologist with experience in hepatic imaging.

Author details

Valentin Ignatov[1], Nikola Kolev[1], Anton Tonev[1], Shteryu Shterev[1], Elitsa Encheva[4], Tanya Kirilova[2], Tsvetelina Teneva[3] and Krassimir Ivanov[1]

1 Department of General and Operative Surgery, University Hospital "St. Marina" – Varna, Bulgaria

2 Department of Gastroenterology, University Hospital "St. Marina"- Varna, Bulgaria

3 Department of Image diagnostics, University Hospital "St. Marina"- Varna, Bulgaria

4 Department of Radiology, University Hospital "St. Marina" – Varna, Bulgaria

References

[1] American Cancer Society. Cancer Facts & Figures 2008. Atlanta: American Cancer Society; 2008.

[2] Jemal A, Siegel R, Ward E, et al. Cancer Statistics – 2008. A Cancer Journal for Clinicians 2008;58 (1):71–96.

[3] Hill M, Morrison B, Bussey H. Etiology of Adenoma Carcinoma Sequence in the Large Bowel. Lancet 1978;1(2):245–247. [PubMed: 74668]

[4] Rickert R, Auerbach O, Garfinkel L, et al. Adenomatous Lesions of the Large Bowel – An autopsy survey. Cancer 1979;43(11):1847–1857. [PubMed: 445371]

[5] Grandqvist S. Distribution of Polyps of the Large Bowel in Relation to Age: A colonoscopic study. Scandinavian Journal of Gastroenterology (SJG) 1981;16(11):1025–1031.

[6] Stryker S, Wolff B, Culp C, et al. Natural History of Untreated Colonic Polyps. Gastroenterology 1987;93(5):1009–1013. [PubMed: 3653628]

[7] Winawer S, Zauber A, Diaz B. The National Polyp Study – Temporal sequence of evolving colorectal cancer from normal colon. Gastrointestinal Endoscopy 1987;33(2): 167.

[8] Fearon E, Vogelstein B. A Genetic Model for Colorectal Tumorigensis. Cell 1990;61(5):759–767. [PubMed: 2188735]

[9] Johnson D, Gurney M, Volpe R, et al. A Prospective Study of the Prevalence of Colonic Neoplasms in Asymptomatic Patients with an Age-Related Risk. American Journal of Gastroenterology (AJG) 1990;85(6):969–974.

[10] Simons B, Morrison A, Lev R, Verhoek-Oftendahl W. Relationship of Polyps to Cancer of the Large Intestine. Journal of the National Cancer Institute (JNCI) 1992;84(5): 962–966.

[11] Potter J, Slattery M. Colon Cancer: A review of the epidemiology. Epidemiologic Reviews 1993;15 (3):499–545. [PubMed: 8174669]

[12] Byers T, Levin B, Rotherberger D, et al. ACS Guidelines for Screening and Surveillance for Early Detection of Colorectal Polyps and Cancer: Update 1997, CA. A Cancer Journal for Clinicians 1997;47(1):154–160.

[13] Winawer S, Fletcher R, Mayer R. Colorectal Cancer Screening: Clinical guidelines and rational. Gastroenterology 1997;112(3):594–642. [PubMed: 9024315]

[14] Robbins D, Itzowitz S. The Molecular and Genetic Basis of Colon Cancer. Medical Clinics of North America (MCNA) 2002;86(6):1467–1495.

[15] Church J. Clinical Significance of Small Colorectal Polyps. Diseases of the Colon and Rectum 2004;47(4):481–485. [PubMed: 14994108]

[16] Lieberman D, Holub J, Eisen G, et al. Prevalence of Polyps Greater Than 9 mm in a Consortium of Diverse Clinical Practice Settings in the United States. Clinical Gastroenterology and Hepatology 2005;3(8):798–805. [PubMed: 16234009]

[17] Odom S, Duffy S, Barone J, et al. The Rate of Adenocarcinoma in Endoscopically Removed Colorectal Polyps. The American Surgeon 2005;71(12):1024–1026. [PubMed: 16447472]

[18] Jass J. Classification of Colorectal Cancer based on Correlation of Clinical, Morphological and Molecular Features. Histopathology 2007;50(1):113–130. [PubMed: 17204026]

[19] Yoo T, Park D, Kim Y, et al. Clinical Significance of Small Colorectal Adenoma Less Than 10 mm: The KASID study. Hepatogastroenterology 2007;54(74):418–21. [PubMed: 17523287]

[20] Smith L. Fibreoptic Colonoscopy: Complications of colonoscopy and polypectomy. Diseases of the Colon and Rectum 1976;11(1):146–150.

[21] Kronberg O, Fenger C, Olsen J, et al. Randomized Study of Screening for Colorectal Cancer with Fecal-Occult-Blood Test. Lancet 1996;348(12):1467–1471. [PubMed: 8942774]

[22] Mandel J, Church T, Bond J, et al. The Effect of Fecal Occult Blood Screening on the Incidence of Colorectal Cancer. The New England Journal of Medicine 2000;343(22): 1603–1607. [PubMed: 11096167]

[23] Allison J, Sskoda I, Ransom L, et al. Screening for Colorectal Neoplasms with New Fecal Occult Blood Tests: Update on performance characteristics. Journal of the National Cancer Institute 2007;99 (11):1462–1470. [PubMed: 17895475]

[24] Imperiale T, Ransohoff D, Itzkowitz S, et al. Fecal DNA verse Fecal Occult Blood for Colorectal Cancer Screening in an Average-Risk Population. The New England Journal of Medicine 2004;351 (26):2704–2714. [PubMed: 15616205]

[25] Ahlquist D, Sargent D, Loprinzi C, et al. Stool DNA and Occult Blood Testing for Screen Detection of Colorectal Neoplasia. Annals of Internal Medicine 2008;149(7): 441–450. [PubMed: 18838724]

[26] Fork F. Double Contrast Enema and Colonoscopy in Polyp Detection. Gut 1981;22:971–977. [PubMed: 7308852]

[27] Morosi C, Ballardini G, Pisani P. Diagnostic Accuracy of the Double-Contrast Enema for Colonic Polyps in Patients with or without Diverticular Disease. Gastrointestinal Radiology 1991;16(2):345–347. [PubMed: 1936780]

[28] Brady A, Stevenson G, Stevenson I. Colorectal Cancer Overlooked at Barium Enema Examination and Colonoscopy: A continuing perceptual problem. Radiology 1994;192(2):373–378. [PubMed: 8029400]

[29] Selby J, Friedman G, Quesenberry C, Weiss N. A Case Control Study of Screening Sigmoidoscopy and Mortality from Colorectal Cancer. The New England Journal of Medicine 1992;326(10):653–657. [PubMed: 1736103]

[30] Elwood J, Sli G, Schlup M, et al. Flexible Sigmoidoscopy or Colonoscopy for Colorectal Screening: A randomized trial of performance and acceptability. Cancer Detection and Prevention 1995;19(4): 337–347. [PubMed: 7553676]

[31] Kewenter J, Breringe H, Engaras B, Haglind E. The Value of Flexible Sigmoidoscopy and Double Contrast Barium Enema in the Diagnosis of Neoplasms in the Rectum and Colon in Subjects with Positive Hemoccult: Results of 1,831 rectosigmoidoscopies and double contrast barium enemas. Endoscopy 1995;27(1):159–163. [PubMed: 7601048]

[32] Newcomb P, Storer B, Morimoto L, et al. Long-Term Efficacy of Sigmoidoscopy in the Reduction of Colorectal Cancer Incidence. Journal of the National Cancer Institute 2003;95(8):622–625. [PubMed: 12697855]

[33] Levin T, Farraye F, Schoen R, et al. Quality in the Technical Performance of Screening Flexible Sigmoidoscopy: Recommendations of an international multi-society task group. Gut 2005;54(6): 807–813. [PubMed: 15888789]

[34] Wolff W, Shinya H. Colonofiberoscopy. Journal of the American Medical Association (JAMA) 1971;217(11):1509–1512.

[35] Hafner M. Conventional Colonoscopy: Technique, indications, limites. European Journal of Radiology (EJR) 2007;61(2):409–414.

[36] Winawer S, Zauber A, Ho M, et al. Prevention of Colorectal Cancer by Colonoscopic Polypectomy. The New England Journal of Medicine 1993;329(27):1977–1981. [PubMed: 8247072]

[37] American Society for Gastrointestional Endoscopy. Appropriate Use of Gastrointestional Endpscopy. Gastrointestinal Endoscopy 2000;52(5):831–837.

[38] Seeff L, Richards T, Shapiro J, et al. How Many Endoscopies are Performed for Colorectal Cancer Screening? Results from CDC's survey of endoscopic capability. Gastroenterology 2004;127(6): 1670–1677. [PubMed: 15578503]

[39] Bartram C. Bowel Preparation – Principles and practice. Clinical Radiology 1994;49(2):365–367. [PubMed: 8045057]

[40] Ristvedt S, McFarland E, Weinstock L, Thyssen E. Patient Preferences for CTC, Conventional Colonoscopy, and Bowel Preparation. American Journal of Gastroenterology 2003;98(4):578–585. [PubMed: 12650790]

[41] "A Consensus Document on Bowel Preparation Prior to Colonoscopy," prepared by a Task Force from American Society of Colon and Rectal Surgeons (ASCRS), the American Society of Gastrointestinal Endoscopy (ASGE), and the Society of American Gastrointestinal and Endoscopic Surgeons (SAGES) on April of 2006.

[42] Cai S, Zhang S, Zhu H, Zheng S. Barriers to Colorectal Cancer Screening: A case-control study. World Journal of Gastroenterology 2009;15(12):2531–2536. [PubMed: 19469005]

[43] Stevenson G, Wilson J, Wilkinson J, et al. Pain Following Colonoscopy: Elimination with carbon dioxide. Gastrointestinal Endoscopy 1992;38(3):564–567. [PubMed: 1397911]

[44] Steine S. Which Hurts the Most? A comparison of pain rating during double-contrast barium enema examinations and colonoscopy. Radiology 1994;191(1):99–101. [PubMed: 8134605]

[45] Orsoni P, Berdah S, Verrier C, et al. Colonic Perforation due to Colonoscopy: A retrospective study of 48 cases. Endoscopy 1997;29(1):160–164. [PubMed: 9201463]

[46] Weitzman E, Zapka J, Estabrook B, Goins K. Risk and Reluctance: Understanding impediments to colorectal cancer screening. Preventive Medicine 2001;32(6):502–513. [PubMed: 11394954]

[47] Rex D, Rahmani E, Haseman J, et al. Relative Sensitivity of Colonoscopy and Barium Enema for Detection of Colorectal Cancer in Clinical Practice. Gastroenterology 1997;112(1):17–23. [PubMed: 8978337]

[48] Bressler B, Paszat L, Vinden C, et al. Colonoscopic Miss Rates for Right-Sided Colon Cancer: A population-based analysis. Gastroenterology 2004;127(2):452–456. [PubMed: 15300577]

[49] Pickhardt P, Nugent P, Mysliwiec P, et al. Location of Adenomas Missed by OC. Archives of Internal Medicine 2004;141(2):352–359.

[50] Heresbach D, Barrioz T, Lapalus M, et al. Miss Rate for Colorectal Neoplastic Polyps: A prospective multi-center study of back-to-back video colonoscopies. Endoscopy 2008;40(4):282–290.

[51] Lieberman D, Moravec M, Holub J, et al. Polyp Size and Advanced Histology in Patients Undergoing Colonoscopy Screening: Implications for CTC. Gastroenterology 2008;135(4):1100–1105. [PubMed: 18691580]

[52] Kim D, Pickhardt P, Taylor A. Characteristics of Advanced Adenomas Detected at CTC Screening: Implications for appropriate polyp size thresholds for polypectomy versus surveillance. American Journal of Roentgenology 2007;188(6):940–944. [PubMed: 17377027]

[53] Lieberman D, de Garmo P, Fleischer D, et al. Colonic Neoplasia in Patients with Non-Specific GI Symptoms. Gastrointestinal Endoscopy 2000;51(6):647–651. [PubMed: 10840294]

[54] Gelfand D. Gastrointestinal Radiology: A short history and predictions for future. American Journal of Roentgenology 1988;150(4):727–730.

[55] Vining, D.; Gelfand, D.; Bechtold, R., et al. Technical Feasibility of Colon Imaging with Helical CT and Virtual Reality. Annual Meeting of American Roentgen Ray Society; New Orleans. 1994. p. 104

[56] Hong, L.; Kaufman, A.; Wei, Y.; Viswambharan, A.; Wax, M.; Liang, Z. IEEE Biomedical Visualization Symposium. IEEE CS Press; CA: 1995. 3D Virtual Colonoscopy; p. 26-32.

[57] Hara A, Johnson C, Reed J, et al. Detection of Colorectal Polyps by CTC: Feasibility of a novel technique. Gastroenterology 1996;110(2):284–290. [PubMed: 8536869]

[58] Hong L, Liang Z, Viswambharan A, et al. Reconstruction and Visualization of 3D Models of Colonic Surface. IEEE Transactions on Nuclear Science (TNS) 1997;44(11): 1297–1302.

[59] Reed J, Johnson C. Automatic Segmentation, Tissue Characterization, and Rapid Diagnosis Enhancements to the CTC Analysis Workstation. Journal of Digital Imaging 1997;10(1):70–73. [PubMed: 9268843]

[60] Wan, M.; Tang, Q.; Kaufman, A.; Liang, Z. Proc IEEE Computer Graphics and Applications. 1999. Volume Rendering Based Interactive Navigation within the Human Colon; p. 397-400.

[61] Coin C, Wollett F, Coin J, et al. Computerized Radiology of the Colon: A potential screening technique. Computed Radiology 1983;7(2):215–221.

[62] Shinners T, Pickhardt P, Taylor A, et al. Patient-Controlled Room Air Insufflation versus Automated Carbon Dioxide Delivery for CTC. American Journal of Roentgenology 2006;186(10):1491–1496. [PubMed: 16714635]

[63] Liang Z, Chen D, Li B, et al. On Segmentation of Colon Lumen for VC. Proc SPIE Medical Imaging 1999;3660:270–278.

[64] Fenlon H, Nunes D, Schroy P, et al. A Comparison of Virtual and Conventional Colonoscopy for the Detection of Colorectal Polyps. The New England Journal of Medicine 1999;341(11):1496–1503. [PubMed: 10559450]

[65] Fletcher J, Johnson C, Welch T, et al. Optimization of CTC Technique: Prospective trial in 180 patients. Radiology 2000;216(4):704–711. [PubMed: 10966698]

[66] Yee J, Akerkar G, Hung R, et al. Colorectal Neoplasia: Performance characteristics of CTC for detection in 300 patients. Radiology 2001;219(4):685–692. [PubMed: 11376255]

[67] Johnson D, Harmsen W, Wilson L, et al. Prospective Blinded Evaluation of CTC for Screen Detection of Colorectal Polyps. Gastroenterology 2003;125(2):311–319. [PubMed: 12891530]

[68] Pickhardt P, Choi R, Hwang I, et al. Computed Tomographic VC to Screen for Colorectal Neoplasia in Asymptomatic Adults. The New England Journal of Medicine 2003;349(12):2191–2200. [PubMed: 14657426]

[69] Johnson C, Chen MH, Toledano A, et al. Accuracy of CTC for Detection of Large Adenomas and Cancers. The New England Journal of Medicine 2008;359(12):1207–1217. [PubMed: 18799557]

[70] Regge D, Laudi C, Galatola G, et al. Diagnostic Accuracy of Computed Tomographic Colonography for the Detection of Advanced Neoplasia in Individuals at Increased Risk of Colorectal Cancer. The Journal of the American Medical Association 2009;301(23):2453–2461.

[71] Brenner D, Georgsson M. Mass Screening with CTC: Should the radiation exposure be of concern? Gastroenterology 2005;129(2):328–337. [PubMed: 16012958]

[72] Neri, E.; Faggioni, L.; Cerri, F., et al. CTC versus Double-Contrast Barium Enema for Screening of Colorectal Cancer: Comparison of radiation burden. 2009. Published online by September 24:

[73] Brenner DJ, Hall EJ. Computed Tomography – An increasing source of radiation exposure. The New England Journal of Medicine 2007;357(11):2277–2284. [PubMed: 18046031]

[74] Lu H, Li X, Li L, Chen D, Xing Y, Wax M, Hsieh J, Liang Z. Adaptive Noise Reduction toward Low-Dose CT. Proc SPIE Medical Imaging 2003;5030:759–766.

[75] Wang J, Li T, Lu H, Liang Z. Penalized Weighted Least-Squares Approach to Sinogram Noise Reduction and Image Reconstruction for Low-Dose X-ray CT. IEEE Transactions on Medical Imaging (TMI) 2006;25:1272–1283.

[76] Wang J, Wang S, Li L, Lu H, Liang Z. VC Screening with Ultra Low-Dose CT & Less-Stressful Bowel Preparation: A computer simulation study. IEEE Transactions on Nuclear Science 2008;55 (5):2566–2575. [PubMed: 19169383]

[77] Rust G, Aurich V, Reiser M. Noise/Dose Reduction and Image Improvements in Screening VC with Tube Currents of 20 mAs with Nonlinear Gaussian Filter Chains. Proc SPIE Medical Imaging 2002;4683:186–197.

[78] Purkayastha S, Tekkis P, Athanasiou T, et al. Magnetic Resonance Colonography versus Colonoscopy as a Diagnostic Investigation for Colorectal Cancer: A meta-analysis. Clinical Radiology 2005;60 (6):980–989. [PubMed: 16124980]

[79] Laks S, Macari M, Bini E. Positional Change in Colon Polyps at CTC. Radiology 2004;231(4):761–766. [PubMed: 15163817]

[80] Liang, Z.; Yang, F.; Wax, M., et al. Inclusion of A Priori Information in Segmentation of Colon Lumen for 3D VC. Conf Record IEEE NSS-MIC, in CD-ROM; 1997.

[81] Liang, Z. Electronic Colon Cleansing Techniques: Past, present, and future. The 11th International Conference on Medical Image Computing and Computer Assisted In-

tervention (MICCAI) Workshop – "New Era of Virtual Colonoscopy"; New York City, NY. September 6; 2008. p. 26-32.

[82] Liang Z, MacFall J, Harrington D. Parameter Estimation and Tissue Segmentation from Multispectral MR Images. IEEE Transactions on Medical Imaging 1994;13(3): 441–449. [PubMed: 18218519]

[83] Summers R, Johnson C, Pusanik L, et al. Automated Polyp Detection at CTC: Feasibility assessment in a human population. Radiology 2001;219(1):51–59. [PubMed: 11274534]

[84] Yoshida H, Nappi J. Three-Dimensional Computer-Aided Diagnosis Scheme for Detection of Colonic Polyps. IEEE Transactions on Medical Imaging 2001;20(8):1261–1274. [PubMed: 11811826]

[85] Wang Z, Liang Z, Li L, et al. Reduction of False Positives by Internal Features for Polyp Detection in CT-Based VC. Medical Physics 2005;32(12):3602–3616. [PubMed: 16475759]

[86] Zhu H, Liang Z, Barish M, Pickhardt P, et al. Increasing Computer-aided Detection Specificity by Projection Features for CTC. Medical Physics, to appear. 2010

[87] Liang Z, Lakare S, Wax M, et al. A Pilot Study on Less-Stressful Bowel Preparation for VC Screening with Follow-up Biopsy by OC. Proc SPIE Medical Imaging 2005;5746:810–816.

[88] Pickhardt, P.; Kim, D. CTC: Principles and practice of virtual colonoscopy. Saunders, Elsevier; Philadelphia, PA, USA: 2009.

[89] Park S, Lee S, Choi E, et al. Flat Colorectal Neoplasma Definition, Importance, and Visualization on CTC. American Journal of Roentgenology 2007;188(5):953–959. [PubMed: 17377029]

[90] Liang Z, Wang S. An EM Approach to MAP Solution of Segmenting Tissue Mixtures: A numerical analysis. IEEE Transactions on Medical Imaging 2009;28(2):297–310. [PubMed: 19188116]

[91] Wang S, Li L, Cohen H, Mankes S, Chen J, Liang Z. An EM Approach to MAP Solution of Segmenting Tissue Mixture Percentages with Application to CT-based VC. Medical Physics 2008;35(12):5787–5798. [PubMed: 19175136]

Chapter 3

Role of Magnetic Resonance Imaging in Locally Advanced Rectal Cancer

Roberta Fusco, Mario Sansone, Mario Petrillo,
Antonio Avallone, Paolo Delrio,
Fabiana Tatangelo and Antonella Petrillo

Additional information is available at the end of the chapter

http://dx.doi.org/10.5772/56831

1. Introduction

This chapter will give an overview of the magnetic resonance imaging (MRI) modalities used in locally advanced rectal cancer (LARC) staging with an emphasis on the role of MRI and its significance for planning an effective therapeutic strategy for the individual patient.

Specifically, the aim of this chapter is to present a brief review about:

1. Methodologies of Magnetic Resonance Imaging in LARC staging
   - a. Morphologic MRI
   - b. Functional MRI
     - i. Dynamic Contrast Enhanced MRI (DCE-MRI)
     - ii. Diffusion Weighted MRI (DW-MRI)
2. The role of MRI in diagnosis, staging, evaluation of response of neoadjuvant treatment, follow-up post surgery.

This chapter will be organised in the following sections. First, in order to better define the role of MRI in LARC management, we will briefly describe the epidemiological scenario and therapeutic options, with an emphasis on issues in which MRI is relevant. Second, we will describe morphologic and functional MRI including DCE-MRI and DW-MRI. Finally, a systematic review of the literature concerning MRI, CT and PET for LARC management will be presented.

2. Epidemiology

Colorectal cancer is the third most common cancer worldwide [1], which includes cancers of the colon, rectum, rectosigmoid junction and anus. Specifically, in men it represents the third commonest neoplasm after prostate and lung cancers while in women it is the second major cause of morbidity and mortality, following breast cancer.

In recent years, mortality rates have decreased due to several factors, including less exposure risk factors, more possibility of prevention and "early diagnosis" followed by an effective management of the disease. In particular, major changes in therapeutic management are given by the standardization of operative procedures and the introduction of adjuvant and neoadjuvant therapy [2-7], able to reduce recurrence risk and tumor size.

Cancers are characterized by profound spatial and temporal heterogeneity in their biologic characteristics. Most invasive cancers typically have alterations in cell physiology that promote malignant growth [2-7]. Rectal cancer is the result of a complex interaction between genetic and environmental factors and it is defined as a tumor whose aboral margin measured with the rigid rectoscope is 16 cm or less from the anocutaneous line. This distance serves to classify rectal cancer into tumours of the upper third (12–16 cm), the middle third (6–12 cm), and the lower third (<6 cm) [26] according to the Union for International Cancer Control (UICC).

The mesorectal fascia is an important anatomic landmark for the diagnostic evaluation of local tumor extent [26]. It is a connective tissue sheath that surrounds the rectum and the perirectal fatty tissue and acts as a natural barrier for tumor spread.

A locally advanced tumor often describes a tumor extending beyond the rectal wall with infiltration to surrounding organs or structures, and/or perforation of the visceral peritoneum. It includes bulky T3 tumors with threatened circumferential margins or T4 tumors, tumors with growth onto the peritoneal surface. A radiological T4 tumor is considered when detected growing outside the mesorectal fascia, while a T3 tumor refers to a tumor invading through muscularis propria [26].

These tumors have traditionally been looked upon as "unresectable", although previous staging, due to the wide tumor extension. However, when it is possible, these tumors cannot be resected without leaving microscopic or gross residual disease at the local site because of tumor adherence or fixation to that site.

3. Therapeutic options

In LARC accurate and detailed anatomic information in tumor extent is essential not only for the selection of the patients for neoadjuvant chemotherapy and radiation therapy to achieve tumor shrinkage but also for the optimal surgical procedure planning. Moreover, the treatment for patients with locally advanced and recurrent rectal cancer differs significantly from patients with rectal cancer restricted to the mesorectum.

http://dx.doi.org/10.5772/56831

Adequate preoperative imaging of the pelvis is therefore important to identify those patients who are candidates for multimodality treatment, including preoperative chemoradiation protocols, intraoperative radiotherapy, and extended surgical resections. Much effort should be made to select patients with these advanced tumors for treatment in specialized referral centers. This has been shown to reduce morbidity and mortality and improve long-term survival rates.

Two main therapeutic options can be considered according to different pathological stages presented [13-35]:

1. Total mesorectal excision (TME): using this surgical technique, the rectum is resected together with all surrounding lymphatic pathways, lymph nodes, mesorectal fatty tissue, and the mesorectal fascia while the parietal pelvis fascia and the pelvic splanchnic nerves are spared. This surgical technique minimizes the chance of tumor being left inside;
2. Adjuvant/neoadjuvant therapy: the aims of adjuvant or neoadjuvant therapy are to enable or facilitate total tumor resection even in advanced disease, to prevent local tumor recurrence, and to minimize the risk of distant metastases.

The majority of patients with primary rectal cancer have a tumor located within the mesorectal fascia, which is generally treated with total mesorectal excision (TME). Results of TME surgery are excellent with a significant reduction in local recurrences when preoperative short-term radiotherapy (5 x 5 Gy) is delivered one week prior to surgery [27]. In ≈10% of all rectal cancer patients the tumor extends into or beyond the enveloping fascia of the mesorectal compartment.

Often these tumors infiltrate adjacent structures and therefore have a higher risk to develop a local recurrence [28].

Patients with these primary locally advanced or recurrent rectal cancer are difficult to treat with surgery alone, but outcome has significantly improved using multimodality treatment. Although preoperative and adjuvant therapy is important in these patients, the mainstay of treatment in rectal cancer is complete surgical removal of the tumor. In both locally advanced and recurrent rectal cancers, this involves not only the removal of the total mesorectum, but en bloc resection of involved structures is often needed.

Although postoperative chemoradiotherapy (CRT) has long been recommended for locally advanced and node positive rectal cancer patients, preoperative treatment is now widely used worldwide. In many European centers, radiotherapy only was used as neoadjuvant treatment for locally advanced rectal cancer, but the addition of chemotherapy has recently demonstrated to improve local control in two large randomized trials [30,31]. Addition of 5-FU and leucovorin to preoperative radiation slightly increased the amount of acute toxicity in T3 to T4 resectable rectal cancer patients [32]. However, it increased the number of complete responses and decreased the local recurrence rate after 5 years.

Not only new chemotherapeutic drugs, but also a vascular endothelial cell growth factor-(VEGF-) specific monoclonal antibody in combination with chemoradiation was recently reported by Willet et al [32] to lead to considerable downstaging of the tumor. Other modalities such as the use of intensity-modulated radiotherapy (IMRT), which has the potential of more accurate delivery of higher radiotherapy dosages, thus avoiding the damage of critical structures surrounding the tumor, are being tested in rectal cancer.

Total pelvic exenteration (TPE) is a widely used technique for resection of locally advanced or recurrent rectal tumors invading the bladder and/or prostate. Longterm survival with excellent local control is possible after TPE for primary locally advanced rectal cancer [33-35]. The majority of resections in primary cancer are without microscopic or macroscopic residual tumor mass, which clearly justifies the use of TPE in selected patients with primary disease. Although current guidelines for colorectal cancer surgery advocate TPE, only one third of the patients in a recent study based on SEER (survival, epidemiology and end results) data underwent the appropriate surgical resection.

These patients had a clinically significant overall survival benefit with no increase in short-term mortality compared with similar patients who did not receive a multi-visceral resection. Local control in rectal cancer patients is related to the dose of irradiation, but because of toxicity to radiosensitive organs (such as small bowels), the external radiation dose should not exceed 60 Gy. A combination of external radiation and intraoperative radiation therapy (IORT) allows the safe delivery of higher effective doses of irradiation than can be delivered with external-beam only techniques. IORT is used when resection margins are narrow or involved with tumor cells and can be applied very specifically to an area at risk, under direct visual control, and with the ability to shield the surrounding structures from radiation. The biological effectiveness of single-dose IORT is considered to be as effective as 2 to 3 times the equivalent dose of fractionated radiotherapy.

3. Role of MRI vs other modalities

3.1. Generalities

Imaging techniques play a pivotal role in the strategies for management of locally advanced rectal cancer patients. The role of diagnostic imaging is to perform a loco-regional staging as accurate as possible in both evaluation of infiltration and extension degrees of disease. Image features also enable preoperative assessment of important prognostic outlines, which may guide patient selection for neoadjuvant therapies. Moreover, imaging plays an important role in therapeutic assessment, surveillance after surgery, and evaluation of suspected disease fall-out. To date, imaging innovations have led to improvements in spatial and contrast resolution, increased data acquisition speeds, and enabled complex image to achieve excellence in anatomic resolution.

There are many different imaging modalities suitable for rectal cancer staging, tumour location and restaging but not all of them have the same accuracy for each indication. An optimal visualization of tumor volume and of its surrounding anatomical structures is necessary for any local cancer treatment. This issue is particularly important for radiotherapy treatment planning in order that a geographical miss can be avoided and the tumor adequately treated.

http://dx.doi.org/10.5772/56831

Among the imaging methods available Magnetic Resonance Imaging (MRI) is currently the modality of choice because of its capacity to perform local staging, since it enables evaluation of anatomic aspects and prognostic factors that are key to choosing the appropriate surgical approach and determining the need for neoadjuvant treatment.

3.2. MRI physical basics

MRI is an imaging technique based on the different magnetic properties of tissues in the body. The exposure to a high intensity magnetic field determines the alignment of the hydrogen nuclei (protons) along the magnetic field axis itself. The emission of radio frequency pulses causes a shift from this alignment, which tends to reconstitute as soon as the impulse is interrupted. This phenomenon leads to a variation in energy level of the charges, which can be translated into a signal whose decoding is the basis of the generation of magnetic resonance images. All this is based on specific parameters that describe these steps of energy levels (including the so-called "relaxation times T1 and T2"), as well as on the concentration of protons within a given tissue.

Pulses sequences are used to obtain the different MR images, sequences consisting of radio frequency pulses with different characteristics in terms of duration, frequency and type of sampling of the resulting signal.

In the various biological tissues, the characteristics of the magnetic resonance signal are influenced mainly by the content of hydrogen atoms (whose nuclei are composed of only one proton). Since water is the most abundant molecule in the body and contains hydrogen atoms, it can be reasonably stated that the increase or the decrease of water in a given tissue is almost always at the basis of changes in signal intensity when using sequences of magnetic resonance imaging.

Where tissue contrast depends primarily on electron density, the tissue contrast obtained by MRI can be extensively varied by imaging the intrinsic tissue properties, as spin-lattice and spin-spin relaxation times, protons density, magnetization transfer, separately or in combination, using a number of pulse sequences, which in turn can be altered by an essentially infinite number of different experimental conditions. These MR parameters can be exploited and tailored to facilitate optimal tumor visualization and evaluation. Another feature of MRI is that cortical bone does not give rise to an MR signal and therefore appears hypointense. This is because cortical bone contains calcium and there are few hydrogen protons to provide an MR signal. Furthermore, MRI can obtain detailed anatomical images in any desired plane, also acquiring 3D or volumetric image sets. Therefore, the superior soft tissue definition provided by MRI, together with its unrestricted multiplanar, volumetric, vascular and functional information has benefits for 3D treatment planning.

3.3. Comparison of MRI and CT

Computed Tomography (CT) scanning is an imaging technique able to reproduce a 3D image of internal organs by irradiating X-ray. In LARC treatment CT shows the effective tumor size and its possible dissemination to internal organs. Although CT imaging provides excellent definition between structures with different electron density or X-ray attenuation characteristics, it distinguishes poorly between structures with similar electron density such as different soft tissue structures, including tumors, unless there is an obvious fat or air interface [60]. The major advantage of MRI compared with CT is in its superior ability to demonstrate and characterize soft tissues that have similar electron densities. In this manner, MRI may provide better delineation not only of the tumor extent, but also of the adjacent critical soft tissue organs. This will allow conformal planning to enhance its therapeutic ratio by more accurately targeting the tumor, avoiding the organs at risk and subsequently improving local control.

3.4. Comparison of MRI and PET/CT

In LARC patient management detection of tumor sites throughout the body is needed with high sensitivity and specificity in order to have accurate information about the local extent. As discussed in the previous section, an accurate tumour visualization can be performing using MRI techniques. An additional value should be given to consider the combination of Positron Emission Tomography (PET) and CT [61]. PET/CT is a diagnostic procedure that allows to obtain morphological images of the human body provided by CT and images of the tissue metabolic processes provided by PET by means of a co-registration system.

Tissues appear differently on PET and on CT images. CT displays anatomy with high spatial resolution, but with low contrast resolution for soft tissues, while PET visualizes pathological sites with high contrast resolution but a limited spatial resolution and surrounding normal anatomical structures are hardly visualized. The combination of metabolic activity with anatomic localization achievable with PET/CT improve accuracy over that of PET or CT alone [62].

4. Role of MRI in LARC

In the recent years MRI has undergone significant transformations resulting from technological innovation that have taken place as the introduction of high-field magnets, powerful gradients, multi-channel phased array coils and endorectal coils improvement. These technological developments have certainly allowed the executing of high quality diagnostic studies due to the high spatial resolution and contrast obtained, to the possibility of identification and distinction of rectal wall layers, and to the possibility of assessing perirectal and sphinteric structures. Mainly, superficial endorectal coils are currently able to identify various layers of lower rectum wall. MRI is thus the ideal technique for rectal cancer staging, combining the capabilities of an accurate loco-regional staging to the outlook and multi-planar properties.

In conclusion, MRI can currently stage with high accuracy the T parameter (related to the degree of tumor infiltration) due to the possibility offered by the endorectal coil to recognize the wall layers, resulting also extremely useful in planning surgery and in prognostic stratification, owing to the ability to accurately identify mesorectum and the distance between mesorectal fascia and neoplasia. Furthermore the high temporal resolution of last generation devices allows to perform perfusion and dynamic studies after gadolinium administration that allow to detection of the residual tumor after neoadjuvant therapy and to diagnose recurrences, distinguishing them from fibrosis.

4.1. Morphological MRI

As regards the topographic relationship of the tumor with the mesorectal fascia can be adequately established with morphologic MRI [26]. The advent of powerful gradient systems and, above all, the development of high-resolution phased array surface coil systems in recent years brought the breakthrough in the staging of rectal cancer by MRI. The use of these phased-array surface coils combines a very high spatial resolution with a large FOV that allows not only detailed evaluation of the intestinal wall but also depicts surrounding anatomy including the mesorectal fascia.

A standard phased-array morphologic MRI protocol for LARC staging (including T-N stage and CRM evaluation) consists of T2-weighted coronal, transversal and sagittal turbospin-echo MR sequences with high spatial resolution (Fig. 1) [26].

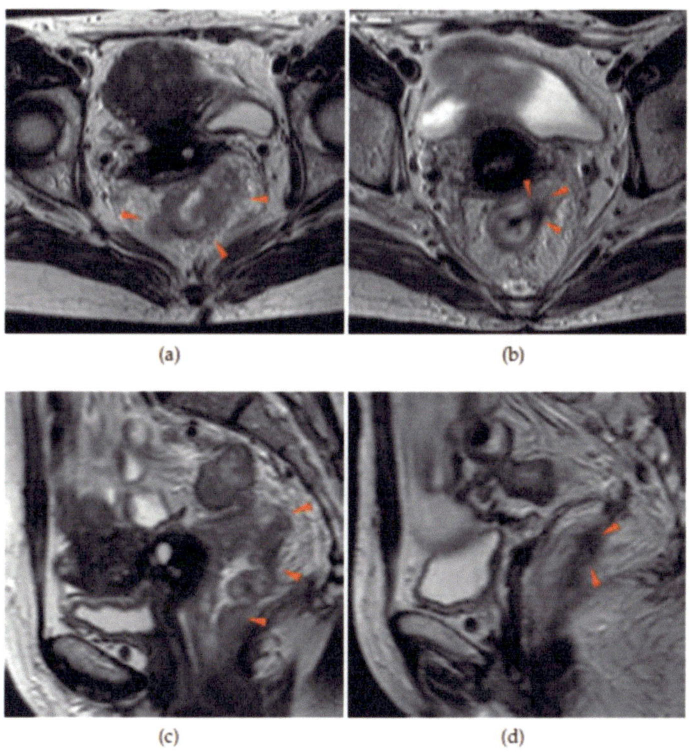

Figure 1. (a) A heterogeneous irregular thickening along the entire rectal wall is well shown on T2w axial pre-pCRT scan (arrowheads). (b) After pCRT, a hypo-intense spiculated area with thin digitations into peri-rectal fat is visible on T2w axial scan (arrowheads). (c) In the same patient, multiple irregular rectal wall thickening are shown on T2w sagittal pre-pCRT scan (arrowheads). (d) A single hypo-intense area, showed also in (b) is pointed by arrowheads, suspecting for a residual post-pCRT tumor focus (arrowheads).

An adequate, state-of-the-art MRI staging classification is capable to predict whether a tumor-free CRM is likely to be achieved or not [26]. In this way one would be able to differentiate patients with minimal mesorectal infiltration in whom neoadjuvant therapy is not mandatory from patients who would definitely benefit from neoadjuvant therapy because the mesorectal fascia is infiltrated or at risk.

The common use of total mesorectal excision (TME) and the shift from a postoperative to a preoperative chemo-radiotherapy (pre-CRT) approach have substantially reduced the risk of local recurrences, increasing curative resection and the rate of anal sphincter preservation and improving local control and overall survival rates [13-18].

4.2. Functional MRI

Although morphological tumour assessment performed by MRI has been repeatedly shown to be the most accurate modality in evaluating the presence of a positive circumferential resection margin (CRM), MRI is considered not to be conclusive in pre-CRT tumor response evaluation since histopathological downstage is not always associated with tumour effective reduction [17]. The main difficulty regarding post-chemoradiation MRI includes discrimination of active tumour and post-treatment fibrosis, particularly when differentiating stage T2 and stage T3 carcinomas, according to different recurrence and overall survival rates between Low Risk (T1/T2N0) and Intermediate Risk (T3/N0) as reported by Gunderson et al. [23-24].

Several studies have shown the potential of functional [diffusion- or perfusion] weighted imaging to predict the response to adjuvant or neoadjuvant therapy [5–7,19].

In fact, it has long been known that the pathophysiology and aggressiveness of a tumor are determined not only by the macroscopic tumor extent but also by other factors such as tumor microcirculation and angiogenesis.

4.2.1. DCE-MRI

Previous considerations support a Dynamic Contrast Enhanced-Magnetic Resonance Imaging (DCE-MRI) approach that could gain a renewed role to MRI adding functional data to the morphological examination. DCE-MRI has been reported by many authors as a tool potentially able to permit an evaluation of pre-CRT effectiveness basing on the strict relationship between tumor growth and angiogenesis [6-7,24-25].

DCE-MRI is gaining a large consensus as a technique for diagnosis, staging and assessment of therapy response for different types of tumours, due to its capability to detect highly active angiogenesis. It is well known that angiogenesis is a key factor in the growth and dissemination of cancer; characterization of the angiogenic status of the tumour on an individual patient basis could allow for a more targeted approach to treatment of rectal cancer [24].

More specifically, in the case of rectal cancer, previous trials have provided the proof of principle that inhibition of angiogenesis has the potential to enhance the effectiveness of the treatment for this disease. In vivo imaging techniques capable to assess tumour perfusion have the potential to improve the management of treatment for patients with rectal cancer [6-7,24-25].

Angiogenesis is a key factor for the growth and dissemination of solid tumors and is a prognostic marker in CRC. Neovascularization arises early in the adenoma–carcinoma sequence via upregulation of vascular endothelial growth factor. Tumor angiogenesis is characterized by structurally abnormal blood vessels that are thin, fragile, tortuous, and hyperpermeable. They have a chaotic, heterogeneous intratumoral distribution. Abnormal vascularity often extends beyond the tumor boundaries into surrounding tissues.

DCE-MRI techniques inform on tissue perfusion and vascular leakage (Fig. 2). T1- or relaxivity-based MR sequences are sensitive to the presence of dilute contrast medium in the extravascular– extracellular space. In most tumors, low-molecular-weight contrast media readily diffuse from the blood into the extravascular– extracellular space at a rate determined by perfusion and the capillary permeability and surface area.

The most commonly used model for analyzing DCE-MRI data uses two compartments where the contrast agent resides (blood plasma and extravascular– extracellular space). K^{trans} (volume transfer constant between the blood plasma and the extravascular–extracellular space, the washin rate, measured in minutes−1) and k_{ep} (rate constant between the extravascular–extracellular space back to the blood plasma, the washout rate, measured in minutes−1) determine the transport between these two compartments.

Physiologically, K^{trans} indicates a variable combination of the flow and permeability properties. For blood vessels where leakage is rapid (that is, when the extraction fraction during the first pass of the contrast agent is high, as typically is found in tumors), perfusion will determine contrast agent distribution and K^{trans} approximates to tissue blood flow per unit volume. There are circumstances in which transport out of the vasculature does not significantly deplete intravascular contrast medium concentration (that is, tissues with lower first-pass extraction fraction). This is typically found after treatment with chemotherapy or late after radiotherapy and in fibrotic lesions, and in these situations, K^{trans} approximates to the product of permeability and the surface area (permeability surface area product).

4.2.2. Diffusion-weighted imaging DWI-MRI

At present, the use of diffusion-weighted imaging (DWI) incorporated into a standard MR protocol is gradually increasing because of its proven benefit not only for tumor detection/characterization but also for monitoring treatment response (8–12). Diffusion-weighted imaging measures water diffusion characteristics, which are dependent on multiple factors such as cell density, vascularity, viscosity of extracellular fluid, and cell membrane integrity (12). By quantifying these properties and expressing them as an apparent diffusion coefficient (ADC), DWI could potentially be used as an imaging biomarker to better select patients with poor prognosis who will truly benefit from a more aggressive neoadjuvant treatment (8-12). In literature it was demonstrated that ADC values of rectal cancers significantly correlate with prognostic factors including the MRF status, the nodal stage and the histological differentiation grade.

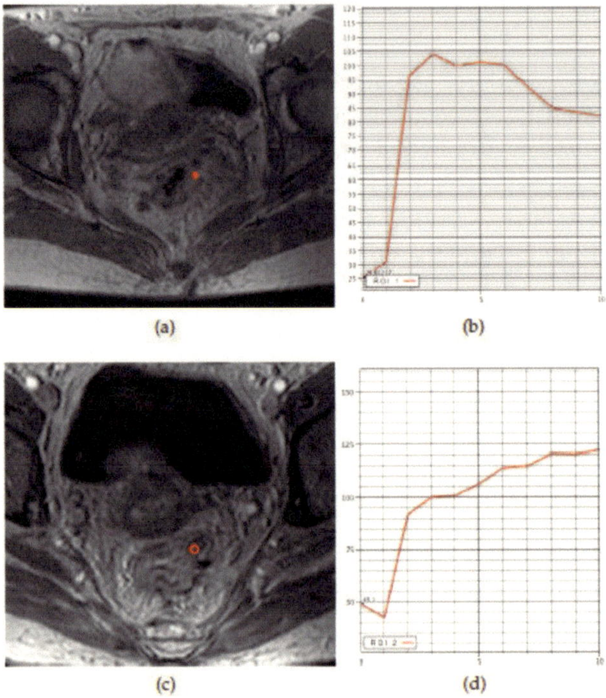

Figure 2. T1w post-contrast scan obtained on the same patient in fig. 8, before (a)-(b) and after (c)-(d) pre-CRT. The analysis of TIC calculated on a ROI, drawn outside the rectal wall where on T2w scans (fig. 8) tumor clearly spreads into peri-rectal fat pad, confirm this suspect showing a rapid CA intake and a fast discharge (b). After pre-CRT, on the same areas showed on T2w scans (fig. 8) no pathological CA uptake is present confirming that hypo-intense tissue visible on T2w scans are tumor nests but only residual inflammation due to pre-CRT. This patient was considered as a Responder. Histopathology showed a TRG 1.

The movement of water molecules in biologic tissues is restricted because their motion is modified and limited by interactions with cell membranes and macromolecules. Water-molecule motion in tissues can be assessed by applying diffusion- weighting gradients to T2-weighted sequences. This process entails the application of two balanced gradients placed symmetrically about a focusing 180° pulse. Water molecules that have not moved during the time taken to apply the first gradient will have acquired phase shifts that are exactly cancelled out by the proceeding second gradient; thus, there is no net additional signal loss induced by the application of the paired diffusion gradients. For water molecules that have moved during the application of the first gradient, however, the acquired phase shifts will not be cancelled out by the second gradient; residual phase incoherence will result in net losses of signal. Hence, the motion of water molecules is detected as attenuation of the measured signal intensity on DWI (Fig. 3).

The sensitivity of the DWI sequence to water motion can be varied by changing the parameter known as the b value (measured in s/mm2), which is proportional to the gradient amplitude, duration of the applied gradient, and time interval between the paired gradients. DWI can be

http://dx.doi.org/10.5772/56831

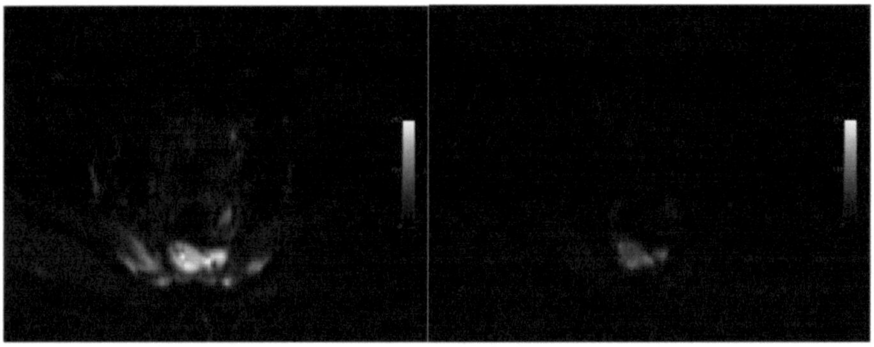

(a) (b)

Figure 3. (a) Axial diffusion weigthed imaging b=0, (b) Axial diffusion weigthed imaging b=800. Hyperintensity diffusion weigthed imaging is consistent with the diagnosis of tumor.

exploited in clinical practice to provide indirect assessments of tissue properties such as cellularity, gland formation, perfusion, and cell death. In general, the greater the cell density per high power field, the more impeded will be tissue water diffusion. Diffusion-weighted signal is derived from the motion of water molecules within the extravascular–extracellular space and intravascular space with some component from intracellular space water. The relative contribution of each space to the derived signal varies from tissue to tissue. In highly vascular tumors, intravascular water diffusion will account for a significant proportion of the diffusion-weighted signal. In highly glandular tissues, such as the pancreas and salivary glands, significant signal contributions arise from glandular water.

By performing DWI using different b values, quantitative analysis is possible with the calculation of the apparent diffusion coefficient (ADC, measured in μm/s). Areas of restricted diffusion show low ADC values. ADC values are inversely correlated with tumor cellularity and reductions in ADC correlate with response to cytotoxic therapy.

Areas retaining high signal intensity on high-b-value images usually (but not always) indicate highly cellular tissues such as tumors. Normal tissues including lymph nodes, spleen, nervous tissues, adrenal glands, bowel mucosa, and endometrium may show the same findings. Lower-signal-intensity regions are seen in most organized normal tissues, cystic spaces, and vessels. However, high signal intensities on high-b-value images are not always reliable indicators of increased cellularity on their own. Occasionally, fluid, edema, or mucinous materials remain of high signal intensity because of high proton density. This observation is called T2-shine through, but this effect can be detected easily by noting corresponding high signal on ADC maps.

There is growing interest in the application of DWI for the evaluation of CRC. DWI aids in detection of lesions, particularly when lesions are small. High-b-value DWI may be a useful tool for detecting and defining tumor extent.

DWI has been shown to be feasible as an early marker of treatment response because cell death and vascular alterations typically occur before size changes. Increases in ADC values with treatment reflect decreases in cellularity and thus provide indirect assessment of chemotherapy induced cell death. It has been reported that transient decreases in ADC may occur early in treatment related to cellular swelling, reduction in blood flow, or reduction in the extravascular– extracellular space due to dehydration. However, early decreases in ADC values are not consistently seen, and it has recently been reported that increases in ADC value with therapy response occur within 3–7 days in responding CRC patients treated with chemotherapy.

Responders had a lower ADC at presentation than non responders. Higher pretreatment ADC values in nonresponders may reflect necrotic tumors that are more resistant to therapy because of concomitant hypoxia. Similarly, for CRC liver metastases, a higher pretreatment ADC is also predictive of poor response.

5. A systematic review

5.1. Methodologies

A systematic literature search was performed to identify English-language studies and articles concerning different diagnostic imaging methodologies available in locally advanced rectal cancer disease after radiation therapy. Data were identified using PubMed database with the following keywords: "locally advanced rectal cancer, magnetic resonance imaging, CT planning, PET imaging". This yielded 309 titles. Articles, reviews and studies that did not present data about specificity and sensibility of tests treated were excluded. Due to the small number of studies for each imaging modality, there was not set a minimum number of patients as an inclusion criteria. For this reason, a total number of 12 titles were considered as studies included in the research.

Details regarding the number of patients, imaging modality investigated, the accuracy values and parameters examined of the studies were recorded. Cascini et al. [41] evaluated ^{18}F-FDG PET to assess the effect of chemoradiation therapy in thirty-three patients with LARC proved disease. They correlate the change in tumor ^{18}F-FDG standardized uptake value (SUV) during and after preoperative radiotherapy with the pathologic response achieved.

The accuracy of CT and MRI in restaging rectal cancer after preoperative chemoradiation in order to plan optimal therapy was performed in Martellucci et al. [42] study, in which thirty-seven consecutive patients undergoing neoadjuvant therapy were evaluated. Considering the depth of invasion after treatment only in neoplasia with stage T3 they found CT agree with histopathology in 19 cases and MRI in 10/12 cases.

Denecke et al. [46] compare CT, MRI and FDG-PET examining a total of twenty-three patients with T3/4 rectal cancer. Response criteria were a change in T category and tumour volume for CT and MRI and a change in glucose uptake for FDG-PET. Their results in sensitivity and specificity suggest that PET is superior to CT and MRI in predicting response to preoperative multimodal treatment of LARC.

A prospective analysis to evaluate tumor response with ^{18}F-FDG PET in twenty-seven patients with biopsy-proven rectal adenocarcinoma was conducted by Leibold et al. [47]. They found

http://dx.doi.org/10.5772/56831

of the total 27 patients, 11 (41%) had pathologic complete response; 16 (59%) had suboptimal response. They evaluate the ability of change in 4 specific PET parameters to predict pathologic response: the maximum SUV in the region of interest, SUV_{max}; the average SUV throughout the entire region of interest, SUV_{avg}; the summed metabolic rate of the tumor, TLG; the virtual graded global assessment of response, VRS.

Chien-Chih Chen et al. [37] evaluated the correlation between pathological verified tumor stage and clinical stage predicted by MRI. The overall predictive accuracy in T stage was 52%, whereas overstaging and understaging occurred in 38% and 10% of patients, respectively. Another study regard the MRI accuracy was conducted by Dresen et al. [45] using T2- weighted MR images obtained before and after radiation therapy and correlating findings with histopathology results.

Kristiansen et al. [39] investigated the possibility of using PET/CT to predict the histopathologic response in 30 patients with LARC treated with a combination of radiotherapy and concurrent Uftoral® and leucovorine. PET/CT correctly identified six of eight patients, specificity 75%, with complete pathologic response.

To evaluate the correlation between the change of SUV_{max} and of apparent diffusion coefficient (ADC) before and after neoadjuvant therapy, thirty patients with locally advanced rectal cancer were recruited in Ippolito et al. [40] analysis, in which all the patients underwent a whole body ^{18}F-FDG PET/CT scan and a pelvic MR examination including DW imaging for staging therapy.

Table 1 summarizes the main characteristics of the examined methodologies in locally advanced rectal cancer studies.

Study	Modality	No.Patients	Parameters
C. C. Chen et al. [37]	MRI	50	TNM
T. Denecke et al. [46]	MRI	23	TNM
	CT	23	TNM
	PET	23	SUV
G. L. Cascini et al. [41]	PET	33	SUV
C. Capirci et al. [38]	PET/CT	45	SUV
C. Kristiansen et al. [39]	PET/CT	30	TRG,SUV
R. Rosenberg et al. [44]	PET/CT	30	SUV
A. Suppiah et al. [36]	MRI	49	TNM
R. C. Dresen et al. [45]	MRI	67	TNM
T. Leibold et al. [47]	PET	27	SUV,TLG,VRS
D. Ippolito et al. [40]	MRI	30	ADC
	PET/CT	30	SUV
J. Martellucci et al. [42]	MRI	20	TNM
	CT	37	TNM
M. J. M. Duréndez et al. [43]	PET/CT	41	SUV

Table 1. Summary of the main characteristics of includes studies about different methodologies used in LARC diseases. Per each study the table reports: imaging modality used; number of patients examined; parameters examined; sensitivity and specificity methodology values.

5.2. Summary ROC curves and Forest Plots

In order to assess individual methodology in LARC treatment, Summary Receiver Operating Characteristic (SROC) curves have been realized, Fig. 4. ROC curves is a statistic technique for displaying, organizing and selecting classifiers based on their performance.

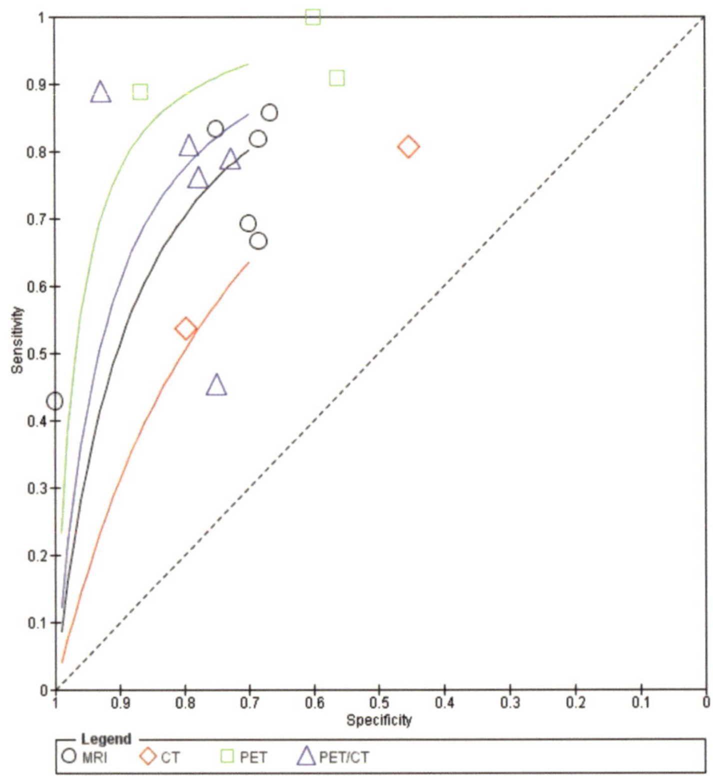

Figure 4. Estimated Summary ROC curves and original data points for four imaging techniques. MRI= magnetic resonance imaging, CT= computed tomography, PET= Positron emission tomography, PET/CT= positron emission tomography and computed tomography.

ROC analysis was performed through the study of the function that links the probability to obtain a true-positive result in the disease like class, i.e. the sensitivity, to the probability to obtain a false-positive result in the non-diseased class, linked to the specificity. In this way a graphical 2D representation that shows the false-positive proportion in x-axis and true-positive proportion in y-axis, relatively to values obtained from each test applied.

For each modality, a model was obtained that was adjusted for significant variables that were set to 1, indicating the ideal design versus 0, as appropriate, Fig. 4. The position of the summary ROC curve indicates the difference in diagnostic performance among the imaging modalities. A summary ROC curve located near the upper left corner indicate rte better diagnostic modality, while a summary ROC curve for a worthless modality is represented by the bisector, also named change line.

Another additional graphical representation realized is the Forest Plot, Fig. 5, which shows the sensitivity and specificity estimates of the results for each study. It is composed of a plot of the measure of effect for each of these studies incorporating confidence intervals represented by horizontal bars. The confidence interval expresses the precision level associated with the parameter estimation: the more is small, the more indicates that the prediction is accurate. In this analysis confidence intervals are computed with a probability of containing the true effect size equal to 95%. The blue square represents the point estimate, i.e. the sensitivity or specificity.

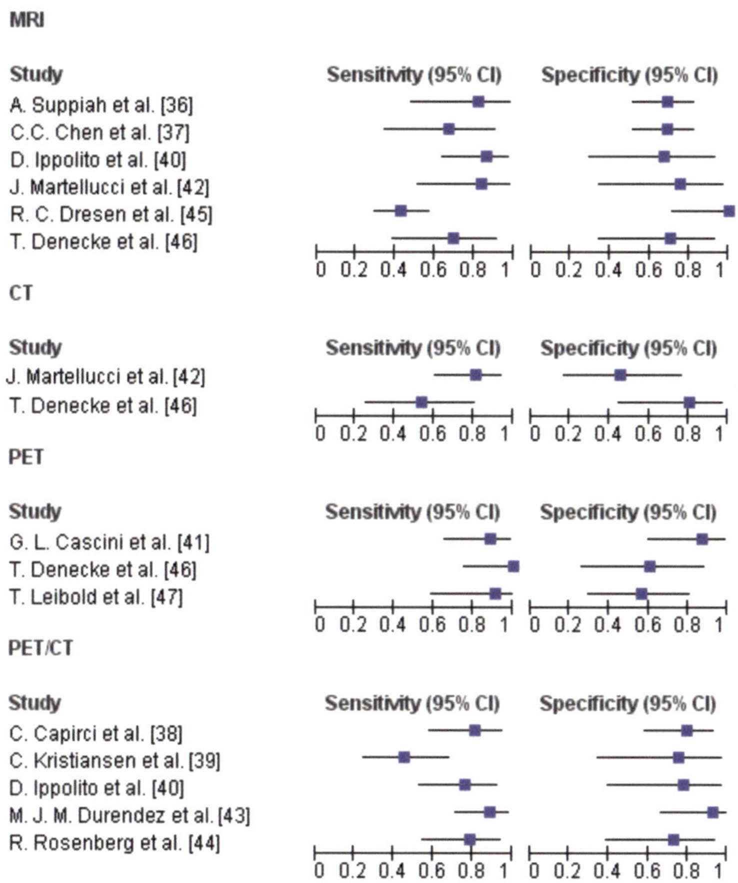

Figure 5. Forest Plot of MRI, CT, PET and PET/CT sensitivity and specificity estimates and their confidence intervals (95%).

5.3. Discussion

The objective of this statistical analysis was to evaluate the diverse methodologies (MRI, PET, PET/CT, CT) in LARC management. In particular, in our analysis we considered the accuracy in assessing the therapy response.

Although, the ROC curves analysis showed that PET has the best accuracy in term of sensitivity and specificity it should be noticed that only three studies have been retrieved from the literature.

However, in agreement with the intuitive considerations MRI and PET/ CT showed a high diagnostic accuracy and their results are also more reliable than PET because the statistical analysis has been carried out on a larger number of studies (6 studies for MRI with a total of 239 patients and 5 studies for PET/CT with a total of 176 patients).

The number of studies for CT is very small to draw detailed conclusions.

In conclusion we could state that a greater number of studies should be performed in the future for each modalities to improve the reliability of any conclusion.

Author details

Roberta Fusco[1,3], Mario Sansone[2], Mario Petrillo[3], Antonio Avallone[4], Paolo Delrio[3], Fabiana Tatangelo[3] and Antonella Petrillo[1]

1 Department of Diagnostic Imaging, Radiant and Metabolic Therapy, "Istituto Nazionale dei Tumori Fondazione G. Pascale " – IRCCS, Naples, Italy

2 Department of Electrical Engineering and Information Technologies University 'Federico II' of Naples, Italy

3 Department of Radiology, Second University of Naples, Italy

4 Gastrointestinal Medical Oncology, "Istituto Nazionale dei Tumori Fondazione G. Pascale " – IRCCS, Naples, Italy

References

[1] Jemal A, Siegel R, Xu J, Ward E. Cancer statistics, 2010. CA Cancer J Clin 2010;60(5): 277–300.

[2] Folkman J Tumor angiogenesis: therapeutic implications. N Engl J Med 1971;285:1182–1186.

[3] Choi HJ, Hyun MS, Jung GJ, Kim SS, Hong SH. Tumor angiogenesis as a prognostic predictor in colorectal carcinoma with special reference to mode of metastasis and recurrence. Oncology 1998; 55:575–581.

[4] Dvorak HF, Brown LF, Detmar M, Dvorak AM. Vascular permeability factor/vascular endothelial growth factor, microvascular hyperpermeability, and angiogenesis. Am J Pathol 1995;146:1029–1039.

[5] Dzik-Jurasz A, Domenig C, George M et al (2002) Diffusion MRI for prediction of response of rectal cancer to chemoradiation. Lancet 360 (9329):307–308

[6] Devries AF, Griebel J, Kremser C et al (2001) Tumor microcirculation evaluated by dynamic magnetic resonance imaging predicts therapy outcome for primary rectal carcinoma. Cancer Res 61(6):2513–2516

[7] DeVries AF, Kremser C, Hein PA et al (2003) Tumor microcirculation and diffusion predict therapy outcome for primary rectal carcinoma. Int J Radiat Oncol Biol Phys 56(4):958–96

[8] Koh DM, Padhani AR. Diffusion-weighted MRI: a new functional clinical technique for tumor imaging. Br J Radiol 2006;79: 633–635.

[9] Koh DM, Collins DJ. Diffusion-weighted MRI in the body: applications and challenges in oncology. AJR Am J Roentgenol 2007; 188:1622–1635.

[10] Patterson DM, Padhani AR, Collins DJ. Technology insight: water diffusion MRI-a potential new biomarker of response to cancer therapy. Nat Clin Pract Oncol 2008;5:220–233.

[11] Padhani AR, Liu G, Koh DM, et al. Diffusion-weighted magnetic resonance imaging as a cancer biomarker: consensus and recommendations. Neoplasia 2009;11:102–125.

[12] deSouza NM, Riches SF, Vanas NJ, et al. Diffusion-weighted magnetic resonance imaging: a potential non-invasive marker of tumour aggressiveness in localized prostate cancer. Clin Radiol 2008;63:774–782.

[13] Avallone A, Delrio P, Guida C, Tatangelo F, Petrillo A, Marone P, Cascini LG, Morrica B, Lastoria S, Parisi V, Budillon A, Comella P. (2006). Biweekly oxaliplatin, raltitrexed, 5-fluorouracil and folinic acid combination chemotherapy during preoperative radiation therapy for locally advanced rectal cancer: a phase I-II study, Brit J Cancer 94(12): 1809–1815.

[14] Avallone A, Delrio P, Pecori B, Tatangelo F, Petrillo A, Scott N, Marone P, Aloi L, Sandomenico C, Lastoria S, Iaffaioli VR, Scala D, Iodice G, Budillon A., Comella P. (2011). Oxaliplatin plus dual inhibition of thymidilate synthase during preoperative pelvic radiotherapy for locally advanced rectal carcinoma: long-term outcome, Int J Radiat Oncol 79(3): 670–676.

[15] Delrio P, Avallone A, Guida C, Lastoria S, Tatangelo F, Cascini GM, Marone P, Petrillo, A, Budillon A, Marzo MD, Palaia R, Albino V, Rosa VD, Parisi V. (2005). Multidis-

ciplinary approach to locally advanced rectal cancer: results of a single institution trial, Suppl Tumori 4(3): S8.

[16] Delrio P, Lastoria S, Avallone A, Ravo V, Guida C, Cremona F, Izzo F, Palaia R, Ruffolo F, Puppio B, Guidetti GM, Cascini GL, Casaretti R, Tatangelo F, Marone P, Rossi GB, Budillon A, Petrillo A, Rosa VD, Comella G, Morrica B, Tempesta A, Botti G, Parisi V. (2003). Early evaluation using PET-FDG of the efficiency of neoadjuvant radiochemotherapy treatment in locally advanced neoplasia of the lower rectum, Tumori 89(4 Suppl): 50–53.

[17] Petrillo A, Catalano O, Delrio P, Avallone A, Guida C, Filice S, Siani A. (2007). Post-treatment fistulas in patients with rectal cancer: MRI with rectal superparamagnetic contrast agent, Abdom Imaging 32(3): 328–331.

[18] Petrillo A, Filice S, Avallone A, Delrio P, Guida C, Tatangelo F, Marone P, Nunziata A, Siani A. (2006). Staging of locally advanced rectal cancer (LARC): proposal of 96 Rectal Cancer – A Multidisciplinary Approach to Management Dynamic Contrast Enhanced Magnetic Resonance Imaging in Rectal Cancer 23 a one-stop magnetic resonance (MR) imaging-based protocol, Eur Radiol Supplements 16: 321–494.

[19] Sansone M, Fusco R, Petrillo A, Petrillo M, Bracale M. (2011). An expectation-maximisation approach for simultaneous pixel classification and tracer kinetic modelling in dynamic contrast enhanced-magnetic resonance imaging, Med Biol Eng Comput 49(4): 485–495.

[20] Fusco R, Sansone M, Petrillo M, Antonella Petrillo. Influence of parameterization on tracer kinetic modeling in DCE-MRI. Journal of Medical and Biological Engineering, Uncorrected Proof Available online 7 Sep 2012, doi: 10.5405/jmbe.1097

[21] Fusco R, Sansone M, Maffei S, Petrillo.A. Dynamic Contrast-Enhanced MRI in Breast Cancer: A Comparison between Distributed and Compartmental Tracer Kinetic Models. Journal of Biomedical Graphics and Computing, Journal of Biomedical Graphics and Computing, vol. 2, no. 2, p. p23, Aug. 2012.

[22] Gunderson LL, Sargent DJ, Tepper JE, O'Connell MJ, Allmer C, Smalley SR, Martenson JA, Haller D. G.,Mayer, R. J., Rich, T. A., Ajani, J. A., Macdonald, J. S. & Goldberg, R.M. (2002). Impact of T and Nsubstage on survival and disease relapse in adjuvant rectal cancer: a pooled analysis, Int J Radiat Oncol 54(2): 386–396.

[23] Gunderson LL, Sargent DJ, Tepper JE, Wolmark N, O'Connell MJ, Begovic M, Allmer C, Colangelo L, Smalley SR, Haller DG, Martenson JA, Mayer RJ, Rich TA, Ajani JA, MacDonald JS, Willett CG, Goldberg RM. Impact of T and N stage and treatment on survival and relapse in adjuvant rectal cancer: a pooled analysis, J Clin Oncol 2004; 22(10): 1785–1796.

[24] Goh V, Padhani AR, Rasheed S. Functional imaging of colorectal cancer angiogenesis, Lancet Oncol 2007; 8(3): 245–255.

[25] Kremser C, Trieb T, Rudisch A, Judmaier W, de Vries A. Dynamic t(1) mapping predicts outcome of chemoradiation therapy in primary rectal carcinoma: sequence implementation and data analysis, JMagn Reson Imaging 2007; 26(3): 662–671.

[26] Beets-Tan RG, Beets GL. Rectal cancer: review with emphasis on MR imaging. Radiology. 2004 Aug;232(2):335-46.

[27] Kapiteijn E, Marijnen CA, Nagtegaal ID, et al. Preoperative radiotherapy combined with total mesorectal excision for resectable rectal cancer. N Engl J Med 2001;345:638–646

[28] Vermaas M, Ferenschild FT, Nuyttens JJ, et al. Preoperative radiotherapy improves outcome in recurrent rectal cancer. Dis Colon Rectum 2005;48:918–928

[29] Gerard JP, Conroy T, Bonnetain F, et al. Preoperative radiotherapy with or without concurrent fluorouracil and leucovorin in T3–4 rectal cancers: results of FFCD 9203. J Clin Oncol 2006;24:4620–4625

[30] Bosset JF, Collette L, Calais G, et al. Chemotherapy with preoperative radiotherapy in rectal cancer. N Engl J Med 2006;355:1114–1123

[31] Bosset JF, Calais G, Daban A, et al. Preoperative chemoradiotherapy versus preoperative radiotherapy in rectal cancer patients: assessment of acute toxicity and treatment compliance. Report of the 22921 randomised trial conducted by the EORTC Radiotherapy Group. Eur J Cancer 2004;40:219–224

[32] Willett CG, Boucher Y, di Tomaso E, et al. Direct evidence that the VEGF-specific antibody bevacizumab has antivascular effects in human rectal cancer. Nat Med 2004;10:145–147

[33] Vermaas M, Ferenschild FT, Verhoef C, et al. Total pelvic exenteration for primary locally advanced and locally recurrent rectal cancer. Eur J Surg Oncol 2007;33(4):452–458

[34] Wiig JN, Poulsen JP, Larsen S, Braendengen M, Waehre H, Giercksky KE. Total pelvic exenteration with preoperative irradiation for advanced primary and recurrent rectal cancer. Eur J Surg 2002;168:42–48

[35] Luna-Perez P, Delgado S, Labastida S, Ortiz N, Rodriguez D, Herrera L. Patterns of recurrence following pelvic exenteration and external radiotherapy for locally advanced primary rectal adenocarcinoma. Ann Surg Oncol 1996;3:526–533

[36] Suppiah A, Hunter IA, Cowley J, Garimella V, Cast J, Hartley JE, Monson JRT. Magnetic resonance imaging accuracy in assessing tumour down-staging following chemoradiation in rectal cancer. Colorectal Disease 22 April 2008;11:249-253.

[37] Chen CC, Lee RC, Lin JK, Wang LW, Yang SH. How Accurate is Magnetic Resonance Imaging in Restaging Rectal Cancer in Patients Receiving Preoperative Combined Chemoradiotherapy? Disease of the Colon & Rectum 17 February 2005;48:722-728.

[38] Capirci C, Rampin L, Erba PA, Galeotti, Crepaldi G, Banti E, Gava M, Fanti S, Mariani G, Muzzio PC, Rubello D. Sequential FDG-PET/CT reliably predicts response of locally advanced rectal cancer to neo-adjuvant chemo-radiation therapy. Nucl Med Mol Imaging 2007;34:1583-1593.

[39] Kristiansen C, Loft A, Berthelsen AK, Graff J, Lindebjerg J, Bisgaard C, Jakobsen A. PET/CT and Histopathologic Response to Preoperative Chemoradiation Therapy in Locally Advanced Rectal Cancer. Disease of the Colon & Rectum 2008;51:21-25.

[40] Ippolito D, Monguzzi L, Guerra L, Deponti E, Gardani G, Messa C, Sironi S. Response to neoadjuvant therapy in locally advanced rectal cancer: assessment with diffusion-weighted MR imaging and 18FDG PET/CT. Abdominal Imaging 20 January 2012.

[41] Cascini GL, Avallone A, Delrio P, Guida C, Tatangelo F, Marone P, Aloj L, De Martinis F, Comella P, Parisi V, Lastoria S. 18F-FDG PET Is an Early Predictor of Pathologic Tumor Response to Preoperative Radiochemotherapy in Locally Advanced Rectal Cancer. The journal of nuclear medicine August 2006;47(8):1241-1248.

[42] Martellucci J, Scheiterle M, Lorenzi B, Roviello F, Cetta F, Pinto E, Tanzini G. Accuracy of transrectal ultrasound after preoperative radiochemotherapy compared to computed tomography and magnetic resonance in locally advanced rectal cancer. Journal of Colorectal Deseases 3 February 2012;27:967-973.

[43] Murcia MJ, Duréndez L, Frutos Esteban J, Luján MD, Frutos G, Valero JL, Navarro Fernández L, Mohamed Salem G, Ruiz Merino MA, Claver Valderas. The value of 18F-FDG PET/CT for assessing the response to neoadjuvant therapy in locally advanced rectal cancer. Nucl Med Mol Imaging 19 October 2012;40:91-97.

[44] Rosenberg R, Herrmann K, Gertler R, Künzli B, Essler M, Lordick F, Becker K, Schuster T, Geinitz H, Maak M, Schwaiger M, Siewert JR, Krause B. The predictive value of metabolic response to preoperative radiochemotherapy in locally advanced rectal cancer measured by PET/CT. Colorectal Disease 3 December 2008;24:191-200.

[45] Dresen RC, Beets GL, Rutten HJT, Engelen SME, Lahaye MJ, Vliegen RFA, de Bruïne AP, Kessels AGH, Lammering G, Beets-Tan RGH. Locally Advanced Rectal Cancer: MR Imaging for Restaging after Neoadjuvant Radiation Therapy with Concomitant Chemotherapy Part I. Are We Able to Predict Tumor Confined to the Rectal Wall? Radiology July 2009;252(1):71-80.

[46] T. Denecke, B. Rau, K.-T. Hoffmann, B. Hildebrandt, J. Ruf, M. Gutberlet, M. Hünerbein, R. Felix, P. Wust, H. Amthauer. Comparison of CT, MRI and FDG-PETin response prediction of patients with locally advanced rectal cancer after multimodal preoperative therapy: Is there a benefit in using functional imaging? European Journal of Radiology 2 April 2005;15:1658-1666.

[47] Leibold T, Akhurst TJ, Chessin DB, Yeung HW, Macapinlac H, Shia J, Minsky BD, Saltz LB, Riedel E, Mazumdar M, Paty PB, Weiser MR, Douglas WW, Larson SM,

Guillem JG. Evaluation of 18F-FDG-PET for Early Detection of Suboptimal Response of Rectal Cancer to Preoperative Chemoradiotherapy: A Prospective Analysis. Official Journal of the society of surgical oncology 2011;18:2783-2789.

[48] Chau I, Allen M, Cunningham D, Tait D, Brown G, Hill M, Sumpter K, Rhodes A, Wotherspoon A, Norman AR, Hill A, Massey A, Prior Y. Neoadjuvant systemic fluorouracil and mitomycin C prior to synchronous chemoradiation is an effective strategy in locally advanced rectal cancer. British Journal of Cancer 2003;88:1017-1024.

[49] Corner C, Khimji F, Tsang Y, Harrison M, Glynne-Jones R, Hughes R. Comparison of conventional and three-dimensional conformal CT planning techniques for preoperative chemoradiotherapy for locally advanced rectal cancer. The British Journal of Radiology !4 December 2009;84:173-178.

[50] Ruby JA, Leibold T, Akhurst TJ, Shia J, Saltz LB, Mazumdar M, Riedel ER, Larson SM, Guillem JG. FDG-PET Assessment of Rectal Cancer Response to Neoadjuvant Chemoradiotherapy Is Not Associated With Long-Term Prognosis: A Prospective Evaluation. Diseases of the colon and rectum 2012;55(4):378-386.

[51] Kuo LJ, Chern MC, Tsou MH, Liu MC, Jian JJM, Chen CM, Chung YL, Fang WT. Interpretation of Magnetic Resonance Imaging for Locally Advanced Rectal Carcinoma After Preoperative Chemoradiation Therapy. Disease of the Colon & Rectum 7 December 2004;48(23-28).

[52] Yeung JMC, Kalff V, Hicks RJ, Drummond E, Link E, Phil D, Taouk Y, Michael M, Ngan S, Lynch AC, Heriot AG. Metabolic Response of Rectal Cancer Assessed by 18-FDG PET Following Chemoradiotherapy is Prognostic for Patient Outcome. Diseases of the colon & rectum 2011;54:518-525.

[53] Mezzi G, Arcidiacono PG, Carrara S, Perri F, Petrone MC, De Cobelli F, Gusmini S, Staudacher C, Del Maschio A, Testoni PA. Endoscopic ultrasound and magnetic resonance imaging for re-staging rectal cancer after radiotherapy. World Journal of Gastroenterology 28 November 2009;44:5563-5567.

[54] Patel UB, Taylor F, Blomqvist L, George C, Evans H, Tekkis P, Quirke P, Sebag-Montefiore D, Moran B, Heald R, Guthrie A, Bees N, Swift I, Pennert K, Brown G. Magnetic Resonance Imaging–Detected Tumor Response for Locally Advanced Rectal Cancer Predicts Survival Outcomes: MERCURY Experience. Journal of Clinical Oncology 2011;1-11.

[55] Johnston DF, Lawrence KM, Sizer BF, Arulampalam THA, Motson RW, Dove E, Lacey N. Locally advanced rectal cancer: histopathological correlation and predictive accuracy of serial MRI after neoadjuvant chemotherapy. The british journal of radiology 2009;82:332-336.

[56] Shanmugan S, Arrangoiz R, Nitzkorski JR, Yu JQ, Li T, Cooper H, Konski A, Farma JM, Sigurdson ER. Predicting Pathological Response to Neoadjuvant Chemoradio-

therapy in Locally Advanced Rectal Cancer Using18FDG-PET/CT. Society of Surgical Oncology 7 March 2012;19:2178-2185.

[57] Itatani Y, Akiyoshi T, Kuroyanagi H, Yamakawa K, Noaki R, Konishi T, Fujimoto Y, Ueno M, Oya M, Suenaga M, Yamaguchi T. Total mesorectal excision of initially unresectable locally advanced rectal cancer infiltrating the pelvic wall after treatment with FOLFOX4 plus bevacizumab and preoperative chemoradiation: report of a case. Surg Today 12 November 2011;42(75-79).

[58] O'Neill BDP, Brown G, Heald RJ, Cunningham D, Tait DM. Non-operative treatment after neoadjuvant chemoradiotherapy for rectal cancer. The lancet oncology July 2007;8:625-633.

[59] Fusco R, Sansone M, Petrillo M, Avallone A, Delrio P, Antonella Petrillo (2011). Dynamic Contrast Enhanced Magnetic Resonance Imaging in Rectal Cancer, Rectal Cancer - A Multidisciplinary Approach to Management, Giulio Aniello Santoro (Ed.), ISBN: 978-953-307-758-1, InTech, Available from: http://www.intechopen.com/books/rectal-cancer-a-multidisciplinary-approach-to-management/dynamic-contrast-enhanced-magnetic-resonance-imaging-in-rectal-cancer.

[60] Beets-Tan RG, Beets GL, Borstlap SC, Oei Tk, Teune TM, von Meyenfeldt MF, et al. Preoperative assessment of local tumour extent in advanced rectal cancer: CT or high- resolution MRI? Abdominal Imaging 2000;25(5):533-41.

[61] Wiering B, Ruers TJ, Oyen WJ. Role of FDG_PET in the diagnosis and treatment of colorectal liver metastases. Expert Rev Anticancer Ther 2004; 4: 607-13.

[62] Park IJ, Kim HC, Yu CS, et al. Efficacy of PET/CT in the accurate evaluation of primary colorectal carcinoma. Eur J Surg Oncol 2006; 32:941-947.

Chapter 4

Role of Tumour Markers in Diagnosis and Follow up of Colorectal Cancer — Potential for Future Research

Robert Partyka

Additional information is available at the end of the chapter

http://dx.doi.org/10.5772/57514

1. Introduction

1.1. Immunodiagnostics of Colorectal cancer — CEA and CA 19-9

Colorectal cancer is the second most common cancer in terms of incidence in men and women. Another concern is the high rate of morbidity and mortality in patients with this cancer. Therefore, researchers are constantly searching for new diagnostic methods that would enable the early detection of recurrent, clinically asymptomatic periods. The development of clinical immunodiagnostics has enriched oncology with the possibility of determining the quantity of glycoproteins and glycolipids in the blood of patients with cancer. These are called neoplastic markers. The usefulness of a neoplastic marker assay has been confirmed in diagnosing alimentary tract neoplasms, mainly in the early post-operative detection of a recurrence of neoplastic disease and in the evaluation of the efficacy of surgery.

According to an account published by The European Group on Tumor Markers (EGTM) of 2003, CEA is the main marker that is used in detecting colorectal cancer. It is important to point out, however, that approximately 10-15 % of patients do not produce CEA at all or that it is secreted in only minimal amounts. In such cases, the normal level of CEA concentration does not exclude the existence of a neoplasm even at an advanced stage. Therefore, the use of CA 19-9 as a tumor marker in diagnostics has been proposed.

1.1.1. Characteristic of CEA tumour marker

Carcinoembryonic antigen is a glycoprotein that contains about 60% carbohydrates. CEAs have epitopes that are specific to the neoplasm and epitopes that connect antibodies against nonspecific cross-reacting antigens (NCA, NCA2, BGP). Its upper normal range is 3 ng/ml [1, 2]

1.1.2. Characteristic of CA 19-9 tumour marker

The CA 19-9 Antigen is associated with gastrointestinal cancers. It occurs in the sialyated Lewis A blood group antigen that is produced in a small amount in the salivary and bronchial glands as well as in the pancreatic and bile ducts. This marker is very useful in the diagnosis of gastrointestinal cancers such as gastric, pancreatic, bile duct cancers and pancreatitis. Its upper normal range is 37 U/ml, but in approximately 1% of healthy people, concentrations reaching 120 U/ml have been detected [1, 2].

1.2. Aim of the study

The purpose of the study was to estimate the usefulness of selected neoplastic markers – conditioned by their location in the pre-operative and post-operative histological evaluations of patients with gastrointestinal cancers.

1.3. Material and methods

256 patients, both won men and women, aged 19-86, in whom colorectal cancer was diagnosed and histopathology was confirmed, were included into the research that was performed between 1991-1998.

Patients were divided into two groups according to the progression of the disease on the TMN scale and patients with a proctologic neoplasm on the Dukes and TMN scales. Neoplasm markers were marked in serum using commercial kits (blood samples were collected from the cubital vein and stored at -20°C after centrifugation). CEA and CA 19-9 were detected using the MEIA method using an Abbott's kit (USA). The upper normal range in healthy subjects is 3 ng/ml for CEA and 37 U/ml for CA 19-9.

The detection of neoplastic markers was performed in the Independent Laboratory of Clinical Immunodiagnostics at State Hospital No. 5 in Sosnowiec, Poland. Blood samples were collected preoperatively, in the first, second and third months after surgery and next after every 3 months for 2-5 years.

1.4. Results

The detection of neoplastic markers was extended about lab tests, abdominal ultrasonography; CT was performed in certain cases. Results were worked out using the t-Student test, the Cochran-Cox test, variance analysis (ANOVA) and the Shapiro-Wilk test for hardly large test.

Table I describes the results of the division of patients according to the stage of the disease on the TNM scale. The pre-operative CEA and CA 19-9 concentrations is presented in Figure 1 and Figure 2.

A pre-operative elevation of the CEA concentration in serum was found in 182 patients (71%). CEA did not exceed the normal range in the Dukes A group. CA 19-9 was increased in 83 (32%) patients in the Dukes C and D groups. The mean concentration of CEA and CA 19-9 changed according to the stage of the disease and were: Dukes A group – CEA ($\bar{x}$=1.82 ng/ml, CA 19-9 $\bar{x}$=12.45 U/ml, Dukes B group – CEA $\bar{x}$=5.97 ng/ml, CA 19-9 $\bar{x}$=15.37 U/ml, Dukes C group – CEA $\bar{x}$=7.42 ng/ml, CA 19-9 $\bar{x}$=55.73 U/ml, Dukes D group – CEA $\bar{x}$=17.97 ng/ml, CA 19-9 70.42 U/ml. In the post-operative follow-up, in which the Dukes D group was excluded, a recurrence was found in 53 patients, an elevation of CEA was found in 47 patients (88.6%) and CA 19-9 was found in 36 patients (67.9%). The recurrence was detected in 100% of the patients when an elevation of CEA CA 19-9 was accepted as a criterion. The results are shown in Figure 3.

Numbers of patients	Dukes scale	TNM scale
8	A	3 – T1N0M0 5 – T2N0M0
61	B	61 – T3N0M0
94	C	37 – T3N1M0 57 – T3N2M0
7	D	2 – T4N2M1 5 – T4N2M1

Table 1. The stages of the disease on the Dukes and TNM scales.

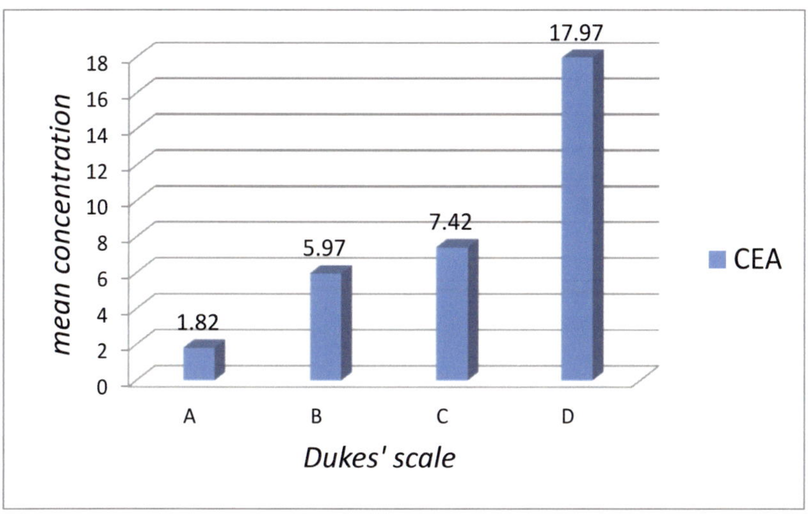

Figure 1. Mean concentration of CEA markers in pre-operative patients.

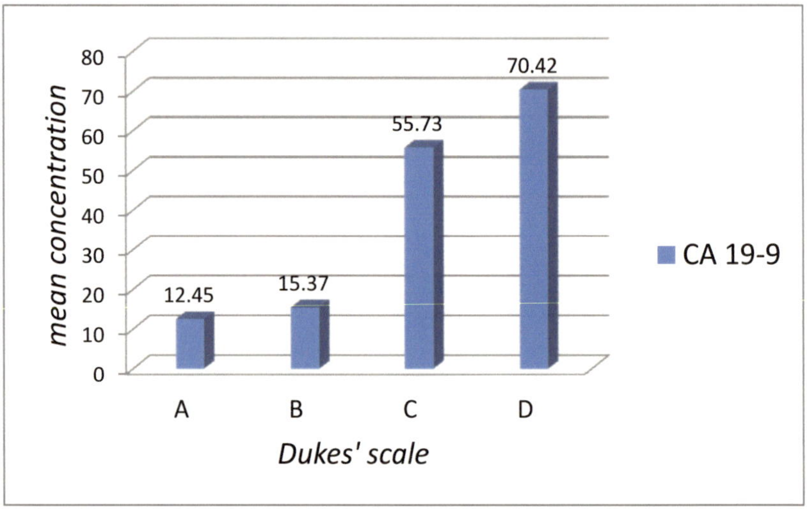

Figure 2. Mean concentration of CA 19-9 markers in pre-operative patients.

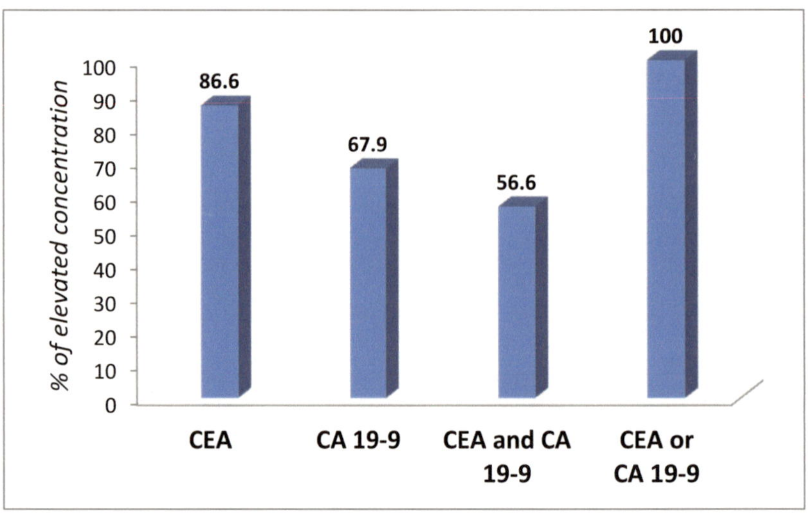

Figure 3. Percentage of CEA and CA 19-9 concentration in patients with a recurrence.

1.5. Discussion

Although the dreams of Bates et al. [3] to find an ideal marker for an active neoplastic process, i.e. that they have a different effect depending on the location of an organ and are absent in healthy people, were frustrated, neoplastic markers are now widely used in clinical diagnostics, usually for patients who have undergone surgery to remove cancerous tissue. Studies that lasted several years revealed that in order to estimate the efficacy of surgery, to detect a recurrence of a neoplastic process in the asymptomatic phase and to estimate the effectiveness of supplementary therapy, a determination of markers in the serum of patients plays a crucial role [1, 2, 4, 5, 6, 7, 8, 9].

Gold and Freedman [10] isolated carcinoembryonic antigen in colon cancer in 1966. They thought that it was specific to colorectal adenocarcinomas. The process of a quantitative determination of CEA in systemic fluids was described shortly thereafter, which indicated that more cancers produce CEA than had been previously thought. Moreover, it was found that its serum concentration may be higher than the normal range in non-neoplastic diseases such as pneumonia, bronchitis, tuberculosis, infections of the urinary tract and also in 30% of smokers [1, 10].

CEA is increased in non-neoplastic diseases of the intestines like colitis ulcerosa and Crohn's disease [1, 4, 11]. This information appeared to reduce the clinical value of a CEA assay; however, the development of monoclonal antibodies against CEA improved the specificity of the assays. This antigen is not present in the serum of all patients, even in a case of a recurrence, which was shown in studies that lasted for several years. Therefore, it is important to enhance clinical immunodiagnostics through the use of other markers (epitopes), which can use the information provided by the assay of CEA. The studies included 256 patients divided according to the stage of the cancer on the Dukes and TNM scales. Two neoplastic cancers CEA and CA 19-9 were determined in all 256 patients. Increased CEA was found in 182 patients (71%) and CA 19-9 was found in 83 patients (32%).

An analysis of the results revealed that in addition to CEA, CA 19-9 is an especially helpful marker. This agrees with the reports of Dienst et al. [12], who found increased concentrations of CEA in 49-58.5% of patients and increased concentrations of CA 19-9 in 21-67% of patients. However, Filela et al. [5] observed increased concentrations of CEA in 61% of patients and increased concentrations of CA 19-9 in 35% of patients. The concentration of both markers changed depending on the stage of the disease. CEA and CA 19-9 concentrations were within normal limits in the Dukes A group; the mean concentration of CEA was above the normal limits, 5.97 ng/ml, and CA 19-9 was within the normal limits in the Dukes B group. In the Dukes C group, the mean concentration of CEA was 7.42 ng/ml and the mean concentration of CA 19-9 was 55.73 U/ml. Similar results can be found in literature. Szymendera [2], Nowacki [7] and Lindmark et al. [13] revealed that in the advanced stages of colon cancer, a percentage of patients have elevated CEA and CEA concentrations. However, about 10-15% of patients do not secrete CEA.

The literature reveals that about 11-13% of patients with histopathologically confirmed colorectal cancer do not "produce" CEA and that an assay of these markers can lead to false negative results [2, 4, 9]. In these cases, the presence of advanced cancer is not excluded by a CEA concentration within the normal limits. CA 19-9 is the marker of first choice in this group of patients. The addition of CA 19-9 to an assay of CEA increased the sensitivity from 71% to 83.6% in our studies; however, 12.5% of patients with CEA within the normal limits had elevated CA 19-9. A positive correlation of CEA, CA 19-9 and the Dukes scale was revealed. Similar results were obtained by other authors. Fillela et al. [5] revealed that multifactoral analysis indicates the prognostic significance of CA 19-9 independent of the Dukes scale. New information about the CA 19-9 antigen has been revealed in recent years. CA 19-9 is sialofucololactotetraosyl and is included in the group of E-selectines. E-selectines enable a rise of remote metastases that is caused by the adhesion of neoplastic cells to epithelial cells in macrocirculation vessels. A pre-operative statistical analysis showed that the probability of recurrence is higher in cases where there is a higher CEA concentration before a treatment. However, Filela et al. [5] revealed that the risk of recurrence is 2.95 times greater in pre-operative patients with an increased concentration of CA 19-9 than in patients with a normal concentration of CA 19-9. 170 of 256 the patients who underwent surgery were tested in the follow-up phase. Patients in the Dukes D group were not tested. A recurrence was observed in 53 of the 170 patients (31%). The mean concentration of CEA was 20.71 ng/ml in the Dukes B group and 20.55 ng/ml in the Dukes C group. The mean concentration of CA 19-9 was 61.61 U/ml and 197.18 U/ml, respectively. A recurrence was detected in 100% of the patients when an increased concentration of CEA or CA 19-9 was used as a criterion. A recurrence was detected in 88.6% of patients when only CEA was estimated and 67.9% of patients when only CA 19-9 was estimated. The differentiation of a local neoplasm and remote metastases is difficult. Szymendera [2] reported that a concentration of CEA that is greater than 20 indicates metastases in the liver, while a small concentration of CEA or CA 19-9 might indicate metastases in the bones or lymph nodes.

1.6. Conclusions

1. Simultaneous detection of CEA and CA 19-9 should be the first immunodiagnostic test in patients suspected of having colorectal cancer.
2. The use of carcinoembryonic antigen is advisable in order to monitor the course of the disease in the case of an increased serum concentration of CEA and CA 19-9.
3. An increased concentration of CA 19-9 along with a normal lack of CEA in the serum of patients with colorectal adenocarcinomas is unfavorable prognostically.

The continuous development of immunodiagnostic methods and the production of monoclonal antibodies can bring new neoplastic markers into diagnostics. One of these is the TPS (Tissue Polipeptide Specific Antigen). Its structure is similar to the TPA (Tissue Polipeptide Antigen). Reports in the last 2-3 years suggest the great value of the determination of TPS in the serum of patients, including patients with gastrointestinal cancers, especially for the early detection of release and estimation of therapy effectiveness. TPS is a marker of cell proliferation and an increase in its concentration in serum often precedes the markers of a tumor

2. Scientific literature indicates interest of a cellular proliferation marker — TPS

A review of medical reports from recent years shows an increasing interest in estimating TPS levels mainly in oncologic diagnostics. Estimating TPS- concentration (which is a marker connected with the proliferation of neoplastic cells) is very important for monitoring patients who have undergone cancer surgery (esp. of the digestive tract, but also for breast and ovarian cancer) proceeding the clinical symptoms of metastasis for 2-7 months.

2.1. Characteristic of tissue polypeptide specific antigen (TPS) — Soluble fragments of cytokeratine 18

TPS (tissue polypeptide specific antigen) is a new marker of cellular proliferation. The antibody directed against TPS enables the determination of the concentration of the soluble fragments of cytokeratin 18 [14]. TPS was introduced into oncological immunodiagnostics by Bjorklund. It has one of the two active epitopes of TPA (tissue polypeptide antigen) that are detectable by the monoclonal antibody M3. TPS is a singular conjugated polypeptide chain that is created in the S and G2 phases of the cellular cycle and is released immediately after mitosis. It has 33 antigen determiners, two of which are connected with the activity of a tumor. TPS is strictly connected with the proliferation of neoplastic cells and is a function of the velocity of cell divisions [15].

2.2. Clinical results of serum concentration of TPS in patients with colorectal cancer

2.2.1. Aim of the study

1. To estimate pre-operative CEA and TPS concentrations in the blood serum of patients with colorectal cancer and rectal carcinomas depending on the advancement of their disease.
2. To attempt to determine whether TPS provides additional information that cannot be obtained from CEA tests only.

2.2.2. Material and methods

178 patients (101 men and 77 women) aged 22-86 years who had been diagnosed with colorectal cancer and had undergone surgery in the years 1991-2002 were included in the study. The patients were being treated at the Department of General Surgery and Coloproctology of the Medical University of Silesia in Sosnowiec. The CEA concentration was determined in the patients' blood serum using the MEIA method and commercial sets from Abbott (USA). TPS was determined using the enzyme-immunological method (EIA) and sets from BEKI (Sweden). The normal concentration of CEA was determined as 3 ng/ml and in the case of TPS – 90 U/l.

The criteria for choosing patients for the research: 178 patients whose pre-operative diagnostics confirmed the existence of a colon or rectal adenocarcinoma in a histopathological examination.

The criteria for excluding patients from the research. The research excluded patients who were diagnosed with:

- an inflammation of the large intestine (colitis ulcerosa, Leśniowski-Crohn disease),
- chronic kidney diseases,

- chronic liver diseases,
- an inflammation of the rheumatoid joints,
- autoimmunological diseases caused by autoimmunity (Hashimoto, Graves-Basedov, thyroid cysts),
- diabetes, or
- chronic infections.

The largest number of patients in the research was in the Dukes C group – 89 patients (50%). The fewest number of patients was in the Dukes A group – 8 patients (10.11%)(Table II)

Numbers of patients	Dukes scale	TNM scale
8	A	3 – T1N0M0 5 – T2N0M0
62	B	62 – T3N0M0
89	C	53 – T3N1M0 36 – T3N2M0
19	D	11 – T4N2M1 8 – T4N2M1

Table 2. The degree of the clinical advancement of colon and rectal carcinomas according to Dukes.

2.2.2.1. Statistical methods

All results were statistically measured using the Statistica 6.0 program from StatSoft Inc.

2.2.3. Results

No increased abnormal CEA concentration was found in any patient in the Dukes A subgroup. An increased amount of CEA was found in 37 cases (59.7%) in the Dukes B subgroup, in 75 patients (83.9%) in the Dukes C subgroup and in 17 cases (89.57%) in the Dukes D subgroup.

Another profile was observed when determining TPS. An increased concentration was found in 3 patients (37.5%) in the Dukes A subgroup. An increased concentration was found in 48 cases (77.4%) in the Dukes B subgroup, in 59 cases (65.5%) in the Dukes C subgroup and in 6 cases (31.6%) in the Dukes D subgroup. (Table III)

Dukes	CEA [%]	TPS [%]
A	0,00	37,5
B	59,68	77,41935
C	83,91	65,51724
D	89,47	31,57895

Table 3. The percentage of patients with an increased abnormal concentration of CEA and TPS in relation to the Dukes scale.

http://dx.doi.org/10.5772/57514

In cases where the division according to the degree of advancement in the whole group of 178 patients was not taken into account, the sensitivity for pre-operative CEA concentration was 72.5% and for TPS – 65.2%. When only cases with increased levels of CEA and TPS concentrations were taken into account, the sensitivity of the test increased to 82.6%.

The concentration of CEA was: 2.34 ng/ml in the Dukes A subgroup, 5.71 ng/ml in the Dukes B subgroup, 8.66 ng/ml in the Dukes C subgroup and 19.97 ng/ml in the Dukes D subgroup, respectively. (Table IV)

Dukes	Number of patients	Average amount	Standard deviation	Standard error	-95% CI	+95% CI
A	8	2,34	0,362284	0,128087	2,03462	2,64038
B	62	5,71	4,385849	0,557003	4,59636	6,82396
C	89	8,66	7,035047	0,745713	7,17906	10,14296
D	19	19,97	9,826148	2,254273	15,23553	24,70763

Table 4. CEA concentration in patients before surgery in relation to the degree of the advancement of the cancer according to Dukes.

Another characteristic was observed in the case of the determination of TPS concentration. The highest average pre-operative TPS concentration was found in the Dukes C subgroup – 226.7 U/l. It was 107.4 U/l in the Dukes A subgroup and 181.2 U/l in the Dukes B subgroup. However, the average amount measured in the Dukes D subgroup was 167.37 U/l, which may be connected with a decrease in proliferation. (Table V)

Dukes	Number of patients	Average amount	Standard deviation	Standard error	-95% CI	+95% CI
A	8	107,41	60,0221	21,22102	57,2328	157,5922
B	62	181,20	75,9138	9,64106	161,9283	200,4853
C	89	226,71	126,6201	13,42170	200,0392	253,3848
D	19	167,37	145,3267	33,34024	97,3295	237,4200

Table 5. TPS concentration in patients before operation in relation to the degree of the advancement of the cancer according to Dukes.

A recurrence of the disease was detected in 47 patients (Dukes B and C). When the concentration of CEA was used, recurrence was detected in 89.4% of patients and when the concentration of TPS was used, recurrence was detected in 80.85% of patients. If the criterion was an elevated concentration of CEA or TPS, recurrence was detected in of 100% patients. The concentration of CEA in patients with a recurrence was $\bar{x}$=12.82 ± 4.73 ng/ml in the Dukes B group and $\bar{x}$=13.5 ± 7.69 ng/ml in the Dukes C group. The concentration of TPS was $\bar{x}$=282.95 ± 56.08 U/l in the Dukes B group and C $\bar{x}$= 313.77 ± 116.62 U/l in the Dukes C group.

2.2.4. Discussion

In diagnosing carcinomas of the digestive system, particularly in the case of colon and rectal carcinomas, the carcinoembryonic antigen (CEA) still remains the "gold standard" [16, 17, 18]. However, great expectations are connected with the introduction of the soluble fragments of cytokeratin 18 (TPS) into the immunodiagnostics of colorectal cancer because TPS reflects the velocity of cell divisions [19].

Our results of pre-operative CEA concentrations are similar to those that have been reported by other researchers. Treska et al. obtained the highest sensitivity of CEA assessment from 45% to 80% depending on the degree of the progression of cancer [20]. Similar results were reported by Turoldo et al. and Marchena et al. [21, 22].

The main aim of the presented research was to estimate the usefulness of determining TPS concentration. The TPS sensitivity was 65.17% in our own clinical research. The highest pre-operative sensitivity equaling 70% was reported by Plebani et al. [23].

We also observed that the sensitivity of the test increased when the results of the determination of TPS and CEA were combined. An abnormal pre-operative CEA concentration was recorded in 129 patients (72.47%). When determining TPS concentration, 116 patients were found to have increased abnormal levels (65.17%). When the established criterion was an increased level of TPS or CEA, then the sensitivity of the test increased to 82.31%. Lindmark et al. using the CEA, CA 19-9, CA 50 and TPS tests proved their correlation with one another; however, only the TPS concentration test had the highest diagnostic sensitivity [18].

It is important to stress that adding TPS determination to the standard tests used for detecting and monitoring colon and rectal carcinomas has recently been approved by the European Group of Tumor Markers. According to the EGTM tests, adding TPS determination to the list of "mass tumor" markers enables an increase in sensitivity, particularly in the earlier stages of colorectal cancer [24].

2.2.5. Conclusions

1. The profile of the activity of pre-operative TPS concentration in the blood serum of patients with colorectal cancer in relation to the degree of the advancement of the cancer is different from that observed for CEA.

2. Determination of TPS concentration in patients with colorectal cancer provides essential information necessary to confirm the cancer, particularly at the earliest stages of its advancement.

http://dx.doi.org/10.5772/57514

3. Apoptosis and proliferation – Bcl-2

The mechanism of malignancy is considered to be an imbalance between apoptosis and the processes of proliferation. A phenotype that is resistant to apoptosis is one of the major features of cancer cells. Recently, attention has been drawn to the function of a number of proteins that inhibit the process of apoptosis within a tumor. To date, only a few works connected with the assessment of apoptosis proteins serum concentrations have been published. Most of the works about apoptosis concern immunohistochemistry studies.

This study attempts to find an answer to the question of whether the serum concentration of antiapoptotic the Bcl-2 protein provides additional information for the post-operative monitoring of patients with colorectal cancer.

3.1. Material and methods

The research was conducted on 46 patients (21 with a B Astler-Coller's stage cancer and 25 with a C Astler-Coller's stage cancer) was it colon cancer, who underwent surgery (resection RO). Their ages ranged from 47 to 85 (average age 67); sex (19 women, 27 men). The patients were divided into 2 groups: I –patients with a recurrence of cancer and II – patients without a recurrence of cancer. The control group consisted of 20 healthy people, mainly medical staff. The average CEA concentration in this group was 1.6 ng/ml+/- 0.43; TPS: 48.67U/l+/- 9.1; Bcl2: 0.31ng/ml+/- 0.13. The period of the observation of the patients and conducting the research was 1-5 years. The recurrence of the disease or the lack of a recurrence was confirmed using a physical examination and additional examinations during the oncological follow-up. Ten ml of venous shunt blood was collected from each patient. The serum was frozen at -20°C after centrifuging-. The blood for testing was collected one day before the surgery and 1, 3, 6 and 12 months after the surgery. CEA was measured using MEIA method and a commercial set from ABBOT (USA). The standard concentration for a healthy person was adopted as 3ng/ml. TPS was measured using the EIA method and sets from Beki Diagnostic Bromma (Sweden). The standard for a healthy person does not exceed 90 U/I. Bcl-2 concentration was labeled using the ELISA method using SORIN-BIOMEDICA tests (Italy). A standard for healthy people is 0.5 ng/ml. The results obtained were analyzed statistically. Calculations were done using Microsoft Excel 2003. The Ethical Committee at the Silesian Medical University approved the studies.

3.2. Results

Of the 46 patients who underwent surgery, a recurrence was detected in 14 patients including 6 with an initial stage of a tumor – B according to the Dukes classification as modified by Astler-Coller and 8 – degree C. The detection time of the recurrence was from 6 to 23 months. Most of the recurrences were distant metastases: 9 in the liver and 2 in the lungs. A local recurrence was observed in the intestinal stapling or retroperitoneal space in 3 patients. (Table VI) and (Figures 4, 5 and 6)

It was established that the Bcl-2 concentration was statistically significantly higher in the recurrence group than in the non-recurrence group when examined 1, 3, 6 and 12 months after the surgery. The TPS concentration was statistically significantly higher in the recurrence group than in the non-recurrence group when examined before and 3, 6 and 12 months after the surgery. The concentration of the antigen, i.e. CEA, was statistically significantly higher in the recurrence group in relation to the non-recurrence group, as was TPS in the pre-operative determinations and 3, 6 and 12 months after the surgery. Bcl-2, TPS and CEA serum concentrations were unrelated to the Astler-Coller stage of colorectal cancer. However, insignificantly higher concentrations of CEA at degree C than at degree B were observed. There was also no dependence related to the sex, the age of a patient, the original location of the tumor and the recurrence. Correlations between the concentrations of the determined parameters in all patients (with a recurrence and without a recurrence) were also noticed. A strong correlation between the concentrations of Bcl-2 and TPS proteins occurred 12 months after the surgery in the recurrence group.

Feature	**No recurrence**				**Recurrence**			
	Average	**SD**	**Min.**	**Max.**	**Average**	**SD**	**Min.**	**Max.**
Bcl2_0	8,09	6,82	0,41	24,39	10,39	6,78	0,57	23,02
Bcl2_1	7,34	6,07	1,74	28,41	8,87	3,17	4,09	14,61
Bcl2_3	7,40	6,58	0,50	29,79	12,15	8,14	0,55	30,00
Bcl2_6	6,97	6,99	0,41	26,40	17,50	7,98	1,98	29,74
Bcl2_12	8,38	7,67	1,47	25,09	20,52	7,03	12,14	29,81
CEA_0	5,26	7,22	1,70	42,60	5,75	2,60	2,30	11,90
CEA_1	2,61	1,00	1,10	6,30	2,46	0,53	1,70	3,00
CEA_3	1,87	0,90	0,40	3,70	4,94	3,88	1,20	17,40
CEA_6	2,21	2,19	0,30	11,90	10,72	5,74	3,70	20,30
CEA_12	2,57	2,97	0,40	14,60	14,86	13,92	1,30	41,00
TPS_0	98,9	19,1	60,4	160,3	118,1	31,1	60,7	168,9
TPS_1	92,8	16,8	64,6	143,7	101,6	17,7	80,3	144,1
TPS_3	95,9	27,0	64,7	188,3	125,2	31,0	90,7	193,7
TPS_6	96,8	35,7	70,3	197,6	152,0	49,0	80,4	279,1
TPS_12	96,6	37,9	70,4	207,4	152,4	34,2	100,0	190,4
Age	66,2	10,9	47,0	85,0	70,4	4,0	64,0	77,0

Table 6. Values of the basic description parameters (0 – preoperative results and 1-, 3-, 6-, and 12 months after the surgery.

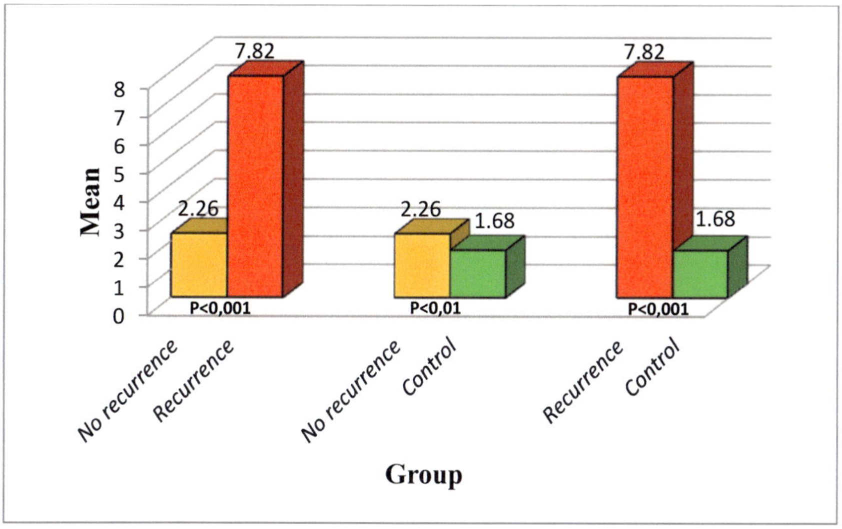

Figure 4. Results of the evaluation of post-operative CEA levels in the group without recurrence, with recurrence and the control group.

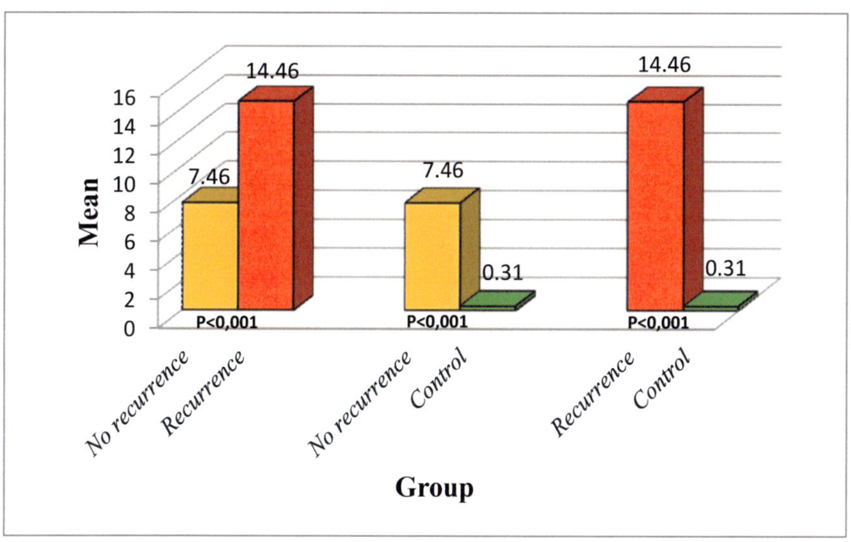

Figure 5. Results of the evaluation of post-operative Bcl-2 levels in the group without recurrence, the recurrence and the control group.

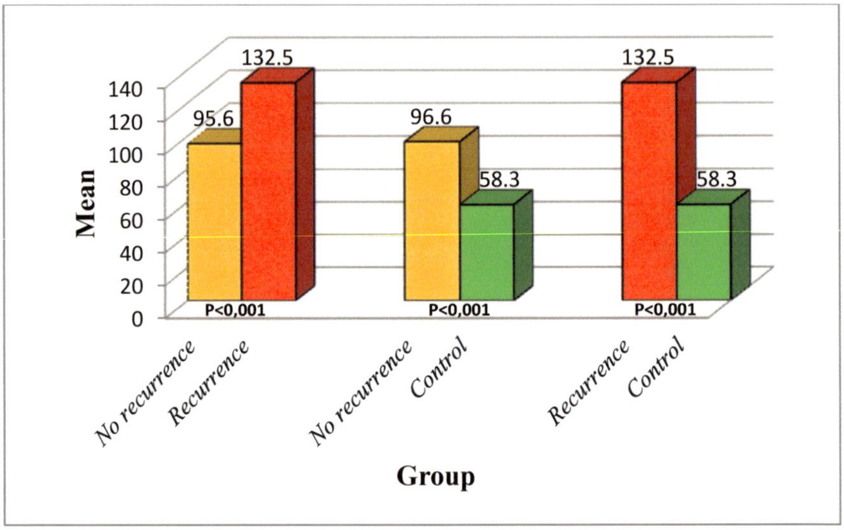

Figure 6. Results of the evaluation of post-operative TPS levels in the group without recurrence, the recurrence and the control group.

3.3. Discussion

The European Tumor Markers Association recommended CEA as a useful clinical marker in the diagnosis and monitoring of patients with colorectal cancer in 2003. To date, many scientific researchers have been shown that the addition of tumor markers in the diagnosis of patients with colorectal cancer is necessary. Colorectal cancer, like breast and lung cancer, reveals a high expression of the antiapoptotic proteins: Bcl-2, Bcl-XL, PED, Il-4, which are secreted by tumor cells, strengthens that expression and protects neoplastic cells by environmental death signals.

A low expression of BAX expression correlates with disease recurrence of the disease in preoperatively irradiated rectal carcinomas and is connected with a worse response. A decrease in the expression of BAX indicates the worst response to chemotherapy and reduces the life expectancy of patients [25, 26, 27].

Our results show that an increase of Bcl-2 in the serum of patients with colorectal cancer is bad prognostically. A high concentration ($\bar{x}$=14.46 ng/ml) was observed in the group with a recurrence of the disease. The concentration of the Bcl-2 protein has been correlated with TPS – a marker of cell proliferation. A high correlation in 12th month after surgery may confirm that the suppression of the apoptosis of cancer cells increases their proliferation.

At the present time the apoptotic process and the process of cell proliferation are the targets of many researchers in different areas of specialization.

3.4. Conclusions

1. A statistically significant excess of Bcl-2 in patients who have a recurrence of colorectal cancer makes information saying about the suppression of cancer cells apoptosis.
2. A statistically significant increase of the concentration of TPS in the group with a recurrence seems to indicate that the suppression of apoptosis is conductive to an excessive proliferation of cancer cells.
3. The findings obtained can mean that the evaluation of Bcl-2 and TPS may be complementary to CEA determinations in the post-operative follow-up of patients with colorectal cancer.

4. Angiogenesis – VEGF

The process of angiogenesis, which is the creation of new blood vessels, plays an important role in the development and metastasis of cancer. It can be initiated by tumor cell hypoxia, tumor suppressor gene mutations and oncogenes. As a result of the accumulation of these processes, tumor cells activate the angiogenic factors. The main factor involved in angiogenesis is VEGF-A. Blocking angiogenesis is one of the ways of preventing the development and metastasis of cancer and is the future of cancer therapy.

4.1. Aim of the study

1. An assessment of the concentration of VEGF-A in the blood serum of patients with colorectal cancer.
2. An attempt to answer the question of whether the determination of VEGF-A provides clinically meaningful information in the post-operative monitoring of patients.

4.2. Material and methods

117 patients underwent surgery for colorectal cancer in the years 2004-2009. Patients were divided according to the Dukes and TNM classifications. The control group consisted of 20 healthy volunteers. A recurrence was detected in 35 patients in the period of 623 months after the surgery, including 11 patients in the Dukes B group and 24 patients in the Dukes C group. Patients with a recurrence were grouped together, while the remaining 71 patients made up the group without a recurrence.

The concentration of CEA and VEGF-A was determined in all of the patients before the surgery and 1, 3, 6 and 12 months after the surgery. CEA was determined by MEIA using Abbott kits (USA); the standard concentration in healthy people is 3 ng/ml. VEGF-A was determined by ELISA using BIOMEDICA Sorin kits (Italy); the standard concentration in healthy people is 350 pg/ml.

The results were analyzed statistically. ROC curves were marked for the diagnostic parameters studied.

4.3. Results

The pre-operative mean CEA concentrations differed significantly in all three degrees of the severity of the disease (p<0.01). In the post-operative control, patients demonstrated statistically significant differences in CEA concentrations 3, 6 and 12 months after surgery with the largest concentration at the month follow-up (p<0,001). (Figure 7).

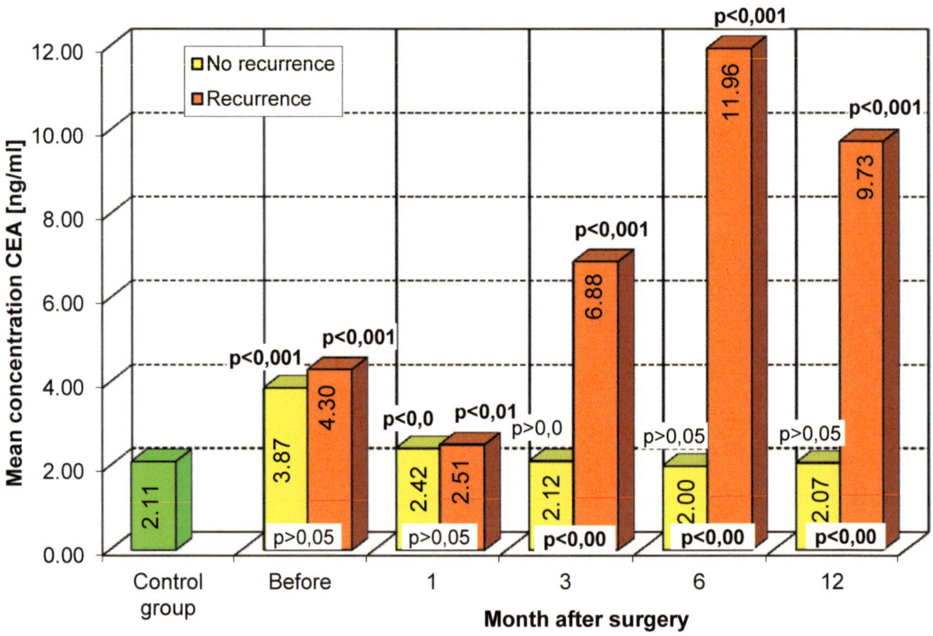

Figure 7. Evaluation of the concentration of CEA in the control group and in the groups of patients with and without a recurrence of a tumor in the subsequent stages of observation.

Most recurrences were detected during this period. The average concentrations of CEA in patients without a recurrence was 2.18 ng/ml and in patients with a recurrence 7.58 ng/ml. The ROC curves analysis showed a concentration of CEA of 3.1 ng/ml as early as 3 months after the surgery, which confirms the recurrence of the cancer (Figure 8).

Pre-operatively, a high concentration of VEGF-A was found in each stage of the disease; however, it showed no difference in levels of statistical significance. Throughout the period of post-operative observation, patients demonstrated a very high statistical significance between the group without a recurrence and those with a recurrence of the neoplastic process (p<0,001). (Figure 9)

The average concentration in patients without a recurrence was 294.24 pg/ml, while in patients with a recurrence it was 501.89 pg/ml. ROC curves showed the usefulness of VEGF-A in detecting a recurrence a month after surgery and a concentration of 412 pg/ml, it is confirmed (Figure 10).

http://dx.doi.org/10.5772/57514

In addition, a high, statistically significant correlation between VEGF-A and CEA was demonstrated 3, 6 and 12 months after surgery (Figure 11 and 12).

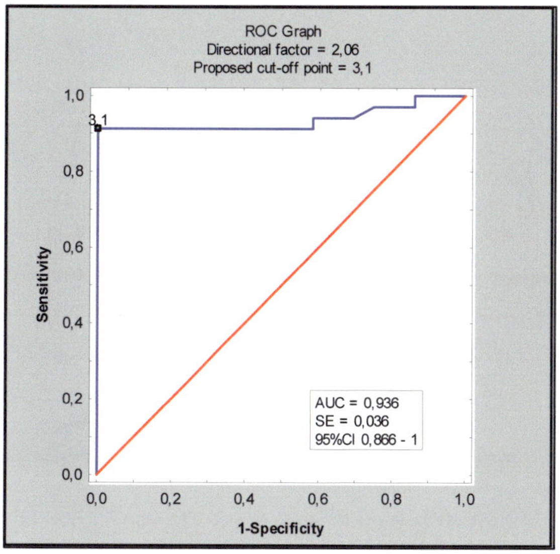

Figure 8. ROC curve for the concentration of CEA determined at the 3-month follow-up.

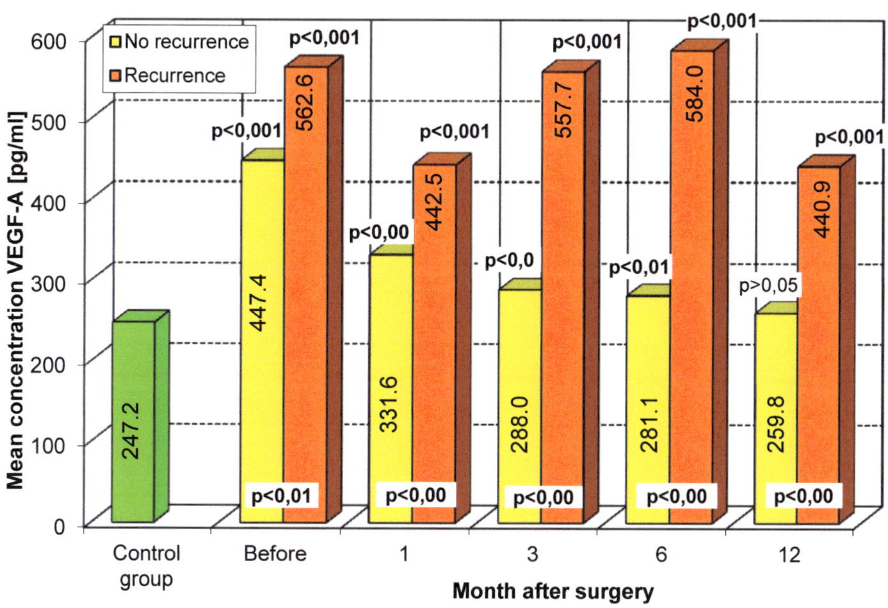

Figure 9. Evaluation of the concentration of VEGF-A in the control group and in the group of patients with and without a recurrence of a tumor in the subsequent stages of observation.

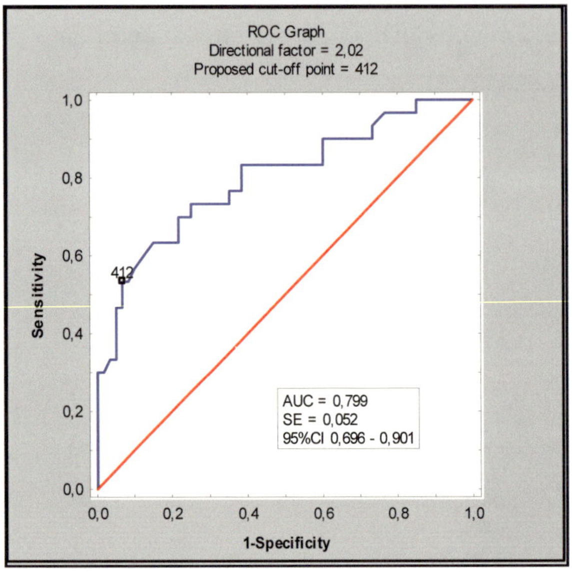

Figure 10. ROC curve for the concentration of CEA determined at a one-month follow-up.

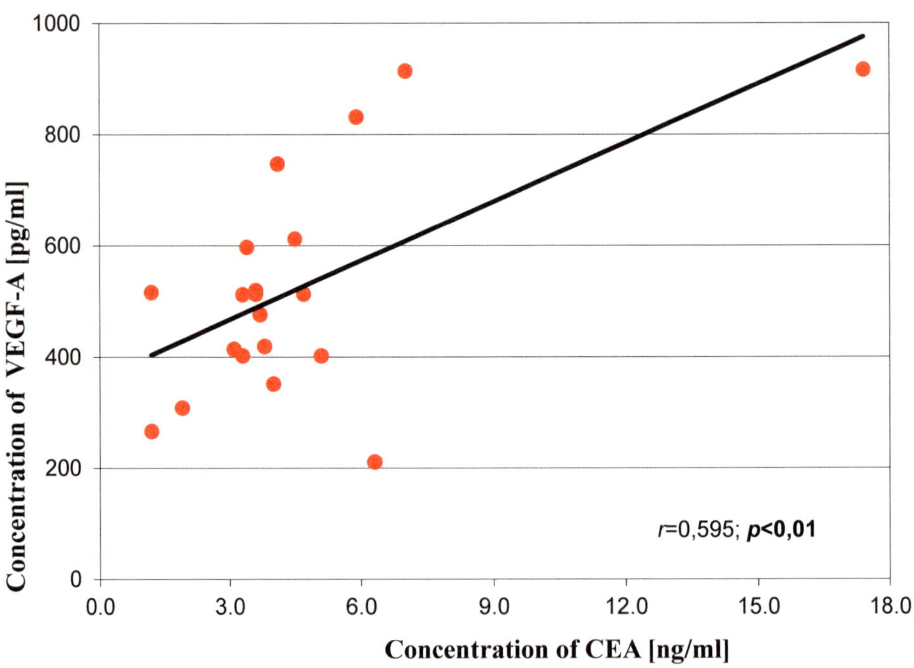

Figure 11. Correlation between the concentrations of CEA and VEGF-A in patients with a recurrence of a tumor 3 months after surgery.

http://dx.doi.org/10.5772/57514

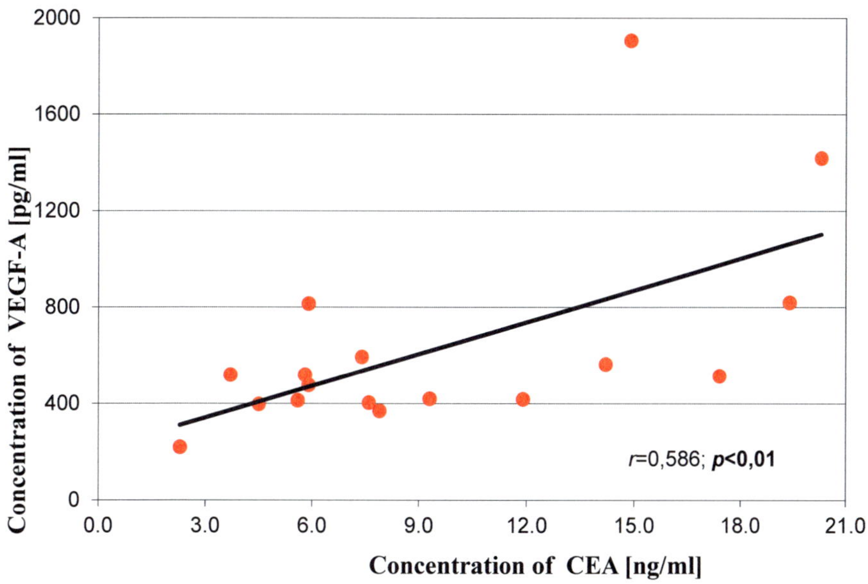

Figure 12. Correlation between the concentrations of CEA and VEGF-A in patients with a recurrence of a tumor 6 months after surgery.

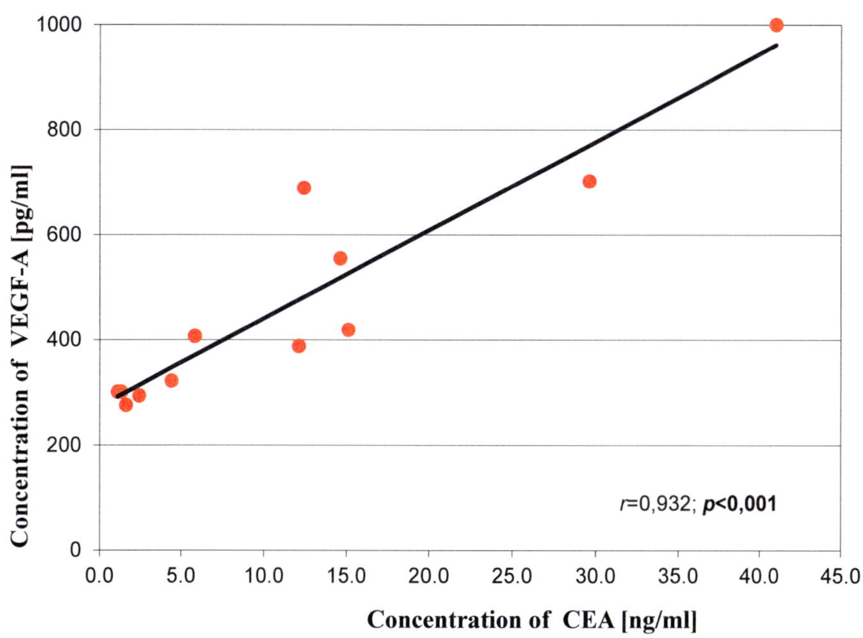

Figure 13. Correlation between the concentrations of CEA and VEGF-A in patients with a recurrence of a tumor 12 months after surgery.

4.4. Discussion

Our results are similar to the results shown by Bombardieri [28], Treska [29], Kokocińska [30] and many others. CEA was discussed in the first part of this chapter. VEGF-A was examined in the blood of patients after the surgery.

We did not find any statistically significant differences between the Dukes classification. In contrast, Fujisaki et al. [31] and Fuhrmann-Benzakein et al. [32] observed such a correlation. The highest concentration of VEGF was observed in patients with a liver metastasis.

Chung et al. [33] and Ohta et al. [34] reported that VEGF may be considered as a proliferation and prognostic factor. A high expression or concentration of VEGF indicates the possibility of the recurrence of a disease in a relatively short time.

Afify et al. [35] also indicated that the concentration of VEGF is very useful in detecting a recurrence of the disease and a metastasis to the liver.

However, Werther et al. and Karatzas et al. [36] reported that A high pre-operative concentration of VEGF suggests liver metastasis in the post-surgery period. Our results confirm those of Afify, Werther and Chung.

The results of our researches show a statistically significantly correlation between VEGF-A and CEA. It is possible that VEGF-A may stimulate the proliferation of tumor cells. To date, only Chung et al. and Ohta et al. have confirmed a connection of VEGF with the proliferation of tumor cells and with the development of cancer [33, 34].

All researches suggest that VEGF-A be added to the immunodiagnostics of CEA in patients with colorectal cancer.

5. Conclusions

1. A statistically significant increase in VEGF-A in patients with a recurrence of a tumor in the early post-operative period supports the usefulness of the inclusion of this marker for monitoring patients, especially in planning their antiangiogenic therapy.
2. The high correlation between CEA and VEGF-A seems to indicate that the concentration of VEGF-A has a close relationship with the proliferation of cells and the development of cancer.

6. Summary

A review of the scientific literature on colorectal diseases over the last 20 years indicates the continued development of Clinical Immunodiagnostics and the "gold standard", which is CEA, but also showed the usefulness and necessity of adding new markers: TPS, Bcl-2, VEGF and their receptors.

In the future, proteins, gene products, phenotyping of patients (determining the phenotype of patients) and molecular cytology should also be added.

Author details

Robert Partyka

Department of Anesthesiology, Intensive Treatment and Emergency Medicine, Medical University of Silesia, Katowice, Poland

The chapter was prepared based on results of research at the Institute of Tumor Markers, which were then compared to the results obtained by other researchers.

References

[1] Kokocińska D.: Przygotowanie składników testu radioimmunologicznego i enzymoimmunologicznego dla oznaczeń progesteronu, oczyszczanie i frakcjonowanie przeciwciał: IgG, F(ab)'2 przeciw progesteronowi i przeciw ferrytynie dla potrzeb diagnostyki klinicznej. Rozprawa habilitacyjna, Katowice, Śl. AM 1993; XVI: 234.

[2] Szymendera JJ, Góźdź S: Rola krążących markerów nowotworowych w diagnostyce I monitorowaniu leczenia chorych na nowotwory. Nowotwory 1995; 45: 369-383.

[3] Bates SH, Longo DL: Use of serum tumor markers in cancer diagnosis and management. Semin Onkol 1987; 14: 102-138.

[4] Dusza D: Dobór oznaczeń markerów nowotworowych u chorych na raka jelita grubego i odbytnicy. Rozprawa doktorska. Śląska AM 1996.

[5] Fillela X, Molina MD, Gran MD et al.: Prognostic value of CA 19-9 levels in colorectal cancer. Ann Surg 1992; 210: 55-59.

[6] Kokocińska D, Kuśmierski S: Antygen CA 72-4 – nowy marker choroby nowotworowej układu pokarmowego. Medycyna 2000 1994; 45(46): 46-47.

[7] Nowacki M: Przydatność kliniczna badań antygenu karcinoembrionalnego (CEA) w surowicy, określenie stopnia zaawansowania, rokowania, leczenia chirurgicznego nowotworów jelita grubego. Nowotwory 1983;1: 13.

[8] Staab HJ, Brummendorf T, Hornung A et al.: The clinical validity of circulating tumor associated antigens CEA and CA 19-9 in primary diagnosis and follow-up patients with gastrointestinal malignancies. Klin Wschr 1985; 63: 106-115.

[9] Wilson MS, Schofieln PF: Markers to study human colonic cell proliferation. Gut 1995; 36(1): 152.

[10] Gold P, Freedman SO: Specific carcinoembryonic antigens in the human digestive system. J Exp Med 1965; 122: 439-462.

[11] Ogata S, Ho J, Chen A et al.: Tumor associated sialylated antigens are constitutively expressed in normal human colonic mucosa. Cancer Res 1995; 1; 36: 1869-1874.

[12] Dienst C, Clodius T, Oldorp T: CA 19-9, CA 50 and CEA bei Pankreas und Gastrointestinaltumoren vergleichende Untersuchungen. Bred Klein 1987; 82: 49-50.

[13] Lindmark G, Bergensrom R, Pahlman I et al.: The association of preoperative serum tumor markers with Dukes' stage and surival in colorectal cancer. Br J Cancer 1995; 71: 1090-1094.

[14] Bonfrer J, Groenveled E, Korse C, Van Dalen A, Oomen LC, Ivanyi D. (1994). Monoclonal antibody M3 used in tissue polypeptide-specific antigen assay for the quantification if tissue polypeptide antigen recognizes keratin 18. Tumor Biol; 15(4): 210-222.

[15] Barak V, Goike H, Panaretakis KW, Einarsson R. Clinical utility of cytokeratins as tumor markers. Clin Biochem 2004; 37(7): 529-540.

[16] Lucsaite R, Sauer-Eppel M, Oremek GM. Value of biomarkers in diagnosis of gastric carcinoma. Clin Exp Med Let 2009; 50(1): 1-4.

[17] Takagawa R, Fujii S, Ohta M, Nagano Y, Kunisaki C, Yamagishi S, Osada S, Ichikawa Y, Shimada H. Preoperative serum carcinoembryonic antigen level as a predictive factor of recurrence after curative resection of colorectal cancer. Ann Surg Oncol 2008; 15(12): 3433-3439.

[18] Lindmark G, Bergstrom R, Pahlman L, Grimelius B. The association of preoperative serum tumor markers with Dukes's stage and survival in colorectal cancer. Brit J of Cancer 1995; 71: 1090-1094.

[19] Barak V, Goike H, Panaretakis KW, Einarsson R. Clinical utility of cytokeratins as tumor markers. Clin Biochem 2004; 37(7): 529-540.

[20] Treska V, Topolcan O, Stanislav K i wsp. Preoperative tumor markers as prognostic factors of colorectal liver metastases. Hepato-Gastroenterology 2009; 56(90): 317-320.

[21] Turoldo A, Balani A, Scaramucci M, Pistan V, Roseano M, Liguori G. Preoperative CEA: prognostic significance in colorectal carcinoma. Tumori 2003; 89(4): 95-97.

[22] Marchena J, Acosta MA, Garcia-Anguiano F, Simpson H, Cruz F. Use of the preoperative levels of CEA in patients with colorectal cancer. Hepatogastroenterology 2003; 50(52): 1017-1020.

[23] Plebani M, De Paoli M, Basso D, Roveroni G, Giacomini A, Galeotti F, Corsini A. Serum tumor markers in colorectal cancer staging, grading, and follow-up. J Surg Oncol 1996; 62(4): 239-244.

[24] Duffy MJ, van Dalen A, Haglund C, Hansson L, Klapdor R, Lamerz R, Nilsson O, Sturgeon C, Topolcan O. Clinical utility of biochemical markers in colorectal cancer:

European Group on Tumor Markers (EGTM) guidelines. Eur J Cancer 2003; 39(6): 718-727.

[25] Paul-Samojedny M, Kokocińska D, Samojedny A i wsp. Expression of cell survival/ death genes: bcl-2 and bax at the rate of colon cancer prognosis. Biochimica et Biophisica Acta 2005; 1741: 25 – 29.

[26] Schelwies K, Sturm I, Grabowski P et al.: Analysis of p53/BAX in primary colorectal carcinoma: low BAX protein expression is a negative prognostic factor In UICC stage III tumors. Int J Cancer 2002; 99 (4): 589-596.

[27] Nehls O, Okech T, Hsieh CJ et al.: Low BAX protein expression correlates with disease recurrence in preoperatively irradited rectal carcinoma. Int J Radiat Oncol Biol Phys 2005; 61(1): 85-91.

[28] Bombardieri E, Saccani JG, Cocciolo MG, Mori M, Rusca M, Seregni E, Becchi G, Fontanesi M, Tardini A et al. Tissue polypeptide antigen and carcinoembryonic antigen in colon tumors: serum levels and immunohistochemical localization. Cancer Detect Prev 1985; 8: 219-226.

[29] Treska V, Topolcan O, Stanislav K, Liska V, Holubec L. Preoperative tumor markers as prognostic factors of colorectal liver metastates. Hepatogastroenterology 2009; 56(90): 317-320.

[30] Kokocińska D, Jarząb B, Kawecki M, Donocik J, Kusmierski S. Antygeny CA 19-9, CEA, CA 50 I ferrytyna w nowotworach przewodu pokarmowego. Pol Przegl Chir 1993; 65: 237-243.

[31] Fujisaki K, Mitsuyama K, Toyonaga A, Matsuo K, Tanikawa K. Circulationg vascular endothelial growth factor in patients with colorectal cancer. Am J Gastroenterol 1998; 93(2): 249-252.

[32] Fuhfmann-Benzakein E, Ma MN, Rubia-Brandt L et al. Elevated levels of angiogenic cytokinez in the plasma of cancer patients. Int J Cancer 2000; 85: 40-45.

[33] Chung Y.S, Maeda K, Sowa M. Prognostic value of angiogenesis in gastrointestinal tumors. Eur J Cancer 1996; 32A(14): 2501-2505.

[34] Ohta Y, Endo Y, Tanaka M, Shimizu J, Oda M, Hayashi Y, Watanabe Y, Sasaki T. Sagnificance of vascular endothelial growth factor messenger RNA expression in primary lung cancer. Clin Cancer Res 1996; 2: 1411-1416.

[35] Afify M, Samy N, Hashim M, Essam T. Clinical significance of vascular endothelial growth factor in Egyptian colorectal cancer patients. Int J Integf Biol 2008; 4(2): 100-107.

[36] Karatzas G. Clinical significance of preoperative serum vascular endothelial growth factor levels in patients with colorectal cancer and effect of tumor surgery. Surgery 2002; 131(5) 548-555.

Section 3

Surgery for colorectal cancer

Chapter 5

Laparoscopy in the Management of Colorectal Cancer

Anton Tonev, Nikola Kolev, Valentin Ignatov,
Vasil Bojkov, Tanya Kirilova and Krassimir Ivanov

Additional information is available at the end of the chapter

http://dx.doi.org/10.5772/56913

1. Introduction

Since the introduction of laparoscopic surgery, minimally invasive techniques have been widely used for benign and malignant diseases. [1, 2] Although many surgeons perform laparoscopic colectomy for benign diseases, its application for colorectal malignancy had slow progress because of oncological considerations. [3] Over time, many randomized controlled trials have been published comparing open to laparoscopic surgery for colorectal cancer, which show that in experienced hands, competent oncology resections can be performed the results are equivalent to open surgery [4-7]. However, the results of the minimally invasive surgery for rectal cancer have not been thoroughly investigated and large multicenter randomized trials are underway.

Large number of randomized controlled trials comparing laparoscopic to open surgery for colon cancer have established better short-term results - less pain, shorter length of stay, faster return of bowel function and equivalent oncological outcomes [2-5]. Laparoscopic rectal surgery is still developing with promising short-term benefit, although depending on the skills and techniques of the surgeon [6]. Surgery of rectal cancer requires more technical skills (total mesorectal excision, low pelvic anastomosis), many fear that the oncological principles could be compromised during laparoscopic resection. In addition to oncological concerns, the widespread of laparoscopic surgery for colorectal cancer is impeded by the significant learning curve.

Hand-assisted techniques introduced in the 1990s were an attempt to overcome some of these limitations and provide an overlap between open and laparoscopic techniques and the transition from open to minimally invasive surgery for many surgeons [1, 8]. Acceptance of minimally invasive procedures by patients and surgeons led to the developent of new technologies to ease the laparoscopic approach. The introduction of single incision laparoscopic surgery (SILS) devices has allowed fewer cuts. [9] The clinical application of endoscopic natural orifice transluminal surgery (NOTES) in colorectal disease is not yet fully accepted, but it was possible great advances in instrumentation and improving techniques for specimen extraction after laparoscopic colectomy [12].

2. Systemic benefits

Basic science studies have demonstrated the better preservation of oncological and immunological functions after laparoscopic surgery before trials on humans [7-9], thus giving hope for better long-term oncologic outcome. Tumor cells are found in systemic blood circulation and in the peritoneal fluid immediately after surgery and if they survive may avoid the immunological defense of the organism. The surgical trauma causes immunological alterations and the organism might be vulnerable during the postoperative period [7-9]. Laparoscopic surgery causes lesser trauma and therefore less effect on the immune system, decreases the proliferation stimuli for cancer cells and neoangiogenesis [7-9, 11]. The changes can last shortly after the operation, but some are observed after months or longer [11]. These potential advantages do not provide better long-term outcomes in human trials, although some report better oncological results after laparoscopic surgery in terms of longer cancer-related survival and less tumor recurrences [10-14].

The rate of conversion to open surgery is still very high, as demonstrated by three multicenter prospective trials - the NCI Clinical Outcomes of Surgical Therapies (COST; 21%), Colon Cancer Laparoscopic or Open Resection (COLOR; 17%), and the Conventional versus Laparoscopic-Assisted Surgery in Colorectal Cancer (CLASICC; 29%) [15, 16]. This could be due to more precautious behavior of the surgeons and their inexperience.

A meta-analysis from 2006 demonstrated intriguing results. It includes 1134 patients after colectomy in two periods – 1996-2000 and 2000-2004. Laparoscopic colectomy was introduced as an option only in the second period. The authors found that 3-year overall survival decreased in the latter, while the overall survival of patients after open colectomy remained the same over the two periods. [17]

Intracorporeal anastomosis for right laparoscopic colectomy improved patient outcome compared with patients who underwent extracorporeal anastomosis. There is found faster recovery of nutrition, faster recovery of intestinal function, and shorter hospitalization. However, there was no difference in average surgery time between the two groups.

According to the differences in age, gender, BMI, ASA class, or abdominal surgical history, in laparoscopic colectomy with extracorporeal anastomosis (laparoscopic-assisted colectomy), the bowel is externalized through a lateral mini-incision. With this approach, bowel mobilization and ligation of vessels is usually laparoscopic, whereas resection of the specimen and creation of the anastomosis is extracorporeal. On the other hand, in laparoscopic right colectomy with intracorporeal anastomosis (totally laparoscopic colectomy), bowel mobilization, ligation of vessels, resection of the specimen, and creation of the anastomosis are totally intracorporeal.

Regarding oncological radicality, there are significant differences in the number of lymph nodes removed. An average of 19 lymph nodes from the intracorporeal group and 14 lymph nodes from the extracorporeal group are reported to be removed. In the literature, some authors have reported no differences in safety, whereas others noted that the only advantage was a smaller incision. On the other hand, other studies affirmed the safety of intracorporeal anastomosis, with the same complication rate as for extracorporeal anastomosis. Because intracorporeal anastomosis is considered more difficult, only a few surgeons have used this kind of technique; however less mobilization is required, and less tension is applied to the bowel and mesentery because the bowel does not need to reach the anterior abdominal wall for externalization. [11] Furthermore, the excessive tension on the mesentery during the mobilization is associated with an increased risk of mesenteric or portal vein thrombosis. Concerning surgical times, there is not a significant difference in surgical time between the two groups. Patients in the intracorporeal group had a shorter hospitalization duration. In some cases, the hospitalization duration was longer possibly because of age (43.2% of patients in the intracorporeal group and 33.4% in the extracorporeal group were over 80 years old). Our results showed a significantly shorter average hospitalization stay in the intracorporeal group. These data agree with a recent Spanish study, although this difference was not significant ($P = 0.5424$) because hospitalization duration is influenced by many patient factors. On the other hand, we found that 71.4% of patients in the intracorporeal group went home within 7 d, and 54.7% of patients in the extracorporeal group went home within this period. [20, 21] Patients in the intracorporeal group and extracorporeal group went home within 7 d. Concerning the recovery of intestinal function, our results found significantly shorter average times for resumption of gas evacuation after 3 d in the intracorporeal group compared to after 3.8 d in the extracorporeal group. Bowel movements occurred after an average of 4.9 d in the intracorporeal group. In the intracorporeal group, the nasogastric tube was removed after 1.8 d, whereas it was removed after 3 d in the extracorporeal group. This difference can be explained by an increased percentage of paralytic ileus in the second group, which is due to the traction of the right colon and terminal ileum through the mini-incision on the pancreas and duodenum. This approach allowed a more rapid recovery of liquid and solid nutrition consumption. [25-27] There are met some major complications, which included severe anemia, occlusion, anastomotic dehisces, and enterocutaneous fistulae. There were no significant differences between the two groups.

In conclusion, our study clearly shows that laparoscopic right colectomy with intracorporeal anastomosis improves patient outcome. Intracorporeal anastomosis resulted in faster recovery of nutrition consumption, faster recovery of intestinal function, and shorter hospitalization duration. The higher number of lymph nodes removed seems to be related to vascular division as the first surgical step as a rule. This confirms that a mini invasive approach improves patient outcome.

3. Port site metastasis

The early trials of laparoscopic colectomy have established high rate of tumor recurrence near the port wounds, which was considered a serious drawback of the new approach. The etiology is unclear, although some authors suggest poor surgical technique and tumor biology as a probable cause. The reported rate in the early trials reached 21%. Recent trials (Hughes et al., 1603 patients, [15] found the rate to be 0.68%. Fleshman et al. [5] reported results based on the NCI COST trial, which demonstrated comparable rates for open and laparoscopic surgery after 5- and 8-year follow up (0.5% and 0.9%, respectively). The Barcelona trials had similar outcome after a median follow-up of 95 months [7]. The European randomized controlled study, the Colon Cancer Laparoscopic or Open Resection (COLOR) trial (2009) established after 53-month median follow-up that the port site metastasis rate was 0.4% after open (n=542) and 1.3% after laparoscopic colectomy (n=534). [19] The location of the recurrences was near the extraction port (n=2) and near the trocar sites (n=5) [5]. Recent studies do not report such high recurrence rates.

Proper training and the use of safe oncologic techniques are essential in the prevention of port site metastases. Such safe techniques are the routing use of wound protectors, less instrument exchange, avoidance of direct trauma to the tumor, avoidance of inadvertent desufflation.

4. Enhanced recovery after surgery

The approach employs a multimodal perioperative care pathway with the aim of attenuating the stress response to surgery and accelerating recovery [21]. Implementation of enhanced recovery protocols has led to improved outcomes across a range of different specialties including reductions in postoperative morbidity and hospital stay [61-65]. The fundamental premise of ERAS is the incorporation of evidence-based practice. It would seem to follow therefore that the evolution of enhanced recovery guidelines should be dynamic, allowing modifications of certain aspects of the program as new data becomes available. Some authors have advocated a rigid adherence to the ERAS protocol, citing study data that demonstrates a proportional relationship between deviation from the protocol and increased morbidity [61]. However, as evidence for components of the ERAS protocol change, it may be that a more flexible and individualised approach should be considered.

5. Perioperative fluid administration

Traditionally, patients undergoing major colorectal surgery have received liberal volumes of intravenous fluids [49]. Excess intravenous fluid during and after surgery has been associated with delayed gut function and increased complication rates [50, 51]. Fluid restriction has been proposed as a possible method of improving recovery and reducing postoperative complications. Brandstrup *et al* [58] found that randomising patients undergoing elective colorectal surgery resection to a restricted fluid protocol reduced cardiopulmonary and wound morbidity. MacKay *et al* [59] found no difference in recovery of gastrointestinal function or time to discharge with postoperative fluid restriction while using a conservative intra-operative protocol. Goal directed fluid therapy *via* oesophageal Doppler (OD) monitoring offers an opportunity to individualise peri-operative fluid administration. OD provides a real time representation of haemodynamic function, and has been shown to be comparable with other methods for estimating cardiac output such as LIDCO. A number of studies have shown that goal-directed fluids reduce morbidity, critical care admissions, and hospital stay [62]. It is not clear however whether these benefits are still significant within an enhanced recovery protocol. Other goal-directed techniques employ central venous oxygen saturation ($ScvO_2$) as a surrogate for mixed venous oxygen saturation. $ScvO_2$ is related to tissue oxygenation and so can be used to titrate oxygen and fluid therapy, particularly in the immediate postoperative period. This approach requires central venous access which is not always available as some groups have developed a less invasive approach to monitoring. While a number of different fluid protocols have been proposed, the optimal approach is still unclear.

6. Evolving postoperative analgesia

Epidural analgesia was considered central to early ERAS protocols, since it reduces the endocrine-mediated stress response [53, 54], and improves postoperative intestinal function [55]. Epidural analgesia also provides superior pain control to systemic opiates, particularly in the first 24-36 h after surgery [56]. Data on the effect of epidural analgesia come predominantly from studies in open surgery while the benefits in laparoscopic surgery are less clear. Levy *et al* [65, 66] performed a meta-analysis to address this question but concluded that there was a paucity of quality data. The authors subsequently performed a study in which patients were randomised to receive epidural, spinal or patient-controlled opiate analgesia following elective laparoscopic colorectal resection. They demonstrated a significantly longer hospital stay, time to return of bowel function and duration of nausea in the epidural group. Intrathecal morphine has been proposed as an alternative [67]. A meta-analysis provides encouraging results in patients undergoing abdominal surgery; reduced post-operative pain in the first 48 h and significantly reduced opiate consumption compared with systemic opiates [68]. Transversus abdominus plane blocks have also been gaining in popularity although comparative data is still lacking [69]. Epidurals can cause vasodilatation and hypotension [70], resulting in excess fluid challenges, third space shift and fluid overload. As studies emerge demonstrating benefits of alternative analgesic techniques, it does raise the question: Should epidural analgesia be the standard technique for all colorectal resections? Perhaps a more individualised approach dependent on the procedure, use of laparoscopy and placement of incisions should be considered. In this way more patients may be able to avoid potential complications while maintaining adequate analgesia and facilitating early mobilisation.

7. Laparoscopic and open surgery in enhanced recovery

The adoption of laparoscopic techniques within colorectal surgery came at a similar time to the introduction of "fast-track" surgery. Early studies examining the effect of laparoscopic surgery showed clear superiority in short term outcomes when compared with open surgery using traditional recovery technique [63, 64]. Patients undergoing laparoscopic surgery have reduced in-patient stays, less morbidity and improved postoperative pain [65, 66]. What is less clear is how much of the benefit is attributable to laparoscopy and how much is an effect of differing perioperative care pathways. Since these early trials there have been a number of small trials comparing laparoscopic and open colorectal surgery within an enhanced recovery setting with conflicting results [55-61]. Most recently a four-armed randomised study of patients undergoing either open or laparoscopic surgery, in an enhanced recovery or standard recovery programme was performed. They demonstrated a significantly faster recovery time following colonic surgery in those patients undergoing laparoscopic procedures within an ERAS programme. What is clear is that there are still a number of areas within the enhanced recovery protocol where the evidence-base continues to change. The relative contributions of different facets of the protocol also remain to be determined. While this is the case we should accept a flexible approach to facilitate the adoption of techniques supported by randomised data. There may also be scope for a degree of individualisation to reflect the wide range of patients and procedures to which enhanced recovery is now being applied. [70]

8. Laparoscopic colectomy

After the initial description in 1991, several reports of laparoscopic colectomy (LC) for colorectal cancer were described. Significant concerns regarding this approach surfaced when minimally invasive techniques applied to colorectal malignancy lead to increased surgical complications and worse cancer outcomes compared to conventional open approaches. An early report, using minimally invasive techniques for benign colorectal disease, showed a significantly high rate of serious complications (18%), including inadvertent enterotomies, intraoperative hemorrhage, anastomotic leaks, and pelvic abscesses. When LC was used to treat colorectal cancer, several papers noted early wound or trocar site recurrences, including one case series documenting a 21% rate. With a less than 1 percent wound implantation rate for open surgery, serious concerns were raised as to the possibility that poor oncologic results were due to a combination of poor technique and abnormal distribution of malignant cells secondary to pneumoperitoneum. Further concerns that laparoscopic techniques may be problematic to cancer patients arose when some studies demonstrated statistically significant worse cancer-specific survival in patients who had conversion from laparoscopic to open surgery. Moloo et al. described decreased survival at 2 years of 76% from 87% for all stages ($P = 0.02$) of colorectal cancer collected from a prospective database of 377 consecutive laparoscopic patients. In the same cohort, at 5 year followup, there was a trend toward decreased overall survival in converted patients (61.9% versus 69.7%, $P = 0.077$). Chan et al. showed an increased local recurrence rate at 3 year followup of 9.8% in the laparoscopically converted group as compared to 2.8% in open patients ($P = 0.03$). The oncological concerns raised in early reports provided a compelling argument to study the question of oncologic equivalence between the open and laparoscopic approach to colorectal cancer in a controlled fashion.

In the early 1990s, several multicenter prospective randomized controlled trials comparing laparoscopic and open surgery for colorectal cancer were initiated. Ultimately, seven large-scale trials compared laparoscopic and open colectomy for colon carcinoma and examined short-term and long-term outcomes. These trials included the Clinical Outcomes of Surgical Therapies (COST) trial funded by the National Cancer Institute in the United States, the Conventional versus Laparoscopic-Assisted Surgery in Colorectal Cancer (CLASICC) trial in the United Kingdom, the Colon Cancer Laparoscopic or Open Resection (COLOR), a multi-center European trial, the Barcelona trial, and several others [20–26]. The main focus of these trials was oncologic outcomes, but short-term outcomes, quality of life, and safety were also evaluated. The CLASICC trial was the only large trial that also evaluated MIS in rectal cancer. Though modest in early studies, the short-term patient-related advantages of laparoscopic surgery have now been confirmed and are significant over the open approach. The Minimally Invasive Colorectal Resection Outcomes (MICRO) review identified 22 randomized controlled trials and 66 cohort series for benign and malignant colorectal disease [27]. Laparoscopic colectomy results in significantly lower pain scores and analgesia requirements, estimated blood loss, return of bowel function, and length of stay. Numerous other trials, including the COST, COLOR, and CLASICC trials, examining short-term outcomes following laparoscopic colectomy for colorectal cancer have confirmed these findings [20–26, 28]. Several studies have also identified a decreased rate of postoperative morbidity including fewer wound infections [21, 23, 27, 29]; this was recently reinforced by a large trial from the National Surgical Quality Improvement Program (NSQIP) database of over 10, 000 patients identifying decreased incidence of wound infection following laparoscopic colectomy (9.5% versus 16.1%, $P < 0.001$) [30]. Quality of life has been assessed in several trials and results varied from no difference to favoring improved quality of life in laparoscopic colectomy [31].

The initially cited oncologic concerns of laparoscopic colectomy for colorectal cancer were later dispelled when surgeons trained in appropriate laparoscopic oncologic resection performed operations in the trial setting. Major trials, including the COST, CLASICC, and COLOR trials, examined tumor specimens and reported long-term data on recurrence and survival. The surgical specimens were evaluated, and parameters such as lymph node yield, circumferential resection margins, and longitudinal margins were quantified. No trial identified statistically significant differences in lymph node yield [20–26] or resection margins [20, 22, 26]. This initial evidence allayed some concerns regarding oncologic resections, but the long-term measures for recurrence and survival were still unknown. Trial data matured, and more evidence accumulated confirming similar recurrence patterns and rates between laparoscopic and open colectomy. Local recurrence, distant recurrence, and wound or port site metastases were the same between groups [4, 5, 7, 24, 32–34]. Disease-free and overall survival in long-term follow-up (up to 7 years) is equivalent [4, 5, 7, 32–34]. The concern that conversion from laparoscopic to open surgery in patients with colon cancer may lead to worse oncologic outcomes was not seen when 5-year COST trial data showed no statistical difference in these two groups.

Despite evidence demonstrating improved short-term outcomes of laparoscopic colectomy and oncologic equivalence, widespread implementation of this technique was slow. The lack of formalized training, outside single-day laparoscopic training courses, and the significant learning curve for straight laparoscopic techniques likely represented significant barriers to adoption. As hand-assisted laparoscopic surgery grew in popularity, a more widespread adaptation with fewer conversions to open surgery occurred in part due to a shorter learning curve with this technique. Three randomized controlled trials have been performed to compare a hand-assisted technique to a laparoscopic technique including patients with both benign and malignant disease, all demonstrating decreased rates of conversion to open surgery [35–37]. A recent meta-analysis compiling 13 studies demonstrated decreased operative times and decreased open conversion rates with a hand-assisted approach [38]. There were no differences in short-term clinical outcomes or oncologic resection results. A recent study by the Mayo Clinic prospectively analyzed the use of hand-assisted surgery in a minimally invasive colorectal practice and found that when applied to a center performing large volumes of laparoscopic surgery, hand-assisted techniques were responsible for more complex procedures to be done laparoscopically [39]. This technique is a minimally invasive approach that has been helpful for surgeons to transition from open to laparoscopic colectomy, especially if they have had little previous laparoscopic experience. Moreover, this technique has allowed a MIS approach in patients otherwise not previously considered candidates (obese, adhesions).

As surgeon experience increased and as more studies demonstrated that laparoscopic colectomy for benign and malignant disease is an acceptable alternative to open surgery, the overall ratio of laparoscopic to open colectomies in the United States has increased. A recent analysis from 2000 through 2004 demonstrated an increasing incidence of laparoscopic colectomy from 3% to 6.5% nationally with increased rates of laparoscopic approaches in urban centers and teaching hospitals [40]. A separate study and database of patients from 2004 through 2006 identified over 32, 000 patients, of which 34% underwent laparoscopic colectomy [41]. This trend toward increased laparoscopy has also been influenced by public knowledge and patient demand for this approach, as well as improved and formalized laparoscopic training in residency programs.

The short-term advantages of laparoscopic surgery over the open approach are confirmed. The minimally invasive approach is characterized by lower pain score and analgesia requirement, estimated blood loss; earlier return of bowel function and shorter length of stay (Minimally Invasive Colorectal Resection Outcomes (MICRO), [20]. The postoperative recovery of pulmonary function is quicker after laparoscopic colectomy. None of the randomized trials have observed significant increase in the anastomotic leakage rate [2-5]. Several studies demonstrated the decreased rate of postoperative morbidity and less wound infections [2-7]. Quality of life after laparoscopic surgery has been evaluated in several trials and the results varied from similar to better QoL than after open surgery [21].

In 2008 Lacy et al. reported the long-term outcomes of Barcelona trial (median follow-up 95 months). The overall survival rate was higher in the laparoscopic (64%) group when compared with the open group (51%) with no statistically significant difference ($p<0.07$). Laparoscopic group demonstrated higher cancer-related survival and lower cancer recurrence in ($p<0.07$ for both). The differences in survival and recurrences between the open and laparoscopic groups were observed for III stage tumors, with significantly better results in terms of overall-survival, cancer-related survival and chances of being free of recurrence. Results for stage I and II did not show any statistical difference. The conclusion is that in a dedicated laparoscopic center, LAC may result in a long-term survival benefit compared with OC, particularly in advanced cases". This oncological advantage can be explained by a preserved cellular immunity, attenuated stress and inflammatory response. [7]

These results seem encouraging and lead the way for laparoscopic surgery, although in a 2007 study by Fleshman (5-year follow-up, COST trial) the data did not demonstrate significant difference in the 5-year overall survival, 5-year disease-free survival, and recurrence rates between the two groups. The pattern of recurrence is also similar. [5] In 2007 Bonjer et al. reported meta-analysis, based on 3-year follow-up data from Barcelona, COST, COLOR and CLASSIC trials. No significant difference in 3-year survival, 3-year disease free survival or tumor recurrence rates between study groups was observed. Analysis by stages did not show any statistical difference in survival between both groups [16].

The hand-assisted laparoscopic surgery is a potential way to decrease operative time and maintain the benefits of the minimally invasive approach. The type of laparoscopic surgery allows introducing a hand through special device in the abdominal cavity, while preserving pneumoperitoneum. This provides proprioception and tactile feedback and ability to perform manual dissection and retraction. A study by Marcell [8] reported the results after multicenter randomized trial. The hand assisted sigmoidectomy group had significantly shorter operative time by 30-minutes when compared with straight laparoscopic group. Both groups had similar short-term outcomes. There were no differences in time to bowel function, pain scores, narcotic use, or time to bowel function. Conversion to open surgery was also significantly less for the hand-assisted group. Incision length was significantly longer for the hand-assisted group, but the difference was small. The authors concluded that hand-assisted surgery results in significantly shorter operative time, while maintaining similar outcomes as straight laparoscopic surgery [17]. Hand-assisted surgery allows to perform more complex procedures and to operate on patients with adhesion or obesity.

9. Laparoscopy for rectal cancer

The use of laparoscopic approach in the treatment of rectal cancer has led to increase of surgical complications and worse cancer outcomes in comparison to the open surgery [6] strong statement to make, may be phrase it differently. Several papers reported increased rate of port-site recurrences, reaching up to 21% [3]. The same parameter for the open approach is 1%. Those results might be explained by poor surgical technique and abnormal distribution of cancer cell due to the pneumoperitoneum [7]. The cancer-specific survival was significantly lower after conversion to open surgery [8, 9].

Based on the data of a prospective trial, including 377 laparoscopic patients [22] the survival decreased from 87% to 76% at 2 years for all stages of colorectal cancer. After a 5-year follow-up the overall survival decreased in converted patients. The local recurrence also proved to be higher: 9.8% and 2.8% for the laparoscopic and open groups, respectively. Several large trials were initiated in the 1990 (Clinical Outcomes of Surgical Therapies (COST) [21]in the

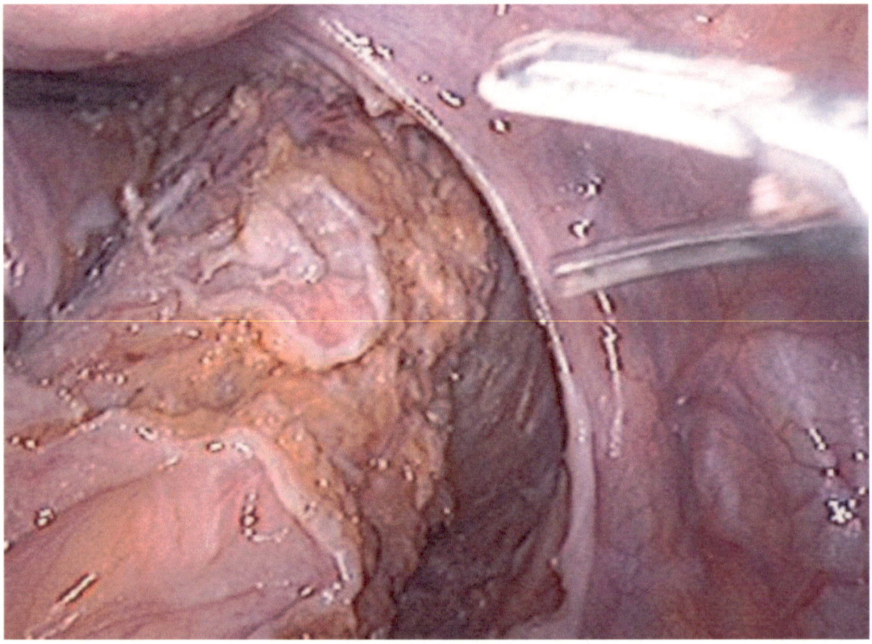

Figure 1. Laparoscopic resection of rectal cancer –anterior mobilization of the rectum

USA, the Conventional versus Laparoscopic-Assisted Surgery in Colorectal Cancer (CLASICC) [6] in the United Kingdom, Colon Cancer Laparoscopic or Open Resection (COLOR) in Europe and the Barcelona trial) [15]. Those trials evaluated laparoscopic and open colectomy for colon carcinoma and examined short-term and long-term outcomes, as well as short-term outcomes, quality of life and safety. Only the CLASSIC trials evaluated minimally invasive surgery for rectal cancer.

The potential benefits of laparoscopic rectal surgery are known and were proven by meta-analysis of studies of non-randomized trials – shorter time of bowel function restoration, shorter length of stay [22]. A characteristic advantage of the laparoscopic surgery is that it provides unobstructed view to the entire surgical team and magnified view of the operating field, thus allowing more accurate dissection. The pneumoperitoneum helps to open the planes of dissection of the mesorectum. The limitations of the laparoscopic rectal surgery are the unsure data on oncological safety [2-5], the concerns about inadequate oncological distant dissection, anastomotic leakage, technical challenges [23, 24].

Significant difficulty poses the obtaining of adequate exposure of the rectum. The narrow pelvis in some patients may cause clashing of the instruments and poor dissection. An experience assistant is required in such cases. The CLASSIC trial reported increased rate of positive circumferential margin after laparoscopic rectal surgery (12%) in comparison to the open group (6%). The distant margin of the tumor is difficult to be identified, as it cannot be palpated. This may cause inadequate distal resection.

http://dx.doi.org/10.5772/56913

The use of laparoscopic stapler requires multiple firings to complete distal rectal resection. In the case of low rectal anastomoses, this increases the anastomotic leakage rate (17% below 12cm from the anal verge [11], 20% below 15cm [23]. The leakage rate after open total mesorectal dissection varies from 4% to 11% [25, 26]. Future improvement of the stapler technology is required.

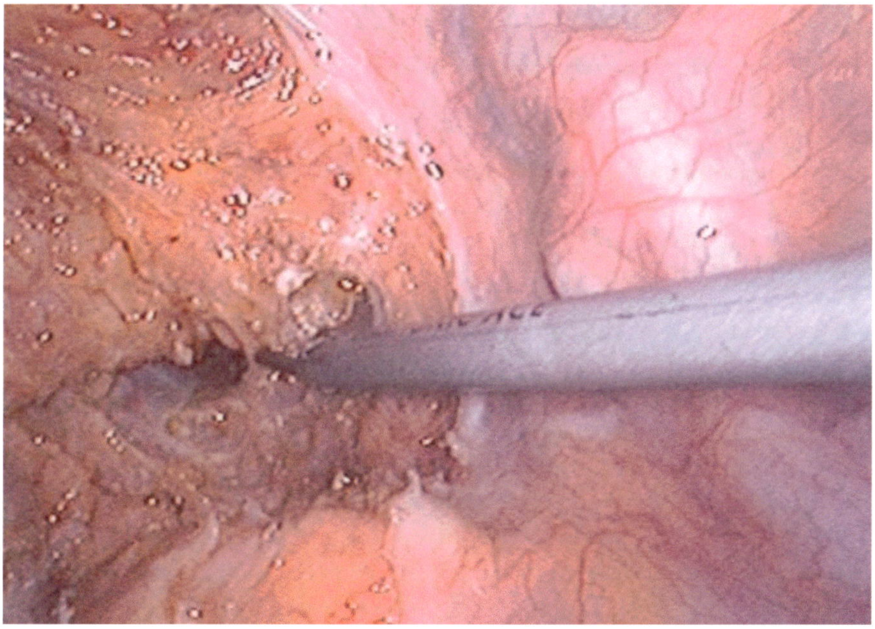

Figure 2. Lymph node dissection in laparoscopic rectal cancer resection

The proven benefits of laparoscopy noted in colon cancer surgery including decreased intraoperative blood loss, smaller length of incision, less postoperative pain, faster recovery of intestinal function, and shorter length of hospital stay likely also apply to rectal cancer surgery [37]. In RCTs the mean operative time for open surgical resection of rectal cancer ranged from 106 to 284 min compared to 120 to 245 min for laparoscopic resection. As expected, duration of operation was significantly longer in the laparoscopic group compared to the open group in 6 of the 8 RCTs [7, 22, 31, 38-40]. Similar results were reported in RCTs of open *vs* laparoscopic resection for colon cancer. Zhou *et al* [24] reported both shorter open and laparoscopic operative times compared to other trials with no significant difference between the two operative approaches (120 min *vs* 106 min for laparoscopic *vs* open resection respectively, P= 0.051). However, no details were provided on tumor stage, conversion rate, or whether the analysis was performed on an intent-to-treat basis. Araujo *et al* [25] was the only RCT to demonstrate significantly shorter operative times with laparoscopic compared to open resection (228 min *vs* 284 min respectively, P = 0.04). However, they attributed these results to fact that the surgical team performing laparoscopic APR was the same whereas open APR was often performed by different surgical teams. In addition, extraction of the specimen from the perineum likely decreased operative time because there was not an abdominal incision to close. Two meta-analyses included operative time as an outcome of interest. Aziz *et al* [17] included 22 studies comparing laparoscopic *vs* open rectal cancer resection in 2071 patients and found that operative time was significantly increased with the laparoscopic group as compared to the open group with a weighted mean difference (WMD) of 40.18 (95% CI, 26.46-56.13). Gao *et al* [26] performed a meta-analysis of short-term outcomes after laparoscopic resection for rectal cancer based on 11 studies and included 643 patients which reported no difference in operating time between open and laparoscopic approaches with a WMD of 1.59 [1.2-1.98]. Intraoperative blood loss was significantly less for the laparoscopic group compared to the open group in 4 of 6 RCTs and ranged from 20 mL to 321.7 mL and from 92 mL to 555.6 mL in the laparoscopic and open groups respectively [31, 35, 38, 40]. Araujo *et al* [25] did not specifically report on the amount of intraoperative blood loss but there was no statistically significant difference in the need for blood transfusions between the two groups which was attributed to the fact that in an APR the majority of blood loss occurs during the perineal portion of the case which is the same regardless of surgical access.

A recent Cochrane review by Breukink *et al* [41] evaluating the safety and efficacy of elective laparoscopic TME for the resection of rectal cancer found that in the majority of studies blood loss was reduced with the laparoscopic approach although this did not translate to fewer blood transfusions. Length of incision was measured in 3 of 8 RCTs and ranged from an average of 5 cm to 10 cm with the laparoscopic approach compared to an average of 19.1 cm to 22 cm with the open approach [7, 38, 40]. Seven of the 8 trials reported a conversion rate which ranged from 0%-34% [7, 38-40]. Conversion to the open approach was commonly defined as length of incision greater than the size needed for tumor extraction or premature abdominal incision to allow improved mobilization. In the majority of studies conversion to open surgery was required because of local tumor invasion or difficult dissection in a narrow pelvis although bulky tumor, dilated small bowel, dense adhesions, bleeding, rectal perforation, difficulty mobilizing the splenic flexure, failure to identify or injury to the ureter, ischemia of the descending colon, and anastomotic failure were also cited. Breukink *et al* [41] reported that 36 of 48 studies assessed conversion and showed a highly variable rate ranging from 0% to 33%. However, they report that the lack of consensus in the definition made results difficult to interpret. In addition, surgeon experience and patient selection criteria were often not mentioned. Two trials reported particularly high rates of conversion. Ng *et al* [37] had a conversion rate of 30.3% but they did not routinely perform preoperative staging with computed tomography scans and therefore frequently converted after diagnostic laparoscopy. Twelve of the 23 patients randomized to laparoscopic surgery were converted to open due to local tumor invasion, bulky tumor, or dilated small bowel which may have been recognized by preoperative imaging. In the CLASICC trial the conversion rate for laparoscopic resection of rectal cancer was reported at 34% and attributed to excessive tumor fixation and uncertainty of tumor clearance [6]. Surgeon learning curve may account for this high rate of conversion as evidenced by the fact that the overall rate of conversion dropped by year of study from 38% in year one to 16% in year six. However, consistent with several non-randomized reports, in the CLASICC trial patients converted to open resection had a higher operative mortality compared to patients in the laparoscopic or open groups (9% *vs* 1% *vs* 5% respectively) [6].

http://dx.doi.org/10.5772/56913

Conversion was also associated with worse oncologic outcomes in nonrandomized comparative and descriptive studies [46].

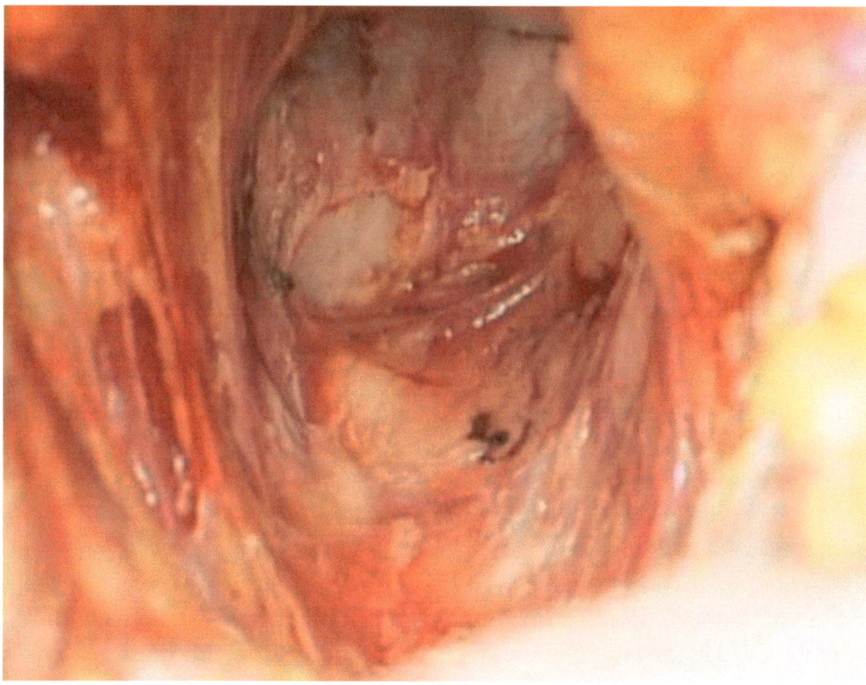

Figure 3. Total mesorectal excision after laparoscopic rectal resection

10. Short-term oncologic outcomes

While the number of lymph nodes retrieved can vary based on age, gender, tumor site, use of pre-operative radiation, and tumor grade, the extent and quality of surgical resection can also have an impact on the number of nodes collected and is therefore often considered a surrogate marker of the oncologic completeness of the resection [37]. The American Joint Committee on Cancer recommends that at least 12 lymph nodes be examined in patients with rectal cancer to confirm the absence of nodal involvement by the tumor [34]. In addition, a number of studies have reported that the number of lymph nodes examined may be associated with patient outcome [25, 26]. Six of the 8 RCTs reported the mean number of lymph nodes retrieved with a range of 5.5 to 17 nodes in the laparoscopic group compared to 11.6 to 18 nodes in the open group [22, 31, 34]. In 4 of the 6 trials the number of lymph nodes isolated was not significantly different based on surgical approach. Araujo *et al* [25] reported a significantly lower yield of lymph nodes with laparoscopic rectal resection compared to open resection (5.5 *vs* 11.9 respectively, $P = 0.04$). They suggested that laparoscopy offered better dissection and accuracy due to better visualization and exposure of structures with less manipulation of the mesorectum especially in a narrow pelvis. Four of the 8 RCTs reported the use of pre-operative chemoradiation. In these trials, the mean number of lymph nodes retrieved ranged from 5.5 to 17 nodes in the laparoscopic group and from 11.6 to 18 nodes in the open group [31, 34, 38, 40]. Some authors [37] found that in the 17 trials that reported the number of lymph nodes retrieved, the mean number of nodes was 10 for the laparoscopic group and 12 for the open group ($P = 0.001$) with the majority of trials reporting a median of 11 or fewer nodes obtained. In 9 of these 17 trials, both groups were treated with preoperative radiation therapy and reported a mean of 10 lymph nodes harvested in the laparoscopic group and 11 in the open group. One of the greatest concerns of laparoscopic TME is that obtaining a complete oncologic resection will be more difficult. Involvement of the circumferential or distal margin is one of the most important prognostic factors in rectal resection with TME and can lead to an increase in local recurrence and a reduction in survival. Radial margins of less than 2 mm are associated with a local recurrence rate of 16% compared to a significantly reduced local recurrence rate of 6% with margins greater than 2 mm [27]. Six of the 8 RCTs reported the involvement of the CRM and no difference was found by surgical approach [7, 31, 38-40, 45]. In the majority of trials the rate of CRM involvement was less than 5%. Patients with positive radial margins often had tumor invading the pelvic side wall or adjacent structure and were frequently converted from a laparoscopic to an open procedure [39]. In the CLASICC study, the only multicenter trial, a positive CRM was identified in 14 of 97 (14%) patients with open surgery and in 30 of 193 (16%) patients with laparoscopic rectal resection [6]. Of patients undergoing anterior resection, the CRM was positive in 16 of 129 (12%) individuals in the laparoscopic group and in 4 of 64 (6%) individuals in the open group. While there is a non-significant higher positivity of the CRM in the laparoscopic anterior resection group, this is once again likely due to the fact that the learning curve was not completed before the start of this study. Two RCTs reported on distal margin status and the incidence of distal margin positivity was not significantly different between the two surgical approaches and in fact was 0% [3, 31]. All 3 meta-analyses and the Cochrane review by Breukink *et al* [41] found no difference in positive margins based on surgical access.

11. Postoperative course

Less postoperative pain, faster recovery of intestinal function, and shorter length of stay are important benefits of laparoscopic colorectal surgery. Only 3 of 8 RCTs compared the exact amount of post-operative pain medication and 2 of these studies reported a significant reduction in analgesic use in the laparoscopic group [39, 40, 45]. Zhou et al [24] did not quantify the exact usage of pain medication, but found no significant difference in the number of days parental analgesics were necessary (4.1 *vs* 3.9 in the open and laparoscopic groups respectively). Resumption of bowel function was usually reported on post-operative days 3 to 5 and ability to tolerate a solid food diet was reported on post-operative days 3 to 6 [7, 31, 35, 39, 40, 45]. In the majority of RCTs earlier bowel movements and diet advancement was reported with the laparoscopic approach. The return of bowel function and reduction in wound pain was thought to contribute to earlier discharge after laparoscopic surgery. While in a majority of trials, the length of stay was not significantly different between surgical approaches, there was a trend toward decreased length of stay with laparoscopic rectal surgery. Breukink *et al* [41] found that laparoscopic TME resulted in earlier return of normal diet, less pain, less narcotic use and a shorter hospital stay.

12. Complications

Rectal cancer surgery is associated with a high rate of morbidity and mortality. Post-operative mortality in RCTs ranged from 1%-4% and demonstrated no statistically significant difference based on surgical approach. The rate of post-operative complications ranged from 6% to 69% and with the exception of Zhou et al [24] did not differ significantly between laparoscopic and open groups. Wound infection and urinary tract infection accounted for the majority of perioperative complications in both groups. There was a higher incidence of wound infection with the open approach however this did not reach statistical significance. Breukink *et al* [41] found no difference in morbidity between the laparoscopic and open groups although there was a trend toward lower morbidity with laparoscopic TME. Aziz *et al* [17] found no difference in perioperative morbidity between the 2 groups while Gao *et al* [26] found that the overall morbidity rate of the laparoscopic group was significantly lower than that of the open group. Anastomotic leak is the most serious complication after sphincter sparing rectal cancer resection especially with neoadjuvant chemoradiation. In addition, development of an anastomotic leak is reported to be associated with decreased long-term survival and higher rates of local recurrence after curative resection for colorectal cancer [39-43]. Operative expertise and selective diversion in high risk patients has resulted in a anastomotic leak rate of 1%-17% in most published series studying laparoscopic resection for rectal cancer [29, 30]. Consistent with reports from non-randomized comparative trials, RCTs demonstrated no significant difference in the incidence of anastomotic leak between the laparoscopic and open technique for the resection of rectal cancer. While the incidence of perioperative morbidity was not different based on surgical access, fewer patients had long-term complications with laparoscopic rectal cancer resection compared to the open approach. Adhesion related bowel obstruction was the most common longterm morbidity. With a median follow-up of greater than 9 years, Ng *et al* [37] found that adhesion-related obstruction requiring hospitalization (18.9% *vs* 2.7%) and reoperation (6.8% *vs* 0%) was higher in the open group. They report a cumulative probability of adhesion-related bowel obstruction at 10 years of 20.5% in the open group and 3.9% in the laparoscopic group. [45] Data on long-term complications was not separated by site of disease but the overall occurrence of incisional hernia (7.9% *vs* 10.9%, P = 0.32) and reoperation for adhesions (1.1% *vs* 2.5%, P = 0.30) was not statistically difference between laparoscopic and open resection. Long-term studies need to be done to determine if laparoscopy decreases the incidence of intra-abdominal adhesion formation by reduced surgical trauma, less tissue handling, and smaller incisions.

13. Long-term outcomes

The initial reports of the long-term outcomes after laparoscopic surgery for rectal cancer were discouraging. Several randomized trials report of the rate of positive circumferential radial margin in the laparoscopic group in comparison to the open group (12-5.9% and 6-4.2%, respectively). The 3-year follow-up did not establish higher local recurrence rate – 7.0% and 7.8%, respectively. The local recurrence rate after laparoscopic and open abdomino-perineal resection were 15.1% and 21.1%, respectively. The overall disease-free survival rate was also similar after laparoscopic and open anterior resection 70.9% and 70.4% and APR – 49.8% and 46.9%. Other data demonstrated 5-year disease survival reaching 83.7% for laparoscopic and 80.4% for open surgery. According to a meta-analysis of 20 laparoscopic rectal cancer studies between 1993 and 2004, including over 2000 patients, there is no significant difference in the number of harvested lymph nodes [22]. Despite the encouraging results, the laparoscopic rectal surgery could be fully evaluated only after long-term results are available. The ongoing studies are the American College of Surgeons Oncology Group (ACOSOG) Z6051 trial from the U.S.; the COLOR II trial from Europe, Canada, and Asia; and the Japanese Japan Clinical Oncology Group (JCOG) 0040 trial.

A number of the clinical trials were performed to determine the safety and feasibility of the laparoscopic approach for rectal adenocarcinoma and therefore the data we have for long-term outcomes is limited [5]. Braga *et al [48]* found no difference in local recurrence (4.0% in the laparoscopic group vs 5.2% in the open group, P= 0.97), overall five-year survival, or disease free five-year survival based on surgical approach. With a median follow-up of 87.2 mo in the laparoscopic group and 90.1 mo in the open group, Ng et al [45] demonstrated that after curative resection, the probability of five-year survival was 75.2% vs 76.5% for laparoscopic vs open APR respectively (P = 0.20). In addition, stage-by-stage comparison for the two groups showed no statistical difference. There were no port site recurrences and overall recurrence rates were not significantly different between the two groups (laparoscopic 20% vs open 25%, P = 0.60). Despite the higher rate of circumferential margin positivity in patients undergoing laparoscopic anterior resection in the CLASICC trial, there was no difference in local recurrence, three- year overall or three-year disease free survival between the two approaches (open OS 66.7% and laparoscopic OS 74.6%, P = 0.17; open DFS 70.4% and laparoscopic DFS 70.9%, P = 0.72; open LR 7.0% and laparoscopic LR 7.98%, P = 0.70) [6]. In addition, there was no significant difference in the rates of local recurrence, three-year overall survival, or three-year disease-free survival in patients undergoing laparoscopic vs open APR [12]. However, the sample size is small and therefore larger studies are needed for conclusive results. Ng et al [37] published results of a randomized trial of laparoscopic vs open anterior resection for upper rectal cancer with a median follow-up of 9 years. No difference in local recurrence, overall survival, or disease-free survival was reported. Although these studies suggest comparative oncologic outcomes between laparoscopic and open rectal cancer resection, they include small sample sizes and are almost all are single institution studies, highlighting the need for large, multi-center RCTs to provide confirmatory data. With a mean follow-up of 35 mo for both groups, overall local recurrence was not statistically different between the 2 groups (laparoscopic 7% vs open 8%, P = NS). Eleven studies provided sufficient data to compare overall survival. Overall survival was 72% for patients undergoing laparoscopic rectal cancer resection and 65% for open resection at an average of 4.4 years (P = 0.5). Subset analysis by [36] demonstrated no significant difference between laparoscopic and open rectal cancer resection in terms of local recurrence (laparoscopic 7.2% vs open 7.8%, P = 0.46), development of distant metastases (laparoscopic 13.5% vs open 9.1%, P = 0.60), or cancer-related mortality (laparoscopic 9% vs open 10%, P = 0.16). While, this data is encouraging, it is no conclusive.

14. Hybrid and hand-assisted laparoscopic rectal surgery

Some authors have introduced a new method of hybrid rectal surgery, aiming to combine the benefits of open and laparoscopic approach. The colonic mobilization is performed laparoscopically, while the rectal dissection is performed through a Pfannenstiel incision. A retrospective review established significantly longer hospital stay after hybrid procedures than after open procedures [27].

Another method is the hand-assisted laparoscopic surgery. A special access device for the hand is introduced in the abdomen. Compared with fully open techniques this method provides shorter operative time. High ligation of vessels, splenic flexure takedown, and lateral mobilization may be accomplished in a shorter period time with a hand-assisted technique. In hand-assisted laparoscopic surgery, rectal exposure and dissection can be either performed directly through the incision using the open techniques or laparoscopically with manual assistance [28]. This method combines the excellent laparoscopic view and the dissection techniques in open surgery and provides tactile sensation.

By performing distal rectal division directly through the incision using the open surgical staplers, hand-assisted laparoscopic rectal surgery may result in a lower anastomotic leakage rate.

15. Summary

After rigorous evaluation the laparoscopic surgery for colon cancer has become the gold standard. Laparoscopic colon resection for cancer, in experienced hands, can be performed safely and reliably with many short-term benefits to the patients while resulting in at least equivalent long-term outcomes as open surgery, which is supported by level 1 data. In conclusion, RCTs have demonstrated that laparoscopy does not adversely affect cancer related survival in patients with adenocarcinoma of the colon. Concerns about the technical difficulty of TME may have contributed to the exclusion of rectal cancer patients from most of these large multicenter RCTs resulting in little data on oncologic outcomes with laparoscopic rectal cancer resection. Laparoscopic rectal dissection is technically more demanding than open and constraints of a narrow pelvis may result in difficulty assessing and obtaining adequate surgical margins. However, there are several proposed benefits of laparoscopic rectal resection. A clear and magnified view of the pelvis provided by the improved optics of laparoscopy may aid sharp dissection for TME and assist in identification of vital pelvic structures including the ureters and autonomic nerves. In addition, pneumoperitoneum may separate the parietal and visceral fascia of the mesorectum facilitating dissection in this plane. Laparoscopic rectal cancer resection has a steep learning curve but increased experience with both open and laparoscopic TME will lead to shorter operating times and decreased morbidity. Current data suggests that laparoscopic rectal cancer resection may benefit patients because of reduced blood loss, earlier return of bowel function, and shorter hospital length of stay. Concerns that laparoscopic rectal cancer surgery may compromise short-term oncologic outcomes including number of lymph nodes harvested and CRM positivity do not appear to be supported by the available literature. However, there is a paucity of data concerning long-term oncologic outcomes and complications with laparoscopic rectal cancer surgery. There are two large, multicenter RCTs that are currently being conducted: the COLOR II trial in Europe and the ACOSOG-Z6051 trial in the United States. Both of these studies are comparing the laparoscopic and open approach for treatment of resectable rectal cancer. Results from these trials will provide information on the long-term outcomes of laparoscopic rectal cancer resection and are eagerly awaited. In view of the lack of level one data on oncologic outcomes, laparoscopic TME for locally advanced, curable rectal cancer should only be performed within the confines of a RCT.

Other potential, but less conclusively demonstrated benefits include better preservation of cell-mediated immune function and reduced tumor cell proliferation. Although a similar level of evidence does not yet exist for the laparoscopic rectal surgery for cancer, the evidence to date suggests that it is likely that the ongoing large randomized trials will demonstrate clinical benefits of laparoscopic rectal cancer surgery. New devices for minimizing of the abdominal trauma are being developed. The steep learning curve, cost and difficult training are still hindrance to the wide use of laparoscopic colon surgery.

Author details

Anton Tonev[1], Nikola Kolev[1], Valentin Ignatov[1], Vasil Bojkov[3], Tanya Kirilova[2] and Krassimir Ivanov[1]

1 Department of General and Operative Surgery, University Hospital “St. Marina”, Varna, Bulgaria

2 Department of Gastroenterology, University Hospital “St. Marina”, Varna, Bulgaria

3 Department of Surgery, University Hospital “St. Marina”, Varna, Bulgaria

References

[1] Reynolds Jr., W. “The first laparoscopic cholecystectomy, ” Journal of the Society of Laparoendoscopic Surgeons, vol. 5, no. 1, pp. 89–94, 2001.

[2] Jacobs M., J. C. Verdeja, and H. S. Goldstein, "Minimally invasive colon resection (laparoscopic colectomy), " Surgical Laparoscopy & Endoscopy, vol. 1, no. 3, pp. 144–150, 1991.

[3] Berends F. J., G. Kazemier, H. J. Bonjer, and J. F. Lange, "Subcutaneous metastases after laparoscopic colectomy, " Lancet, vol. 344, no. 8914, p. 58, 1994.

[4] Buunen M. et al., "Survival after laparoscopic surgery versus open surgery for colon cancer, long-term outcome of a randomized clinical trial, " The Lancet Oncology, vol. 10, no. 1, pp. 44–52, 2009.

[5] Fleshman J., D. J. Sargent, E. Green et al., "Laparoscopic colectomy for cancer is not inferior to open surgery based on 5-year data from the COST Study Group trial, " Annals of Surgery, vol. 246, no. 4, pp. 655–662, 2007.

[6] Jayne D. G., P. J. Guillou, H. Thorpe et al., "Randomized trial of laparoscopic-assisted resection of colorectal carcinoma: 3-year results of the UK MRC CLASICC trial group, " Journal of Clinical Oncology, vol. 25, no. 21, pp. 3061–3068, 2007.

[7] Lacy M., S. Delgado, A. Castells et al., "The long-term results of a randomized clinical trial of laparoscopy-assisted versus open surgery for colon cancer, " Annals of Surgery, vol. 248, no. 1, pp. 1–7, 2008.

[8] Cima R. R., J. Pattana-arun, D. W. Larson, E. J. Dozois, B. G. Wolff, and J. H. Pemberton, "Experience with 969 minimal access colectomies: the role of hand-assisted laparoscopy in expanding minimally invasive surgery for complex colectomies, " Journal of the American College of Surgeons, vol. 206, no. 5, pp. 946–950, 2008.

[9] Froghi F., M. H. Sodergren, A. Darzi, and P. Paraskeva, "Single incision laparoscopic surgery (SILS) in general surgery: a review of current practice, " Surgical Laparoscopy, Endoscopy and Percutaneous Techniques, vol. 20, no. 4, pp. 191–204, 2010.

[10] Pigazzi A., F. Luca, A. Patriti et al., "Multicentric study on robotic tumor-specific mesorectal excision for the treatment of rectal cancer, " Annals of Surgical Oncology, vol. 17, no. 6, pp. 1614–1620, 2010.

[11] Zimmern A., L. Prasad, A. Desouza, S. Marecik, J. Park, and H. Abcarian, "Robotic colon and rectal surgery: a series of 131 cases, " World Journal of Surgery, vol. 34, no. 8, pp. 1954–1958, 2010.

[12] Dozois E. J., D. W. Larson, S. C. Dowdy, V. P. Poola, S. D.- Holubar, and R. R. Cima, "Transvaginal colonic extraction following combined hysterectomy and laparoscopic total colectomy: a natural orifice approach, " Tech Coloproctol. 2008 Sep;12 (3):251-4. doi: 10.1007/s10151-008-0428-4. Epub 2008 Aug 5

[13] Heald RJ, Moran BJ, Ryall RD, Sexton R, MacFarlane JK. Rectal cancer: the Basingstoke experience of total mesorectal excision, 1978-1997. Arch Surg 1998;133 (8):894–899

[14] Southall JC, Lee SW, Allendorf JD, Bessler M, Whelan RL. Colon adenocarcinoma and B-16 melanoma grow larger following laparotomy vs. pneumoperitoneum in a murine model. Dis Colon Rectum 1998;41 (5):564–569

[15] Clinical Outcomes of Surgical Therapy Study Group. A comparison of laparoscopically assisted and open colectomy for colon cancer. N Engl J Med 2004;350 (20): 2050–2059

[16] Bonjer HJ, Hop WC, Nelson H, et al; Transatlantic Laparoscopically Assisted vs Open Colectomy Trials Study Group. Laparoscopically assisted vs open colectomy for colon cancer: a meta-analysis. Arch Surg 2007;142 (3): 298–303

[17] Aziz O, Constantinides V, Tekkis PP, et al. Laparoscopic versus open surgery for rectal cancer: a meta-analysis. Ann Surg Oncol 2006;13 (3):413–424

[18] Hughes ESR, McDermott FT, Polglase AL, Johnson WR. Tumor recurrence in the abdominal wall scar tissue after large-bowel cancer surgery. Dis Colon Rectum 1983;26 (9): 571–572

[19] Veldkamp R, Khury E, Hop WC, et al. Colon Cancer Laparoscopic or Open Resection Study Group (COLOR). Laparoscopic surgery versus open surgery for colon cancer;short-term outcomes of a randomized trial. Lancet Oncol 2005;6:477–484

[20] Noel JK, Fahrbach K, Estok R, Cella C, Frame D, Linz H, Cima RR, Dozois EJ, Senagore AJ. Minimally invasive colorectal resection outcomes: short-term comparison with open procedures. J Am Coll Surg. 2007 Feb;204 (2):291-307. Epub 2006 Dec 12.

[21] Stucky CC, Pockaj BA, Novotny PJ, Sloan JA, Sargent DJ, O'Connell MJ, Beart RW, Skibber JM, Nelson H, Weeks JC. Long-term follow-up and individual item analysis of quality of life assessments related to laparoscopic-assisted colectomy in the COST trial 93-46-53 (INT 0146). Ann Surg Oncol. 2011 Sep;18 (9):2422-31.

[22] Moloo H, Mamazza J, Poulin EC, Burpee SE, Bendavid Y, Klein L, Gregoire R, Schlachta CM. Laparoscopic resections for colorectal cancer: does conversion survival? Surg Endosc. 2004 May;18 (5):732-5. Epub 2004 Apr 6.

[23] Leroy J, Jamali F, Forbes L, et al. Laparoscopic total mesorectal excision (TME) for rectal cancer surgery: long-term outcomes. Surg Endosc 2004;18 (2):281–289

[24] Liang JW, Zhang XM, Zhou ZX, Wang Z, Bi JJ. Learning curve of laparoscopic-assisted surgery for rectal cancer].Zhonghua Yi Xue Za Zhi. 2011 Jun 28;91 (24):1698-701.

[25] Araujo SE, da Silva eSousa AH Jr, de Campos FG, Habr-Gama A, Dumarco RB, Caravatto PP, Nahas SC, da Silva J, Kiss DR, Gama-Rodrigues JJ. Conventional approach x laparoscopic abdominoperineal resection for rectal cancer treatment after neoadjuvant chemoradiation: results of a prospective randomized trial. Rev Hosp Clin Fac Med Sao Paulo. 2003 May-Jun;58 (3):133-40.

[26] Gao F, Cao YF, Chen LS. Meta-analysis of short-term outcomes after laparoscopic resection for rectal cancer. Int J Colorectal Dis. 2006 Oct;21 (7):652-6.

[27] Allendorf JDF, Bessler M, Kayton ML, et al. Increased tumor establishment and growth after laparotomy vs laparoscopy in a murine model. Arch Surg 1995;130 (6): 649–653

[28] Lee SW, Feingold DL, Carter JJ, et al. Peritoneal macrophage and blood monocyte functions after open and laparoscopic-assisted cecectomy in rats. Surg Endosc 2003; 17 (12):1996–2002

[29] Martin JK Jr, Goellner JR. Abdominal fluid cytology in patients with gastrointestinal malignant lesions. Mayo Clin Proc 1986;61 (6):467–471

[30] Shantha Kumara HM, Feingold D, Kalady M, et al. Colorectal resection is associated with persistent proangiogenic plasma protein changes: postoperative plasma stimulates in vitro endothelial cell growth, migration, and invasion. Ann Surg 2009;249 (6): 973–977

[31] Law WL, Lee YM, Choi HK, Seto CL, Ho JW. Impact of laparoscopic resection for colorectal cancer on operative outcomes and survival. Ann Surg 2007;245 (1):1–7

[32] Lee SW, Gleason NR, Bessler M, Whelan RL. Port site tumor recurrence rates in a murine model of laparoscopic splenectomy decreased with increased experience. Surg Endosc 2000;14 (9):805–811

[33] Milsom JW, Bo°hm B, Hammerhofer KA, Fazio V, Steiger E, Elson P. A prospective, randomized trial comparing laparoscopic versus conventional techniques in colorectal cancer surgery: a preliminary report. J Am Coll Surg 1998; 187 (1):46–54; discussion 54–55

[34] Marcello PW, Fleshman JW, Milsom JW, et al. Handassisted laparoscopic vs. laparoscopic colorectal surgery: a multicenter, prospective, randomized trial. Dis Colon Rectum 2008;51 (6):818–826

[35] Lacy AM, Garcı´a-Valdecasas JC, Delgado S, et al. Laparoscopy-assisted colectomy versus open colectomy for treatment of non-metastatic colon cancer: a randomised trial. Lancet 2002;359 (9325):2224–2229

[36] Leung KL, Kwok SP, Lam SC, et al. Laparoscopic resection of rectosigmoid carcinoma: prospective randomised trial. Lancet 2004;363 (9416):1187–1192

[37] Ng SS, Leung KL, Lee JF, Yiu RY, Li JC. MRC CLASICC trial. Lancet 2005;366 (9487): 713; author reply 713–714

[38] Wexner SD, Cohen SM. Port site metastases after laparoscopic colorectal surgery for cure of malignancy. Br J Surg 1995; 82: 295-298

[39] Milsom JW, Böhm B, Hammerhofer KA, Fazio V, Steiger E, Elson P. A prospective, randomized trial comparing laparoscopic versus conventional techniques in colorec-

tal cancer surgery: a preliminary report. J Am Coll Surg 1998; 187: 46-54; discussion 54-55

[40] Kemp JA, Finlayson SR. Outcomes of laparoscopic and open colectomy: a national population-based comparison. Surg Innov 2008; 15: 277-283

[41] Breukink S, Pierie J, Wiggers T. Laparoscopic versus open total mesorectal excision for rectal cancer. Cochrane Database Syst Rev 2006; (4): CD005200

[42] Kim SH, Park IJ, Joh YG, Hahn KY. Laparoscopic resection for rectal cancer: a prospective analysis of thirty-month follow-up outcomes in 312 patients. Surg Endosc 2006; 20: 1197-1202

[43] Laurent C, Leblanc F, Gineste C, Saric J, Rullier E. Laparoscopic approach in surgical treatment of rectal cancer. Br J Surg 2007; 94: 1555-1561

[44] Quirke P, Steele R, Monson J, Grieve R, Khanna S, Couture J, O'Callaghan C, Myint AS, Bessell E, Thompson LC, Parmar M, Stephens RJ, Sebag-Montefiore D. Effect of the plane of surgery achieved on local recurrence in patients with operable rectal cancer: a prospective study using data from the MRC CR07 and NCIC-CTG CO16 randomised clinical trial. Lancet 2009; 373: 821-828

[45] Nagtegaal ID, Quirke P. What is the role for the circumferential margin in the modern treatment of rectal cancer? J Clin Oncol 2008; 26: 303-312

[46] Rullier A, Gourgou-Bourgade S, Jarlier M, Bibeau F, Chassagne-Clément C, Hennequin C, Tisseau L, Leroux A, Ettore F, Peoc'h M, Diebold MA, Robin YM, Kleinclaus I, Mineur L, Petitjean C, Mosnier JF, Soubeyran I, Padilla N, Lemaistre AI, Bérille J, Denis B, Conroy T, Gérard JP. Predictive factors of positive circumferential resection margin after radiochemotherapy for rectal cancer: The French randomised trial ACCORD12/0405 PRODIGE 2. Eur J Cancer 2012 Aug 18

[47] Marijnen CA, Nagtegaal ID, Kapiteijn E, Kranenbarg EK, Noordijk EM, van Krieken JH, van de Velde CJ, Leer JW. Radiotherapy does not compensate for positive resection margins in rectal cancer patients: report of a multicenter randomized trial. Int J Radiat Oncol Biol Phys 2003; 55: 1311-1320

[48] Braga M, Frasson M, Vignali A, Zuliani W, Capretti G, Di Carlo V Laparoscopic resection in rectal cancer patients: outcome and cost-benefit analysis. Dis Colon Rectum. 2007 Apr;50 (4):464-71.

[49] Kehlet H. Multimodal approach to control postoperative pathophysiology and rehabilitation. Br J Anaesth 1997; 78: 606-617

[50] Lassen K, Soop M, Nygren J, Cox PB, Hendry PO, Spies C, von Meyenfeldt MF, Fearon KC, Revhaug A, Norderval S, Ljungqvist O, Lobo DN, Dejong CH. Consensus review of optimal perioperative care in colorectal surgery: Enhanced Recovery After Surgery (ERAS) Group recommendations. Arch Surg 2009; 144: 961-969

[51] Spanjersberg WR, Reurings J, Keus F, van Laarhoven CJ. Fast track surgery versus conventional recovery strategies for colorectal surgery. Cochrane Database Syst Rev 2011; (2): CD007635

[52] Teeuwen PH, Bleichrodt RP, de Jong PJ, van Goor H, Bremers AJ. Enhanced recovery after surgery versus conventional perioperative care in rectal surgery. Dis Colon Rectum 2011; 54: 833-839

[53] Arumainayagam N, McGrath J, Jefferson KP, Gillatt DA. Introduction of an enhanced recovery protocol for radical cystectomy. BJU Int 2008; 101: 698-701

[54] Gustafsson UO, Hausel J, Thorell A, Ljungqvist O, Soop M, Nygren J. Adherence to the enhanced recovery after surgery protocol and outcomes after colorectal cancer surgery. Arch Surg 2011; 146: 571-577

[55] Lowell JA, Schifferdecker C, Driscoll DF, Benotti PN, Bistrian BR. Postoperative fluid overload: not a benign problem. Crit Care Med 1990; 18: 728-733

[56] Lobo DN, Bostock KA, Neal KR, Perkins AC, Rowlands BJ, Allison SP. Effect of salt and water balance on recovery of gastrointestinal function after elective colonic resection: a randomised controlled trial. Lancet 2002; 359: 1812-1818

[57] Tambyraja AL, Sengupta F, MacGregor AB, Bartolo DC, Fearon KC. Patterns and clinical outcomes associated with routine intravenous sodium and fluid administration after colorectal resection. World J Surg 2004; 28: 1046-1051; discussion 1051-1052

[58] Brandstrup B, Tønnesen H, Beier-Holgersen R, Hjortsø E, Ørding H, Lindorff-Larsen K, Rasmussen MS, Lanng C, Wallin L, Iversen LH, Gramkow CS, Okholm M, Blemmer T, Svendsen PE, Rottensten HH, Thage B, Riis J, Jeppesen IS, Teilum D, Christensen AM, Graungaard B, Pott F. Effects of intravenous fluid restriction on postoperative complications: comparison of two perioperative fluid regimens: a randomized assessor-blinded multicenter trial. Ann Surg 2003; 238: 641-648

[59] MacKay G, Fearon K, McConnachie A, Serpell MG, Molloy RG, O'Dwyer PJ. Randomized clinical trial of the effect of postoperative intravenous fluid restriction on recovery after elective colorectal surgery. Br J Surg 2006; 93: 1469-1474

[60] Conway DH, Mayall R, Abdul-Latif MS, Gilligan S, Tackaberry C. Randomised controlled trial investigating the influence of intravenous fluid titration using oesophageal Doppler monitoring during bowel surgery. Anaesthesia 2002; 57:845-849

[61] Liu S, Carpenter RL, Neal JM. Epidural anesthesia and analgesia. Their role in postoperative outcome. Anesthesiology 1995; 82: 1474-1506.

[62] Park WY, Thompson JS, Lee KK. Effect of epidural anesthesia and analgesia on perioperative outcome: a randomized, controlled Veterans Affairs cooperative study. Ann Surg 2001; 234: 560-569; discussion 560-569

[63] Rodgers A, Walker N, Schug S, McKee A, Kehlet H, van Zundert A, Sage D, Futter M, Saville G, Clark T, MacMahon S. Reduction of postoperative mortality and mor-

bidity with epidural or spinal anaesthesia: results from overview of randomized trials. BMJ 2000; 321: 1493

[64] Wu CL, Cohen SR, Richman JM, Rowlingson AJ, Courpas GE, Cheung K, Lin EE, Liu SS. Efficacy of postoperative patient-controlled and continuous infusion epidural analgesia versus intravenous patient-controlled analgesia with opioids: a meta-analysis. Anesthesiology 2005; 103: 1079-1088; quiz 1109-1110

[65] Levy BF, Tilney HS, Dowson HM, Rockall TA. A systematic review of postoperative analgesia following laparoscopic colorectal surgery. Colorectal Dis 2010; 12: 5-15

[66] Levy BF, Scott MJ, Fawcett W, Fry C, Rockall TA. Randomized clinical trial of epidural, spinal or patient-controlled analgesia for patients undergoing laparoscopic colorectal surgery. Br J Surg 2011; 98: 1068-1078

[67] Virlos I, Clements D, Beynon J, Ratnalikar V, Khot U. Shortterm outcomes with intrathecal versus epidural analgesia in laparoscopic colorectal surgery. Br J Surg 2010; 97: 1401-1406

[68] Meylan N, Elia N, Lysakowski C, Tramèr MR. Benefit and risk of intrathecal morphine without local anaesthetic in patients undergoing major surgery: meta-analysis of randomized trials. Br J Anaesth 2009; 102: 156-167

[69] Charlton S, Cyna AM, Middleton P, Griffiths JD. Perioperative transversus abdominis plane (TAP) blocks for analgesia after abdominal surgery. Cochrane Database Syst Rev 2010; (12):CD007705

[70] Marret E, Remy C, Bonnet F. Meta-analysis of epidural analgesia versus parenteral opioid analgesia after colorectal surgery. Br J Surg 2007; 94: 665-673

Chapter 6

Single-Incision Laparoscopic Colectomy: A New Era in the Treatment of Colorectal Cancer?

Fabio Cianchi, Fabio Staderini and Benedetta Badii

Additional information is available at the end of the chapter

http://dx.doi.org/10.5772/56871

1. Introduction

The laparoscopic technique has been enthusiastically applied to the resection of colorectal cancer for more than 15 years [1]. There is evidence that laparoscopy for colorectal cancer offers the opportunity for a meticulous dissection of the mesocolon and mesorectum under direct vision while facilitating a true no-touch technique [2]. Additional benefits, such as less postoperative pain, reduced need for postoperative analgesia, less ileus, shorter hospital stay, less blood loss, and better cosmesis are also well documented [3,4].

During recent years, great effort has been made to minimize parietal trauma for cosmetic reasons and to further reduce surgery-related pain and morbidity. New techniques, such as natural orifice transluminal endoscopic surgery (NOTES) [5] have been developed in order to reach the goal of "scarless" surgery. Although NOTES actually allows for no scarring of the body surface, it has several disadvantages and limitations with the currently available instruments, including limited access, less familiar working angles and operative approaches. Furthermore, it is associated with possible complications caused by opening of the stomach, colon or vagina, and may not be fully suitable or safe for advanced procedures, such as colectomies [6].

Single incision laparoscopic surgery (SILS) is currently regarded as the next major advance in minimally invasive surgical approaches to colorectal disease that is more feasible for generalized use [7-10]. SILS reduces the invasiveness of laparoscopic conventional surgery (LCS) by decreasing the number of incisions and ports through the abdominal wall. This theoretically could provide important clinical advantages, including less postoperative pain, reduction of port-site associated morbidity (such as wound infection, bleeding, visceral injury and port site herniation), quicker recovery and shorter hospital stay. The small incision through the abdominal wall allows for "scarless" surgery as the wound is usually hidden within the umbilicus, thus providing potentially better cosmesis. Moreover, SILS permits surgeons to use familiar standard laparoscopic instruments but also perform complex procedures, such as colorectal operations, which require extraction of large surgical specimens or intestinal anastomosis.

2. Technical aspects of SILS

SILS was first reported in 1992 by gynecologists who performed single-incision hysterectomy [11]. The performance of the first transumbilical cholecystectomy was published in 1999 [12] and the first single-incision appendectomy was reported in 1998 [13]. The use of SILS in colorectal surgery was first reported in 2008 by Remzi and co-workers [8] and Bucher and colleagues [14].

Since these first reports, it has been evident that SILS raises a number of specific new challenges compared with LCS. The skills required for SILS are different from those needed in conventional multiport laparoscopy, even for experienced laparoscopic surgeons [15]. The handling of straight instruments in parallel with the laparoscope through a small single incision decreases the freedom of movement for the surgeon, and complicates the holding of the laparoscope for the assistant and instruments for the surgeon. The most outstanding technical challenges involved in SILS are the following:

1. Loss of triangulation with straight instruments: the loss of this dogmatic principle of laparoscopic surgery often imposes the need to operate with crossed hands and does not allow an ergonomically favorable position for the surgeon and assistants. The inherent technical challenge is that the visual axis becomes more axial or in-line, so a movement of the camera often results in a inadvertent movement of an adjacent instrument, thus increasing the difficulty of performing even relatively simple tasks.

2. Restricted number of working instruments and thus difficulty of achieving correct exposure and the necessary traction to tissues.

3. Restricted external working space: the multiple instruments and laparoscopes required for a procedure are competing for the same space at the fulcrum of the entry port, causing external hand collisions and difficulty with instrument tip manipulation internally.

4. Difficulty in maintaining pneumoperitoneum.

5. Requirement of training and adjustment.

New operative hardware is being developed to facilitate the technique [16]. Many of the big healthcare manufacturers have developed multilumen access devices to allow for the insertion of several instruments through a single large fascial incision (Figure 1).

Initially, these devices offered three openings with limited gas inflow and outflow, but we are now seeing revision of the devices, incorporating more access ports so standard laparoscopic dissection techniques can be utilized. Newly designed equipment, such as

http://dx.doi.org/10.5772/56871

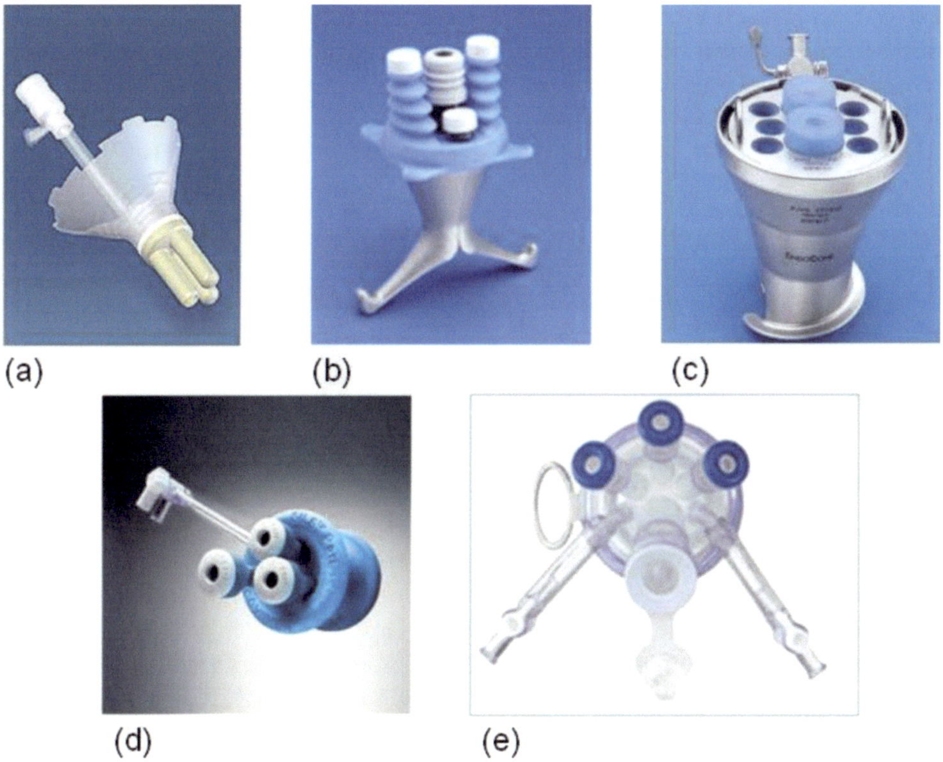

Figure 1. Single port systems: (a) Uni-x (Pnavel Systems, Morganville, New Jersey, USA); (b) X-Cone (Karl Storz, Tuttlingen, Germany); (c) Endo-Cone (Karl Storz, Tuttlingen, Germany); (d) SILS Port (Covidien, Norwalk, Connecticut, USA); (e) Olympus TriPort + (Advanced Surgical Concepts, Bray, Ireland.

articulating or curved instruments and flexible scopes, have been introduced to recreate triangulation (Figure 2).

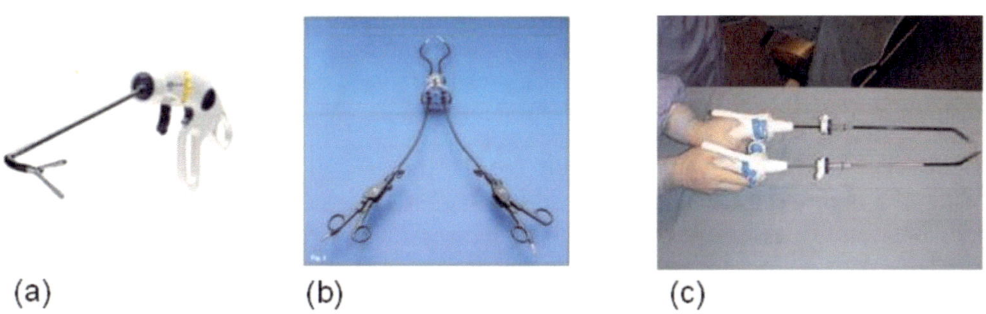

Figure 2. Articulating and curved instruments for SILS: (a) SILS Hand Instrument (Covidien, Norwalk, Connecticut, USA); (b) The Cuschieri Coaxial Deviating Instruments (Karl Storz, Tuttlingen, Germany); (c) Cambridge Endo Instruments (Cambridge Endoscopic Devices, Framingham, Massachusetts, USA).

Moreover, the introduction of an extra-long, 5 mm laparoscope allows placement of the camera on a different plane from the other instruments and help in moving the operator's hand further apart to avoid handle collision (Figure 3) [17]. All these devices have made single site surgery easier and more efficient.

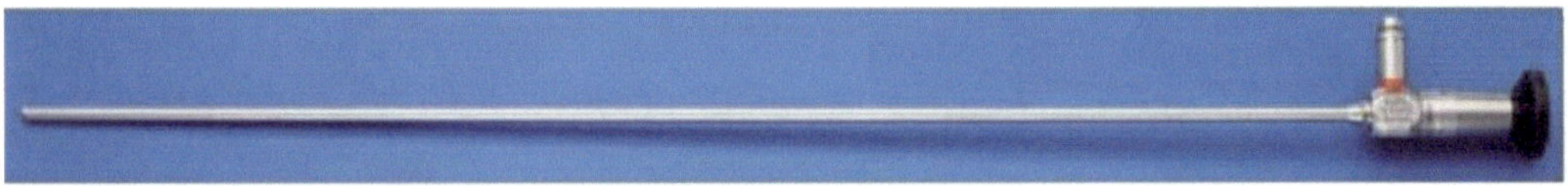

Figure 3. Extra-long, 5 mm, 30° laparoscope (Karl Storz, Tuttlingen, Germany).

3. Feasibility and safety of single-incision colectomy

All the challenges encountered with single-port surgery are magnified with colorectal procedures. Unlike laparoscopic cholecystectomy or appendicectomy, which involve surgery in only one abdominal quadrant, single-incision laparoscopic colectomy often requires operating in different abdominal quadrants. In addition, the need for adequate oncological margins and the creation of a tension-free anastomosis are essential. Although the use of this new approach for complex colorectal procedures might understandingly be viewed as difficult to implement, over the past few years there has been significant interest in SILS for colonic resections in both benign and malignant conditions. In fact, between 2008 and 2012, a nearly 7-fold increase occurred in the number of articles related to single-port colorectal surgery [18-20]. Unfortunately, the currently available literature relating to the technique includes mostly case reports or small case series describing the feasibility, safety and technical difficulties of different operations [21-42]. There are very few studies comparing SILS to LCS and there is a need for randomized controlled trials to definitively establish that SILS is no different from standard laparoscopic surgery in terms of completion rates, complications and oncological adequacy but with the advantage of being more cosmetic with subsequently reduced morbidities including pain [43]. The studies published to date have a number of other flaws limiting their impact. These include low sample size, selection bias and difficulty in blinding the patients enrolled. The vast majority of studies involve a very carefully selected SILS cohort of uncomplicated cases, which significantly limits their generalization.

The most significant datum emerging from the literature is that colonic SILS has been offered to date to a highly selected group of patients [18,19]. This selection is based on two main parameters: body mass index (BMI) that is an indirect measure of visceral fat, and tumor site, that is directly linked to the type of surgical procedure.

It is well known that visceral fat is one the most critical factors in the identification of the correct surgical plane in laparoscopic surgery [44]. This concept is obviously amplified in SILS and visceral obesity is reported as the primary cause of conversion to multiport laparoscopy in most studies [45]. Therefore it is understandable that most patients who are candidates for this type of surgery had a low BMI. Makino et al. [18] have reviewed 23 studies with a total of 378 patients undergoing single-port colectomy. The mean value of BMI was 25.5 kg/m^2 in these patients. Similar results have been found by Fung et al. [19] in their recent review. These authors have analyzed 38 colonic SILS articles containing 565 patients and the median BMI was 25.8 kg/m^2. On the basis of these findings, some studies have suggested the use of preoperative abdominal computed tomography to predict accurately the pattern of visceral fat, allowing better selection of patients for SILS colectomy and reducing the number of conversions [44].

The other factor that has markedly influenced the currently available data on SILS for colorectal cancer is the type of surgical procedure. Makino et al. [18] have reported that 279 (73.8%) of the 378 procedures analyzed in their review were right hemicolectomy, followed by sigmoidectomy (n = 27), performed essentially for diverticular disease, and anterior resection of the rectum (n = 20). Moreover, a high number of published studies have specifically limited the analysis of safety, feasibility and short-term results to only single-port right hemicolectomy [14,25,32-38,42,45-48], thus demonstrating that this type of procedure is the least complex to perform with the single-port technique at the beginning of the experience. Actually, right hemicolectomy involves surgery only in one/two quadrants while left procedures require operating in a multitude of different and opposite abdominal quadrants, from the hypochondrium for splenic flexure mobilization to the pelvis for a total mesorectal excision (TME). Moreover, in right hemicolectomy the surgeon has the possibility of creating an extracorporeal intestinal anastomosis through umbilical access while in left colectomies and anterior resection of the rectum the anastomosis is intracorporeal, thus augmenting the complexity of the procedure.

These considerations clearly show that there is an inevitable case-selection bias in assessing the outcomes of colo-rectal SILS from published studies. Although randomized controlled trials comparing single-port and multi-port right hemicolectomy have not been reported yet, the most significant data available to date relate to this type of procedure. In 2012, the two largest experiences with single-port right hemicolectomies in a single institution have been reported. Waters et al. [49] analyzed the short-term outcomes with single-incision right hemicolectomy in 100 patients. Operative indications were oncological in 92 patients, 57 for adenocarcinoma and 35 for polyps not suitable for endoscopic removal. Morbidity (13%) and mortality (1%) rates were acceptable as well as operative time (median value, 105 minutes) and conversion rate to multiport or open procedures (2% and 4%, respectively). Most importantly, there was no compromise of oncological adequacy with no positive tumor margins and a mean number of 18 lymph nodes retrieved and examined in the surgical specimens. Interestingly, patients with a wide range of BMI measurements were offered single-incision right hemicolectomy, with the largest approaching superobesity at a BMI of 46 kg/m^2 and a mean patient BMI of 28. Unfortunately, no results regarding postoperative pain, cosmetic results or direct comparison with the multi-port laparoscopic approach were reported.

Chew et al. [50] have reported the short outcomes of single-incision laparoscopic hemicolectomy in 40 consecutive patients. These results were compared with those of 104 conventional laparoscopic hemicolectomies. Indications for surgery were oncological in the majority of patients in the two groups. The authors found that single-incision right hemicolectomy is a feasible and safe procedure with equivalent outcomes in terms of operative time, oncological adequacy, postoperative morbidity, and conversions when compared with conventional laparoscopic right hemicolectomy. In particular, there were no differences in lymph node retrieval (median value of 18 and 19 lymph nodes for multi-port and single-port surgery, respectively) and resection margin clearance.

The data regarding left sided procedures, in particular anterior resection of the rectum for cancer, are much more limited. This is mainly due to the complexity of these procedures, in particular some surgical steps such as mobilizing the splenic flexure and dissection of the mesorectum. The fairly great distance of the spleen and the deep pelvis from the umbilicus amplify the difficulty of creating instrument triangulation, especially when standard, straight laparoscopic instruments are used. Even adequate traction of the rectum and stapling procedures have been associated with technical difficulties and adjunctive methods of traction and suspension such as transparietal suture, are frequently needed to achieve adequate surgical exposure [51-56]. Bulut et al. [57] have recently reported their early experience in single-incision surgery for rectal cancer treatment. This study was conducted on 10, highly selected patients: the mean tumor diameter was very small (3.2 cm), BMI was ≤25 in all patients and 8 of them were females, thus providing the advantages of a wide pelvis and relative lack of visceral fat. Although the authors stated that single-incision surgery for rectal cancer can be performed safely in this kind of patient, the overall mean operation time was quite long (240 min) and 6 patients received stomas (4 had diverting ileostomy after anterior resection of the rectum and 2 had colostomy after Hartmann procedure and abdominoperineal resection). Moreover, mesorectum excision was classified as nearly complete in 4 patients and the median number of examined lymph nodes was quite low, namely 14.

One of the most challenging maneuvers in single-incision rectal surgery is maintaining an adequate operative field during TME. Uematsu et al. [54] have proposed a new rectum-suspending system composed of a suspending bar and a bowel clamp with an extracorporeal magnetic tool. This apparatus, along with single access through the right iliac fossa instead of the umbilicus, allowed the authors to perform TME and transect the rectum by ensuring a proper tension. Nevertheless, the proposed new technique is actually complex and, as the authors stated, is not recommended for males with narrow pelvis or obese individuals or when mobilization of the splenic flexure is required because of the distance between the spleen and the single access through the right iliac fossa. Altogether, these data clearly show that some unresolved issues still remain in performing SILS for the treatment of rectal cancer.

There are more data, which are somewhat more reliable regarding other less complex left-sided procedures, such as left hemicolectomy or sigmoidectomy [52,58-60]. In fact, sigmoidectomy is the most frequent procedure performed for benign left-side pathology, predominantly diverticular disease or large colonic polyps not suitable for endoscopic removal. Recently, Vestweber et al. [61] have reported the largest series of patients undergoing single-incision colorectal surgery in a single institution. One hundred and fifty out of 244 procedures were sigmoidectmy (n = 145) with left hemicolectomies (n = 4) and high anterior resection of the rectum (n = 1). Most of these patients were operated on for diverticular disease (n = 142) followed by colonic polyps (n = 4) and colonic cancer (n = 4). The mean operative time for left-sided procedures was 146 ± 48 min and in all cases standard straight, non-articulating laparoscopic instruments along with ultrasonic or radiofrequency dissector/sealer were used. It seems that the authors did not experience any particular technical problems in performing these types of procedures that do not actually need wide splenic flexure mobilization or mesorectal dissection. The fairly higher incidence of early postoperative complications (12.6%) than rates stated in the literature, was imputed to the high rate of severe, complicated diverticular disease rather than to the complexity of single-incision procedure.

The literature concerning subtotal colectomy or proctocolectomy (with or without ileoanal anastomosis), at this time consists only of case reports and a few small case series [62-68]. The predominant indication for this type of operation has been ulcerative colitis followed by polyposis coli [64,65,67]. Overall, 36 single-incision total colectomies have been reported in the literature: these studies have demonstrated the feasibility and safety of single-incision technique even in these more complex colonic procedures but cannot provide any comparative results with traditional laparoscopy. It is likely that cosmetic results will be magnified by single-incision total colectomy since patients suffering from ulcerative colitis or polyposis coli are usually young and may prefer a small incision hidden in the umbilicus. If an ileostomy is scheduled, the single incision is usually performed in the right lower quadrant of the abdomen and the terminal ileum is brought out through this port-site, thus minimizing the traumatic and cosmetic impact of the procedure.

4. Comparison between single-incision and conventional laparoscopic colectomy

As all these data indicate, there are still several limitations to an analysis of the adequacy of single-incision technique in the treatment of colorectal cancer. The most important limiting factor in the interpretation of reported outcomes is the careful selection of patients, with an almost 3-fold predominance of right-sided pathology, a low to average BMI and non-bulky colonic disease. If this case-selection bias is taken into account and the oncological adequacy of a single-incision procedure is hypothetically accepted, this innovation would be justified only in the presence of clear short-term benefits over conventional laparoscopic colonic surgery. These benefits should comprise a lower complication rate, reduced postoperative pain, faster recovery and better cosmesis.

To date, only two randomized trials have compared short-term outcomes after single-incision and conventional laparoscopic colectomies for colon cancer. In 2011, Huscher et al. [69] reported the results of a study conducted on 32 patients, with 16 in the single-incision and 16 in the conventional laparoscopic group. Although the authors confirmed the safety and technical feasibility of single-incision colectomy, they did not show any superiority of the procedure over conventional laparoscopy in terms of postoperative morbidity, resumption of oral liquid/solid food intake and length of hospital stay.

More recently, Poon et al. [70] reported findings from a randomized controlled trial, which enrolled 50 patients, 25 in each study group. As expected, the patients were carefully selected in regard to BMI (median value, 23.2 kg/m^2) and tumor size (< 4 cm). On the contrary, there was a predominance of left-sided procedures, with 14 anterior resections, 1 sigmoidectomy, 2 left hemicolectomies and only 8 right hemicolectomies in the single-incision group. The authors did not find any statistically significant difference in operative outcome and oncological adequacy between the single-incision and the conventional laparoscopic group. Interestingly, they found a lower postoperative pain score and shorter median hospital stay in the single-incision group. Although these findings emerge from a randomized controlled trial, they cannot be considered definitive due the low number of patients involved in the study.

Two recent meta-analyses have addressed the issue of comparison between SILS and LCS for both benign and malignant colorectal diseases [71,72]. Both studies have been published in 2012 and thus have included all the comparative studies published to date with the exception of the above mentioned randomized trial by Poon et al. Notwithstanding the heterogeneity of the analyzed studies (14 by Zhou et al. and 15 by Yang et al) in terms of type of procedures performed, indication for surgery, different patient inclusion and exclusion criteria, neither meta-analysis found any significant difference in the incidence of postoperative complications or operative time between single-incision and conventional laparoscopic colectomy. Importantly, they show that patients undergoing single-incision colectomy had a significantly shorter length of hospital stay, significantly shorter incision length, significantly less estimated blood loss, and significantly more lymph nodes harvested during oncological resections. Unfortunately, the two pooled analyses were not able to compare the pain score due to lack of data, the differences in scoring methods and in postoperative care and pain management in the available reported data. However, at least three studies [48,73,74] show a significant decrease in pain scores for patients undergoing single-incision colectomy compared to conventional laparoscopy. The decreased pain score is likely due to less surgical trauma as a consequence of eliminating the additional ports at separate sites on the abdominal wall. There is no meta-analysis regarding cosmetic results due to absence of adequate information on this interesting outcome in the individual studies. Only one study reported cosmetic score results with an advantage for SILS over LCS [23]. However, it is logical to assume that a shorter final incision length in single-incision surgery results in improved cosmetic satisfaction for the majority of the patients.

Another important issue emerging from the literature data is that experienced laparoscopic surgeons have performed almost all single-incision colectomies. This implies that SILS is offered not only to a select group of patients but is also performed by a select group of surgeons. It might appear premature to propose a complex and technically challenging evolution of conventional laparoscopy colectomy when this has yet to be fully accepted as a gold standard in the treatment of colorectal cancer [75]. It must be considered that in 2010, only about 20% of colorectal resections in England and in other countries were performed laparoscopically [76]. Therefore, although the principles of SILS are highly attractive, they might not, at this moment, be transferable and proposed to the general community of surgeons.

The last but not least important concern about single-incision colectomy regards the costs. It is logical to expect an initial increase in costs associated with SILC over conventional laparoscopic surgery since the additional equipment such as single-incision access ports or flexible/articulating instruments are still relatively new. In their analysis of single-incision right-hemicolectomy, Waters et al. [46] found a marginal increase in direct operative cost of US $310 to $410 per case. If patients have a shorter length of hospital stay, and consequently, a quicker return to work and normal activity after single-incision surgery, it is likely there will be an improvement in the cost-effectiveness of SILS in the future.

5. Conclusion

Most of the current studies on single-incision colectomy for cancer are observational and lack statistical power due to the relatively low number of patients studied. Although meta-analyses can increase the statistical power by pooling results of all available trials, only randomized, controlled studies can provide high levels of evidence. To date, only two randomized controlled studies have compared short-term results between single-incision and conventional laparoscopic surgery and, unfortunately, even these studies have enrolled a very low number of patients. Bearing in mind these limitations, we can still glean several important factors from these published series:

1. Colonic SILS is technically demanding but the introduction of new specialized equipment including multilumen ports, angled scopes, articulated instruments and instruments of variable length, will eventually reduce this difficulty.

2. Principles of colonic SILS are attractive and applicable in carefully selected groups of patients, namely with right-sided pathology, low BMI and non-bulky tumors.

3. In the hands of experienced laparoscopic surgeons, colonic SILS in the above mentioned patients has been demonstrated to be safe and feasible with rates of surgery-related complications and mortality, operative time and oncological adequacy comparable with those of conventional laparoscopy.

4. Two meta-analyses and one randomized controlled study provide evidence in support of some advantages of SILS over conventional laparoscopy, namely, shorter length of hospital stay, significantly shorter incision length and significantly less estimated blood loss; other hypothesized benefits, such as reduction in postoperative pain and improvement of cosmesis remain unproven.

Further high-powered randomized studies comparing SILS and LCS by using standardized outcome assessment tools are needed to confirm or not the above-mentioned results. But one thing is certain: we will not see the same dramatic clinical advantages with the passage from LCS to SILS as we saw with the advent of laparoscopic technique over open surgery.

Furthermore, the more complex the procedure performed by single-incision surgery, the more likely are there to be advantages in comparison with conventional laparoscopic procedures.

In this prospective, a possible field of investigation might be the assessment of systemic stress response of single-incision versus conventional laparoscopy in colorectal surgery. The reduced parietal trauma and manipulation of the peritoneum could decrease the postoperative inflammatory response to surgical stress and as a consequence, more efficient immunocompetency against tumor cells might be maintained since the earliest postoperative days [77,78]. All these factors might influence the long-term oncological results of SILS with a potential improvement in survival rates of patients operated on for colorectal cancer.

Author details

Fabio Cianchi[1,2*], Fabio Staderini[1,2] and Benedetta Badii[1,2]

*Address all correspondence to: fabio.cianchi@unifi.it

1 Department of Surgery and Translational Medicine, Center of Oncological Minimally Invasive Surgery, University of Florence, Italy

2 Unit of Endocrine and Minimally Invasive Surgery, AOU Careggi, Florence, Italy

References

[1] Jacob BP, Salky B. Laparoscopic colectomy for colon adenocarcinoma: an 11-year retrospective review with 5-year survival. Surg Endosc 2005;19 (5) 643-649.

[2] Lujan HJ, Plasencia G, Jacobs M, Viamonte M 3rd, Hartmann RF. Long-term survival after laparoscopic colon resection for cancer: complete five-year follow-up. Dis Colon Rectum 2002;45 (4) 491-501.

[3] Guillou PJ, Quirke P, Thorpe H, Walker J, Jayne DG, Smith AM, Heath RM, Brown JM; MRC CLASICC trial group. Short-term end points of conventional versus laparoscopic-assisted surgery in patients with colorectal cancer (MRC CLASSICC trial): multicentre, randomized controlled trial. Lancet 2005;365 (9472) 1718-1726.

[4] Clinical outcomes of surgical therapy (COST) study group. A comparison of laparoscopically assisted and open colectomy for colon cancer. N Engl J Med 2004;350 (20) 2050-2059.

[5] Gumbs AA, Fowler D, Milone L, Evanko JC, Ude AO, Stevens P, Bessler M. Transvaginal natural orifice transluminal endoscopic surgery cholecystectomy: early evolution of the technique. Ann Surg 2009;249 (6) 908-912

[6] Brunner W, Schirnhofer J, Waldstein-Wartenberg N, Frass R, Weiss H. Single incision laparoscopic sigmoid colon resections without visible scar: a novel technique. Colorectal Dis. 2010;12(1) 66-70.

[7] Romanelli JR, Earle DB. Single-port laparoscopic surgery: an overview. Surg Endosc 2009;23 (7) 1419-1427.

[8] Remzi FH, Kirat HT, Kaouk JH, Geisler DP. Single port laparoscopy in colorectal surgery. Colorectal Dis 2008;10 (8) 823-826.

[9] Bucher P, Pugin F, Morel P. Transumbilical single incision laparoscopic sigmoidectomy for benign disease. Colorectal Dis 2009;12 (1) 61-65

[10] Curcillo PG 2nd, Podolsky ER, King SA. The road to reduced port surgery: from single big incisions to single small incisions, and beyond. World J Surg 2011;35 (7) 1526-1531

[11] Pelosi MA, Pelosi MA 3rd. Laparoscopic supracervical hysterectomy using a single-umbilical puncture (mini-laparoscopy). J Reprod Med. 1992;37(9) 777-784.

[12] Bresadola F, Pasqualucci A, Donini A, Chiarandini P, Anania G, Terrosu G, Sistu MA, Pasetto A. Elective transumbilical compared with standard laparoscopic cholecystectomy. Eur J Surg. 1999;165(1) 29-34.

[13] Esposito C. One-trocar appendectomy in pediatric surgery. Surg Endosc. 1998;12(2)177-178.

[14] Bucher P, Pugin F, Morel P. Single port access laparoscopic right hemicolectomy. Int J Colorectal Dis. 2008;23(10) 1013-1016

[15] Islam A, Castellvi AO, Tesfay ST, Castellvi AD, Wright AS, Scott DJ. Early surgeon impressions and technical difficulty associated with laparoendoscopic single-site surgery: a Society of American Gastrointestinal and Endoscopic Surgeons learning center study. Surg Endosc 2011:25 (8) 2597-2603.

[16] Chew MH, Wong MT, Lim BY, Ng KH, Eu KW. Evaluation of current devices in single-incision laparoscopic colorectal surgery: a preliminary experience in 32 consecutive cases. World J Surg. 2011;35(4) 873-880.

[17] Dhumane P, Diana M, Leroy J, Marescaux J. Minimally invasive single-site surgery for the digestive system: a technological review. J Minim Access Surg 2011;7 (1) 40-51.

[18] Makino T, Milsom JW, Lee SW. Feasibility and safety of single-incision laparoscopic colectomy: a systematic review. Ann Surg. 2012;255(4) 667-676.

[19] Fung AK, Aly EH. Systematic review of single-incision laparoscopic colonic surgery. Br J Surg. 2012;99(10) 1353-1364.

[20] Diana M, Dhumane P, Cahill RA, Mortensen N, Leroy J, Marescaux J. Minimal invasive single-site surgery in colorectal procedures: Current state of the art. J Minim Access Surg. 2011;7(1) 52-60.

[21] Bucher P, Pugin F, Morel P. Single-port access laparoscopic radical left colectomy in humans. Dis Colon Rectum 2009;52 (10) 1797–1801.

[22] Brunner W, Schirnhofer J, Waldstein-Wartenberg N, Frass R, Weiss H. Single incision laparoscopic sigmoid colon resections without visible scar: a novel technique. Colorectal Dis 2010;12 (1) 66–70.

[23] Lee SW, Milsom JW, Nash GM. Single-incision versus multiport laparoscopic right and hand-assisted left colectomy: a case-matched comparison. Dis Colon Rectum 2011;54(11) 1355–1361.

[24] Gash KJ, Goede AC, Chambers W, Greenslade GL, Dixon AR. Laparoendoscopic single-site surgery is feasible in complex colorectal resections and could enable day case colectomy. Surg Endosc 2011;25(3) 835–840.

[25] Keshava A, Mackenzie S, Al-Kubati W. Single-port laparoscopic right colonic resection. ANZ J Surg 2010; 80(1-2) 30–32.

[26] Ross H, Steele S, Whiteford M, Lee S, Albert M, Mutch M et al. Early multi-institution experience with single-incision laparoscopic colectomy. Dis Colon Rectum 2011;54 (2) 187–192.

[27] Lu CC, Lin SE, Chung KC, Rau KM. Comparison of clinical outcome of single incision laparoscopic surgery using a simplified access system with conventional laparoscopic surgery for malignant colorectal disease. Colorectal Dis 2012;14 (4) 171–176

[28] Gaujoux S, Bretagnol F, Ferron M, Panis Y. Single-incision laparoscopic colonic surgery. Colorectal Dis 2011;13 (9) 1066–1071

[29] Geisler D, Garrett T. Single incision laparoscopic colorectal surgery: a single surgeon experience of 102 consecutive cases. Tech Coloproctol 2011; 15 (4) 397–401.

[30] Ramos-Valadez DI, Patel CB, Ragupathi M, Bokhari MB, Pickron TB, Haas EM. Single-incision laparoscopic colectomy: outcomes of an emerging minimally invasive technique. Int J Colorectal Dis 2011;26 (6) 761–767.

[31] van den Boezem PB, Sietses C. Single-incision laparoscopic colorectal surgery, experience with 50 consecutive cases. J Gastrointest Surg 2011;15 (11) 1989–1994.

[32] Adair J, Gromski MA, Lim RB, Nagle D. Single-incision laparoscopic right colectomy: experience with 17 consecutive cases and comparison with multiport laparoscopic right colectomy. Dis Colon Rectum 2010;53 (11) 1549–1554.

[33] Boni L, Dionigi G, Cassinotti E, Di Giuseppe M, Diurni M, Rausei S et al. Single incision laparoscopic right colectomy. Surg Endosc 2010;24 (12) 3233–3236.

[34] Keshava A, Young CJ, Mackenzie S. Single-incision laparoscopic right hemicolectomy. Br J Surg 2010;97 (12) 1881–1883.

[35] Lim YK, Ng KH, Eu KW. Single site laparoscopic right hemicolectomy: an oncological feasible option. World J Surg Oncol 2010;8 (8) 79.

[36] Pietrasanta D, Romano N, Prosperi V, Lorenzetti L, Basili G, Goletti O. Single-incision laparoscopic right colectomy for cancer: a single-centre preliminary experience. Updates Surg 2010; 62(2) 111–115.

[37] O'Connor DJ, Feinberg E, Jang J, Vemulapalli P, Camacho D. Single-incision laparoscopic-assisted right colon resection for cancer. JSLS 2010;14 (4) 558–560.

[38] Ramos-Valadez DI, Patel CB, Ragupathi M, Bartley Pickron T, Haas EM. Single-incision laparoscopic right hemicolectomy: safety and feasibility in a series of consecutive cases. Surg Endosc 2010;24 (10) 2613–2616.

[39] Cianchi F, Qirici E, Trallori G, Mallardi B, Badii B, Perigli G. Single-incision laparoscopic colectomy: technical aspects and short-term results. Updates Surg 2011;64(1) 19-23.

[40] Katsuno G, Fukunaga M, Nagakari K, Yoshikawa S, Ouchi M, Hirasaki Y. Single-incision laparoscopic colectomy for colon cancer: early experience with 31 cases. Dis Colon Rectum 2011;54 (6) 705–710.

[41] Papaconstantinou HT, Thomas JS. Single-incision laparoscopic colectomy for cancer: assessment of oncologic resection and short-term outcomes in a case-matched comparison with standard laparoscopy. Surgery 2011;150 (4) 820–807.

[42] Saber AA, El-Ghazaly TH. Single-incision transumbilical laparoscopic right hemicolectomy using SILS port. Am Surg 2011;77 (2) 252–253.

[43] Arezzo A, Morino M. Endoscopic surgery through single-port incision: time for a trial?. Surg Endosc. 2011; 25(6) 1709-1711.

[44] Tsujinaka S, Konishi F, Kawamura YJ, Saito M, Tajima N, Tanaka O et al. Visceral obesity predicts surgical outcomes after laparoscopic colectomy for sigmoid colon cancer. Dis Colon Rectum 2008;51 (12) 1757–1765.

[45] Chen WT, Chang SC, Chiang HC, Lo WY, Jeng LB, Wu C et al. Single-incision laparoscopic versus conventional laparoscopic right hemicolectomy: a comparison of short-term surgical results. Surg Endosc 2011;25 (6) 1887–1892.

[46] Waters JA, Guzman MJ, Fajardo AD, Selzer DJ, Wiebke EA, Robb BW et al. Single-port laparoscopic right hemicolectomy: a safe alternative to conventional laparoscopy. Dis Colon Rectum 2010;53 (11) 1467–1472.

[47] Wong MT, Ng KH, Ho KS, Eu KW. Single-incision laparoscopic surgery for right hemicolectomy: our initial experience with 10 cases. Tech Coloproctol 2010;14 (3) 225–258.

[48] Papaconstantinou HT, Sharp N, Thomas JS. Single-incision laparoscopic right colectomy: a case-matched comparison with standard laparoscopic and hand-assisted laparoscopic techniques. J Am Coll Surg 2011;213 (1) 72–80.

[49] Waters JA, Rapp BM, Guzman MJ, Jester AL, Selzer DJ, Robb BW, Johansen BJ, Tsai BM, Maun DC, George VV. Single-port laparoscopic right hemicolectomy: the first 100 resections. Dis Colon Rectum. 2012;55(2) 134-139

[50] Chew MH, Chang MH, Tan WS, Wong MT, Tang CL. 1.Conventional laparoscopic versus single-incision laparoscopic right hemicolectomy: a case cohort comparison of short-term outcomes in 144 consecutive cases. Surg Endosc. 2012 18. [Epub ahead of print].

[51] Uematsu D, Akiyama G, Magishi A, Nakamura J, Hotta K. Single-access laparoscopic left and right hemicolectomy combined with extracorporeal magnetic retraction. Dis Colon Rectum 2010;53 (6) 944–948.

[52] Takemasa I, Sekimoto M, Ikeda M, Mizushima T, Yamamoto H, Doki Y, Mori M. Video. Transumbilical single-incision laparoscopic surgery for sigmoid colon cancer. Surg Endosc 2010; 24 (1) 2321.

[53] Law WL, Fan JK, Poon JT. Single incision laparoscopic left colectomy for carcinoma of distal transverse colon. Colorectal Dis 2010;12 (7) 698–701.

[54] Uematsu D, Akiyama G, Narita M, Magishi A. Single-access laparoscopic low anterior resection with vertical suspension of the rectum. Dis Colon Rectum 2011;54 (5) 632–637.

[55] Co CS, Cheung HY, Yau KK, Chung CC, Li M. Combined single-port and endoluminal technique for laparoscopic anterior resection. Surg Laparosc Endosc Percutan Tech 2010;20 (4) 253–256.

[56] Kawahara H, Watanabe K, Ushigome T, Noaki R, Kobayashi S, Yanaga K. Umbilical incision laparoscopic surgery with one assist port for anterior resection. Dig Surg 2010;27 (5) 364–366.

[57] Bulut O, Nielsen CB, Jespersen N. Single-port access laparoscopic surgery for rectal cancer: initial experience with 10 cases. Dis Colon Rectum. 2011; 54(7) 803-809

[58] Remzi FH, Kirat HT, Geisler DP. Laparoscopic single-port colectomy for sigmoid cancer. Tech Coloproctol 2010;14 (3) 253–255.

[59] Uematsu D, Akiyama G, Matsuura M, Hotta K. Single-access laparoscopic colectomy with a novel multiport device in sigmoid colectomy for colon cancer. Dis Colon Rectum 2010;53 (4) 496–501.

[60] Ramos-Valadez DI, Ragupathi M, Nieto J, Patel CB, Miller S, Pickron TB et al. Single-incision versus conventional laparoscopic sigmoid colectomy: a case-matched series. Surg Endosc 2012;26 (1) 96–102.

[61] Vestweber B, Galetin T, Lammerting K, Paul C, Giehl J, Straub E, Kaldowski B, Alfes A, Vestweber KH. Single-incision laparoscopic surgery: outcomes from 224 colonic resections performed at a single center using SILS™. Surg Endosc. 2013; 27 (2) 434-442.

[62] Geisler DP, Condon ET, Remzi FH. Single incision laparoscopic total proctocolectomy with ileopouch anal anastomosis. Colorectal Dis 2010;12 (9) 941–943.

[63] Nagpal A, Soni H, Haribhakti S. Single-incision laparoscopic restorative proctocolectomy with ileal pouch anal anastomosis for ulcerative colitis: first Indian experience and literature review. Int J Colorectal Dis 2011;26 (4) 525–526.

[64] Fichera A, Zoccali M, Gullo R. Single incision ('scarless') laparoscopic total abdominal colectomy with end ileostomy for ulcerative colitis. J Gastrointest Surg 2011;15 (7) 1247–1251.

[65] Cahill RA, Lindsey I, Jones O, Guy R, Mortensen N, Cunningham C. Single-port laparoscopic total colectomy for medically uncontrolled colitis. Dis Colon Rectum 2010;53 (8) 1143–1147.

[66] Geisler DP, Kirat HT, Remzi FH. Single-port laparoscopic total proctocolectomy with ileal pouch–anal anastomosis: initial operative experience. Surg Endosc 2011;25 (7) 2175–2178.

[67] Leblanc F, Makhija R, Champagne BJ, Delaney CP. Single incision laparoscopic total colectomy and proctocolectomy for benign disease: initial experience. Colorectal Dis 2011;13 (11) 1290–1293.

[68] Paranjape C, Ojo OJ, Carne D, Guyton D. Single-incision laparoscopic total colectomy. JSLS. 2012;16(1) 27-32.

[69] Huscher CG, Mingoli A, Sgarzini G, Mereu A, Binda B, Brachini G, Trombetta S. Standard laparoscopic versus single-incision laparoscopic colectomy for cancer: early results of a randomized prospective study. Am J Surg. 2012;204(1) 115-120.

[70] Poon JT, Cheung CW, Fan JK, Lo OS, Law WL. Single-incision versus conventional laparoscopic colectomy for colonic neoplasm: a randomized, controlled trial. Surg Endosc. 2012;26(10) 2729-2734.

[71] Zhou YM, Wu LP, Zhao YF, Xu DH, Li B. Single-incision versus conventional laparoscopy for colorectal disease: a meta-analysis. Dig Dis Sci. 2012;57(8) 2103-2112.

[72] Yang TX, Chua TC. Single-incision laparoscopic colectomy versus conventional multiport laparoscopic colectomy: a meta-analysis of comparative studies. Int J Colorectal Dis 2013;28 (1) 89-101.

[73] Kim SJ, Ryu GO, Choi BJ, Kim JG, Lee KJ, Lee SC, Oh ST. The short-term outcomes of conventional and single-port laparoscopic surgery for colorectal cancer. Ann Surg. 2011;254(6) 933-940

[74] Vasilakis V, Clark CE, Liasis L, Papaconstantinou HT. Noncosmetic benefits of single-incision laparoscopic sigmoid colectomy for diverticular disease: A case-matched comparison with multiport laparoscopic technique. J Surg Res 2013; 180 (2) 201-207.

[75] Hassan I, Advani V. Single incision laparoscopic colon surgery. Is the ride worth the curve? Colorectal Dis 2010;12 (9) 847–848.

[76] National Institute for Health and Clinical Excellence (NICE). NICE Implementation Uptake Report: Laparoscopic Surgery for Colorectal Cancer, 2010; http:// www.nice.org.uk/ media/B4D/4A/UptakeReportColorectalCancer.pdf

[77] Sammour T, Kahokehr A, Chan S, Booth RJ, Hill AG. The humoral response after laparoscopic versus open colorectal surgery: a meta-analysis J Surg Res. 2010;164(1) 28-37.

[78] Huang C, Huang R, Jiang T, Huang K, Cao J, Qiu Z. Laparoscopic and open resection for colorectal cancer: an evaluation of cellular immunity. BMC Gastroenterol. 2010;28(10) 127.

Chapter 7

Robotic Colorectal Cancer Surgery

Ray Swayamjyoti, Jim Khan and Amjad Parvaiz

Additional information is available at the end of the chapter

http://dx.doi.org/10.5772/58350

1. Introduction

A robot is a mechanical or virtual agent, usually an electro-mechanical machine that is guided by a computer program or electronic circuitry. Robots have been linked with the future and modern civilization but have been around for more than 2000 years since ancient Greek automata. Their real surgical application has been in the last 20 years [1, 2].

Robots were first used in medicine to help people with disabilities to aid in their rehabilitation process. The Edinburgh Modular Arm System [3] was one of the first bionic arm which was engineered by Dr. David Gow in the early eighties.

The National Aeronautics and Space Administration (NASA) developed the first telemanipulator robot in 1985 at the behest of the Defense Department of the United States of America with the aim to decrease war casualties using telerobotic surgery [4].

It was believed that robots could have prevented more than a third of the soldiers from dying during the Vietnam War secondary to haemorrhage [5].

Robotic colorectal operations have gained considerable interest after successful implementation in the field of urology and gynaecology. The advantages of a stable platform, better vision and better access has made this an attractive tool in many specialities. [6] Pelvic and rectal resections are best suited for robotic operations [6].

2. The Da Vinci surgical robotic system

The Federal Drug and Administration approved the use of the da Vinci robotic system for surgical treatment in 2000 and it was first used at the Ohio State University Hospital for oesophageal and pancreatic surgery [22].

Year	Milestones
1985	• PUMA 560 was used under computerised tomography guidance to orient a needle for brain biopsy [7]
1992	• PROBOT - developed at Imperial College, London and was used to perform prostatic surgery at Guy's and St Thomas' Hospital, London [8] • The ROBODOC developed by Integrated Surgical Systems was used to curve out accurate fittings in the femur for hip replacement [8]
1998	• Zeus robotic surgical system – used for reconstruction of the Fallopian tube performed at the Ohio State University Medical Center [9]
1999	• Robotics assisted closed chest bypass on a beating heart was performed at the London Health Sciences Centre [10]
2000	• **FDA approval of da Vinci robotic system**[11]
2002	• Robotic cholecystectomy [12] • **Robotic Right Hemicolectomy** [13] • Robotic bowel resections [14]
2006	• Unassisted robotic surgery using artificial intelligence to correct atrial fibrillation at a hospital in Milan [15]
2007	• Denervation of spermatic cord for testicular pain using robotic assisted microsurgery performed at Winter Haven Hospital and University of Florida [16]
2008	• Magnetic Resonance guided neurosurgical procedure performed at University of Calgary [17] • Microsurge developed by German Aerospace Center [18]
2010	• Sophie Surgical System developed by Eindhoven University of Technology [19] • Femoral reconstruction [20] • World's first all robotic operation i.e. prostatectomy using the da Vinci robot along with McSleepy robot used for anaesthesia at McGill University Hospital, Canada [21]

Table 1. Development of Robotics to aid in Surgical Procedures.

At present it is extensively used throughout the world and has sold over 2000 units worldwide in 2013. It is estimated then more than 200,000 operations have been performed in 2012 [23, 24].

The initial model of da Vinci was released in the year 1999, later this was updated to "S" in 2007 and in 2009 Si was released with improved functions and better performance. The author uses the da Vinci "Si" robotic system for his colorectal operations.

The da Vinci system consists of a surgeon's console and four interactive robotic arms attached to the robotic cart controlled by the surgeon from the console. One of the arms carries an endoscopic camera via a 12mm port. The camera has two lenses, which gives a 3D image with stereoscopic vision when the surgeon looks through the eyepiece in the console. The three other arms are used to hold tools and tissues i.e. scissors, bovies, electrocautery. The arms are maneuvered using two-foot pedals and two hand controllers.

http://dx.doi.org/10.5772/58350

Unlike laparoscopy the da Vinci system allows the surgeon to perform operation seated at the console, with the hands and eyes positioned in line with the instruments. The operating surgeon is able to control the movements of the camera using the foot pedal rather than relying on an assistant. The system is able to filter and decipher surgeon's hand movements into steady and precise micro movements.

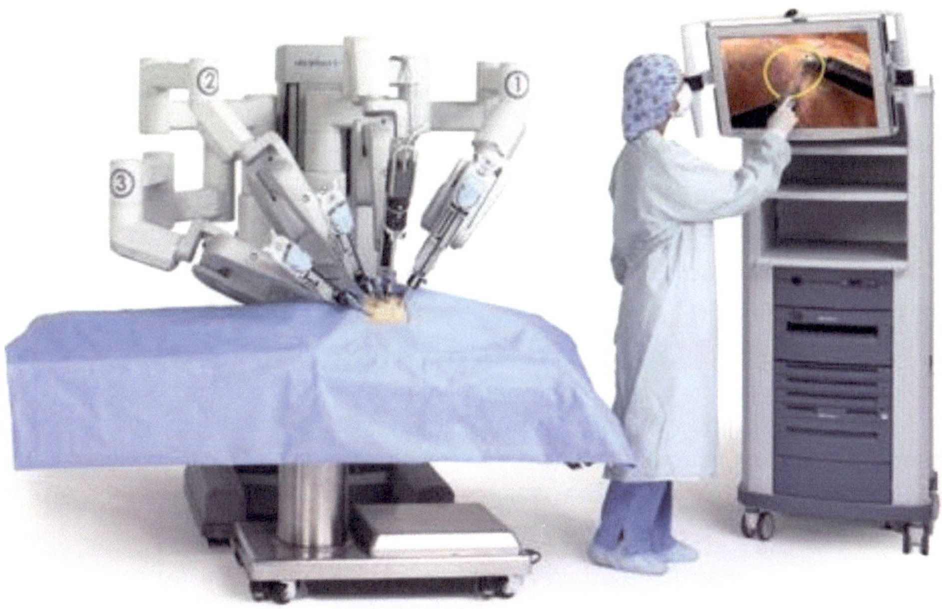

Figure 1. [25]: showing the robotic stack/cart and the monitor used by the assistant to follow the operation

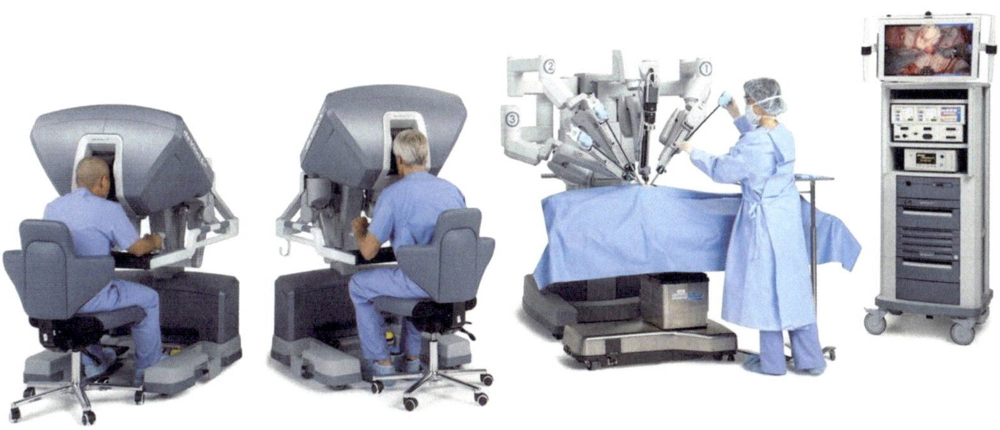

Figure 2. [26] : showing robotic and vision carts and the surgeon's console with an additional teaching console

3. Evidence of robotics in colorectal surgery

Robotic colorectal surgery is gaining widespread interest worldwide and in the continent. Data collected in 2012 suggests that most of the reported or published data shows that majority of the robotic colorectal operations have been performed in the United States (32%) followed by South Korea (20%), Italy (15%), Canada, Germany and Netherlands accounted for 5% and the rest of the world less than 2% [13].

The first colorectal surgical publication was published by Weber et al in 2002 [27] and since then there has been a tenfold rise in publication in colorectal surgery [13]. The important landmark studies are summarized in table 2.

Laparoscopic colorectal operations have many advantages over conventional open operations. The benefits in terms of short term outcomes are well established and include shorter hospital stay, faster return to work, better cosmesis, less post operative pain, less risk of bleeding and ileus. Long term outcomes including cancer specific and disease free survival have been subject of many well-designed trials.

The COLOR (COlon cancer Laparoscopic or Open resection) trial (330 stated that laparoscopic colectomy was associated with less significant blood loss, earlier recovery of bowel function, use of fewer analgesics and with a shorter hospital stay when compared with open colectomy. It however took half an hour longer than open operations and had 19% chances of converting to open operation. The reasons for conversion were mainly attributed to tumour size of more than 6cms and in patients who had involvement of adjacent structures.

There were concerns regarding tumour recurrence associated with laparoscopic colectomy. The meta-analysis of four randomized control trials (CLASICC trial, COST trial, Barcelona trial and COLOR trial) where patients with colonic cancers were randomised to either open or laparoscopically assisted colectomy concluded that the positive margins were found in specimens after open operations were 2.1% as compared to 1.3% after laparoscopic operation. The overall disease free survival at three years was 83.5% for open operations and 82.2% for laparoscopic operations [34]. Hence, the evidence shows that laparoscopic colonic operation is oncologically safe and viable with comparable outcomes to open surgery [34, 35].

The safety and viability for rectal cancers is still less clear especially with the higher circumferential margin (CRM) involvement with laparoscopic rectal operations when compared to open rectal operations as mentioned in the CLASSIC trial [34]. There was however, no difference in local recurrence at three years [36]. There was a higher conversion rate in the laparoscopic rectal subgroup (34%) in comparison to laparoscopic colonic group (25%). Conversions to open operations led to higher mortality and morbidity [34, 37]. Conversions were mainly attributed to bulky tumours [33] and increased technical difficulty [37]. The robot promises to abolish some of these technical problems faced during dissection of rectal tumours using laparoscopy and the ROLARR (RObotic versus LAparoscopic Resection for Rectal cancer) trial results are awaited. It is an international, multicentre, prospective, randomised, and controlled, unblinded, parallel-group trial of robotic-assisted versus laparoscopic surgery for the curative treatment of rectal cancer [37].

Year	Reference	Country	Study type	Number of patients
2002	Weber et al.	USA	Case series	2,
				3,
	Hashizume et al.	Japan		18
	Talamini et al.	USA		
2003	Vibert et al.	France	Case series	3,
	Giulianotti et al.	Italy		16
2004	Hubens et al.	Belgium	Case series,	8,
	Anvari et al.	Canada	Prospective Comparative	10,
	D'Annibale	Italy	Comparative	53
2005	Woeste et al.	Germany	Comparative,	6,
	Bonder et al.	Austria	Case series,	14,
	Ruurda et al.	Holland	Case series	23
2007	Heemskerk et al.	Netherlands	Comparative	19
2008	Baik et al.	Korea,	Randomized trial,	18,
	Spinoglio	Italy,	Comparative,	50,
	Huettner et al.	USA,	Comparative,	70,
	Soravia et al.	Switzerland	Case series	40
2009	Baik et al.	Korea	Comparative,	56,
	DeHoog et al.	Netherlands	Case control	20
2010	Tsoraides et al.	USA,	Retrospective,	102,
	Kim and kang	Korea,	Comparative,	100,
	Bianchi et al.	Italy,	Comparative,	56,
	Pernazza and Morpurgo	Italy,	Case series,	50,
	DeSouza et al.	USA,	Case control,	40,
	Zimmern et al.	USA,	Case series,	131,
	Popescu et al.	Romania	Comparative	122
2011	Kang and kim	Korea	Retrospective	204
2012	Antoniou SA et al [28]	Germany	Case series	39
2013	Casillas MA Jr et al [29]	USA	Case series	344
	Germain A et al [30]	France	Case Series	77
	Barrie J et al [31]	UK	Comparative	34
	Wormer BA et al [32]	USA	Comparative	1809

Table 2. [13]

The skills required for laparoscopic operations are different to open operations.

Limitations of laparoscopic surgery include loss of depth perception, reduced tactile feedback and a declined range of motion [33]. The author believes that limited space in the pelvis, with two-dimensional visions and a bulky specimen can make laparoscopic operations very difficult.

Laparoscopic TME rectal resections have a steep learning curve [38], requiring precise pelvic dissection with preservation of autonomic nerves. There is higher incidence of male sexual dysfunction due to inadvertent injury to the nerves following TME resections [39]. It is estimated that 50% of colorectal surgeons perform laparoscopic colorectal operations in the UK and only a quarter of them perform laparoscopic TME resections [40]. Approximately 50-70 cases are needed to surmount the laparoscopic colorectal learning curve [35, 38, 41].

The COREAN trail [42] trial compared open surgery with laparoscopic surgery for mid or low rectal cancer after neoadjuvant chemoradiotherapy. There was a conversion rate of 1.2% in the COREAN trial as compared to 34% in the CLASSIC trial. The low conversion rate in the COREAN trial was attributed to greater experience of the surgeons who has performed an average of seventy laparoscopic operations as compared to twenty per average surgeon in the CLASSIC trial [43].

The learning curve for performing robotic colorectal operations is shorter and is achieved after 15-20 cases [37, 38]. There are three phases that has been identified in the learning curve for robotic colorectal operations [44, 45, 46]

- Phase 1 – initial learning (1-15 cases)
- Phase 2 – increased competence (15-25 cases)
- Phase 3 – period of highest skill (>25 cases)

The other advantages of robotic colorectal resections are that

- It is superior in narrow areas like the pelvis and it's safe and feasible [47] with good three dimensional view and zoom magnification [37]
- It has 7 degrees of freedom of movement [37]
- It is associated with lower conversion rates to open operation [48]
- It has better pathologic and functional outcomes. It is associated with less complication rates, shorter duration of hospital stay, time to recover to normal bowel function or first flatus and time to start diet. It also causes less postoperative pain [49].
- Hospitals who perform high-volume robotic colorectal operations have significantly lower rates of postoperative bleeding and ileus [50]
- the double console that comes with the robotic cart allow trainees to take part actively at the surgical procedure and learn from it [51]
- simulators are available than can be attached to the console which provides a platform for surgical trainees to practice their skills before actually performing the procedures

There are however some limitations of the da Vinci system. In particular

- there is a definite learning curve for this technique
- loss of tactile feedback although partly compensated by better vision, still can have its effects on the performance and outcomes
- Hospitals that perform less robotic colorectal operations had more complications with longer length of hospital stay causing higher cost for the hospital. [19]
- High cost of purchasing as well as maintaining the robotic system [22]

	LNs (mean N)			Distal margin(mean, cm)			Positive CRM (%)		
	ROB	LAP	*p*	ROB	LAP	*p*	ROB	LAP	*p*
Park et al, 2010	17.3	14.2	*0.06*	2.1	2.3	ns	4.9	3.7	0.5
Kim et al, 2010	14.7	16.6	*ns*	2.7	2.6	0.09	3	2	ns
Kwak et al, 2011	20	21	*0.7*	2.2	2.0	0.8	1.7	0	>0.9
Baek et al, 2011	13	16	*0.07*	3.6	3.8	0.6	2.4	4.9	1
Bianchi et al, 2010	18	17	*0.7*	2	2	1.0	0	4	0.9
Baik et al, 2009	18.4	18.7	*0.8*	4	3.6	0.4	7	8	0.7
Patriti et al, 2009	10.3	11.2	*>0.05*	2.1	4.5	>0.05	0	0	ns

(LNs: lymph nodes, CRM: circumferential resection margin, ns: not significant, ROB: robotic procedure, LAP: laparoscopic procedure.)

Table 3. Oncologic results of robotic and laparoscopic surgery for rectal cancer [52].

	LNs (mean)			Distal margin (mean, cm)			Positive CRM (%)		
	ROB	OPEN	*p*	ROB	OPEN	*p*	ROB	OPEN	*p*
De Souza et al], 2011	15	16.8	0.26	na	na		0	3	0.25
Kim et al, 2012	20	19.6	0.7	2.7	1.9	0.001	1	1	1
Park et al, 2011	19.4	18.5	0.06	2.8	2.3	0.002	1	2	0.9

(LN: lymph nodes, CRM: circumferential resection margin, na: not assessed, ROB: robotic procedure, OPEN: laparoscopic procedure.)

Table 4. Oncologic results of open and robotic surgery for rectal cancer [52].

4. Patient selection

Patient selection is the key especially in the early stages of the learning curve. The author would recommend choosing patients with

- ASA grade 1-3
- BMI <30
- Age <75 years
- No previous pelvic or intra-abdominal surgery
- T1/T2 tumours
- Tumors that are at or just above the peritoneal reflection of the rectum
- Avoid patients who received neo-adjuvant chemo-radiotherapy and
- Avoid patients who for medical reasons will not be able to tolerate Trendelenburg position

5. Patient preparation

- Bowel preparation – phosphate enema for left sided operations. Bowel preparation not necessary for right sided colonic operations.

Bowel preparation is controversial in colorectal surgery. Surgeons differ in their approach. Mechanical bowel preparation results in a colon that is clear of feces. However, it can leave liquid stool in the bowel that is more likely to contaminate the operative field and the pelvis in the event of an anastomotic leak. In our experience, bowel preparation also results in small bowel distension that can make operations more difficult. The authors do not use bowel preparation for right-sided colonic resections. Two-phosphate enemas are used for left sided colorectal resections.

- low residue diet 3-4 days before operation
- 4 high calorie drinks to be taken the night before operation
- Eating and drinking normally up to 6 hours before operation
- 2 high calorie drinks to be taken up to 2 hours before operation
- Intra-operative fluids are restricted to 500 mL per hour as tolerated by the patient. This minimizes the risk of edema of the face and neck that can occur due to the steep Trendelenburg position and excessive fluids. Goal directed therapy is the standard approach using esophageal Doppler.

http://dx.doi.org/10.5772/58350

6. Operating room configuration

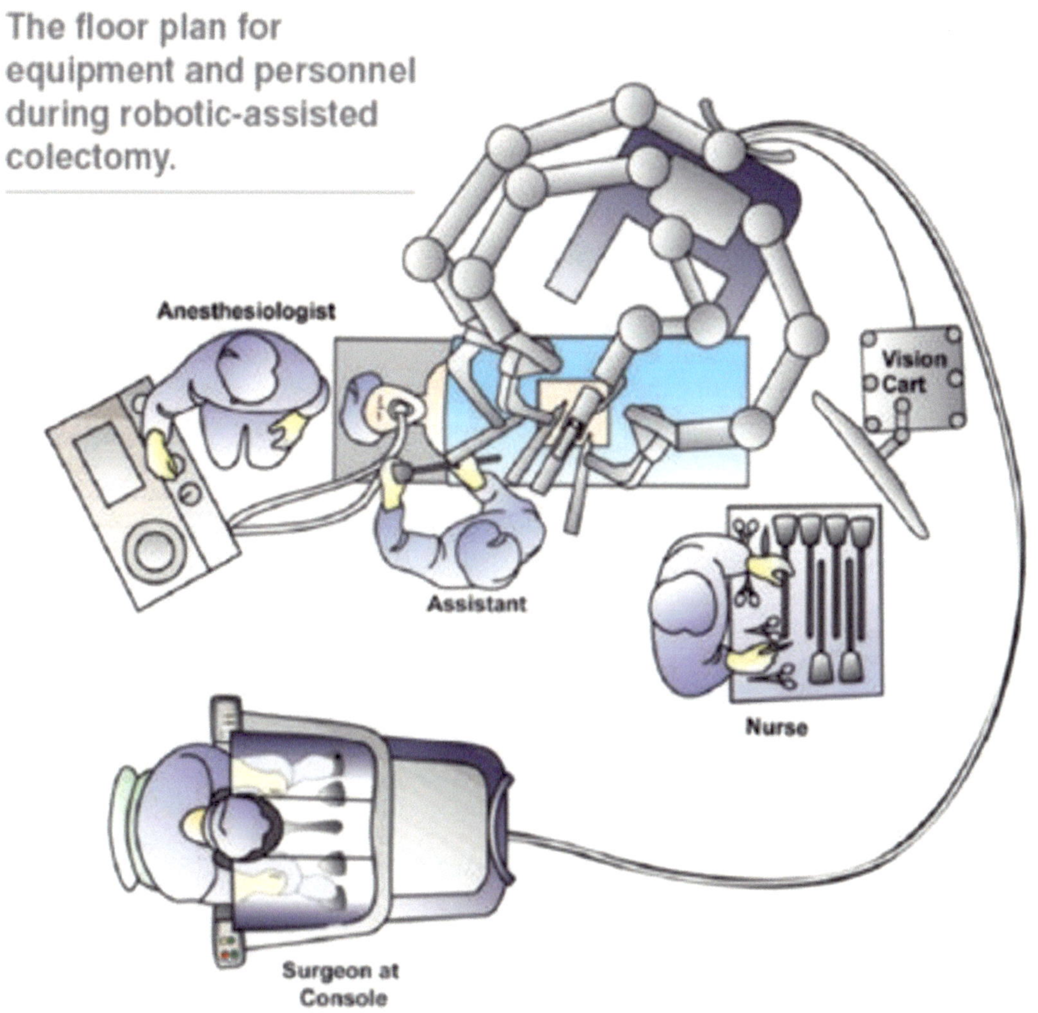

Figure 3. [53]: showing operating room set up during colectomy

7. Positioning

- Patient is positioned supine in a modified lithotomy position with legs wrapped around adjustable stirrups
- Legs are abducted and slightly flexed at the knees

- Patient's arms are wrapped alongside the body to reduce possibility of shoulder injury and additional shoulder harness can be placed to support Trendelburg's position
- Pressure points and bony prominences are padded and the body position is secured with vacuum-mattress device, especially lateral on the right side.
- Secure the patient to the table to avoid any shifting with the Trendelenburg position.
- Patient is tilted right side down and adjust the angle during initial exposure
- A body warmer (bear hugger) is applied to prevent patient hypothermia.
- Sequential compression devices (Flowtrons) are applied to the legs for DVT prophylaxis.
- After positioning, padding, securing and preparing the patient in the supine position, the table is then placed in a Trendelenburg position, whereby the steepness should be adjusted as per exposure needs during the initial exposure step.

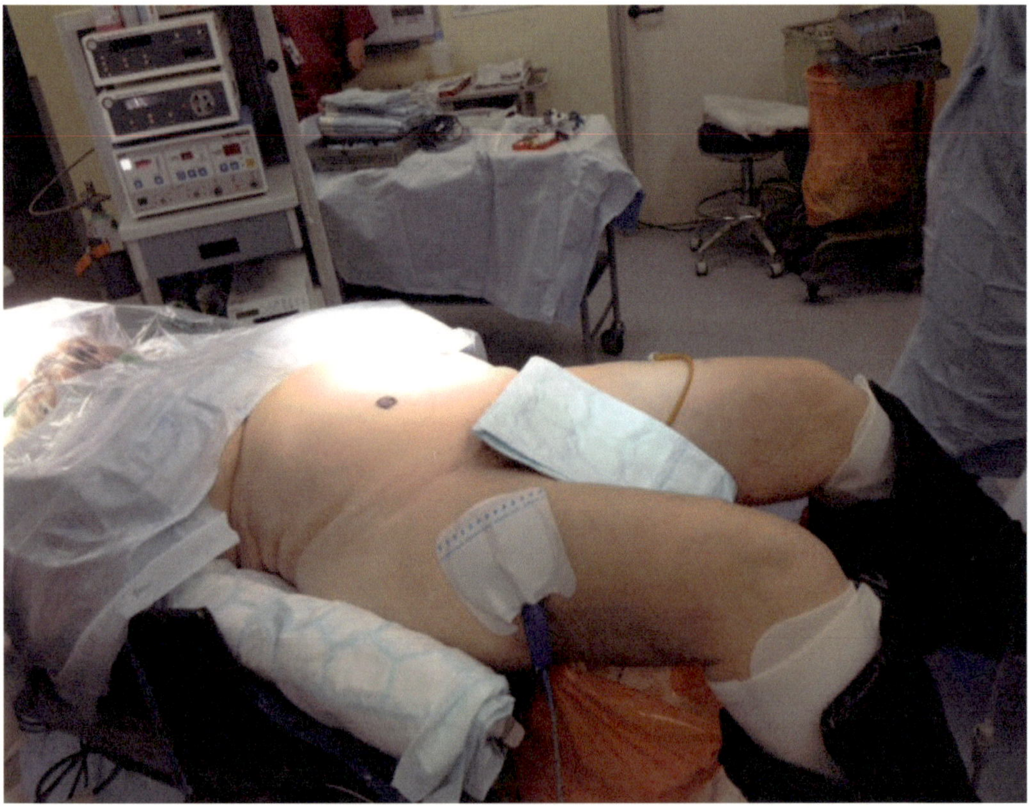

Image 1. Showing positioning of patient

http://dx.doi.org/10.5772/58350

8. Right-sided operations

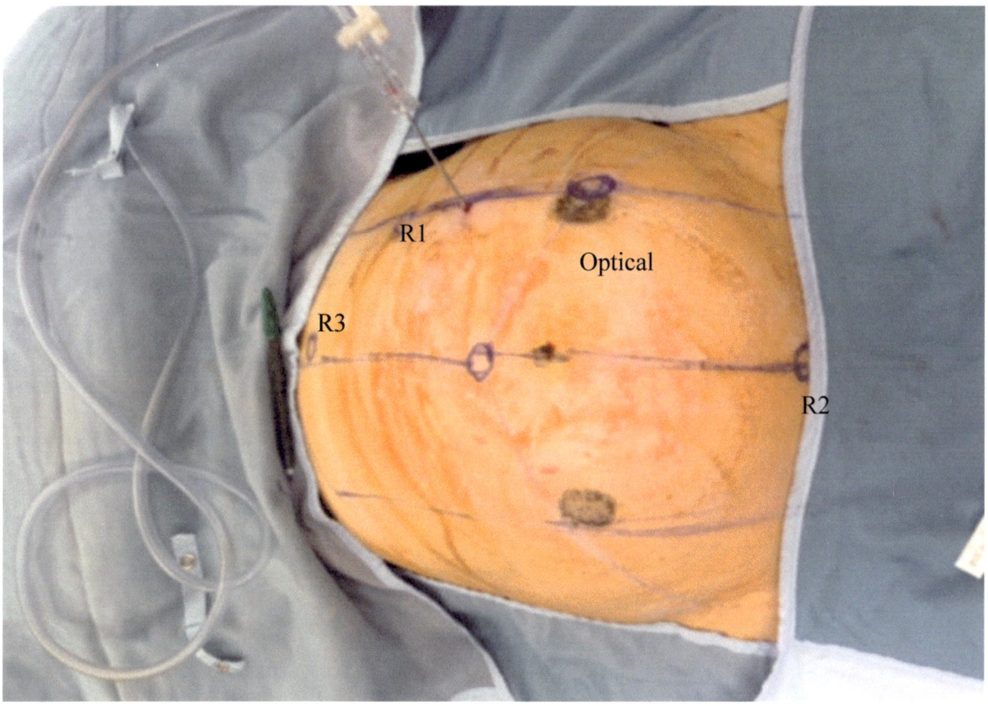

Image 2. Showing marking for Right Colonic resections. Insufflation via Veress needle at LUQ.

9. Port placements

9.1. Preparing for port placement

- Port placement is the key for a successful robotic procedure. Narrow space between the ports will result in clashing of the arms and poor ergonomics. We recommend marking of the abdomen for port placement after CO2 insufflation.
- The initial pneumopertioneum can be established with a Veress needle or Hassan's technique at LUQ or at camera port site.
- Initial assessment of entire anatomy of the abdomen focusing on adhesions, peritoneal seedlings and liver metastasis is carried out once the camera port is inserted. Place remaining ports under endoscopic vision avoiding injury to the inferior epigastric vessels.

9.2. Instrument port placements for left sided colorectal operations [54]

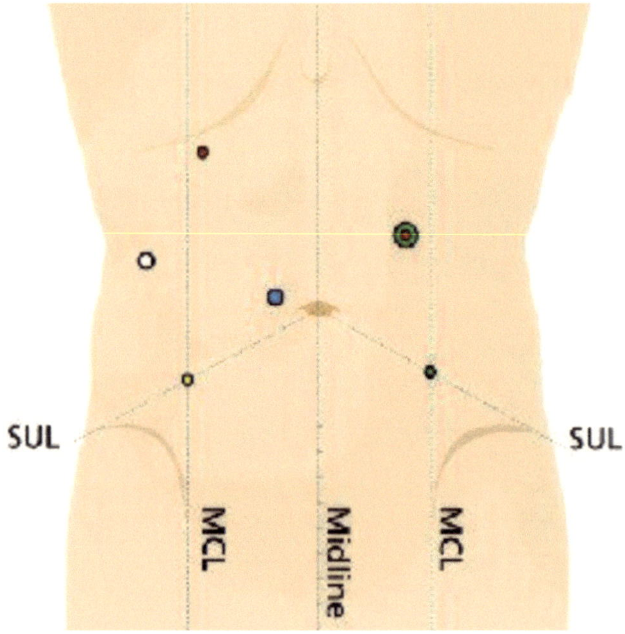

Diagram 1 Showing post placements for left sided colorectal operations

- **Robotic camera port, 12 mm (Blue):** Place the port 3-4 cm right and 3-4 cm above umbilicus. Distance to symphysis pubis should be ~22-24 cm.
- **Robotic instrument arm port, 8 mm (Yellow):** Place the port a minimum of 8 cm from the camera port, on the right spinoumbilical line (SUL) at the crossing of the mid-clavicular line (MCL). Distance to symphysis pubis should be ~14-16 cm. Linear stapler can be used from this port.
- **Robotic instrument arm port, 8 mm (Green):** Place the port a minimum of 8 cm from the camera port, on the left spinoumbilical line (SUL) at the crossing of the mid-clavicular line (MCL). The distance to the symphysis pubis should be ~14-16 cm.
- **Robotic instrument arm port, 8 mm (Red):** Place the port ~ 3 cm sub-xyphoid and ~ 2 cm medial to the right MCL
- **Robotic instrument arm port, 8 mm (Green-Red):** Place the port 7-8 cm below the left costal margin, slightly medial to the left MCL. Place the port a minimum of 8 cm from the other instrument ports and the camera port.
- **Assistant port, 5 mm (White):** Place the port 8-10 cm cephalad to the instrument arm port and ~ 4 cm lateral to the right MCL (a minimum of 8 cm from the camera port). This port is used for suction/irrigation, ligation and retraction.

http://dx.doi.org/10.5772/58350

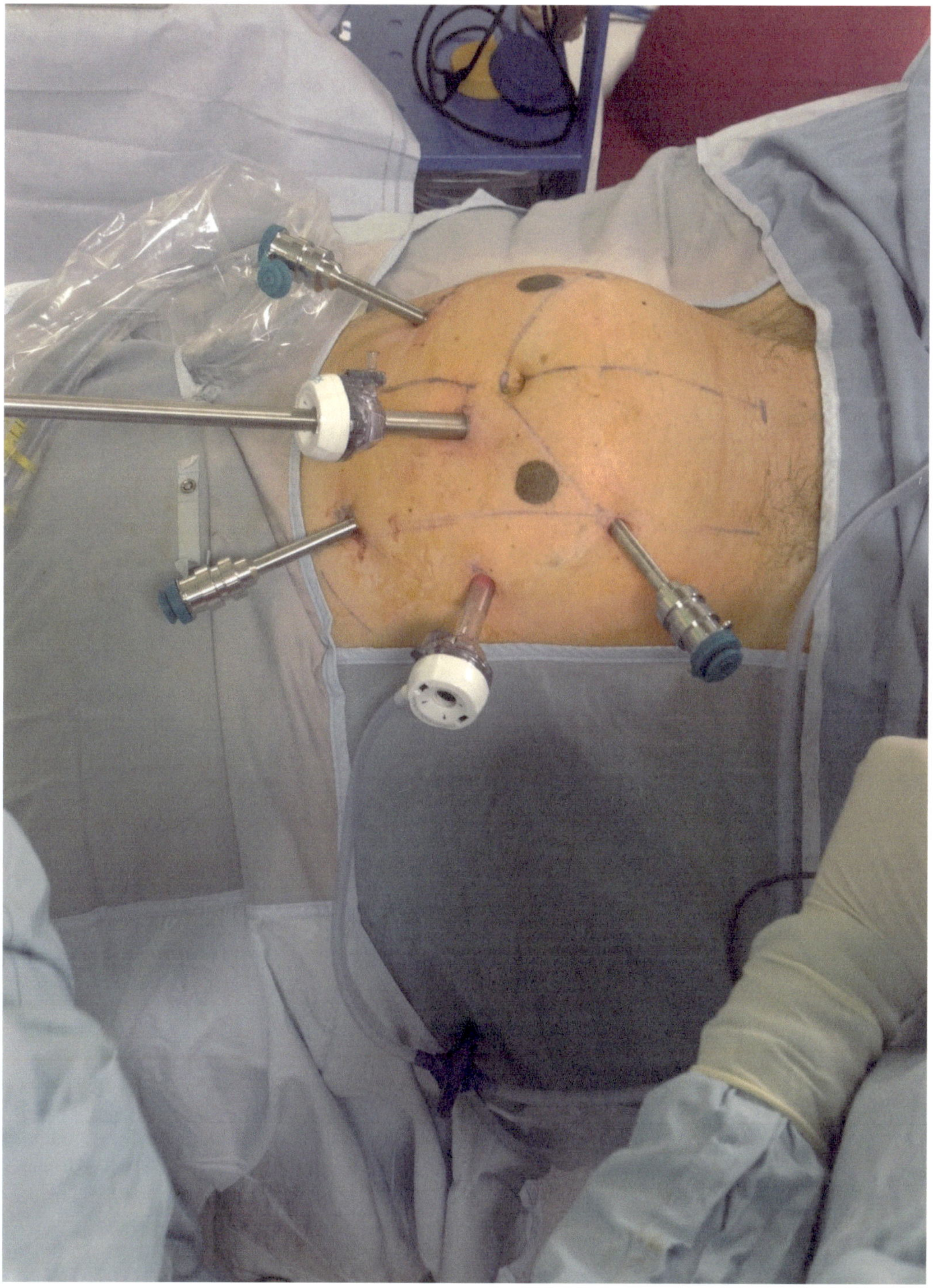

Image 3. Showing port placements for left sided colorectal operations

9.3. Port placement for right sided colonic resections

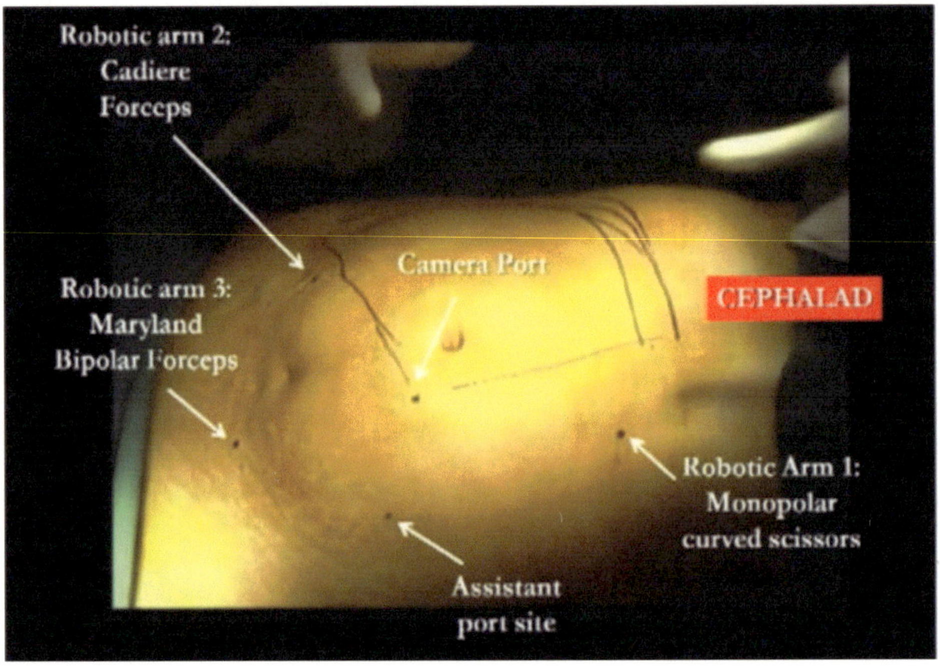

Image 4. [74]: showing port placements for right sided colonic resections

9.4. Instrument port placements for right sided colorectal operations

- Camera port 12mm, at left spinoumbilical line (SUL)
- Robotic arm port 1, 8mm, at left mid-clavicular line (MCL) 8cms below costal margin
- Robotic arm port 2, 8mm, is placed in at right SUL 2cms lateral to right MCL
- Robotic arm port 3, 8mm, is placed in midline 3 cms from pubic symphysis
- Assistant port, 5mm, place at LIF lateral to left MCL

9.5. Operative steps for left sided colorectal operations

- Initial exposure is acquired by cephalad retraction of the omentum to expose the transverse colon and by moving the small bowel out of the pelvis. Loops of small bowel can be stacked in the right upper quadrant to expose the Inferior Mesenteric Vein (IMV). A small swab placed against the small bowel loops can sometimes help by preventing the bowel from slipping into the operative area.
- Primary vascular control is achieved by ligating the Inferior Mesenteric Artery (IMA) and IMV earlier in the operation. Disposable locking clips are used to secure these vessels before division.

http://dx.doi.org/10.5772/58350

- Medial to lateral mobilization of sigmoid and descending colon is carried out towards the left sidewall and superiorly towards the spleen. The plane between mesocolon and Gerota's fascia is developed. Left ureter and gonadal vesssels should be identified at this stage.
- Splenic flexure mobilization (SFM) is not mandatory. However, if the anastomosis is likely to be at tension, SFM is strongly recommended. If SFM is needed, IMV is divided high and the plane above the pancreas is developed which can lead the surgeon into the lesser sac. Gastrocolic omental division from above can complete this step safely.
- Rectal dissection and division – Total Mesorectal Excision (TME) is carried out to the pelvic floor for a mid to low rectal cancer or to the peritoneal reflection for an upper rectal cancer. Great care is taken to avoid injury to the parasympathetic nerves.
- Anastomosis - Rectal division and anastomosis is performed using surgical staplers. Care should be taken not to damage the pelvic floor at this stage. For rectal division, stapler can be inserted through the assistant port or the R1 can be disabled and undocked and the port changed to a 12 mm port to allow the stapler to pass through. In patients with a very narrow pelvis, a supra-pubic port can be used to divide the rectum anteroposteriorly. We perform a routine flexible sigmoidoscopy to check for anastomotic bleeding, viability of the colon and rectum and at the same time perform a leak test to check for anastomotic leak.

9.6. Operative steps for right sided colonic resections

- The patient is positioned in modified Lloyd –Davis position with slight Trendelenberg tilt. The ileocolic and Superior Mesenteric Artery (SMA) pedicles are exposed by retraction of the small bowel and appropriate traction and counter traction on the mesentry. Dissection along the Superior Mesenteric Vein (SMV) will expose the ileocolic vein and artery that are then divided after clipping. Duodenum is identified early and dissection carried out towards the liver to enter the lesser sac.
- Lateral to medial mobilization allows the right colon to be freed up. Sub ileal dissection completes this dissection allowing the whole specimen to come to the midline. Gastrocolic omental division results in complete mobilization of the heaptic flexure.
- Ileocolic anastomosis can be performed intra or extra corporeally depending upon the surgeons preference. Specimen is extracted either through a midline or suprapubic incision.

9.7. Post-operative management — (Enhanced Recovery Programme [55])

Day of operation:

- Pain management with epidural followed by PCA and then oral/IV/IM analgesia
- Post-operatively the patients are transferred to Surgical High Care for close monitoring
- All patients should have DVT (unless contraindicated) and antibiotic prophylaxis
- Patients encouraged to sit out of bed and encouraged to drink straight after the operation including 2 protein drinks

First post-operative day:

- The patient will have an epidural and urinary catheter
- Will be encouraged to drink 2 litres of fluid and drink 4 high protein drinks
- Will be encouraged to eat normal food
- Will be encouraged out of bed for 8 hours and take 3 walks of 50 meters each with help from the physiotherapists

Second post-operative day:

- Epidural and urinary catheter removed. Pain management using PCA.
- Will be encouraged to drink 2 litres of fluid and drink 4 high protein drinks
- Will be encouraged to eat normal food
- Will be encouraged out of bed for 8 hours and take 3 walks of 50 meters each with help from the physiotherapists

Post-operative days 3-5:

- The patient is discharged from the hospital if stable in three to five days i.e. passed flatus and or opening bowels
- Pain controlled with oral medications
- Able to mobilize and physiotherapists happy with progress

Outpatient follow-up:

- Follow up at OPD 2-3 weeks post-operatively
- All Cancer patients are discussed at Multidisciplinary Team Meeting, regarding additional therapy or adjuvant radiation with or without chemotherapy as indicated.

10. Future developments

10.1. Role of ICG in bowel anastomosis and lymph node mapping using da Vinci robot

Indocyanine green (ICG) is a cyanine fluorescent dye that absorbs near infrared wavelengths of light. It binds to plasma proteins and travels in the vascular system [56]. ICG emits an infrared signal when excited by laser light *in situ,* which can be detected with near-infrared fluorescence camera system (NIRF) [57].

The image from NIRF gives visual assessment of blood vessels, blood flow, and tissue perfusion. ICG has been widely used by the ophthalmologists to visualise retinal blood vessels [58] and the technique has been amalgamated into the da Vinci Si robotic system.

Water soluble ICG can be given intravenously during surgical procedure. The surgeon is able switch into fluorescence imaging modes from normal white light mode by pressing pedals in the console and is able to view infrared images of blood flow in the microvasculature as well as tissue perfusion in real time. This is particularly useful during bowel anastomosis and improving patient outcomes [59].

Lymph nodes harvesting can be a difficult procedure to perform in cancer surgery.

The use of ICG is an attractive method to facilitate visualisation of lymphatic vessels, sentinel nodes, and metastatic lymph nodes. It was first introduced by Lim and Soter [60].

ICG has been used in the recent past to harvest lymphnodes for cutaneous rectal carcinoma metastasis [61] and cutaneous Kaposi's sarcoma [62] with successful outcome.

It has also been used in transcutaneous Sentinel Lymph Node detection in vulvar cancer patients [63] and for identification of lymphatic pathway involved in the spreading of prostate cancer [64].

10.2. Robotic Single Incision Laparoscopic Surgery (SILS) or Colectomy (SILC)

Single incision laparoscopic colectomy (SILC) is well established. SILC is associated with shorter post-operative length of hospital stay and smaller skin incision. There is no difference in operating time or in conversion rate when compared to multiport laparoscopic colorectal operations [65]. The main drawback with SILC is exposure, conflict of instruments, ease of instrumentation, camera operation and ergonomics [66].

Robotic single incision laparoscopic surgery may be the answer to some of the problems associated with SILC. The author believes that robotic single incision colectomy will result in less abdominal wall trauma, less pain, needing fewer analgesics, early mobilisation and decreased length of hospital stay. It will have better cosmetic result due to fewer numbers of incisions. There is good evidence to suggest that multiple laparoscopic port incisions can cause port site hernias even with 5mm ports [67, 68].

Early experience with robotic SILC performing right hemicolectomy is safe and feasible [69]. We need more studies to validate robotic SILC for left sided operations.

Other surgical specialties where robotic SILS is gaining interest are listed below:

- Spinioglio G et al mentioned that it took them less time to perform robotic single port laparoscopic cholecystecomies than laparoscopic SILS [70].
- Robotic single-port trans-umbilical total hysterectomy is technically feasible in selected patients with gynaecological disease [71].
- Hahn Tran et al have successfully performed robotic single-port inguinal hernia repair without any complications [72].
- The authors believe that robots will also play a role in natural orifice endoscopic surgery and specimen retrieval via the natural orifice in the near future

The perfect robotic platform should have a low external profile, which can be deployed through a single access site. It should be able to restore intra-abdominal triangulation while maintaining the maximum degree of freedom for accurate maneuvers and strength for reliable traction. Several purpose-built robotic prototypes for single-port surgery are being tested [73].

The author believes that robots will also play a role in natural orifice endoscopic surgery and specimen retrieval via the natural orifice in the near future.

11. Summary

In summary the developments of surgical robotics over the last decade has been very exciting. The technology is improving rapidly. Robots certainly allow the surgeons to perform better operations with improved safety. In colorectal surgery robotics will find its place in pelvic and rectal cancer surgery. The cost of instruments and the system are the biggest barrier to the widespread uptake of robotic surgery by the surgical community. The future applications of this technology may result in further benefits that will offset the cost issue.

Author details

Ray Swayamjyoti, Jim Khan and Amjad Parvaiz

Portsmouth Hospitals NHS Trust, Queen Alexandra Hospital, Portsmouth, UK

References

[1] Ewing DR, Pigazzi A, Wang Y, Ballantyne GH. Robots in the operating room--the history. *Semin Laparosc Surg.* 2004 Jun;11(2):63-71.

[2] Valero R, Ko YH et al Robotic surgery: history and teaching impact. *Actas Urol Esp.* 2011 Oct;35(9):540-5. doi: 10.1016/j.acuro.2011.04.005. Epub 2011 Jun 22.

[3] Dharia SP, Falcone T. Robotics in reproductive medicine. Fertil Steril 2005; 84: 1–11. 4)

[4] Prem N Kakar, Jyotirmoy Das, Preeti Mittal Roy, and Vijaya Pant Robotic invasion of operation theatre and associated anaesthetic issues: A review Indian J Anaesth. 2011 Jan-Feb; 55(1): 18–25. doi: 10.4103/0019-5049.76577

[5] Satava R, Richard M. Surgical robotics: The early chronicles: A personal historical perspective. Surg Laparosc Endosc Percutan Tech. 2002;12:6–16.

[6] Robot-assisted right colectomy: surgical technique and review of the literature Wojciech Witkiewicz, Marek Zawadzki, Marek Rząca, Zbigniew Obuszko, Videosurgery Miniinv 2013; 8 (3): 253–257 DOI:10.5114/wiitm.2011.33761

[7] Kwoh YS, Hou J, Jonckheere EA, Hayati S. A robot with improved absolute positioning accuracy for CT guided stereotactic brain surgery. IEEE Trans Biomed Eng 1988; 35: 153–60.

[8] http://www.robot.md/publications/robodoc-surgical-robot-sucess-story.pdf

[9] McConnell, PI; Schneeberger, EW; Michler, RE (2003). "History and development of robotic cardiac surgery". Problems in General Surgery 20 (2): 20–30.

[10] http://biomed.brown.edu/Courses/BI108/BI108_2000_Groups/Heart_Surgery/Robotics.html Biomed.brown.edu. Retrieved 13/11/2013

[11] http://en.wikipedia.org/wiki/Da_Vinci_Surgical_System

[12] Marescaux J, Smith MK, Fo◎lscher D, Jamali F, Malassagne B, Leroy J. Telerobotic laparoscopic cholecystectomy: initial clinical experience with 25 patients. Ann Surg 2001;234:1-7.

[13] Robotic Colorectal Surgery: A Systematic Review, Sami AlAsari and Byung Soh Min, *ISRN Surg.* 2012; 2012: 293894. Published online 2012 May 13. doi: 10.5402/2012/293894

[14] Robotic gastrointestinal surgery: early experience and system description. Talamini M, Campbell K, Stanfield C. *J Laparoendosc Adv Surg Tech A.* 2002 Aug;12(4):225-32.

[15] http://www.engadget.com/2006/05/19/robot-surgeon-performs-worlds-first-unassisted-operation/

[16] http://www.roboticinfertility.com/main.html

[17] http://www.ucalgary.ca/news/may2008/neuroArm

[18] Hagn, U., Nickl, M., Jörg, S., Tobergte, A., Kübler, B., Passig, G., Gröger, M., Fröhlich, F., Seibold, U., Konietschke, R., Le-Tien, L., Albu-Schäffer, A., Grebenstein, M., Ortmaier, T. & Hirzinger, G. (2008). "DLR MiroSurge – towards versatility in surgical robotics". Proceedings of CURAC 7: 143–146.

[19] http://w3.wtb.tue.nl/nl/nieuws/artikel/?tx_ttnews%5Btt_news%5D=10041&tx_ttnews%5BbackPid%5D=465&cHash=ebb243e7ff

[20] http://med.over.net/clanek/php?full=1&id=25545&title=V_UKC_Ljubljana_prvi___na_svetu_uporabili___ilnega_robota_za_posege_na_femoralnem___ilju#.UoN3TaWc9MI

[21] http://www.smartplanet.com/blog/smart-takes/worlds-first-all-robotic-surgery-performed-in-canada/

[22] Melvin, W. S.; Needleman, B. J.; Krause, K. R.; Ellison, E. C. (February 2003). "Robotic Resection of Pancreatic Neuroendocrine Tumor". Journal of Laparoendoscopic & Advanced Surgical Techniques 13 (1): 33–36. doi:10.1089/109264203321235449.

[23] Babbage Science and technology (18 January 2012). "Surgical robots: The kindness of strangers" (http://www.economist.com/blogs/babbage/2012/01/surgical-robots). *The Economist*. Retrieved 21 February 2013.

[24] "da Vinci Products FAQ" (http://www.intuitivesurgical.com/products/products_faq.html#18). Intuitive Surgical. Retrieved 21 February 2013.

[25] http://intuitivesurgical.com/company/media/images/davinci_si_images.html

[26] http://intuitivesurgical.com/company/media/images/systems-si/Si_0185_%20two_male_surgeons_lookin_in_sm.jpg

[27] Weber PA, Merola S, Wasielewski A, Ballantyne GH, Delaney CP. Telerobotic-assisted laparoscopic right and sigmoid colectomies for benign disease. *Diseases of the Colon and Rectum*. 2002; 45(12):1689–1696.

[28] Robot-assisted laparoscopic surgery of the colon and rectum. Antoniou SA, Antoniou GA, Koch OO, Pointner R, Granderath FA. Surg Endosc. 2012 Jan;26(1):1-11. doi: 10.1007/s00464-011-1867-y. Epub 2011 Aug 20.

[29] Improved perioperative and short-term outcomes of robotic versus conventional laparoscopic colorectal operations. Casillas MA Jr, Leichtle SW, Wahl WL, Lampman RM, Welch KB, Wellock T, Madden EB, Cleary RK. *Am J Surg*. 2013 Oct 23. pii: S0002-9610(13)00608-9. doi: 10.1016/j.amjsurg.2013.08.028.

[30] Long-term outcome of robotic assisted laparoscopic rectopexy for full-thickness rectal prolapse in elderly patients. Germain A, Perrenot C, Scherrer ML, Ayav C, Brunaud L, Ayav A, Bresler L. Colorectal Dis. 2013 Dec 5. doi: 10.1111/codi.12513.

[31] Attaining Surgical Competency and Its Implications in Surgical Clinical Trial Design: A Systematic Review of the Learning Curve in Laparoscopic and Robot-Assisted Laparoscopic Colorectal Cancer Surgery. Barrie J, Jayne DG, Wright J, Murray CJ, Collinson FJ, Pavitt SH. Ann Surg Oncol. 2013 Nov 12.

[32] The first nationwide evaluation of robotic general surgery: a regionalized, small but safe start. Wormer BA, Dacey KT, Williams KB, Bradley JF 3rd, Walters AL, Augenstein VA, Stefanidis D, Heniford BT. Surg Endosc. 2013 Nov 7.

[33] Wittich P, Kazemier G, Schouten WR, Jeekel J, Lange JF, Bonjer HJ. The 'Colon cancer laparoscopic or open resection' (COLOR) trial. *Ned Tijdschr Geneeskd.* 1997 Sep 27;141(39):1870-1. 34)

[34] Bonjer, H. J., et al. "Laparoscopically assisted versus open colectomy for colon cancer: a meta-analysis." *Arch Surg* 142 (2007): 298-303.

[35] Nelson H, Sargent DJ, Wieand HS, et al. A comparison of laparoscopically assisted and open colectomy for colon cancer. *New England Journal of Medicine*. 2004;350(20): 2050–2059.

[36] Jayne DG et al. J Clin Oncol 2007; 25: 3061-8.

[37] ttp://www.eme.ac.uk/projectfiles/085201protocol.pdf

[38] Jayne DG, Guillou PJ, Thorpe H, et al. Randomized trial of laparoscopic-assisted resection of colorectal carcinoma: 3-Year results of the UK MRC CLASICC trial group. *Journal of Clinical Oncology*. 2007;25(21):3061–3068.

[39] 8. Jayne DG et al. Br J Surg. 2005; 92: 1124-32.

[40] Schwab KE, Dowson HM, Van Dellen J, Marks CG, Rockall TA. The uptake of laparoscopic colorectal surgery in Great Britain and Ireland: a questionnaire survey of consultant members of the ACPGBI. *Colorectal Disease*. 2009;11(3):318–322.

[41] Neutel CI, Gao RN, Wai E, Gaudette LA. Trends in in-patient hospital utilization and surgical procedures for breast, prostate, lung and colorectal cancers in Canada. *Cancer Causes and Control*. 2005;16(10):1261–1270.

[42] Sung-Bum Kang, et al. Open versus laparoscopic surgery for mid or low rectal cancer after neoadjuvant chemoradiotherapy (COREAN trial): short-term outcomes of an open-label randomised controlled trial. Lancet Oncol. 2010;11:637–45. doi: 10.1016/S1470-2045(10)70131-5.

[43] Paolo Pietro Bianchi, Fabrizio Luca, Wanda Petz, Manuela Valvo, Sabine Cenciarelli, Massimiliano Zuccaro, and Roberto Biffi, The role of the robotic technique in minimally invasive surgery in rectal cancer, *Ecancermedicalscience.* 2013; 7: 357. Published online 2013 September 26. doi: 10.3332/ecancer.2013.357

[44] Malak B. Bokhari, Chirag B. Patel, Diego I. Ramos-Valadez, Madhu Ragupathi, and Eric M. Haas, Learning curve for robotic-assisted laparoscopic colorectal surgery, *Surg Endosc.* 2011 March; 25(3): 855–860. Published online 2010 August 24. doi: 10.1007/s00464-010-1281-x

[45] Jiménez-Rodríguez RM, Díaz-Pavón JM, de la Portilla de Juan F, Prendes-Sillero E, Dussort HC, Padillo J. Learning curve for robotic-assisted laparoscopic rectal cancer surgery. Int J Colorectal Dis. 2013 Jun;28(6):815-21. doi: 10.1007/s00384-012-1620-6. Epub 2012 Dec 15.

[46] Sng KK, Hara M, Shin JW, Yoo BE, Yang KS, Kim SH. The multiphasic learning curve for robot-assisted rectal surgery. Surg Endosc. 2013 Sep;27(9):3297-307. doi: 10.1007/s00464-013-2909-4. Epub 2013 Mar 19.

[47] Halabi WJ,Kang CY,Jafari MD,Nguyen VQ,Carmichael JC,Mills S,Stamos MJ,Pigazzi A, Robot-assisted laparoscopic colorectal surgery. Alimoglu O, Atak I, Orhun K, Eren

T, Minerva Chirurgica, October 2013, vol./is. 68/5(471-8), 0026-4733;0026-4733 (2013 Oct)

[48] Robotic-assisted Colorectal Surgery in the United States: A Nationwide Analysis of Trends and Outcomes. World Journal of Surgery, 12 2013, vol./is. 37/12(2782-90), 0364-2313;1432-2323 (2013 Dec)

[49] Kim CW, Baik SH, Robotic rectal surgery: what are the benefits?. Minerva Chirurgica, October 2013, vol./is. 68/5(457-69), 0026-4733;0026-4733 (2013 Oct)

[50] Deborah S. Keller, Lobat Hashemi, Minyi Lu, and Conor P. Delaney, Short-Term Outcomes for Robotic Colorectal Surgery by Provider Volume, Journal of the American College of Surgeons, 2013-12-01, Volume 217, Issue 6, Pages 1063-1069.e1

[51] Bertani E, Chiappa A, Ubiali P, Cossu ML, Arnone P, Andreoni B, Robotic colectomy: is it necessary?, Minerva Chirurgica, October 2013, vol./is. 68/5(445-56), 0026-4733;0026-4733 (2013 Oct)

[52] http://www.gastroendonews.com/ViewArticle.aspx?d_id=187&a_id=13617

[53] https://www.davincisurgerycommunity.com/

[54] http://www.colorectal-surgeon.com/enhanced-recovery-programme.htm

[55] http://www.cancer.gov/

[56] Jarmo T. Alander, Ilkka Kaartinen, Aki Laakso, Tommi Pätilä, Thomas Spillmann, Valery V. Tuchin, Maarit Venermo, and Petri Välisuo, A Review of Indocyanine Green Fluorescent Imaging in Surgery. Int J Biomed Imaging. 2012; 2012: 940585. Published online 2012 April 22. doi: 10.1155/2012/940585

[57] Flower RW. Injection technique for indocyanine green and sodium fluorescein dye angiography of the eye. Investigative Ophthalmology. 1973;12(12):881–895.

[58] Bae, Se Jin Baek, Hyuk Hur, Seung Hyuk Baik, Nam Kyu Kim, and Byung Soh Min, Intraoperative Near Infrared Fluorescence Imaging in Robotic Low Anterior Resection: Three Case Reports Sung Uk, Yonsei Med J. 2013 July 1; 54(4): 1066–1069. Published online 2013 May 14. doi: 10.3349/ymj.2013.54.4.1066

[59] Lim H, Soter N. *Clinical Photomedicine*. New York, NY, USA: Marcel Dekker Inc.; 1993.

[60] Karrer S, Abels C, Bäumler W, Steinbauer M, Landthaler M, Szeimies RM. Photochemotherapie von kutanen Rektumkarzinom- Metastasen mit Indocyaningrun [photochemotherapy with indocyanine green in cutaneous metastases of rectal carcinoma] *Deutsche medizinische Wochenschrift*. 1997;122(37):1111–1114.

[61] Abels C, Karrer S, Bäumler W, Goetz AE, Landthaler M, Szeimies R-M. Indocyanine green and laser light for the treatment of AIDS-associated cutaneous Kaposi's sarcoma. *British Journal of Cancer*. 1998;77(6):1021–1024.

[62] Crane LMA, Themelis G, Arts HJG, et al. Intraoperative near-infrared fluorescence imaging for sentinel lymph node detection in vulvar cancer: first clinical results. *Gynecologic Oncology*. 2011;120(2):291–295.

[63] Inoue S, Shiina H, Arichi N, et al. Identification of lymphatic pathway involved in the spreading of prostate cancer by fluorescence navigation approach with intraoperatively injected indocyanine green. *Journal of the Canadian Urological Association*. 2011;5(4):254–259.

[64] Maggiori L, Gaujoux S, Tribillon E, Bretagnol F, Panis Y., Single-incision laparoscopy for colorectal resection: a systematic review and meta-analysis of more than a thousand procedures. Colorectal Dis. 2012 Oct;14(10):e643-54. doi: 10.1111/j.1463-1318.2012.03105.x.

[65] Ross H, Steele S, Whiteford M, Lee S, Albert M, Mutch M, Rivadeneira D, Marcello P. Early multi-institution experience with single-incision laparoscopic colectomy. Dis Colon Rectum. 2011 Feb;54(2):187-92. doi: 10.1007/DCR.0b013e3181f8d972.

[66] Khurshid N, Chung M, Horrigan T, Manahan K, Geisler JP., 5-millimeter trocar-site bowel herniation following laparoscopic surgery. JSLS. 2012 Apr-Jun;16(2):306-10.

[67] Yamamoto M, Minikel L, Zaritsky E., Laparoscopic 5-mm trocar site herniation and literature review. JSLS. 2011 Jan-Mar;15(1):122-6. doi: 10.4293/108680811X13022985131697.

[68] Ostrowitz MB, Eschete D, Zemon H, DeNoto G., Robotic-assisted single-incision right colectomy: early experience. Int J Med Robot. 2009 Dec;5(4):465-70. doi: 10.1002/rcs.281.

[69] Spinoglio G, Lenti LM, Maglione V, Lucido FS, Priora F, Bianchi PP, Single-site robotic cholecystectomy (SSRC) versus single-incision laparoscopic cholecystectomy (SILC): comparison of learning curves. First European experience., Grosso F, Quarati R. Surg Endosc. 2012 Jun;26(6):1648-55. doi: 10.1007/s00464-011-2087-1. Epub 2011 Dec 17.

[70] Eun Ji Nam, Sang Wun Kim, Maria Lee, Ga Won Yim et al, Robotic single-port transumbilical total hysterectomy: a pilot study, *Gynecol Oncol.* 2011 June 30; 22(2): 120–126. Published online 2011 June 30. doi: 10.3802/jgo.2011.22.2.120. *PMCID:* PMC3152752

[71] Hanh Tran, Robotic Single-Port Hernia Surgery, F *JSLS.* 2011 Jul-Sep; 15(3): 309–314. doi: 10.4293/108680811X13125733356198. *PMCID:* PMC3183567

[72] Autorino R, Kaouk JH, Stolzenburg JU, Gill IS, Mottrie A, Tewari A, Cadeddu JA.Current status and future directions of robotic single-site surgery: a systematic review. *Eur Urol.* 2013 Feb;63(2):266-80. doi: 10.1016/j.eururo.2012.08.028. Epub 2012 Aug 23.

[73] Mathew R, Kim SH. Robotic right hemicolectomy with D3 lymphadenectomy and complete mesocolic excision: Technical detail. OA Robotic Surgery 2013 Jun 01;1(1):6. http://www.oapublishinglondon.com/article/710,

Chapter 8

Surgical Strategies for Liver Metastases from Colorectal Cancer

Nikola Kolev, Valentin Ignatov, Anton Tonev,
Tanya Kirilova, Georgi Ivanov,
Alexander Zlatarov and Krassimir Ivanov

Additional information is available at the end of the chapter

http://dx.doi.org/10.5772/56915

1. Introduction

Colorectal carcinoma is one of the more common types of cancer around the world. For patients in UICC stage I (i.e., those who have pT1/2 tumors and do not have any lymph node metastases), the probability of surviving 5 years is 90% [2]. The prognosis of patients in stages II (pT3/4 tumors without lymph node metastases) and III (tumors with lymph node metastases) has improved steadily in recent years. At present, the 5-year survival in these two groups is 80% and 60% [1].

Approximately, 1.2 million cases of CRC occur yearly worldwide, with 412, 900 new cases diagnosed in Western Europe alone and 150, 000 in the United States. [1, 2] Resection of colorectal liver metastases (CRLM) is the only treatment offering the possibility of cure and has been shown to provide clear survival benefits. [3] Unfortunately, only 10% to 20% of patients with CRLM are eligible for this procedure upfront. On the other hand, during the last 10 years, major advances in the management of CRLM have taken place involving principally three different fields: oncology (new and more effective chemotherapeutic agents), interventional radiology (portal embolization and radiofrequency), and surgery (better instruments and newer techniques). These advances as part of a multidisciplinary team approach have gradually but effectively increased the resectability rate to 20%-30% of cases with a 5-year survival of 35%-50%. [3]

Nonetheless, distant metastases eventually arise in about 20% of patients who are stage II or III at the time of diagnosis [3]. About 35% of all patients already have distant metastases when the diagnosis is made. Patients with untreated hepatic metastases have a very poor prognosis.

In a prospective, observational study carried out on 484 patients from 1980 to 1990, the median time to death was 6.9 months [4]. Adson and colleagues, in the 1970's, were the first to show that patients could be cured by the resection of hepatic metastases [5]. Since then, resection has become established as a standard treatment. For this review, we selectively searched the literature for articles containing the words "colorectal liver metastases, " "chemotherapy, " and "surgery, " paying special attention to studies carried out on larger groups of patients and to randomized clinical trials. [6]

Most favorable outcomes were observed in patients with pedicle lymph node involvement (5-year survival rate 25% vs 0% for patients with celiac and/ or para-aortic lymph node metastases), and in patients younger than 40 years (5-year survival rate 45% vs 10% for older patients). [7, 8] In relation to our results and those reported by others, we recommend combining hepatectomy with lymphadenectomy only for young CLM patients presenting with pedicle lymph node involvement, in the absence of disease progression after preoperative chemotherapy. On the other hand, patients presenting with celiac or para-aortic lymph node involvement should not be subjected to this oncosurgical treatment strategy. Even concomitant pulmonary metastases should not be considered a contraindication to surgery. Patients with only pulmonary metastases as a site of extrahepatic disease have a particularly good outcome after complete metastasectomy of both liver and lung disease. Five-year survival rates ranged from 22% to 50% in patients with metastases limited to the lungs. [8] Also, selected patients with complex multiorgan metastases have been associated with prolonged survival after a multimodality treatment. Patients with simultaneous hepatic and extrahepatic disease (EHD) do, however, need to be selected for surgery. Elias et al stated that EHD, when resectable, is no longer a contraindication to hepatectomy. [18] More importantly, the total number of metastases, whatever their location, has a strong prognostic effect than the site of the metastases. In addition, a study conducted at our centre demonstrated that patients with concomitant EHD who were resected experienced a lower 5-year survival than those without EHD (28% vs 55%, $P<.001$). Five poor prognostic factors were identified with multivariate analysis: EHD location other than lung metastases, EHD concomitant to colorectal liver metastases recurrence, CEA-level>10 ng/ml, >6 colorectal liver metastases and right colon cancer. The five-year survival ranged from 64% (0 factors) to 0% (>3factors). [19]

We aim to report the new trends in strategies about surgical treatment of colorectal liver metastases and our experience according to surgical and oncological outcome in patients, operated for IV stage colorectal cancer.

2. Criteria for resectability

Currently available data have led to a change in the indications for resecting hepatic metastases of colorectal carcinoma. Previously, the indication was based on tumor-biological and clinical characteristics. The new criterion is the feasibility of complete resection of both intra- and extrahepatic disease. R0-resectable hepatic metastases, in patients without any extrahepatic metastases, should be resected. [12] As the determination of resectability is becoming ever more complex, all patients with hepatic metastases of colorectal carcinoma should be presented to an experienced hepatobiliary surgeon before the beginning of treatment. Postoperative hepatic function can be predicted more precisely with the aid of CT volumetry. This technique enables prediction of the remaining volume of hepatic tissue after surgery to within 10% of the actual value. [9, 11]

Metastases are considered resectable when the following criteria are met:

- exclusion of a non-resectable extrahepatic tumor manifestation,
- parenchymal involvement <75%,
- <3 hepatic veins and <7 hepatic segments involved,
- no hepatic insufficiency, no Child B or C cirrhosis,
- no severe accompanying diseases.

Metastases are considered non-resectable or marginally resectable when an R0 resection is not possible. Metastases are also considered marginally resectable in the setting of, for example, extra-hepatic tumor manifestations, technical impediments to surgery, or inadequate expected residual liver mass. For these patients, intensified preoperative chemotherapy can be considered. The feasibility of secondary resection should be evaluated at each re-staging under chemotherapy. [15]

3. New treatment strategies

Today, patients with metastatic CRC should be treated by multidisciplinary teams including surgeons, oncologists and radiologists. Evidence of the benefit of perioperative chemotherapy over surgery alone [22] and the potential benefit of adjuvant chemotherapy (after liver resection) [23] caused a rethink among the experts particularly in terms of the timing of the administration of chemotherapy for CRC patients with initially resectable liver and lung metastases. Poor prognostic factors for patients with liver metastases are multiple metastases, >5 cm in diameter, synchronous presentation, lymph node-positive primary and high tumor marker levels. [17] Thus, even when the metastases are technically resectable (in terms of number, location and size), when facing a patient with more than one of the poor prognostic factors listed above, the current trend is to refer patients for neoadjuvant chemotherapy before surgery. The data from the EORTC study showed quite clearly that nearly all patients were able to tolerate neo-adjuvant chemotherapy. Also, analysis of the PFS curves from the EORTC–EPOC trial shows that the main difference comes after the first 2 months when the curves drop down and then move out in parallel, suggesting that the benefit conferred by perioperative chemotherapy might be a consequence of a reduction in the occurrence of early cancer relapse as a consequence of preoperative chemotherapy. [16] An exception to preoperative chemotherapy is, however, those patients with a single resectable metachronous metastasis who could be directly referred to surgery, [14] with the recognition that this accounts for <10% of patients seen in routine clinical practice. All other patients with resectable metastases should be treated up front with chemotherapy, with the caveats that the patient is able to receive chemotherapy and the position of the lesion is not going to be lost. On the other hand, it has also become a standard strategy to give postoperative adjuvant chemotherapy to all resected patients (if possible) based on the data for the resected patients in the EORTC–EPOC trial. [22] For patients who are non-responders, there are two treatment strategies available: 1) change to a new chemotherapy protocol or 2) liver resection before the metastatic disease becomes unresectable. At this point it is important to mention that, the decision to perform either treatment strategy should always be decided by a multidisciplinary. Currently, it has become mandatory to select the systemic therapy regimen based on biological predictive factors, such as KRAS mutation status. This strategy has had a double impact: first of all, it has helped to optimize the choice of first-line treatment, in turn decreasing the risk of immediate disease progression; secondly, it has also helped to better select the second-line 'rescue' treatment strategies with the possibility of resection. [27] However, considering that surgery is still the only treatment that has curative potential per se, in some situations this can be the treatment of choice, even if resistance to medical treatment generally means that the patient has a unfavorable tumor biology. The situation is much simpler for patients whose metastases are initially unresectable, where systemic therapy is administered until an adequate response has been achieved. [24]

4. Primarily resectable hepatic metastases

For operable hepatic metastases, hepatic resection is the treatment of choice. The reported 5-year-survival rates that have been achieved after the resection of isolated hepatic metastases with curative intent range from 25% to 50% [1–4, 6–8]. Hepatic metastases, however, are primarily resectable in only about 20% of patients [4]. For the remaining 80%, resection is contraindicated by the presence of diffuse hepatic metastases, non-resectable extra-hepatic disease, or impaired liver function. It is now generally accepted that the contraindications for hepatic resection that were defined in the 1980's are no longer applicable. At that time, the presence of 4 or more tumor nodules, metastases exceeding 5 cm in size, extra-hepatic disease, or a tumor-free resection margin of less than 1 cm [9] was held to contraindicate hepatic resection. Many subsequent studies have confirmed that these are, indeed, relevant prognostic factors for survival after the resection of hepatic metastases of colorectal carcinoma, yet long-term survival is still possible when hepatic resection is performed despite the presence of these supposed contraindications. There have also been technical improvements in the treatment of hepatic metastases of colorectal carcinoma. Diagnostic assessment has become markedly more sensitive through the use of modern types of CT and MRI scanners and the introduction of PET-CT (5, 10–14]. Furthermore, surgical dissecting techniques and the development of potent systemic chemotherapy protocols have been optimized [15–18]. As a result, 5-year survival rates after the resection of hepatic metastases of colorectal carcinoma have improved markedly. [6] Today, even patients with more than three metastases or with metastases larger than 5 cm in diameter can be cured with appropriate surgical treatment, as found in a recent analysis [7]. One hundred and two patients were tumor-free 10 years after the resection of hepatic metastases of colorectal carcinoma, and only one patient among them developed a recurrent tumor thereafter.

http://dx.doi.org/10.5772/56915

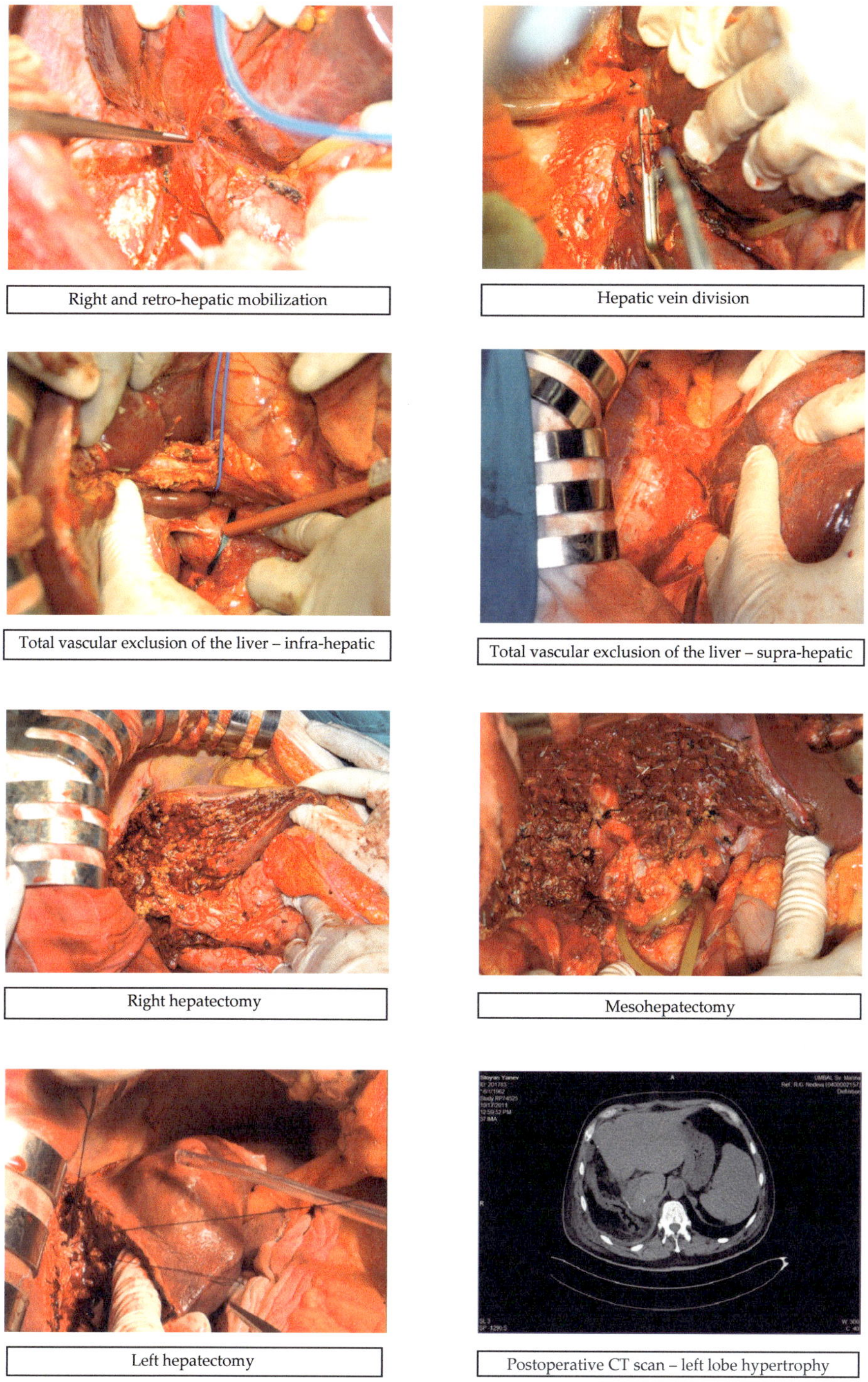

Figure 1. Different types of liver resections

5. Perioperative complications

Hepatic resections can now be performed safely and effectively. The mortality of hepatic resection was about 5% as late as 1990, while recent articles on the subject generally document figures between 1% and 2%. This reduction of mortality has been achieved even though the resections themselves have become ever more extensive. [3]

6. Long-term results after hepatic resection

More than 40% of appropriately selected patients with colorectal carcinoma who undergo the resection of hepatic metastases survive for at least 5 years thereafter [5, 6, 8, 9]. This is particularly true of patients whose surgery was performed more recently. As many as two-thirds of patients later develop a recurrent tumor, and half of them have a recurrent tumor in the liver [23]. In one of the largest studies performed to date, which included 1001 patients, showed that the benefit of surgery extends not just to patients who have undergone an R0 resection (5-year survival: 37%), but also to those who have undergone an R1 resection, i.e., a resection with positive margins, up to 20% of whom are still alive 5 years after surgery. [31]

7. Prognostic parameters

Many different prognostic scores are used to predict the patient's risk of recurrence and chances of long-term survival on the basis of preoperatively measured parameters. The three most commonly used scoring systems in hepatic surgery are those of Nordlinger, Fong, and Iwatsuki [2, 9, 24]. Although these scoring systems differ with respect to certain individual parameters, they share the common feature that a low score (i.e., the presence of no more than a few risk factors) is correlated with a low risk of recurrence, while the chance of long-term survival is less than 10% when all risk factors are present. No preoperatively measurable prognostic parameter can identify with any certainty the patients who will not benefit from surgical treatment. The most important prognostic factor, according to all studies, is a tumor-free resection margin [10, 11, 25, 26].

8. Expanded application of resection for CRLM

Liver resection is the current preferred treatment for CRLM patients and should be undertaken whenever feasible and potentially curative (R0), regardless of prognostic factors and presence of extra hepatic metastases. The main limiting factors to perform curative resection of CRLM are: presence of bilobar or bulky disease and presence of extra hepatic disease. Resection in patients with multiple or bulky lesions may result in insufficient residual hepatic tissue (i.e., less than 30% functional parenchyma). [19]

9. Neoadjuvant chemotherapy in patients with resectable CRLM

Despite major survival improvements achieved with successful primary hepatectomy for CRLM, [7-13, 20] many of these patients experience disease recurrence. Data indicate that pre or post-operative chemotherapy may provide a meaningful benefit, although controlled trials are needed. Tanaka et al [21] reported a retrospective analysis of patients with multiple CRLMs, wherein use of neoadjuvant chemotherapy was an independent predictor of survival by multivariate analysis. In 71 patients undergoing hepatectomy for more than five bilobar liver tumors, 3- and 5-year survival rates were superior (*P*<.05, log-rank) in the neoadjuvant chemotherapy group (n=48; 67.0% and 38.9%) than in the hepatectomy-alone group (n=23; 51.8% and 20.7%). Furthermore, neoadjuvant treatment reduced the need for extended (>4 segments) hepatectomies (39 of 48 neoadjuvant vs 23 of 23 control patients). Data from the LiverMetSurvey [5] also indicate a survival improvement with neoadjuvant treatment. In 207 patients with more than five metastases resected, 5-year survival was better with neoadjuvant treatment, although not significantly (20% vs 15%) and among 1, 045 patients who had only one liver metastasis resected, 5-year survival rates were 49% and 57% with and without neoadjuvant chemotherapy, respectively. Similar results were reported in a metanalysis by Mitry et al, [22] which showed a strong trend toward better diseasefree survival with adjuvant 5-FU treatment (HR 0.76, *P*=5.8), and a trend toward favorable overall survival (HR 0.76, *P*=9.8). In addition, a phase III randomized study (The EORTC Intergroup) examined perioperative FOLFOX4 (5-fluorouracil (5-FU), leucovorin, oxaliplatin) chemotherapy for patients with potentially resectable CRLM.23 A total of 364 patients with up to four CRLM were randomized between perioperative FOLFOX4 (oxaliplatin 85 mg/mI and LV5FU2), six cycles before and six cycles after surgery (CT), vs surgery alone (S). Eleven of 182 patients were ineligible in each arm, mostly due to more advanced disease; 31 and 30 patients in the CT and S arms, respectively, could not undergo resection. At a median follow-up of 3.9 years, progression-free survival (PFS) was significantly better with CT in the group of resected patients, although the trial was formally not positive in the intentionto- treat (ITT) analysis (HR 0.79, *P*=.058). In terms of postoperative chemotherapy in resectable patients with CRLM data from United States and Europe show better survival in patients receiving adjuvant chemotherapy after resection of CRC liver metastases. [24] Use of adjuvant or neoadjuvant systemic treatment is widely recognized as standard of care in cases of liver resection, and was the focus of single-center studies with XELOX/FOLFOX25 and XELOX plus bevacizumab.26 So far, only one study has as yet shown a clear benefit. [27] In this randomized trial, 109 patients (75 assessable) with one to three hepatic lesions received hepatic arterial floxuridine plus intravenous 5-FU (n=30) or no further therapy (n=45) after hepatectomy. The 4-year recurrence-free rates (46% vs 25%) and 4-year liver recurrence-free rates (67% vs 43%) were significantly better in the adjuvant therapy group. Median survival differences were not statistically significant (64% vs 49%), however, the trial was insufficiently powered to evaluate overall survival. [33]

10. Strategies for improving resectability

At present, only 10% to 20% of patients with hepatic metastases of colorectal carcinoma can be considered candidates for resective surgery. Opportunities for resection are often limited by an unfavorable anatomical site of the metastasis (-es), poor function of the remaining hepatic parenchyma, and/or the patient's poor general condition. Multiple strategies have been developed in order to increase the percentage of patients whose metastases are resectable.

Liver surgery has progressed in parallel to the improvements in chemotherapy and interventional radiology. Bad-located tumors (situated deeply or close to critical vascular or biliary structures) can now be safely resected thanks to the availability of sophisticated instruments such as the ultrasonic dissector, argon gas diathermy and new techniques such as the one of low-central venous pressure anaesthesia that allows an almost bloodless field. With the routine use of intraoperative ultrasound examination precise localization of liver lesions and planning of the resection is done aiming at removing all possible lesions with a clear margin and at the same time preserve the maximum of liver parenchyma. This improvement in surgical planning and techniques has been directly responsible for the low hospital mortality. The risk of liver resection for CRLM has decreased in specialized hepatobiliary centres probably below the figures observed after colorectal surgery. The mortality of elective liver resection on non-cirrhotic livers is estimated to be around 1% [35, 36] at a time when patients' age and disease complexity are increasing, in addition to the associated changes of SOS and CASH often present in chemotherapy patients undergoing surgery. The experience of the centre has a major impact on outcome: the mortality and morbidity of liver resections decreased inversely to the number of cases performed in the institution. [37] It has been shown in US that patients resected at high volume centres (>25 cases/year) for liver cancer have not only a better perioperative outcome, but also a better long-term survival, [38] and similar results concerning the correlation between high volume surgery and specialization and outcome were observed in Europe. [39]

11. Preoperative chemotherapy ("down-staging")

When hepatic metastases of colorectal carcinoma are unresectable, systemic chemotherapy is indicated. About 20% of metastases respond to treatment with 5-fluorouracil (5-FU) and folic acid [4]. When these are used in combination with newer drugs, such as oxaliplatin or irinotecan (CPT-11), the response rate rises as high as 60% [29]. Folprecht et al. reviewed the available studies on the "down-staging" of hepatic metastases of colorectal carcinoma and found that resectionrates are correlated with response rates [4]. The first major clinical series of this type was published in 1996 by Bismuth et al. [13] and updated in the years thereafter [14, 30]. The 5-year-survival was 40% (95% confidence interval: 33% to 68%) and was thus comparable to that of patients with primarily resectable hepatic metastases. A major bias in the studies of neoadjuvant chemotherapy published to date arises from patient selection. In the available prospective studies of patients with "isolated" hepatic metastases (i.e., no extrahepatic metastases), the criteria for nonresectability differ from one study to another and are often poorly defined. The hepatotoxicity of all currently used chemotherapeutic drugs argues against their use as neoadjuvant treatment for patients with primarily resectable hepatic metastases. Oxaliplatin can cause sinusoidal obstruction ("blue liver"), while irinotecan can induce fatty liver or steatohepatitis [31–34]. These changes are associated with significantly more frequent perioperative complications. Vauthey et al. found that steatohepatitis after irinotecan use is associated with a significantly higher 90-day mortality [15].

12. Systemic chemotherapy in patients with non-resectable CRLM

Systemic chemotherapy is currently the main treatment approach for non-resectable CRLM. Incorporation of drugs such as oxaliplatin and irinotecan have led to an improvement of median survival as well as response rates compared with those achieved previously with 5-fluoracil (5-FU)/leucovorin-based regimens. Development of oral fluoropyrimidines has also improved treatment options in these patients. Median survival duration after systemic chemotherapy alone is approximately 20 months, [28, 29] however, only 1% to 2% of such patients remain alive at 5 years. [3, 30] On the other hand, the improved efficacy of newer regimens in down staging tumors is rendering more patients resectable. [14]

13. Accompanying chemotherapy

There is no longer any doubt that patients benefit from hepatic resections that are performed with curative intent. The current discussion concerns the question whether they also benefit from accompanying adjuvant or neo-adjuvant chemotherapy. The first encouraging data on adjuvant chemotherapy after hepatic resection were published by Kemeny et al., who compared local intra-arterial therapy combined with systemic 5-FU chemotherapy to adjuvant treatment with 5-FU alone. A trend was found toward improved progression-free survival in the group that additionally received regional therapy (37.4 versus 17.2 months, $p = 0.06$) [20, 44]. Nonetheless, the overall survival was no better in this group. This finding could not be replicated in a German study of intraarterial chemotherapy administered in the hepatic artery [21]. There are currently two further options for systemic chemotherapy: neo-adjuvant and adjuvant postoperative chemotherapy. For adjuvant chemotherapy, data are only available on 5-FU based treatment. Portier et al., in the AURC 9002 trial, describe an improved 5-year tumor-free survival of 33.5% among patients receiving adjuvant 5-FU bolus therapy, compared to 26.7% treated with resection alone [22]. These 5-FU patients' overall survival was no better than that of their counterparts without 5-FU, but the study size was, in any case, inadequate to detect a moderate benefit. An unplanned subgroup analysis revealed that patients with a greater tumor burden (diameter >5cm, or 3 or more tumor nodules) survived longer if they received adjuvant chemotherapy. Likewise, a pooled analysis of a number of studies, including the FFCD study, found a trend toward a benefit from adjuvant 5-FU treatment, in terms of both progression-free survival and overall survival [23]. These data appear promising, especially because there have been further improvements in chemotherapeutic regimens since they were published. Further evidence that adjuvant 5-FU treatment confers a survival benefit after the resection of hepatic metastases of colorectal carcinoma comes from a cohort study of 792 patients by Parks et al. [24]: The median survival time was 47 months, compared with 36 months without 5-FU. This year (2010), Nordlinger et al. have published the results of the

EORTC 40 983 trial, in which neoadjuvant therapy with FOLFOX (folic acid, 5-FU, and oxaliplatin) before and after hepatic resection was compared with resection alone. There were 182 patients in each of the study's two groups (with and without neoadjuvant therapy). The declared study endpoint of a significantly improved progression-free 3-year survival was not met in the intent-to-treat analysis. Tumor-free survival was 28.1% after surgery alone and 35.4% in the FOLFOX group [25]. The study did, however, show a significantly improved tumor-free 3-year survival when all patients whose data could be completely evaluated were taken into account (as opposed to the intent-to-treat analysis). Data on overall survival are currently unavailable. It should also be mentioned that the chemotherapy group had a higher rate of postoperative complications, but their postoperative mortality was no higher. Thus, in our view, preoperative chemotherapy should remain reserved, at least for now, to patients whose hepatic metastases are marginally resectable. This group includes patients whose tumor burden is high because of multiple hepatic metastases and extrahepatic tumor manifestations. Our view is founded on the documented survival benefit that can be achieved in patients who have a large burden of initially unresectable hepatic metastases by down-staging their tumors with chemotherapy, in order to render them resectable. [29]

14. Portal-vein embolization

In some cases, the resection of one or more hepatic metastases is technically feasible, yet cannot be performed because the amount of liver tissue remaining after resection would be too small. To minimize the risk of postoperative hepatic insufficiency, ipsilateral hepatic atrophy and contralateral hepatic hypertrophy can be induced preoperatively by selective embolization of the hepatic portal vein, or else by ligation of the branch of the portal vein that leads to the hepatic lobe containing the metastasis.

14.1. Definitions

Future liver remnant (FLR) is the liver that will be left in place after surgery and that was not targeted by embolization. The FLR must hypertrophy after portal vein embolization (PVE). Most teams wait 4 weeks before surgery. FLR hypertrophy must be measured by way of computed axial tomography (CAT) examination after injection of iodine with volumetric measurements of the FLR segments, with the results compared with the measurements performed before PVE using the same technique. Hypertrophy can be quantified as FLR hypertrophy, which is defined as the difference between FLR after a waiting period from 3 to 6 weeks after PVE minus FLR before PVE divided by FLR before PVE. The waiting period must be long enough to allow hypertrophy and as short as possible to avoid tumor growth, which precludes surgery. Hypertrophy can also be quantified by increased FLR ratio. The FLR ratio is defined as (FLR volume—tumor in the FLR)/ (total liver volume—total tumor volume) [8]. Technical success of PVE is defined by a complete occlusion of portal branches feeding the future resected liver segments. Branches of the FLR must be patent with hepatopetal flow. In the late phase of control portography, parenchymography must be visible only in the FLR. Clinical success is considered to occur when the patient reaches the volumetric criteria for liver resection. Patients with Tumors that Developed in Normal Underlying Liver Parenchyma PVE is recommended when the FRL-to-total liver ratio is 25 to 30 [7, 10, 11]. The indication of PVE can be extended to a 40% FLR ratio in patients having received chemotherapy or showing abnormal indocyanine green test results (or other abnormal liver function tests) [10, 12, 13]. Portal-vein embolization should always be considered when the residual hepatic volume without it would be less than 30% of the normal size of the liver, and when at least two contiguous hepatic segments are free of metastases. For technical surgical reasons, the left lateral segments 2 and 3 are particularly suitable for this approach. As long as the liver is not cirrhotic, portal-vein embolization results in a 40% to 60% hypertrophy of the contralateral hepatic lobe. It remains unclear at present whether the stimulus to hypertrophy that portal-vein embolization provides might also accelerate the growth of tumor nodules [16, 35]. In any case, the data regarding morbidity, mortality, and long-term survival are comparable to those of standard hepatic resections [16, 36–39].

Patients with Tumors that Develop in Chronic Liver Disease and Cirrhosis States

In such cases, the decision is based either on liver volume or on liver volume plus estimation of overall liver function by indocyanin green retention rate at 15 min. An FRLR of 40% is recommended when the ICCG 15 is between 10% and 20%. When the ICCG 15 is[20%, an FRLR of 50% is recommended [12–14].

Patients with Tumors Invading the Biliary Tree Associated with Cholestasis

Because biliary obstruction has impaired liver regeneration and hypertrophy, the biliary tree of the FRL must be drained first, and PVE can be performed secondarily. The indication is an FRLR\40% [15].

Contraindication for PVE [11]

PVE is contraindicated in the following types of patients:

1. Tumors invading the portal vein

2. Portal hypertension (blocked to free hepatic veinpressure gradient[12 mmHg)

3. Coagulation disorders (PT\60%, platelet count\50 G/l)

4. Even if previous transarterial chemoembolization (TACE) may improve PVE results [16], a minimum of 3-week delay between TACE and PVE is recommended.

Patients should be informed that this procedure is not an antitumoral treatment but a treatment made to increase safety or to enable a surgical procedure. Minor complications are encountered in 20% to 25% of cases and are mainly associated with slight fever and abdominal discomfort and pain. Major complications are infrequent and mainly include infection and subcapsular hematoma, hemobilia, and portal vein thrombosis 9\2% of cases). Mortality due to PVE has not been reported. When tumors (usually small nodules) are present in the nonembolized lobe, it must be explained to the patient that those lesions might increase in size more quickly due to PVE [17]. Patients must also be told that the efficacy of the procedure can be estimated approximately 4 weeks after

PVE by way of CAT with injection of contrast media and liver volumetry.

14.2. Embolization method

Access to the portal system should be done under ultrasound guidance to puncture a peripheral branch [8]. Access can be obtained by way of controlateral approach (i.e., puncture of the left portal branch and embolization of theright portal branches) or ispsilateral approach (puncture of the right portal branch to embolize right portal branches. The advantage of the controlateral approach is easier catheterization, but there is a risk of damage to the FLR. Five-French materials (catheter or introductory sheath) are usually recommended. The catheter should be placed at the splenomesenteric confluence to perform a portography to visualize portal anatomy, including its variations, and to localize segment IV branches. Measurement of portal pressure is not routinely performed in patients with normal liver. In cirrhotic patients, measuring the portal and central venous pressures is useful to determine whether the patient has a portostemic gradient[12 mmHg in, which case the patient is at major risk of perisurgical complications [18, 19]. These patients are not eligible for PVE. The aim of embolization is complete obstruction of the targeted branches and redistribution of flow to the FLR branches only. Final portography is mandatory to verify this objective. A final pressure measurement should be obtained at the end of the procedure in patients with chronic liver disease to document portal pressure increase, which is usually approximately 3 mmHg. Embolization of segment IV branches is recommended in patients with tumors who are undergoing extended right hepatectomy. However, if embolization of that segment causes risk of reflux into the portal branch of the FRL, such embolization must not be performed because any major reflux into FRL portal branches might preclude surgery.

15. Two-stage hepatic resection

A further way of enabling curative resection of patients with extensive bilobar hepatic metastases of colorectal carcinoma is so-called two-stage hepatic resection [17]. This technique is suitable for patients with bilateral hepatic metastases who can undergo neither complete tumor resection, nor tumor resection combined with a local ablative procedure, because of the risk of postoperative hepatic insufficiency. Most, but not all, of the tumor burden is resected in a first operation, and then the remaining tumor nodules are resected in a second one, after liver tissue has regenerated. The decision whether to operate in one or two stages depends on the quantity and quality of the extratumoral hepatic tissue. The second operation is usually performed three to four weeks after the first, to allow time for the residual liver tissue to become adequately hypertrophic. [40]

16. Extreme liver surgery

Involvement of major vascular structures (vena cava or hepatic veins) by liver metastases has been considered as a contraindication to surgery for colorectal liver metastases. However, at

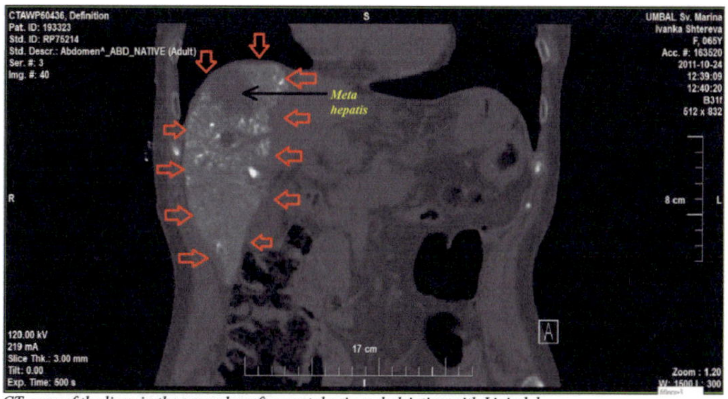

CT-scan of the liver in the same day after portal vein embolsiation with Lipiodol.

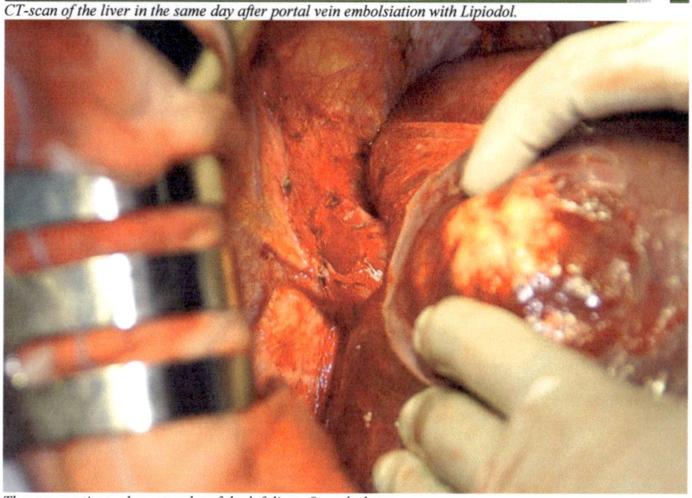

The same patient – hypertrophy of the left liver, 8 weeks later

Figure 2. Portal vein embolization and liver hypertrophy.

the present time this clinical situation is no longer considered as contraindication due to the experience gained with total vascular exclusion (TVE) of the liver combined with vascular reconstruction. These techniques have made the surgery possible even for this group of patients, without exposing them to the risk of massive intraoperative blood loss and gas embolism. TVE consists on hepatic inflow and outflow occlusion. [46-48] This can be achieved by clamping the portal vein/ hepatic artery as well as the supra and infra hepatic vena cava. Alternatively, the hepatic veins are isolated and clamped in addition to the vascular portal structures. The latter technique is more advantageous as it can preserve the caval flow, however, in cases of caval infiltration by metastatic lesion/s this technique is not feasible. On the other hand, if hemodynamic instability is encountered while the vena cava is clamped, a veno-venous bypass should be installed to overcome this complication. Although, it is believed that the hepatic blood flow can be interrupted safely up to 60 minutes, when vascular resection/ reconstruction is necessary, a 60 minute duration of ischemia may be not sufficient. [47] Hence, hypothermic perfusion of the liver should be instituted. The combination of TVE with in situ hypothermic perfusion was evaluated in our center. [68] It is found that this combination was

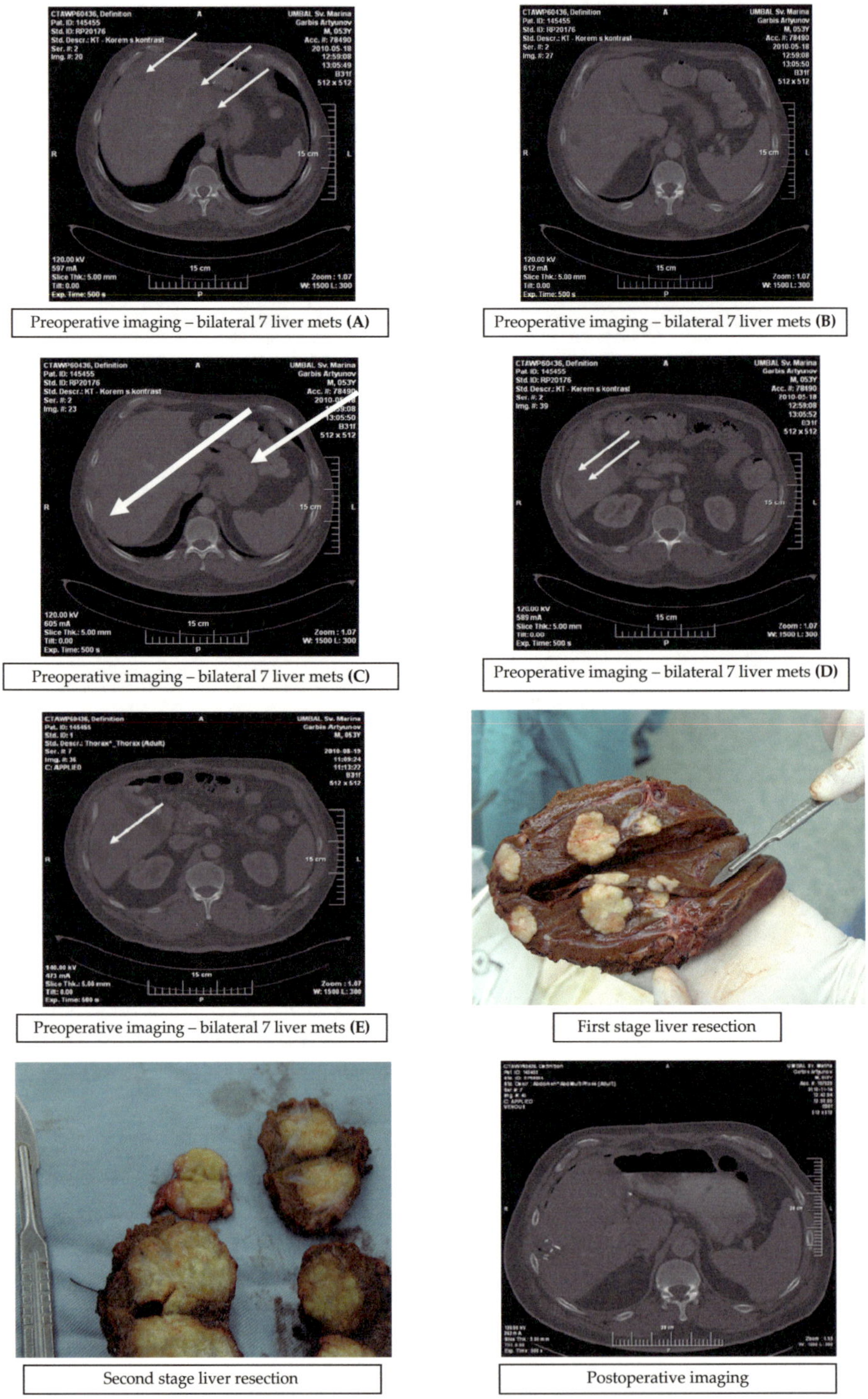

Figure 3. Two stage hepatectomy.

http://dx.doi.org/10.5772/56915

associated with a better liver tolerance to ischemia, a better liver function, and a significantly lower rate of complications compared to standard TVE >60 min. In some cases, a combined liver and vascular resection may be required. An experience with such cases (combined liver and vena cava resection) has shown that a 5-year survival of 38.3% can be obtained even for this group of patients. [49] In conclusion, using TVE and vascular reconstruction techniques, surgery in cases with involvement of the vena cava or hepatic veins is not necessarily contra-indicated. However, a very careful evaluation and selection of the cases should be done, making sure that the risks involved do not counterbalance the desired benefits. [42]

17. Timing of surgery

Optimal duration chemotherapy and timing of liver surgery in responding patients have not been definitively established. For patients not considered resectable, in the clinical setting, most surgeons perform liver resection as soon as metastases become operable. Similarly, there is still debate, whether chemotherapy should precede resection when metastases are synchronous, particularly when the primary tumor is in place and the surgery involves the resection of the primary tumor as well as a simultaneous major liver resection. At the present, many surgeons believe that the chemotherapy is a better choice for patients with synchronous liver metastases, although these conclusions come from retrospective or surgical series from a single center. Capussotti and colleagues have published several papers on this topic. [40-43] There is only one randomized study [23] which has evaluated the results of preoperative chemotherapy and demonstrating an absolute difference in favor of chemotherapy. However, this study has a drawback as it was not possible to separate the benefits of preoperative chemotherapy from those of adjuvant postoperative chemotherapy. Another issue is the impact which the disease progression while on chemotherapy has on the timing of surgery. Disease progression during neoadjuvant chemotherapy indicates a poor prognosis. In a cohort of 131 patients undergoing rescue hepatectomy, 5-year survival rates were 8% if disease progressed during preoperative chemotherapy, 30% if disease was stable, and 37% in responders. [14] These findings suggest that hepatectomy for CRC metastases should be undertaken as soon as technically feasible and underscore the importance of collaboration between medical oncologists and surgeons in achieving that goal. Medical oncologists should be referring patients for surgery before tumor progression, and surgeons need to consider tumor evolution in addition to resectability. Thus, patients with biologically aggressive tumors unlikely to benefit from resection may be spared surgery upfront and can instead consult with the medical oncologist for a better regimen likely to induce tumor response or stabilization. [44]

18. Local tumor destruction and hybrid techniques

In recent years, local ablative methods such as cryotherapy and radiofrequency ablation (RFA) have come into more common use for the *in situ* destruction of hepatic metastases. Among these methods, RFA has been studied the best. It can be performed percutaneously, laparoscopically, or at open surgery and is currently used for tumors up to 5 cm in diameter. Lencioni et al. recently reported a multicenter study of 423 patients with a total of 615 metachronous metas - tases of colorectal carcinoma who were treated with RFA. The average tumor size was 2.7 cm [18]. In this patient group, 25% had local tumor progression, and the 1-, 3-, and 5-year survival rates were 86%, 47%, and 24%. These figures correspond to those of Abdalla et al., who found that tumor progression is more probable after RFA than after surgical resection [19, 43]. In general, RFA is associated with low morbidity and mortality. As no prospective data are yet available for a comparison of local ablative techniques to hepatic resection with curative intent, the procedure cannot be recommended as an alternative to hepatic resection, though it does play a role as an additional, complementary method of achieving complete tumor destruction in patients whose lesions are not otherwise R0-resectable.

19. Radiofrequency thermal ablation (RFA)

RFA is the most widely used technique for local destruction of CRLM and has gained popularity because of its relative easy usage, and its effectiveness as an adjuvant treatment.48 For the treatment of CRLM, RFA can be used as: 1) a definitive treatment per se; 2) a complementary procedure to surgery, or 3) in the treatment of recurrent metastatic disease after surgery. Results so far show that RFA must be restricted to cases in which the size of the dominant lesion is less than 3 cm or when a maximum of three tumours are present.49 In a study on percutaneous RFA for CRLM, local control was achieved in 78% of tumours <2.6 cm, but only in 47% of tumours 2.6-4.0 cm and 32% of tumours >4.0 cm.42 The anatomic location of a metastasis is an additional limitation of RFA. In the vicinity of a large hepatic vessel, the heat sink effect significantly increases the risk of incomplete ablation. Also, the risk of thermal injury is increased when nodules are close to main biliary structures or to extrahepatic organs. In these cases, new RFA techniques or additional procedures, such as hepatic inflow occlusion or intraductal cooling, have to be considered. [50, 51] Because of the high local recurrence rates, and of the anatomical limitations described above, there is still no place for RFA in patients with resectable colorectal metastases. Surgical RFA for small resectable CRLM could only be acceptable in a randomized trial comparing resection with surgical RFA, [52] and it was shown that hepatic resection is still the treatment of choice for CRLM and that RFA alone provides survival only slightly superior to non-surgical treatment. [53] This is the case also for patients with solitary liver metastases who are treated with RFA (higher LR rate and shorter recurrence free and overall survival). [54] Radiofrequency ablation has been proposed to treat a limited number of small metastases, simultaneously with right PVE. [46, 47] Although this strategy is theoretically appealing because it limits the number of surgical operations, its effectiveness compared to two-step hepatectomies is doubtful. The place of RFA in the treatment of CRM is limited: it is most useful for early recurrences detected as small lesions after resection, because it is not mandatory to stop the chemotherapy, except for the use of bevacizumab, and because RFA allows a ''test of time'' that helps to select out patients with very aggressive/ disseminated disease that would not benefit from repeated surgery.

19.1. Frequency of complications

19.1.1. Mortality

A total of 21 deaths were reported in 11 series, [41] with overall mortality varying from 0% to 5.2%. Four deaths were related to cirrhosis. Eleven occurred in patients undergoing resections, eight of which were major hepatectomies. Eight deaths were related to liver failure, four of which were subsequent to major hepatectomy with IRFA on the remnant liver for bilobar disease. Five deaths were caused by myocardial infarct; one of these related to a carcinoid crisis and another to a haemorrhage. Four deaths resulted from portal thrombosis, three of which occurred in cirrhotic patients. One of these patients had been treated by IRFA alone. Four deaths were related to septic complications; two of these referred to pulmonary infections, one to infection of the ascites and one to multiple deep abscesses. Lastly, three deaths were reported after postoperative haemorrhaging; one was caused by liver failure after an intrahepatic haematoma in a cirrhotic setting, one resulted from myocardial infarction following a haemorrhage in a large metastasis treated by IRFA, and one patient was treated by major hepatectomy and two IRFA sessions and died of cardiac arrest after postoperative bleeding.31

19.1.2. Infections

Abdominal infections were reported in 49 patients in 21 series. [41] Diagnosis of infection was delayed by up to 5 months. Seventeen liver abscesses were reported, of which one was fatal and were related to IRFA. Only one case of biliary digestive anastomosis was observed. Ten cases of perihepatic abscesses at resection sites were reported. Twelve were following digestive system-associated procedures. These abscesses were treated by percutaneous drainage and antibiotics. One patient needed re-operation and died from septic shock. Seven cases of wound infection were reported; two were re-operated. Lastly, one case of peritonitis after infection of the ascites was reported and was fatal.

19.1.3. Biliary complications

Twenty-five early (30 postoperative days) and 14 delayed (sometimes for >4 months18) biliary complications [42] were reported in 10 series. Twelve biliary leakages occurred, 10 of which were early. Six occurred in resection combined with IRFA. One early leakage was caused by a prophylactic cholecystectomy, but two delayed leakages were associated with a biliary stenosis. Fifteen intrahepatic bile collections were described, one of which induced duodenal compression. One article gave details of the treatment of eight biliomas: all eight were drained percutaneously and two recurred after drain clamping. Two were related to biliary stenoses and were treated by intrahepatic stenting; the other six patients underwent endoscopic sphincterotomy. Eleven biliary stenoses associated with jaundice and biliary dilatation were reported, of which five were early. These were complicated by biliomas, biliary leakage and cholangitis. In their prospective study, some authors [43] did not observe a correlation between central or peripheric localization of the tumour and the frequency of biliary complications.

19.1.4. Liver failure

Liver failure was reported in 24 patients in 11 articles [41] and was fatal in eight patients. Fourteen liver failures occurred after IRFA combined with major resection. Six liver failures occurred in cirrhotic patients; three of these failures occurred after IRFA alone. Two liver failures were subsequent to portal thrombosis.

19.1.5. Vascular complications

Different types of vascular complication were described in in a total of 22 patients. Associated procedures such as cholecystectomy or colectomy induced six haemorrhages, two of which were fatal and one required re-operation after prophylactic cholecystectomy. Three haemorrhages from the needle track were treated during surgery by compression. In three cirrhotic patients, haemorrhage occurred in the necrosis induced by the IRFA; one patient died as a result. [25]

Treatment of two juxta-portal lesions induced haemorrhages from arterial injuries. 25, 26 In one patient, an arterio-portal fistula appeared in an area of necrosis 6 weeks later and was treated by a transfemoral embolization. [18] Similarly, a false aneurysm occurred in one patient 6 months after IRFA and led to a haemorrhage. Five portal thromboses were reported, [19, 25, 34] four of which were complete and fatal. Three of these occurred in cirrhotic patients treated with Pringle vascular occlusion.

19.1.6. Skin burns

Eight dispersive pad skin burns were reported in four articles. Skin burns occurred when RFA ran for >30 min on high power and within large and multiple skin pads. One skin burn occurred in a patient with bilateral hip prostheses.30 One third-degree skin burn required surgical treatment. [38]

19.1.7. Visceral damage

Two instances of thermal gastric damage [41] and one of acute cholecystitis near the gallbladder were observed after IRFA during surgery and were treated immediately.

19.1.8. Comparison with hepatectomy

The morbidity of hepatectomy depends on the extent and complexity of the hepatic resection. Intraoperative RFA as a standalone treatment is indicated for unresectable tumours in patients in whom major hepatectomy would leave a low level of functional hepatic reserve. Mortality and morbidity rates in major hepatic resection are 0–5% and 20–50%, respectively. [45] Rates of liver failure after major hepatectomy preceded by portal embolization are 4–10% vs.2.6% after IRFA [46, 47] combined with hepatic resection. There is reported mortality of 2.3% and morbidity of 19.8% in patients treated by resection and combined IRFA, and estimates their results to be comparable with those of resection alone. [31] Morbidity rates after major hepatic

http://dx.doi.org/10.5772/56915

resection and IRFA combined with hepatic resection are comparable, even if IRFA is indicated in tumours unresectable by hepatectomy alone. [48]

The past 10 years have represented a period of learning for surgeons who deal with liverme-tastases with the aim of treating more patients by combining IRFA with resection. The benefit: risk ratio is now well known and surgeons have access to the knowledge they need to make more informed choices about whether to resect, ablate or renounce treatment on a lesion-by-lesion basis. Surgeons who are skilled in intraoperative ultrasound diagnosis and guidance are now not only able to choose whether or not to perform surgery, but are also able to perform IRFA and do not need to involve a radiologist. Specific complications related to IRFA are rare, especially if the lesion is <35 mm in diameter and is located far from a main biliary duct and no additional septic procedures are used. The surgeon can decide to ablate a lesion in a more difficult situation, but this carries greater risk. Combining resection with IRFA leads to higher morbidity, especially in difficult patients with numerous bilateral lesions, but this may be necessary to achieve R0 (microscopically negative) resection margins.

20. Hepatic re-resection in case of recurrent tumor

The resection of hepatic metastases of colorectal carcinoma is followed by tumor recurrence in up to two thirds of cases, and about half of these recurrences are found in the liver [12, 23, 27, 28]. In general, whenever there is a chance of a curative resection, resection should be considered for recurrent tumors as well. The operative morbidity and mortality of hepatic reresection in experienced centers are no greater than those of primary resection. In a study on second operations in 94 patients with recurrent hepatic metastases of colorectal carcinoma, 38% of the patients were alive 5 years after surgery [12]. Thus, whenever complete resection of the tumor is possible, surgery is indicated even for patients with recurrent hepatic metastases.

21. Conclusion

The results of surgical treatment of metastatic colorectal carcinoma have improved markedly in recent years. The reasons for this include developments in medical imaging, in perioperative and surgical treatment, and in chemotherapy, with the introduction of potent new protocols. Clinicopathological factors such as tumor size, number of tumor nodules, and extrahepatic tumor manifestations no longer contraindicate hepatic resection. The main consideration at present is the need to achieve a complete R0 resection. Accompanying chemotherapy should be considered, especially for patients with an unfavorable risk profile. Neoadjuvant chemotherapy is reserved for patients with marginally resectable metastases. The resectability or nonresectability of hepatic metastases is a matter that must be evaluated by a surgeon who is experienced in the treatment of hepatic metastases. Hepatic resection of colorectal liver metastases after downsizing by chemotherapy provides the only chance of long term survival for patients with initially unresectable colorectal liver metastases. Additional surgical techniques can be combined to chemotherapy to further improve resectability. The only absolute contraindication for resection is the inability to completely resect all metastases, avoiding postoperative liver failure by leaving enough functional liver parenchyma. The presence of poor prognostic factors no longer limits the indications for resection. Neoadjuvant treatment with chemotherapeutic agents such as irinotecan and oxaliplatin, hepatic artery infusion combined with systemic therapy and biologic agents (bevacizumab, cetuximab) play an important role in increasing the number of patients eligible to secondary resection. However, with the progressive use of neoadjuvant chemotherapy further studies are necessary to answer questions such as the risk: benefit ratio in maximizing response rates versus vascular changes in the liver (current opinion still divided concerning their importance). These questions remain challenging and should not be underestimated. The perfecting of surgical techniques together with safer procedures, as well as the improvement in chemotherapy regimens have allowed doctors to offer patients with liver metastasis the possibility of curative treatment or longterm survival. Factors that were previously considered contraindications for the surgery, such as number of metastases, synchronous metastases and even the presence of extrahepatic disease, must be considered only as prognostic factors and must not prevent the patient from having the opportunity of being treated.

Author details

Nikola Kolev[1], Valentin Ignatov[1], Anton Tonev[1], Tanya Kirilova[2], Georgi Ivanov[1], Alexander Zlatarov[1] and Krassimir Ivanov[1]

1 Department of General and Operative Surgery, University Hospital "St. Marina", Varna, Bulgaria

2 Department of Gastroenterology, University Hospital "St. Marina", Varna, Bulgaria

References

[1] Jemal A, Murray T, Ward E, Hao Y, Xu J, Murray T, et al. Cancer statistics, 2005. CA Cancer J Clin. 2005;55:10-30.

[2] International Agency for research on cancer: GLOBOCAN 2002 data. [Accessed 2006 Nov 16]. Available from: http:// www-dep.iarc.fr

[3] Stangl R, Altendorf-Hofmann A, Charnley RM, Scheele J. Factors influencing thenatural history of colorectal liver metastases. Lancet. 1994;343:1405-10.

[4] Mentha G, Majno P, Terraz S, Rubbia-Brandt L, Gervaz P, Andres A, et al. Treatment strategies for the management of advanced colorectal liver metastases detected synchronously with the primary tumour. EJSO. 2007;33:76-83.

[5] Livermetsurvey. International registry of liver metastases of colorectal cancer. [Accessed 2010 Mar].

[6] Choti M, Sitzmann J, Tiburi M, Sumetchotimetha W, Rangsin R, Schulick RD, et al. Trends in long term survival following liver resection for hepatic colorectal metastases. Ann Surg. 2002;235:759-66.

[7] Abdalla EK, Vauthey JN, Ellis LM, Ellis V, Pollock R, Broglio KR, et al. Recurrence and outcomesfollowing hepatic resection, radiofrequency ablation, and combined resection/ablation for colorectal liver metastases. Ann Surg. 2004;239:818-27.

[8] Fong Y, Fortner J, Sun RL, Brennan MF, Blumgart LH. Clinical score for predicting recurrence after hepatic resection for metastatic colorectal cancer: analysis of 1001 consecutive cases. Ann Surg. 1999;230:309-18.

[9] Nordlinger B, Jaeck D, editors. Traitment de metastases hépatiques as cancers colorectaus. Paris: Springer-Verlag; 1992.

[10] Gayowski TJ, Iwatsuki S, Madariaga JR, Selby R, Todo S, Irish W, et al. Experience in hepatic resection of colorectal cancer – analysis of clinical and pathological risk factors. Surgery. 1994;116:703-71.

[11] Minagawa M, Maltuuchi M, Torzilli G, Takayama T, Kawasaki S, Kosuge T, et al. Extension of the frontiers metastases from colorectal cancer: Long-term results. Ann Surg. 2000;231: 487-99.

[12] Ercolani G, Grazi GL, Ravaioli M, Cescon M, Gardini A, Varotti G, et al. Liver resection for multiple colorectal metastases: influence of parenchymal involvement and total tumor volume versus number or location on long term survival. Arch Surg. 2002;137:1187-92.

[13] Scheele J, Stangl R, Altendorf-Hofmann A. Hepatic metastases from colorectal carcinoma: impact of surgical resection on the natural history. Br J Surg. 1990;77:1241-6.

[14] Adam R, Delvart V, Pascal G, Valeanu A, Castaing D, Azoulay D, et al. Rescue surgery for unresectable colorectal liver metastases downstaged by chemotherapy: a model to predict longterm survival. Ann Surg. 2004;240:644-58.

[15] Rodgers M, Mccall J. Surgery for colorectal liver metastases with hepatic lymph node involvement: A Systematic review. Br J Surg. 2000;87:1142-55.

[16] Adam R, De Haas RJ, Wicherts DA, Aloia TA, Delvart V, Azoulay D, et al. Is hepatic resection justified after chemothera- py in patients with colorectal liver metastases and lymph node involvement? J Clin Oncol. 2008;26:3672-80.

[17] Pfannschmidt J, Dienemann H, Hoffmann H. Surgical resection of pulmonary metastases from colorectal cancer: a systematic review of published series. Ann Thorac Surg. 2007;84:324-38.

[18] Elias D, Liberale G, Vernerey D, Pocard M, Ducreux M, Boige V, et al. Hepatic and extrahepatic colorectalmetastases: when resectable, their localization does not matter, but their total number has a prognostic effect. Ann Surg Oncol. 2005;12: 900-9.

[19] Adam R, Haas RJ, Wicherts D, et al. Concomitant extrahepatic in patients with colorectal liver metastases: when is there a place for surgery? Ann Surg. 2011. In press.

[20] Adam R, Pascal G, Azoulay D, Tanaka K, Castaing D, Bismuth H. Liver resection for colorectal metastases: the third hepatectomy. Ann Surg. 2003;238:871-83.

[21] Tanaka K, Adam R, Shimada H, Azoulay D, Lévi F, Bismuth H. Role of neoadjuvant chemotherapy in the treatment of multiple colorectal metastases to the liver. Br J Surg. 2003;90:963-9.

[22] Mitry E, Fields AL, Bleiberg H, Labianca R, Portier G, Tu D, et al. Adjuvant chemotherapy after potentially curative resection of metastases from colorectal cancer: A pooled analysis of two randomized trials. J Clin Oncol. 2008;26:4906-11.

[23] Nordlinger B, Sorbye H, Glimelius B, Poston GJ, Schlag PM, Rougier P, et al. Perioperative chemotherapy with FOLFOX4 and surgery versus surgery alone for resectable liver metastases from colorectal cancer (EORTC Intergroup trial 40983): a randomised controlled trial. Lancet. 2008;371: 1007-16.

[24] Parks R, Gonen M, Kemeny N, Jarnagin W, D'Angelica M, DeMatteo R, et al. Adjuvant chemotherapy improves survival after resection of hepatic colorectal metastases: analysis of data from two continents. J Am Coll Surg. 2007;204:753-61.

[25] Gruenberger B, Scheithauer W, Punzengruber R, Zielinski C, Tamandl D, Gruenberger T. Importance of response to neoadjuvant chemotherapy in potentially curable colorectal cancer metastases. BMC Cancer. 2008;8:120.

[26] Kemeny MM, Adak S, Gray B, Macdonald JS, Smith T, Lipsitz S, et al. Combined-modality treatment for resectable metastatic colorectal carcinoma to the liver: Surgical resection of hepatic metastases in combination with continuous infusion of chemotherapeutic-An Intergroup Study. J Clin Oncol. 2002;20:1499-505.

[27] Thirion P, Wolmark N, Haddad E, Buyse M, Piedbois P. Survival impact of chemotherapy in patients with colorectal metastases confined to the liver: A reanalysis of 1458 non-operable patients randomized in 22 trials and 4 meta-analysis. Meta-Analysis Group in cancer. Ann Oncol. 1999;10:1317-20.

[28] Hobday TJ, Kugler JW, Mahoney MR, Sargent DJ, Sloan JA, Fitch TR, et al. Long-term survivors of metastatic colorectal cancer treated with chemotherapy only: A North central Cancer Treatment group review. J Clin Oncol. 2002;20: 4574-80.

[29] Giacchetti S, Itzhaki M, Gruia G, Adam R, Zidani R, Kunstlinger F, et al. Long-term survival of patient with unresectable colorectal cancer liver metastases following infusional chemotherapy with 5-fluorouacil, leucovorin, oxaliplatin and surgery. Ann Oncol. 1999;10:663-9.

[30] Folprecht G, Grothey A, Alberts S, Raab HR, Kuhne CH. Neoadjuvant treatment of unresectable colorectal liver metastases: Correlation between tumor response and resection rates. Ann Oncol. 2005;16:1311-9.

[31] Ychou M, Viret F, Kramar A, Desseigne F, Mitry E, Guimbaud R, et al. Tritherapy with fluorouracil/leucovorin, irinotecan and oxaliplatin (FOLFIRINOX): a phase II study in colorectalcancer patients with non-resectable liver metбstases. Cancer Chemother Pharmacol. 2008;62:195-201.

[32] Van Cutsem E, Kцhne CH, Hitre E, Zaluski J, Chang Chien CR, Makhson A, et al. Cetuximab and chemotherapy as initial treatment for metastatic colorectal cancer. N Engl J Med. 2009;360:1408-17.

[33] Bokemeyer C, Bondarenko I, Makhson A, Hartmann JT, Aparicio J, De Braud F, et al. Fluorouracil, leucovorin, and oxaliplatin with and without cetuximab in the first-line treatment of metastatic colorectal cancer. J Clin Oncol. 2009;27:663-71.

[34] Ocvirk J, Brodowicz T, Wrba F, Ciuleanu TE, Kurteva G, et al. Cetuximab plus FOLFOX6 or FOLFIRI in metastatic colorectal cancer: CECOG trial. World J Gastroenterol. 2010;16:3133-43.

[35] Folprecht G, Gruenberger T, Bechstein WO, Raab HR, Lordick F, Hartmann JT, et al. Tumour response and secondary respectability of colorectal liver metastases following neoadjuvant chemotherapy with cetuximab: the CELIM randomized phase 2 trial. The Lancet Oncol. 2010;11:38-47.

[36] Adam R, Aloia T, Levi F, Wicherts DA, De Haas RJ, Paule B, et al. Hepatic resection after rescue cetuximab treatment for colorectal liver metastases previously refractory to conventional systemic therapy. J Clin Oncol. 2007;25: 4593-602.

[37] De Baere T, Roche A, Elias D, Lasser P, Lagrange C, Bousson V. Preoperative portal vein embolization for extension of hepatectomy indications. Hepatology. 1996;200:559-63.

[38] Madoff DC, Abdalla EK, Gupta S, Wu TT, Morris JS, Denys A, et al. Transhepatic ipsilateral rightportal vein embolization extended to segment IV: improving hypertrophy and resection outcomes with spherical particles and coils. J Vasc Interv Radiol. 2005;16:215-25.

[39] Abdalla EK, Barnett CC, Doherty D, Curley SA, Vauthey JN. Extended hepatectomy in patients with hepatobiliary malignancies with and without preoperative portal vein embolization. Arch Surg. 2002;137:675-80.

[40] Razafindratsira T, Isambert M, Evrard S Complications of intraoperative radiofrequency ablation of liver metastases. HPB (Oxford). 2011 Jan;13 (1):15-23.

[41] Vauthey JN, Chaoui A, Do KA, Bilimoria MM, Fenstermacher MJ, Charnsangavej C, et al. Standardized measurement of the future liver remnant prior to extended liver resection: methodology and clinical associations. Surgery. 2000;127: 512-9.

[42] Azoulay D, Castaing D, Smail A, Adam R, Cailliez V, Laurent A, et al. Resection of nonresectable liver metastases from colorectal cancer after percutaneous portal vein embolization. Ann Surg. 2000;231:480-6.

[43] Madoff DC, Abdalla EK, Vauthey JN. Portal vein embolization in preparation for major hepatic resection: evolution of a new standard of care. J Vasc Interv Radiol. 2005;16:779-90.

[44] Elias D, De Baere T, Roche A, Ducreux M, Leclere J, Lasser P. During liver regeneration following right portal embolization the growth rate of liver metastases is more rapid than that of the liver parenchyma. Br J Surg. 1999;86:784-8.

[45] Kokudo N, Tada K, Seki M, Ohta H, Azekura K, Ueno M, et al. Proliferative activity of intrahepatic colorectal metastases after preoperative hemihepatic portal vein embolization. Hepatology. 2001;34:267-72.

[46] Elias D, Santoro R, Ouellet JF, Osmak L, De Baere T, Roche A. Simultaneous percutaneous right portal vein embolization and left liver tumour radiofrequency ablation prior to a major right hepatic resection for bilateral colorectal metastases. Hepatogastroenterology. 2004;51:1788-91.

[47] Terraz S, Constantin C, Majno P, Spahr L, Mentha G, Becker CD. Image-guided multipolar radiofrequency ablation of liver tumours: initial clinical results. Eur Radiol. 2007;17:2253-61.

[48] Lencioni R, Cioni D, Crocetti L, Franchini C, Pina CD, Lera J, et al. Early-stage hepatocellular carcinoma in patients with cirrhosis: long-term results of percutaneous image-guided radiofrequency ablation. Radiology. 2005;234:961-7.

[49] Berber E, Pelley R, Siperstein AE. Predictors of survival after radiofrequency thermal ablation of colorectal cancer metastases to the liver: a prospective study. J Clin Oncol. 2005;23:1358-64.

[50] Solbiati L, Livraghi T, Goldberg SN, Ierace T, Meloni F, Dellanoce M, et al. Percutaneous radiofrequency ablation of hepatic metastases form colorectal cancer: long-term results in 117 patients. Radiology. 2001;221:159-66.

[51] De Baere T, Bessoud B, Dromain C, Ducreux M, Boige V, Lassau N, et al. Percutaneous radiofrequency ablation of hepatic tumors during temporary venous occlusion. Am J Roentgenol. 2002;178:53-9.

[52] Elias D, Sideris L, Pocard M, Dromain C, De Baere T. Intraductal cooling of the main bile ducts during radiofrequency ablation prevents biliary stenosis. J Am Coll Surg. 2004;198:717-21.

[53] Mulier S, Ni Y, Jamart J, Ruers T, Marchal G, Michel L. Local recurrence after hepatic radiofrequency coagulation. Multivariate meta-analysis and review of contributing factors. Ann Surg. 2005;242:158-71.

[54] Aloia TA, Vauthey JN, Loyer EM, Ribero D, Pawlik TM, Wei SH, et al. Solitary colorectal liver metastases: resection determines outcome. Arch Surg. 2006;141:460-7.

[55] Wicherts DA, Miller R, de Haas RJ, Bitsakou G, Vibert E, Veihan LA et al. Long-term results of two-stage hepatectomy for irresectable colorectal cancer liver metastases. Ann Surg. 2008;248:994-1005.

[56] Martin R, Paty P, Fong Y, Grace A, Cohen A, De Matteo R et al. Simultaneous liver and colorectal resections are safe for synchronous colorectal liver metastasis. J Am Coll Surg. 2003;197:233-41; discussion 41-2.

[57] Reddy SK, Pawlik TM, Zorzi D, Gleisner AL, Ribeiro D, Assumpção L et al. Simultaneous resections of colorectal cancer and synchronous liver metastases: a multi-institutional analysis. Ann Surg Oncol. 2007;14:3481-91.

[58] Brouquet A, Mortenson MM, Vauthey JN, Abdalla EK. Surgical strategies for synchronous colorectal liver metastases in 156 consecutive patients: classic, combined or reverse strategy? J Am Coll Surg. 2010;210:934-41.

[59] Mentha G, Majno PE, Andres A, Rubbia-Brandt L, Morel P, Roth AD. Neoadjuvant chemotherapy and resection of advanced synchronous liver metastases before treatment of the colorectal primary. Br J Surg. 2006;93:872-8.

[60] Poultsides GA, Servais EL, Saltz LB, Patil S, Kameny NE, Guillem JG et al. Outcome of primary tumor in patients with synchronous stage IV colorectal cancer receiving combination chemotherapy without surgery as initial treatment. J Clin Oncol. 2009;27:3379-84.

[61] Tebbutt NC, Norman AR, Cunningham D, Andreyev J. Intestinal complications after chemotherapy for patients with unresected primary colorectal cancer and synchronous metastases. Gut. 2003;52:568-73.

[62] Adam R, Pascal G, Castaing D, Azoulay D, Delvart V, Paule B et al. Tumor progression while on chemotherapy: a contraindication to liver resection for multiple colorectal metastases? Ann Surg. 2004;240:1052-61; discussion 61-4.

[63] Herman P, Machado MAC, Diniz AL, Coimbra FJF, Sallum RA, Montagnini AL. Surgical treatment of colorectal cancer hepatic metastases; experience of A. C. Camargo Cancer Hospital - São Paulo. Appl Cancer Res. 2006;26:88-93.

Chapter 9

Management of Non-Hepatic Metastatic Disease in Colorectal Cancer

C. Alberto Blanco, R. Sánchez, F. Piniella,
D. Pescador, G. Borobio, A. García and C. Cano

Additional information is available at the end of the chapter

http://dx.doi.org/10.5772/57487

1. Introduction

Colorectal cancer is one of the most frequent malignant tumors and a leading cause of cancer-related death. One third of the patients develop a metastasis during the course of the disease. Because of that, it is very important to know about the evolution of the illness, how to make a quick diagnosis and how to provide an appropriate treatment depending on the tumor and the location of the metastases.

Management of patients with colorectal metastases without the intervention of a multidisciplinary team specialized in the liver can lead to patients being denied potentially curative treatments.

1.1. Metastatic disease

It´s necessary to have a protocol before the treatment of metastatic disease:

- Physical examination
- Laboratory test: The serum carcinoembryonic antigen (CEA) level is a valuable marker in patients with recurrent colorectal cancer. It must be remembered that about 25% of tumors do not secrete CEA.
- Imaging: Radiologic imaging is a critical component of the preoperative research on a patient with colorectal liver metastasis. In fact, it is often used to determine whether the patient should be further considered for resection.
- Surgical indications: the patient must be in acceptable health to tolerate the physiologic consequences of the surgery. Next, the primary colorectal cancer must be resected and the

presence of other extrahepatic disease must be ruled out. Preoperative workup should include a recent colonoscopy, chest X-ray and chest CT.

- Complications: Successful outcome in hepatic surgery depends largely upon minimizing intraoperative blood loss. Excessive blood loss is not only associated with increased perioperative morbidity but also with a shorter time to recurrence and decreased survival rates after resection of colorectal liver metastases.
- Survival

2. Non hepatic disease in colorectal cancer

2.1. Lung metastases

2.1.1. Lung metastases in CRC

Colon cancer is a systemic disease in 19% of the patients, and the liver and lungs are the most common locations for a metastasis. Colorectal adenocarcinoma is the most common cancer leading to pulmonary metastasectomy

2.1.1.1. Symptoms

Most pulmonary metastases are asymptomatic and they are detected incidentally during the initial diagnostic staging study for a primary tumor or in the monitoring imaging studies afterwards, generally during a thoracic CT scan. Symptoms such as coughing, pain or hemoptysis mainly appear in patients with hilar involvement.

2.1.1.2. Preoperative evaluation

A solitary pulmonary nodule in a patient with a previous cancer can be bening or malignant (primary or secondary); although in most cases will be malignant (Mery et al. 2004). When there are multiple nodules, the probability of metastatic disease increases significantly.

There are no pathognomonic radiological features that distinguish the metastasis of primary tumors, even though metastasis is generally well circumscribed, spherical with smooth margins and are mainly subpleurales or periferics. However, primary lung cancers are single lesions, with irregular edges, asociated linear densities and are often more central.

Although the background and radiographic features of a lesion can provide clues as to whether an individual lesion is bening or malignant, it is not posible to distinguish reliably a metastasis from a primary lung cancer. The resection of the nodule is the most reliable method to establish the diagnosis.

The presence of pulmonary metastasis makes it necessary to carry out a complete staging. The extent of the required pulmonary resection will guide the preoperative evaluation of the patients: patients who require a pneumonectomy will need a higher level of cardiopulmonary

http://dx.doi.org/10.5772/57487

reserve compared with patients who only require wedge resections (Villeneuve and Sundaresan 2009). The key for a successful surgical resection of pulmonary metastases is an adequate selection of the patient through a preoperative evaluation and a precise surgical planning. To do so, we can use the following diagnostic tests:

High-resolution helical CAT scan is a basic tool which detects approximately 20-25% more nodes that standard CT, and the detection is reliable in nodes of 2-3 mm (Remy-Jardin et al. 1993; Collie et al. 1994).

PET – An examination with Positron Emission Tomography (PET-FDG) is recommended to optimize the selection of patients who are candidates for pulmonary metastasectomy. However, we have to take into account the fact that PET has a limited sensitivity for lesions <1 cm in size (Reinhardt et al. 2006). It is very useful to assess the intra-thoracic node involvement (hilar or mediastinal), local hidden recurrence of the primary tumor or in other locations such as the abdomen or the pelvis (Villeneuve and Sundaresan 2009).

The main value of PET is its high sensitivity to detect an extra-thoracic disease. In general terms, metastasectomy must not be performed unless all the deposits or foci of the disease are treatable (except when the patient is included in a specific protocol such as a clinical trial for a vaccine or symptomatic lesions that cannot be treated otherwise). In any case, a positive extra-thoracic result in a PET examination is not enough evidence to rule a patient out from surgery for pulmonary metastases. All suspicious extra-thoracic FDG-highlighted areas must be biopsied before surgery.

Preoperative biopsy – In patients with highly suspicious lesions in imaging tests, the final diagnosis is often achieved after the surgical removal of the metastases. However, in many cases, a preoperative biopsy with CT-guided fine needle aspiration is a useful and less invasive method to obtain a pathological diagnosis, particularly if the diagnosis of the metastatic disease is not clear, if the patient is not a good candidate for surgery or if the patient has a primary tumor (such as testicular germ-cell cancer or lymphoma) for which surgery may not be required.

Bronchoscopy (with or without endobronchial ultrasound) is indicated as part of the evaluation in cases of lesions that are centrally located in the CT scan, patients with symptoms of involvement of the respiratory tract and some types of tumors prone to endobronchial involvement, such as breast cancer, colon cancer and renal cell carcinoma [36]. Bronchoscopy is performed before surgery, when a positive result may contraindicate an operation.

The presence of pathological mediastinal adenopathies requires a **biopsy** with a mediastinoscopy or ultrasound-guided endobronchial needle **aspiration cytology**. Most authors consider mediastinal node involvement (N2) as a contraindication for resection.

2.1.1.3. Treatment

Management of patients with pulmonary metastases, according to the guidelines of the National Comprehensive Cancer Network (NCCN) will depend on the form of presentation along time and on whether the metastases can be resected or not. Synchronous resectable metastases are treated with chemotherapy with or without later resection; and if they cannot be resected, then chemotherapy is indicated. Metachronous resectable metastases can be resected with or without neoadjuvant chemotherapy, and chemotherapy is indicated when they cannot be resected. The evaluation of patients in treatment with chemotherapy that can be transferred to surgery is carried out every 2 months in the selected cases (2013).

Although the quality of the currently available evidence on pulmonary **metastasectomy** in cases of colorectal cancer is not enough to draw conclusions on the effectiveness of this kind of surgery (Pfannschmidt et al. 2007; Fiorentino et al. 2010; Pfannschmidt et al. 2010; Salah et al. 2012; Gonzalez et al. 2013), pulmonary metastasectomy in cases of selected patients with metastatic colorectal cancer is a general practice and it is included in the clinical guidelines (Poston et al. 2011). The objective is to limit surgery only for patients who have the highest chances to benefit from it, either with longer survival rates or symptom relief, and to optimize the time of the operation.

The **resectability criteria** admitted by the main groups are the following (Ehrenhaft et al. 1958; Martini and McCormack 1998; Greelish and Friedberg 2000; Jaklitsch et al. 2001; Pfannschmidt et al. 2003; Kondo et al. 2005):

- Complete anatomical resection maintaining an adequate pulmonary function (McAfee et al. 1992; Regnard et al. 1998; Inoue et al. 2000; Sakamoto et al. 2001)
- Removal of the primary tumor without persistence of residual disease (R0)
- The existence of resectable extra-pulmonary metastases does not contraindicate pulmonary resection (Yano et al. 1993; Ambiru et al. 1998; Irshad et al. 2001; Rena et al. 2002); in this case, the metastases must be treatable with surgery or other therapeutic approach.
- Resectable metastases can be treated with a synchronous resection or a sequential approach.

The resection of one or more pulmonary lesions may also be indicated in a patient with a known malignant tumor when:

- A new primary lung cancer cannot be ruled out
- There are symptomatic metastases (such as bronchial obstruction with distal suppuration) that cannot be treated in any other way
- Tissue is required for a new therapeutic strategy (such as an autologous vaccine), preferably in the framework of a clinical trial.

The approach depends on the number, size, location and estability during the time in TC. In general, Video-assisted thoracoscopic surgery (VATS) is ideal for peripheral metastases single or few, stable and smaller than 3 cm. The central lesions are likely to require a segmentectomy or lobectomy and is best addressed by open thoracotomy.

Video-assisted thoracoscopic surgery has the advantage that it is less painful, postoperative recovery is faster, hospitalization is shorter and lower long-term morbidity, especially intrathoracic recurrences (Saisho et al. 2009). Recurrence rates appear to be similar to the approach using thoracotomy (Saisho et al. 2009). There are no randomised trials comparing results between open resections and thoracoscopic surgery, although retrospectively patients treated by VATS have similar results to patients treated by conventional open thoracotomy (Carballo et al. 2009)

Concerning the number of metastasis, it is clear that technically the fewer there is, the better. Although there is no general consensus, ideally from technical and oncologic point of view, it would be less than five (Hellman and Weichselbaum 1995; Weichselbaum and Hellman 2011) however it is true that in the majority of cases, unique pulmonary metastasectomies are conducted and in these patients there is a greater survival advantage (Fiorentino et al. 2010). Metastases in both lungs are not a contraindication for surgery.

For some patients with metastatic CRC, repeated pulmonary metastasectomy offers an excellent opportunity for long-term survival, and it is associated with a low operative mortality rate. Patients with more than 2 metastatic nodes and a maximum diameter of the metastatic pulmonary node of more than 3 cm present a significantly lower survival rate (Hendriks et al. 2001; Salah et al. 2013).

In the case of patients who do not meet the criteria for a metastasectomy, there are alternative ablative techniques to locally control the lesion, such as **stereotactic radiotherapy** and **radiofrequency ablation** or **cryoablation**. The experience with these ablation techniques is limited, but the initial results look promising (Pennathur, Abbas et al. 2009). The role of **chemotherapy** is not yet defined for pulmonary metastases with a colorectal origin, because traditionally, these lesions do not show a good response to adjuvant treatments. Currently, chemotherapy has shown very good responses in primary CRC with regimens such as FOLFOX (fluorouracil, leucovorin and oxaliplatin) and FOLFIRI (fluorouracil, leucovorin and irinotecan), with or without the addition of biological agents such as bevacizumab (anti-vascular endothelial growth factor, VEGF), cetuximab and panitumumab (anti-epidermal growth factor, EGFR). These therapies have not yet been systematically studied, and they may become the most effective treatment for pulmonary metastases. As a last resort, patients whose functional state is poor are candidates for palliative treatment only (Villeneuve & Sundaresan 2009).

External radiotherapy can be an option in very specific cases or in clinical trials, provided that the tumors are not potentially resectable.

2.1.2. Prognostic factors

There are many factors that have an influence on survival after a metastasectomy. The presence of one or more factors for poor prognosis does not represent an absolute contraindication for a metastasectomy (Quiros and Scott 2008). Unfavourable prognostic factors include number and size of the metastasis, inability to completely resect the entire metastatic disease, a short disease-free interval after treatment for the primary tumor and thoracic node involvement. For its part, the histology of the tumor also influences the results.

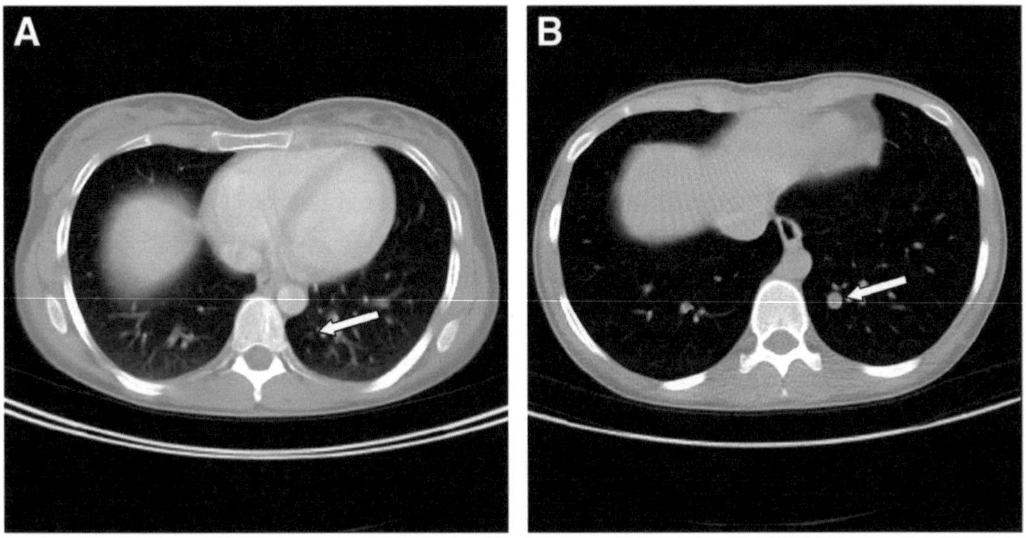

Figure 1. Comparison of chest scanning during shallow breathing (A) and chest scanning with additional low-dose CT during maximal inspiration (B). (A) Lung metastasis from colorectal cancer is only barely visible during shallow breathing (arrow). Also note blurred lung vessels and congested lung parenchyma in this image. (B) Metastasis can be clearly detected by low-dose CT during maximal inspiration (arrow). Additionally, lung parenchyma is well inflated, and lung vessels are displayed sharply. http://jnm.snmjournals.org/content/48/1_suppl/45S/F2.expansion.html

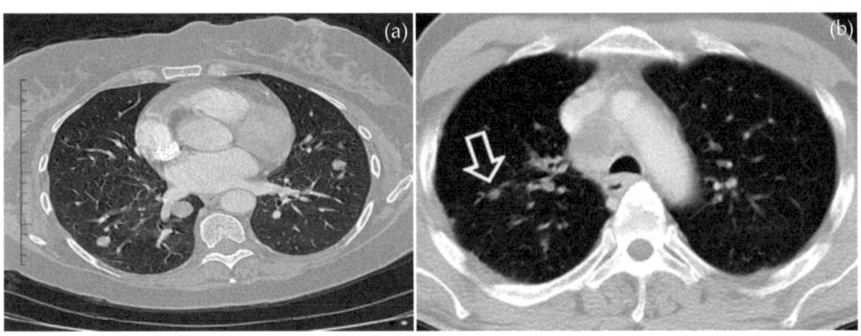

Figure 2. Multiple metastases Multiple pulmonary metastases from colorectal carcinoma. http://radiopaedia.org/articles/pulmonary-metastases, TC/PET metastases from colorectal cancer

3. Node metastases

3.1. Definition and physiopathology

Node metastases are, like with other cancers, the most important dissemination route for colorectal cancers. This makes lymph node involvement the most important factor in the prognosis and therapeutic approach for colorectal cancer.

http://dx.doi.org/10.5772/57487

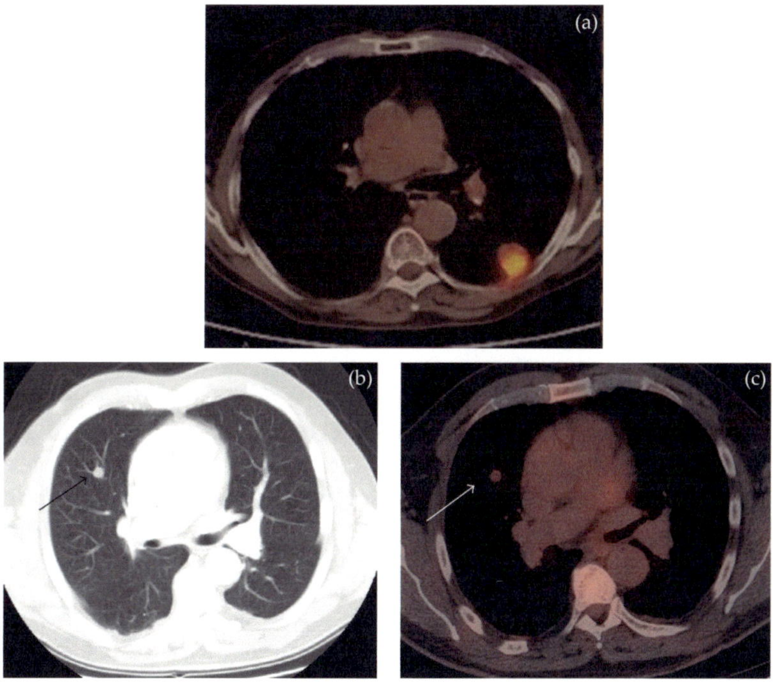

Figure 3. Patient with rectal carcinoma and mildly FDG avid metastases to lung. (a) There is a suspicious right upper lobe lung nodule (arrow) on CT in a patient with prior history of rectal carcinoma. (b) The lesion is only mildly FDG avid (arrow) on fused PET-CT. Based on these images the lesion is not definitively malignant. This may be due to the limited resolution of PET and the small lesion size or reduced cellularity. (c) Lung biopsy was subsequently performed confirming that the lesion (arrow) represented a metastatic deposit from rectal carcinoma. http://www.hindawi.com/journals/ijso/2011/846512/fig7/

The first metastases usually appear in the paracolic nodes closest to the primary tumor they are draining, and frequently only one or two nodes close to the tumor are involved. However, as the disease evolves, node propagation is larger and affects a variable amount of nodes located further away, on the arteriovenous system that depends on the intestinal segment involved. As the neoplasm moves forward, nodes from the main colic vessels that drain the intestinal neoplastic area are invaded, and the process gradually spreads upwards through the node chain that accompanies the vessels until it finally reaches the nodes that depend on the large mesenteric vessels (and, in the case of the rectum, the nodes that depend on the iliac vessels through the hemorrhoidal venous system). In short, it is known that here is a correlation between each segment of the colon and its venous and lymphatic drainage which, although there may be individual alterations, essentially depends on the superior mesenteric venous system up to the splenic flexure of the colon and, from there, up to the superior rectal vein which depends on the inferior mesenteric vein. Both are affluent to the portal vein and the structure of the lymph drainage system is essentially the same. In the area of the rectum, it has been traditionally accepted that the superior rectal venous system depends on the inferior mesenteric system, that the middle rectal system depends on the inferior mesenteric system and the internal iliac system, and that the inferior rectal system depends on the internal and external iliac system.

On the other hand, there are evidences that show that there are factors of the tumor cells which increase angiogenesis and lymphomagenesis, and which lead to an increased rate of node metastasis and a worse prognosis. Specifically, vascular endothelial growth factor C (VEGF-C) and cyclooxygenase-2 (COX-2) (Coexpression of VEGF-C and Cox-2 in Human Colorectal Cancer and its Association With Lymph Node Metastasis Soumaoro et al. Dis Colon Rectum, March 2006 392-398).

Node involvement plays a fundamental role in the correct definition of the extent of tumor spread, together with the depth of the involvement through the wall of the colon or the rectum, the size of the tumor or the presence of metastases. The number of involved nodes and their distance to the tumor is the basis of some classic classifications, such as Dukes, Astler and Coller and the more modern TNM, whose description is already analyzed elsewhere. All decisions on the treatment must be adopted with reference to the TNM classification, instead of the old Dukes system or the modified Astler-Coller staging system (Colon and rectum. In: Edge SB, Byrd DR, Compton CC, et al., eds.: AJCC Cancer Staging Manual. 7th ed. New York, NY: Springer, 2010, pp 143-64).

Given the importance of the whole number of involved nodes in a proper staging and in order to obtain a reliable and comparable prognosis, it is necessary to establish a set of minimum quality criteria for lymphadenectomy. Otherwise, the scenario might be undervalued. Patients in stage I or II (that is, without node involvement) show five-year survival rates of 75%; in contrast to survival rates with N1, which are only 45-60%. Also, the higher the number of nodes studied by the pathologist (and indirectly, resected by the surgeon), the higher the staging accuracy; if that number is low, there is an undervaluing of the tumor dissemination state. (Staging accuracy in colorectal carcinoma. Wong et al. Journal of Clinical Oncology. Vol 17. nº 9 1999pp2896-2900).

A panel sponsored by the American Joint Committee on Cancer (AJCC) and the National Cancer Institute of the USA and presented at the World Conference on Gastroenterology of Sydney in 1990 (J. Gastroenterol Heptol 6:325-244. 1991) has recommended that at least 12 lymph nodes be examined in patients with colon and rectal cancer in order to confirm the lack of node involvement due to the tumor. Wong et al. recommend at least the analysis of 14 nodes in pT2 and pT3 tumors.

There is a special situation with staging patients with rectal cancer and neoadjuvant chemotherapy with ypT0-2. In these cases, staging based on the surgical specimen usually shows a decrease in size and in the involvement of the wall of the intestine of the tumor, but if this is taken into account together with the reduction in the number of existing nodes in the specimen removed from the rectum, it could lead to an undervaluing with negative consequences for the patient's survival (Comparative Analisis of Limph Node Metastasis in Patients UIT ypT0-2 Rectal Cancers. Park et al. Disease of the Colon and Rectum. Volume 56: 2 (2013). Here, it is necessary to insist on the fact that, just as the primary treatment of node metastases in CRC must spread as much as possible (total mesorectal excision, or TME); in the case of patients who have undergone neoadjuvant treatment with chemotherapy it is also essential to perform a TME.

The studies that want to ensure the diagnosis of node involvement have researched the presence of micrometastastases or metastases that have been diagnosed with immunohistochemical techniques in patients in stages I and II (that is, without node involvement in microscopical terms), and they have found that the presence of micrometastastases in these patients does not affect the prognosis and must not be taken into account when treating CRC (Are Lymph Node Micrometastastases of any Clinical Significance in Dukes Stages A and B Colorectal Cancer? Oberg et al. Dis Colon Rectum, October 1998 ol. 41, No. 10 1244-1249).

3.2. Sentinel lymph node

In tumors with a metastasis that takes place through the lymphatic system (breast cancer and melanoma, mainly), there has been a great success in mapping the dissemination of the primary tumor with the so called sentinel lymph node biopsy technique. In view of this situation, several studies have started to analyze it, because lymphadenectomy is an important part in the primary treatment of CRC, both from the staging point of view and in order to prevent recurrence of the tumor if there are infiltrated lymph nodes left. Having a map of lymph dissemination similar to the one obtained with breast cancer would mean knowing the minimum required level of lymphadenectomy, or even of visceral resection. This would allow the medical team to apply an adequate surgical treatment from an oncological perspective but with the minimum morbidity and mortality. Unfortunately, it does not seem that this technique shows reliable results with colorectal cancer ("Técnica del ganglio centinela…". Sardon Ramos et al. CIR ESP. 2013 91(6) 366-371.1).

The identification of the sentinel lymph node shows a low sensitivity in the detection of metastasis and micrometastasis. Approximately one half of the adenopathies are lost if a lymphadenectomy is performed based on the results of the sentinel lymph node study. Faerden et al: sentinel node mapping in colonic cancer Disease of the colon & rectum. Volume 51: 891–896 (2008).

3.3. Treatment of lymphatic metastasis

Treatment of lymphatic metastasis, given its close relation with the growth of the primary tumor, is the same as for the original lesion: primary resection with exeresis of the nodes of the lymphatic area that drain the tumor. If there is a tumor recurrence in the nodes, the patient is classified as stage IV, which means that there will be the corresponding treatment: chemotherapy and surgery and radiotherapy, which will be provisionally palliative.

4. Bone metastases

4.1. Introduction

Bone metastases from colorectal cancer are uncommon (10-23% in autopsy cases). They usually appear late in the natural history of metastatic disease and are associated with liver or lung metastasis. Acrometastasis is reported to be 0.3-3% of all bone metastases. Cancers of the rectum and cecum are accompanied by bone metastasis more frequently than cancers of other portions of the colon. Signet ring cell carcinoma shows a high incidence of bone metastasis.

Pain is the most common symptom of bone metastasis. As a result of the loss of bone density affected bones become prone to fracture and injury.

Testing for bone metastasis includes X-ray and bone scanning. Open biopsy is necessary to establish the diagnosis, exclude osteomyelitis and allow treatment. Early diagnosis is important for improving quality of life in these patients.

Therapeutic management of this condition includes chemotherapy, radiotherapy and surgery, but because survival after onset of bone metastasis is very poor, palliative treatment is the main objective.

4.2. Physiopathology

Bone destruction secondary to metastasis is not caused by the tumor cells, but by the activation of the osteoclasts. The tumor cells secrete an osteoclast activating factor, and the osteoclasts induce the loss of cortical bone and trabecular bone. This process is divided in four stages (Mundy & Yoneda, 1995):

1. The tumor cells adhere to the basement membrane (laminin, E-cadherin, integrins).
2. The tumor cells produce proteolytic enzymes that damage the basement membrane.
3. The tumor cells migrate via the basement membrane under the specific control of chemotactic factors.
4. The tumor cells can stimulate the activity of the osteoclasts.

Clohisy et al. have described four mechanisms that stimulate osteoclast-mediated bone destruction (Clohisy et al., 2000):

a. Stimulation of the union between the osteoclasts and the bone.

b. Stimulation of the osteoclast-mediated bone resorption.

c. Extension of the survival time of osteoclasts.

d. Acceleration of the production of osteoclasts by precursor cells.

4.3. Clinical presentation

a. *Constitutional symptoms*: Some patients report anorexia, nausea, vomiting, asthenia, malaise, and weight loss.

b. *Symptoms derived from the primary location*: Colorectal carcinoma usually presents itself accompanied by an alteration of the intestinal rhythm and by the expulsion of blood originated in the rectum. In advanced stages of the disease, the patient presents constipation, and a transabdominal mass can be perceived on palpation. A rectal examination needs to be performed, because tumors of the lower part of the rectum can be easily found.

http://dx.doi.org/10.5772/57487

c. *Symptoms derived from the metastatic disease*: Regardless of the symptoms that metastases may produce on other regions, bone metastases can lead to:

a. PAIN in the affected area, or referred pain, which may be of insidious, and either progressive or sudden onset, and it may be slight and intermittent or continuous and activity-related. Night pain is a typical symptom, and it does not always disappear with oral analgesics, unlike the pain that derives from degenerative processes, such as osteoarthritis, which increases with loads and articular mobility. When pain affects a long bone, it is easily located by the patient, but when it affects the pelvis or the spinal column, the pain makes it difficult to properly locate the lesion. When it affects the femur or the tibia (load-bearing bones), patients report pain when walking, although the pain usually appears when the bone destruction levels are over 50% and they indicate an imminent fracture.

b. SWELLING: It may be a sign of lesion aggressiveness when the tumor invades the cortical bone and affects soft tissue. This presentation is characteristic from colorectal carcinoma, renal carcinoma and melanoma.

c. FUNCTIONAL DEFICIT: it appears as a consequence of pain. It may be a result of a medullary or radicular involvement in the case of spinal metastases.

d. IMMINENT FRACTURE: It is a fracture that can appear as a result of a physiological load. Anamnesis and plain X-ray are necessary for the diagnosis, and the cortical involvement, the location and characteristics of the lesion (lytic, sclerotic or mixed) and the existence of fracture lines must be assessed. Permeating and lytic lesions of the proximal third of the femur are prone to fractures. Pain after radiation is also a sign of an imminent fracture. In cases in which an imminent fracture is expected on an active patient, a prophylactic fixation is recommended, especially in load-bearing bones.

4.4. Diagnostic assessment

In the context of colorectal carcinoma, bone metastases normally appear when the disease is already in an advanced stage (with metastases on other areas), and when the diagnosis has already been established. For this reason, a histological diagnosis is not usually necessary, and a treatment can be planned in advance. However, we must also take into account the fact that in 1-2% of the cases, the osteolytic lesion is unrelated to the primary tumor, which means that a biopsy is advisable.

4.4.1. Complete physical examination

Including the thyroid gland, breasts, lungs and digestive system.

4.4.2. Laboratory analyses

1. COMPLETE BLOOD COUNT: Anemia, leukopenia or thrombocytopenia may be a sign of medullary involvement.

2. ESR: High levels may indicate a myeloma or an active process.

3. ELECTROPHORESIS OF SERUM PROTEINS: They can show a monoclonal gammopathy and they can confirm a possible myeloma diagnosis.

4. BIOCHEMICAL ANALYSIS: It can rule out hyperparathyroidism.

5. ALKALINE PHOSPHATASE: It shows high levels in cases of advanced metastatic disease. Very high levels show an unfavourable prognostic factor.

6. CARCINOEMBRYONIC ANTIGEN: Its levels are high in digestive or hepatocellular carcinomas.

7. PROSTATE-SPECIFIC ANTIGEN: It can detect a prostate carcinoma.

8. HEPATIC ENZYMES AND SERUM ELECTROLYTES: They can show bone and liver involvement.

4.4.3. Imaging tests

1. ANTEROPOSTERIOR AND LATERAL X-RAYS OF THE LESION: In order to assess an imminent fracture and to analyse the information they provide.

2. THORACIC X-RAY: In order to see the existence of carcinoma or lung metastases.

3. THORACIC AND ABDOMINAL CT SCAN: In order to assess the existence of possible visceral metastases.

4. Tc99m BONE SCINTIGRAPHY: In order to assess bone lesions.

Data from the clinical record, an exhaustive physical examination, blood tests and imaging tests identify more than 85% of all the primary tumors that appear as a bone metastasis. The following tests could also be performed, albeit only when required:

- NMR: It is seldom recommended in cases of isolated bone lesions (fig. 1), but it may be useful in cases of a single metastasis in which a resection can be performed, in order to rule out *skip metastases* or metastases inside the bone and on the vertebrae, due to its excellent properties for the exploration of the bone marrow.

- POSITRON EMISSION TOMOGRAPHY (PET): This imaging technique is becoming more and more important in the field of orthopaedic oncology. It uses [18F]2-fluoro-2-deoxy-Dglucose (FDG) as a tracer. This is a glucose analog which is taken to the cells by a group of proteins. This marker is absorbed by malignant tissue with an increased metabolic activity. PET scans have a very high sensitivity, and it is an important technique for the identification of primary lesions and other metastases. It can establish the difference between a local recurrence and a scar, and it is also useful in the assessment of response to treatment.

4.4.4. Biopsy

Puncture biopsy is an excellent way to confirm a diagnosis of bone metastasis. CT-guided fine-needle aspiration and thick- or trephine-needle biopsies are very precise techniques, and they are easy to use. The orthopaedic surgeon must choose the exact location, taking into account the location of the lesion, viable access routes and, whenever possible, the final incision line of the operation, in case of resection surgery, excising the entire area of the biopsy, because it might be contaminated.

When finding certain locations (usually on the pelvis), a CT scan may be necessary in order to identify the best point and route of access that will reach the metastatic area and to avoid regions with reactive sclerotic bone, because these parts may not have tumor cells.

If colorectal carcinoma presents itself with a bone metastasis and the lesion is biopsied, the biopsy may not always provide a diagnosis for the primary tumor, because a tissue compatible with adenocarcinoma does not always tell the difference between primary tumors of the digestive system, prostate, breast and lung.

4.5. Supportive measures

4.5.1. Analgesic therapy

Around 70% of all patients with a bone metastasis report pain at some point along the course of the disease. The physiopathological pain may be due to medullary compression, distension of the periosteum or peripheral neurovascular involvement, as well as to pathological fractures, whenever they are present and mediated by substances such as histamine, substance P or other cytokines.

4.5.2. Bisphosphonates

Metastatic osteolysis is caused by the stimulation of osteoclast activity. For this reason, bisphosphonates can play an important role in this process, because they inhibit the osteoclast activity. They bind with the mineral bone matrix and they have a great physicochemical impact on the hydroxyapatite crystals.

Some authors have suggested that they are not only useful in the treatment of pain and the prevention of osteolytic complications, but that they can also modify the natural course of evolution of cancer in some cases, due to the effect they have on some intermediate products, such as growth factors.

Ross et al. carried out a systematic review of all randomized essays on patients with bone metastasis. It is a meta-analysis based on 18 randomized studies in which different bisphosphonates have been compared with a placebo or between themselves. Most of these studies were performed on patients with breast carcinoma (Ross et al, 2004). The review showed a decrease in the incidence and an increase in the time until the appearance of bone complications, with a better evolution of pain and functional capacity, with regard to the control group who received a placebo. Treatment with oral bisphosphonates (clodronate, etidronate) caused a decrease in the number of spinal and non-spinal fractures, but it had no effect on the indications of radiotherapy or in hypercalcaemia.

4.5.3. Treatment of hypercalcaemia

Hypercalcaemia affects 10-40% of cancer patients at some point, and it causes anorexia, nausea, vomiting, polydipsia, polyuria, dehydration, constipation, confusion and coma.

It is the result of PTHrP production, which activates bone metabolism and induces an excess of osteoclast activity. Osteoclasts are then stimulated by local factors produced by tumor cells, such as interleukin 6. Moreover, calcium levels are also increased due to lower levels of renal calcium elimination, because PTHrP acts on the renal receptors of the parathyroid hormone and it increases calcium resorption on the renal tubule. Polyuria and reduction of intravascular volume appear as a consequence, and for this reason, the initial treatment with these patients is rehydration with intravenous saline serum in order to balance the intravascular volume and to improve glomerular filtration and renal secretion of calcium.

Calcitonin inhibits osteoclasts and it has a rapid effect, although for a brief period of time. For this reason, it is mainly used in emergency treatments.

Plicamycin normalizes calcium levels in up to 50% of the cases, but its serious adverse effects make it unadvisable to use it.

4.6. Non-surgical treatment

4.6.1. Treatment of metastatic bone disease secondary to colorectal carcinoma

The treatment of bone metastases derived from colorectal tumors is the same as the treatment for other metastases caused by other tumors. Surgical resection of the primary tumor, together with chemotherapy and radiotherapy for the rectal cancer is the treatment of choice, depending on the cases.

4.6.2. Radiotherapy

Radiotherapy is the most widely used palliative treatment for bone metastasis. It is the treatment of choice for painful lytic bone metastases without short-term risk of fracture, and it is combined with surgery when there is an imminent fracture or when the fracture has already taken place. It leads to the necrosis of tumor cells, which makes it possible for the bone tissue to regenerate afterwards. The result is pain relief and, later on, a re-calcification of the destroyed areas of the bone, which is important for the functional recovery of the patient and the prevention of pathological fractures.

4.6.3. Surgical treatment

Surgery for bone metastases requires a previous complete general and local assessment. It presents its own indications, objectives, techniques and means, and it is associated to a program for postoperative radiotherapy that follows the lines that have been previously described.

http://dx.doi.org/10.5772/57487

5. Brain metastases

The increasing incidence of brain metastases in patients with metastatic colorectal cancer has been attributed to the longer survival rates seen with newer systemic therapies. Compared to the era when 5-fluorouracil was the primary agent for metastatic disease, median survival has increased markedly with the introduction of oxaliplatin, irinotecan, and biologic therapies (from 6 to 7 to approximately 24 months).

However, the incidence of brain metastases in metastatic colorectal cancer is still low, 2.3 percent in one of the series. Brain metastases are usually a late-stage phenomenon, and the vast majority of patients have metastases in other sites, particularly the lung. Outcomes are poor, despite aggressive treatment.

The most common mechanism of metastasis to the brain is by hematogenous spread. Metastases are usually located directly at the junction of the gray matter and white matter where blood vessels decrease in diameter and act as a trap for clumps of tumor cells. Brain metastases also tend to be more common at the terminal "watershed areas" of arterial circulation. The distribution of metastases roughly follows the relative weight and blood flow in each area:

- Cerebral hemispheres — approximately 80 percent
- Cerebellum — 15 percent
- Brainstem — 5 percent

Different primary tumors may have a predilection for metastasis to different areas within the brain. Gastrointestinal tumors more commonly metastasize to the posterior fossa.

5.1. Clinical presentation

Brain metastases have highly variable clinical features and should be suspected in any cancer patient who develops neurologic symptoms or behavioural abnormalities. However, multiple other causes can also be responsible. In the majority of patients, a gradually expanding tumor mass and its associated edema cause symptoms. Less commonly, intratumoral hemorrhage, obstructive hydrocephalus, or embolization by tumor cells result in symptoms.

Headache: Headaches occur in approximately 40 to 50 percent of patients with brain metastases. The frequency is higher when multiple lesions are present or a metastasis is located in the posterior fossa.

Focal neurologic dysfunction: Focal neurologic dysfunction is the presenting symptom of 20 to 40 percent of patients. Hemiparesis is the most common complaint but the manifestations depend upon the location of the metastases.

Cognitive dysfunction: Cognitive dysfunction, including memory problems and mood or personality changes, is the presenting problem in 30 to 35 percent of patients.

Seizures: New onset of seizures is the presenting symptom in 10 to 20 percent of patients. Seizures in patients with brain metastases are almost exclusively associated with supratentorial disease.

Stroke: Another 5 to 10 percent present acutely due to stroke caused by hemorrhage into a metastasis, hypercoagulability, invasion or compression of an artery by tumor, or embolization of tumor cells.

5.2. Diagnosis

Imaging studies provide useful information but brain biopsy is necessary in some cases for a definitive diagnosis.

Contrast-enhanced MRI is the preferred imaging study for the diagnosis of brain metastases.

Biopsy should be performed when the diagnosis of brain metastases is in doubt. This is particularly important in patients with a single lesion.

Positron emission tomography (PET) may also be useful in these patients by finding other sites of metastatic disease.

5.3. Treatment

Patients with BM from CRC have a poor prognosis, because they often have substantial extracranial metastatic disease.

Traditionally, the therapeutic goal in many of these patients has been to palliate debilitating neurologic symptoms, because most of these patients die of systemic disease. However, new advances in metastatic CRC management—including the incorporation of monoclonal antibody therapies bevacizumab, cetuximab, and panitumumab— are enhancing the outcomes of patients with systemic disease.

6. Ovarian metastases

Isolated ovarian metastases from primary CRC occur with a low frequency. The incidence of ovarian metastases (synchronous or metachronous) in patients with CRC is 1 to 14 percent. Bulky ovarian metastases are often symptomatic and less responsive to systemic chemotherapy than are other sites of disease. Resection is associated with fairly low morbidity and, in some cases, may improve quality of life and prolong survival, even in the setting of widespread extraovarian metastatic disease. There is a debate regarding prophylactic oophorectomy at the time of curative resection for primary CRC.

There is a rare variety of ovarian metastasis known as Krukenberg tumor (KT), which has been the focus of extensive research due to its poor prognosis. Although the age range of patients is highly variable, KT usually appears in premenopausal women, and for some authors, the diagnosis of primary tumor after KT is a factor for poor prognosis. They are usually large bilateral lesions, solid and bulbous, and they have a gastrointestinal origin in more than 90% of the cases. Although the form of presentation and the treatment are not different from the rest of metastatic ovarian lesions secondary to a primary tumor with a digestive origin, the prognosis is worse. It has been proven that a combined therapy of radical surgery and radiochemotherapy can achieve a slight improvement in long-term survival rates.

7. Peritoneum metastases

7.1. Definition and physiopathology

Colorectal cancer is a pathological process that spreads through the lymphatic channels through hematogenous ways and through the invasion of the intestine wall. These mechanisms result in metastases to the lymph nodes, liver and also peritoneal dissemination. Although the spread to the lymph and venous systems implies the existence of a local invasive process, peritoneal dissemination can appear in tumors with high as well as low malignancy. The dissemination of the cancer that leads to liver and lymph node metastases takes place before the surgical resection of the primary colorectal neoplasm. Peritoneal dissemination, as well as dissemination in the resection area (local recurrence) can also take place as a result of the surgical trauma associated to the resection of the primary neoplasm. The filtration of malignant cells through the severed lymph channels can also be a mechanism in this intraoperative phenomenon of cancer dissemination. Dissemination inside the peritoneal cavity is one of the most severe forms of carcinomatous dissemination from the colon, because it rapidly takes away —provisionally— all hope for a surgical resection of the lesion. Together with lymphatic and hematogenous dissemination, transcoelomic spread is one of the routes of tumor dissemination. In the early stages of peritoneal invasion, transcoelomic spread may be limited to the neighbouring structures just around the primary tumor, with a potential development of isolated carcinoid plaques in the adjacent peritoneum. It is of course a possibility that some of these nodes are not originated in a transperitoneal spread but in a dissemination of the subperitoneal lymph nodes, as Miles proposes (1926). In a later stage, peritoneal metastases spread until there is a diffuse peritoneal carcinomatosis in which there are tumor nodes that spread through the entire parietal peritoneum, greater omentum and adjacent viscera, and abundant ascites appears (Cirugía del ano, recto y colon. John Golligher 2ª edición). For Hara (Hara *et al*. Comparative analysis of intraperitoneal minimal free cancer cells between colorectal and gastric cancer patients using quantitative RT-PCR: possible reason for rare peritoneal recurrence in colorectal cancer. Clin Exp Metastasis 2007;24:179–89), peritoneal metastases take place in two stages: first of all, the tumor cells detach themselves from the serosal surface of the primary tumor and are transported in the peritoneal cavity, and in the second stage, malignant cells in the peritoneum adhere to places like the omentum and the mesenterium, and they grow and spread through the peritoneal cavity afterwards.

Four characteristics have been identified as risk factors for tumor cell exfoliation in the peritoneal cavity: 1. Depth of the invasion, 2. Involvement of lymph nodes, 3. Lymph node invasion, and 4. Venous invasion (Peritoneal cytology in colorectal cancer. Noura *et al*: Diseases of the Colon & Rectum. volume 52: 7 2009).

The identification of these tumor cells with preoperative peritoneal washing cytology can identify those patients at risk of presenting a peritoneal recurrence of the tumor process.

Peritoneal carcinomatosis is a common form of recurrence, and it is frequently the only one, after surgical curative treatment in digestive and gynecological tumors. It is logical to think that the dissemination of tumor cells by the tumor is a common previous mechanism for peritoneal carcinomatosis of abdominal tumors.

There are studies about the mechanisms and incidence of intraperitoneal dissemination of CRC that have contributed to a better comprehension and a different perception of the pathological basis of peritoneal carcinomatosis. Although the incidence rates for the presence of tumor cells during the resection of primary tumors widely vary, the presence of free tumor cells in the peritoneal cavity (similar to the micrometastases in the blood or the bone marrow) is not an independent prognostic factor, and it seems possible that these tumor cells can effectively contribute to the failure of the treatment at an intraperitoneal level. In fact, two studies found a correlation between the presence of free tumor cells in the peritoneal cavity and the recurrence of the tumor in the peritoneal cavity (Peritoneal Carcinomatosis of Colorectal Origin. M.J. Koppe. Ann Surg 2006 Febrero. 243("): 212-222).

Approximately 50% of the patients with CRC stage IV present peritoneal carcinomatosis, and approximately 25% of the patients present a recurrence of their tumor in the peritoneal cavity (peritoneal carcinomatosis), without a clear involvement of the liver or the lungs (Chu DZ, Lang NP, Thompson C, et al. Peritoneal carcinomatosis in nongynecologic malignancy: a prospective study of prognostic factors. *Cancer*. 1989;63:364–367. Sugarbaker PH, Cunliffe WJ, Belliveau J, et al. Rationale for integrating early postoperative intraperitoneal chemotherapy into the surgical treatment of gastrointestinal cancer. *Semin Oncol*. 1989;16:83–97).

Local or peritoneal metastases are factors that represent a poor prognosis for colorectal cancer (Graf et al, 1991; Mahteme et al, 1996; Shepherd et al, 1997; Assersohn et al, 1999) and their treatment is still an important challenge.

The EVOCAPE study shows an average survival of 5.2 months in patients with peritoneal carcinomatosis of colorectal origin. (Sadeghi B, Arvieux C, Glehen O, et al. Peritoneal carcinomatosis from non-gynecologic malignancies: results of the EVOCAPE Multicentric prospective study. *Cancer*. 2000;88:358–363.).

Patients with peritoneal metastases or locally advanced tumors without distance metastases can benefit from cytoreductive surgery with intraperitoneal chemotherapy (Mahteme et al. British Journal of Cancer (2004) 90 403-407).

The average survival rate for patients with carcinomatosis treated with chemotherapy is around 6-12 months (Gramont er al.2000), although this does not factor the modern therapeutic approaches that include immunomodulating agents, which have not yet been evaluated enough and appeared after the year 2000.

7.2. Peritoneal cytology

In this situation, peritoneal cytology before the resection of the primary tumor and, when needed, cytoreduction, is a useful tool to assess the prognosis of the patients (both with and without peritoneal carcinomatosis). And it can also be useful when deciding whether to choose systemic or intraperitoneal chemotherapy.

In a multivariate analysis, peritoneal cytology appears as an independent predictor for survival in patients with tumors pT3 or pT4 (Peritoneal cytology in colorectal cancer. Noura *et al*: Diseases of the Colon & Rectum. volume 52: 7 2009). Patients with negative cytology results show better five-year survival rates in cases in which at least the serosal layer is affected by the tumor than patients with positive results (68% vs. 20.6%). These results are also reflected in the fact that patients with positive cytology results present a higher rate of peritoneal dissemination than patients with negative cytology results. Some patients with macroscopic peritoneal dissemination and negative cytology have been proven to have survived for a long time (more than 10 years, in some cases); whereas patients with peritoneal dissemination and positive cytology results show five-year survival rates close to zero. When the peritoneal cytology results are positive, monitoring has to be particularly careful in order to obtain an early detection of recurrence (Peritoneal Cytology in Colorectal Cancer. Nishikawa et al. Disease of the Colon and Rectum. Volume 52:12 (2009). All these promising results with regard to peritoneal cytology must be included in the evaluation, prognosis and therapeutic approach, and this requires subsequent prospective studies that homogenize the way in which the cytology is performed (technique, staining, etc.) and its inclusion in the different studies, such as its inclusion in the selection protocols to perform Sugarbaker technique.

7.3. Treatment

Peritoneal carcinomatosis and ascites are usually signs of advanced colorectal cancer, and survival rates, as we have said, are low. However, a more aggressive approach for surgical cytoreduction of the peritoneal disease has been used as in the treatment for ovarian cancer, primary peritoneal cancer and appendicular mucinous tumors such as pseudomyxoma and cystadenocarcinoma, and it shows better results than palliative surgery and conventional chemotherapy by themselves. The extrapolation of these therapies to the treatment of CRC seems inappropriate, because these tumors are biologically different, and they are mainly of a low grade. The arrival of intraperitoneal chemotherapy combined with peritoneal debulking seems to offer an increased survival rate in selected patients with colorectal carcinomatosis. Sugarbaker described in 1995 the surgical techniques that lead, when this is not possible, to a complete resection of the peritoneal neoplastic disease. As in other scenarios of resectable metastatic disease, it is advisable to consolidate the results obtained thanks to surgery with a complementary treatment that eradicates the residual microscopic disease. The intraperitoneal administration of certain cytostatic drugs leads to a higher exposure of the peritoneal surface to the drugs than with the usual systemic administration. The perioperative administration (hypertermia-modulated intraoperative administration and/or early postoperative administration) avoids the difficulties that have been traditionally associated with the intraperitoneal administration of cytostatic drugs (difficulty of access, erratic distribution, pain…), which have been one of the main causes of its poor reception by specialists in medical oncology.

This way, and after decades of preclinical and clinical efforts, cytoreductive surgery combined with preoperative hyperthermic intraperitoneal chemotherapy (HIPEC) appear in this new century as an indissoluble and feasible multimodal strategy with proven effectiveness in the treatment of selected cases of peritoneal carcinomatosis in colorectal cancer, although, as we have said before, it can also be useful for other tumors (González-Moreno S. Cirugía citoreductora y quimioterapia intraperitoneal perioperatoria para las neoplasias con diseminación peritoneal: ha llegado el momento. Cir Esp. 2005;78(6):341-3)(Sugarbaker PH, Mora JT, Carmignani P, Stuart OA, Yoo D. Update on chemotherapeutic agents utilized for perioperative intraperitonealchemotherapy. Oncologist. 2005;10:112-22.)(Treatments and Outcomes of Peritoneal Surface Tumors Through a Centralized National Service (United Kingdom) S. Rout, Diseases Of The Colon & Rectum Volume 52: 10 (2009).

There are protocols for the selection of patients which, among other things, try to establish the mass of the tumor and its location by mapping the abdominal cavity in order to assess the size of the tumor and the possibility of achieving an adequate cytoreduction. Laparoscopy is a technique that is currently included in the treatment protocols when there is suspicion or preoperative evidence of peritoneal carcinomatosis. After obtaining a laparoscopic diagnosis of the affected areas (including images obtained during the process, if possible), the patient is sent to a health centre with experience in cytoreductive surgery and HIPEC in order to assess the procedure (commonly referred to as Sugarbaker technique).

The prognosis and results depend on the level of cytoreduction. It is necessary to take into account the fact that this cytoreduction goes through a peritonectomy and the resection of visceral metastases that sometimes involve several days of surgery, with the corresponding increase of morbidity and mortality. For this reason, it is essential to have specialized or experienced centres when assessing the results.

As we have said, the level of cytoreduction is directly related to the prognosis. The success rate of cytoreduction has been established according to different systems, although it is generally classified as CCR 0 (Completeness of Cancer Resection) when there is no microscopic tumor, CCR 1 when there are no nodes larger than 0.5 cm and CCR 2 when there are clearly visible tumors (more than 0.5 cm). Average survival is 33 months for CCR 0, 12.5 months for CCR 1 and 8.5 months for CCR 2 (Glehen O, Cotte E, Schreiber V, Sayag-Beaujard AC, Vignal J, Gilly FN. Intraperitoneal chemohyperthermia and attempted cytoreductive surgery in patients with peritoneal carcinomatosis of colorectal origin. *Br J Surg*. 2004;91:747–754).

The most commonly used chemotherapeutic agents are mitomycin C and cisplatin combined with 5-FU. These agents are heated to 47-59 ºC and inserted in the peritoneal cavity, which lets the surgeon spread it to all necessary spaces. They are left in the cavity for one hour and a half to two hours, and then they are drained. The catheters are left in place for postoperative drainage (Royal RE, Pingpank JF Jr. Diagnosis and management of peritoneal carcinomatosis arising from adenocarcinoma of the colon and rectum. *Semin Oncol*. 2008;35:183–191).

Morbidity rates in the procedure of cytoreduction and HIPEC are around 30% and 60%, and mortality is less than 2%. Logically, covering the logistic needs for intensive care, chemotherapy and trained surgeons with an established protocol allow for an adequate morbidity and mortality. This therapy must be applied to patients in whom a complete or almost complete cytoreduction can be achieved. With these conditions, the existing studies (although retrospective) show an important improvement of survival, with some results showing a five-year survival rate of 49% when cytoreduction is complete. (Yan TD, Black D, Savady R, Sugarbaker PH. Systematic review on the efficacy of cytoreductive surgery combined with perioperative intraperitoneal chemotherapy for peritoneal carcinomatosis from colorectal carcinoma. *J Clin Oncol*. 2006;24: 4011–409).

It is possible to apply delayed and repeated intraperitoneal systemic chemotherapy after the cytoreduction with acceptable morbidity rates. It is also possible to administer delayed intraperitoneal chemotherapy in up to 83% of the patients who had previously undergone cytoreduction (Delayed Repeated Intraperotoneal Chemotherapy. Fajardo et al. Diseases of Colon and Rectum. Volumen 55.: 10 (2012)).

On the other hand, there are reasons to be optimistic about the use of immunomodulating treatments (targeted monoclonal antibodies) which, when combined with other 'traditional' chemotherapeutic approaches, are showing some really promising results. We still need more studies that let us know what conditions lead to a successful outcome (such as the KRAS status of the primary tumor) and also whether they have a beneficial effect in peritoneal carcinomatosis.

Chemotherapy and targeted therapies: There are currently eight active and approved drugs for patients with metastatic colorectal cancer which are used separately or combined with other drugs:

5-FU, Capecitabine, Irinotecan., Oxaliplatin, Bevacizumab, Cetuximab, Aflibercept and Panitumumab.

These chemotherapeutic agents, some of which are monoclonal antibodies, can be combined in different ways and represent an encouraging future for patients with peritoneal metastases who were previously called 'terminally ill'.

7.4. Treatment of metastatic disease

Initial management of the primary site in patients who present with stage IV disease is controversial, and there are no data from prospective randomized studies to guide treatment. In general, the choice and sequence of treatment is guided by the presence or absence of symptoms from the primary tumor and whether or not the metastases are potentially resectable.

Surgery provides a potentially curative option for selected patients who present with limited metastatic colorectal cancer.

Management in patients with unresectable metastatic disease: systemic and hepatic arterial infusion chemotherapy may be useful treatment options in patients with unresectable disease.

Other established treatment is radiofrequency ablation.

Author details

C. Alberto Blanco[1*], R. Sánchez[2], F. Piniella[3], D. Pescador[3], G. Borobio[3], A. García[3] and C. Cano[3]

*Address all correspondence to: titoberto2002@hotmail.com

1 Hospital Santos Reyes, Aranda de Duero (Burgos), Spain

2 Health Care Centers of Aranda de Duero (Burgos), Ávila, Spain

3 Health Care Centers of Aranda de Duero (Burgos), Salamanca, Spain

References

[1] Hara et al. Comparative analysis of intraperitoneal minimal free cancer cells between colorectal and gastric cancer patients using quantitative RT-PCR: possible reason for rare peritoneal recurrence in colorectal cancer. Clin Exp Metastasis 2007;24:179–89.

[2] Noura et al. Peritoneal cytology in colorectal cancer.: Dis Colon Rectum. Vol 52: 7 (2009)

[3] Koppe et al. Peritoneal carcinomatosis of colorectal origin.. Ann Surg 2006 243: 212-222.

[4] Chu et al. Peritoneal carcinomatosis in nongynecologic malignancy: a prospective study of prognostic factors. *Cancer*. 1989;63:364–367.

[5] Sugarbaker et al. Rationale for integrating early postoperative intraperitoneal chemotherapy into the surgical treatment of gastrointestinal cancer. *Semin Oncol.* 1989;16:83–97.

[6] Sadeghi et al. Peritoneal carcinomatosis from non-gynecologic malignancies: results of the EVOCAPE Multicentric prospective study. *Cancer*. 2000;88: 358–363.

[7] Wagner et al. Eartly postoperative intraperitoneal chemotherapy folloeonng cytoreductive surgery for appendiceal mucinous neoplasms with isolated peritoneal metastasis. Dis Colon Rectum Vol 55: 4 (2012) 407-415.

[8] Mahteme et al. Improve survival in patients with peritoneal metastases from colorectal cancer: a preliminary study. British Journal of Cancer (2004) 90 403-407.

[9] Nishikawa et al. Peritoneal Cytology in Colorectal Cancer.. Dis Colon Rectum. Vol 52:12 (2009)

[10] González-Moreno S. Cirugía citoreductora y quimioterapia intraperitoneal perioperatoria para las neoplasias con diseminación peritoneal: ha llegado el momento. Cir Esp. 2005 ;78(6):341-343

[11] Sugarbaker et al.. Update on chemotherapeutic agents utilized for perioperative intraperitonealchemotherapy. Oncologist. 2005;10:112-22

[12] Rout et al. Treatments and Outcomes of Peritoneal Surface Tumors Through a Centralized National Service (United Kingdom) Dis Colon Rectum Volume 52: 10 (2009)1705-1715.

[13] Glehen et *al.* Intraperitoneal chemohyperthermia and attempted cytoreductive surgery in patients with peritoneal carcinomatosis of colorectal origin. *Br J Surg.* 2004;91:747–754.

[14] Royal et al.. Diagnosis and management of peritoneal carcinomatosis arising from adenocarcinoma of the colon and rectum. *Semin Oncol.* 2008;35:183–191

[15] Yan et al. Systematic review on the efficacy of cytoreductive surgery combined with perioperative intraperitoneal chemotherapy for peritoneal carcinomatosis from colorectal carcinoma. *J Clin Oncol.* 2006;24: 4011–409.

[16] Fajardo et al. Delayed repeated intraperotoneal chemotherapy.. Dis Colon Rectum. Vol 55.: 10 (2012);1044-1052

[17] Soumaoro et al. Coexpression of VEGF-C and Cox-2 in Human Colorectal Cancer and its Association With Lymph Node Metastasis Dis Colon Rectum, March 2006 vol 49, nº 3; 392-398.

[18] Óberg, A. e*t al.* Are lymph node micrometastases of any clinical significance in Dukes stages A and B colorectal cancer? Dis Colon Rectum, October 1998 Vol 41, No. 10 1244-1249.

[19] Edge SB, Byrd DR, Compton CC, et al., eds.: AJCC Cancer Staging Manual. 7th ed. New York, NY: Springer, 2010, pp 143-64.

[20] Wong et al. Staging accuracy in colorectal carcinoma. Journal of Clinical Oncology. Vol 17. nº 9 (1999) 2896-2900.

[21] Wang et al. Curative resection of T1 colorectal carcinoma: risk of lymph node metastasis and long-term prognosis. Dis Colon Rectum June 2005. Vol 48, No. 6, 1182-1192.

[22] Kelder et al. Impact of the number of histologically examined lymph nodes on prognosis in colon cancer: a population-based study in the Netherlands. Dis Colon Rectum. Vol. 52 (2009); 260-267.

[23] J. Gastroenterol Heptol 6:325-244. 1991

[24] Park et al. Comparative analisis of limph node metastasis in patients with ypT0-2 rectal cancers after neoadjuvant chemoradiotherapy. Dis Colon Rectum. Vol 56: 2 (2013).135-141.

[25] Sardon et al. Técnica del ganglio centinela en el cáncer de colon. Experiencia en 125 casos.CIR ESP. 2013; 91(6) 366-371

[26] Watanabe et *al*. Heterogeneity of KRAS status may explain the subset of discordant KRAS status between primary and metastatic colorectal cancer. Dis Colon Rectum Vol 54: 9(2011) 1170-1178.

[27] Faerden et al. Sentinel node mapping in colonic cancer Dis Colon Rectum. Vol 51: (2008) 891–896

[28] (2013). "Rectal Cancer." *National Comprehensive Cancer Network (NCCN) guidelines* Retrieved Jun 30, 2013, from www.nccn.org.

[29] Ambiru, S., M. Miyazaki, H. Ito, K. Nakagawa, H. Shimizu, A. Kato, S. Nakamura, H. Omoto and N. Nakajima (1998). "Resection of Hepatic and Pulmonary Metastases in Patients with Colorectal Carcinoma." *Cancer* 82(2): 274-278.

[30] Carballo, M., M. S. Maish, D. E. Jaroszewski and C. E. Holmes (2009). "Video-Assisted Thoracic Surgery (Vats) as a Safe Alternative for the Resection of Pulmonary Metastases: A Retrospective Cohort Study." *J Cardiothorac Surg* 4: 13.

[31] Collie, D. A., A. R. Wright, J. R. Williams, B. Hashemi-Malayeri, A. J. Stevenson and C. M. Turnbull (1994). "Comparison of Spiral-Acquisition Computed Tomography and Conventional Computed Tomography in the Assessment of Pulmonary Metastatic Disease." *Br J Radiol* 67(797): 436-444.

[32] Ehrenhaft, J. L., M. S. Lawrence and D. M. Sensenig (1958). "Pulmonary Resections for Metastatic Lesions." *A.M.A. archives of surgery* 77(4): 606-612.

[33] Fiorentino, F., I. Hunt, K. Teoh, T. Treasure and M. Utley (2010). "Pulmonary Metastasectomy in Colorectal Cancer: A Systematic Review and Quantitative Synthesis." *J R Soc Med* 103(2): 60-66.

[34] Gonzalez, M., A. Poncet, C. Combescure, J. Robert, H. B. Ris and P. Gervaz (2013). "Risk Factors for Survival after Lung Metastasectomy in Colorectal Cancer Patients: A Systematic Review and Meta-Analysis." *Ann Surg Oncol* 20(2): 572-579.

[35] Greelish, J. P. and J. S. Friedberg (2000). "Secondary Pulmonary Malignancy." *Surg Clin North Am* 80(2): 633-657.

[36] Hellman, S. and R. R. Weichselbaum (1995). "Oligometastases." *J Clin Oncol* 13(1): 8-10.

[37] 10. Hendriks, J. M., S. Romijn, B. Van Putte, E. Eyskens, J. B. Vermorken, E. Van Marck and P. E. Van Schil (2001). "Long-Term Results of Surgical Resection of Lung Metastases." *Acta Chir Belg* 101(6): 267-272.

[38] Inoue, M., Y. Kotake, K. Nakagawa, K. Fujiwara, K. Fukuhara and T. Yasumitsu (2000). "Surgery for Pulmonary Metastases from Colorectal Carcinoma." *Ann Thorac Surg* 70(2): 380-383.

[39] Irshad, K., F. Ahmad, J. E. Morin and D. S. Mulder (2001). "Pulmonary Metastases from Colorectal Cancer: 25 Years of Experience." *Can J Surg* 44(3): 217-221.

[40] Jaklitsch, M. T., C. M. Mery, J. M. Lukanich, W. G. Richards, R. Bueno, S. J. Swanson, S. J. Mentzer, B. D. Davis, E. N. Allred and D. J. Sugarbaker (2001). "Sequential Thoracic Metastasectomy Prolongs Survival by Re-Establishing Local Control within the Chest." *J Thorac Cardiovasc Surg* 121(4): 657-667.

[41] Kondo, H., T. Okumura, Y. Ohde and K. Nakagawa (2005). "Surgical Treatment for Metastatic Malignancies. Pulmonary Metastasis: Indications and Outcomes." *Int J Clin Oncol* 10(2): 81-85.

[42] Martini, N. and P. M. McCormack (1998). "Evolution of the Surgical Management of Pulmonary Metastases." *Chest Surg Clin N Am* 8(1): 13-27.

[43] McAfee, M. K., M. S. Allen, V. F. Trastek, D. M. Ilstrup, C. Deschamps and P. C. Pairolero (1992). "Colorectal Lung Metastases: Results of Surgical Excision." *Ann Thorac Surg* 53(5): 780-785; discussion 785-786.

[44] Mery, C. M., A. N. Pappas, R. Bueno, S. J. Mentzer, J. M. Lukanich, D. J. Sugarbaker and M. T. Jaklitsch (2004). "Relationship between a History of Antecedent Cancer and the Probability of Malignancy for a Solitary Pulmonary Nodule." *Chest* 125(6): 2175-2181.

[45] Pfannschmidt, J., H. Dienemann and H. Hoffmann (2007). "Surgical Resection of Pulmonary Metastases from Colorectal Cancer: A Systematic Review of Published Series." *Ann Thorac Surg* 84(1): 324-338.

[46] Pfannschmidt, J., H. Hoffmann and H. Dienemann (2010). "Reported Outcome Factors for Pulmonary Resection in Metastatic Colorectal Cancer." *J Thorac Oncol* 5(6 Suppl 2): S172-178.

[47] Pfannschmidt, J., T. Muley, H. Hoffmann and H. Dienemann (2003). "Prognostic Factors and Survival after Complete Resection of Pulmonary Metastases from Colorectal Carcinoma: Experiences in 167 Patients." *J Thorac Cardiovasc Surg* 126(3): 732-739.

[48] Poston, G. J., D. Tait, S. O'Connell, A. Bennett and S. Berendse (2011). "Diagnosis and Management of Colorectal Cancer: Summary of Nice Guidance." *BMJ* 343: d6751.

[49] Quiros, R. M. and W. J. Scott (2008). "Surgical Treatment of Metastatic Disease to the Lung." *Semin Oncol* 35(2): 134-146.

[50] Regnard, J. F., D. Grunenwald, L. Spaggiari, P. Girard, D. Elias, M. Ducreux, P. Baldeyrou and P. Levasseur (1998). "Surgical Treatment of Hepatic and Pulmonary

Metastases from Colorectal Cancers." *Ann Thorac Surg* 66(1): 214-218; discussion 218-219.

[51] Reinhardt, M. J., N. Wiethoelter, A. Matthies, A. Y. Joe, H. Strunk, U. Jaeger and H. J. Biersack (2006). "Pet Recognition of Pulmonary Metastases on Pet/Ct Imaging: Impact of Attenuation-Corrected and Non-Attenuation-Corrected Pet Images." *Eur J Nucl Med Mol Imaging* 33(2): 134-139.

[52] Remy-Jardin, M., J. Remy, F. Giraud and C. H. Marquette (1993). "Pulmonary Nodules: Detection with Thick-Section Spiral Ct Versus Conventional Ct." *Radiology* 187(2): 513-520.

[53] Rena, O., C. Casadio, F. Viano, R. Cristofori, E. Ruffini, P. L. Filosso and G. Maggi (2002). "Pulmonary Resection for Metastases from Colorectal Cancer: Factors Influencing Prognosis. Twenty-Year Experience." *Eur J Cardiothorac Surg* 21(5): 906-912.

[54] Saisho, S., M. Nakata, S. Sawada, M. Yamashita, H. Saeki, A. Kurita and S. Takashima (2009). "Evaluation of Video-Assisted Thoracoscopic Surgery for Pulmonary Metastases: 11-Years of Experience." *Surg Endosc* 23(1): 55-61.

[55] Sakamoto, T., N. Tsubota, K. Iwanaga, T. Yuki, H. Matsuoka and M. Yoshimura (2001). "Pulmonary Resection for Metastases from Colorectal Cancer." *Chest* 119(4): 1069-1072.

[56] Salah, S., K. Watanabe, J. S. Park, A. Addasi, J. W. Park, J. Zabaleta, F. Ardissone, J. Kim, M. Riquet, K. Nojiri, M. Gisabella, S. Y. Kim and K. Tanaka (2013). "Repeated Resection of Colorectal Cancer Pulmonary Oligometastases: Pooled Analysis and Prognostic Assessment." *Ann Surg Oncol* 20(6): 1955-1961.

[57] Salah, S., K. Watanabe, S. Welter, J. S. Park, J. W. Park, J. Zabaleta, F. Ardissone, J. Kim, M. Riquet, K. Nojiri, M. Gisabella, S. Y. Kim, K. Tanaka and B. Al-Haj Ali (2012). "Colorectal Cancer Pulmonary Oligometastases: Pooled Analysis and Construction of a Clinical Lung Metastasectomy Prognostic Model." *Ann Oncol* 23(10): 2649-2655.

[58] Villeneuve, P. J. and R. S. Sundaresan (2009). "Surgical Management of Colorectal Lung Metastasis." *Clin Colon Rectal Surg* 22(4): 233-241.

[59] Weichselbaum, R. R. and S. Hellman (2011). "Oligometastases Revisited." *Nature reviews. Clinical oncology* 8(6): 378-382.

[60] Yano, T., N. Hara, Y. Ichinose, H. Yokoyama, T. Miura and M. Ohta (1993). "Results of Pulmonary Resection of Metastatic Colorectal Cancer and Its Application." *J Thorac Cardiovasc Surg* 106(5): 875-879.

[61] Igor T. Gavrilovic and Jerome B. PosnerJournal of Neuro-Oncology (2005) 75: 5–14 _ Springer 2005

[62] Tim J. Kruser, Samuel T. Chao,Paul Elson, Gene H. Barnett,Michael A. Vogelbaum, Lilyana Angelov, Robert J. Weil, Robert Pelley, John H. Su CANCER July 1, 2008 / Volume 113 / Number 1

[63] Germán Borobio León, Asunción García Plaza, Roberto González Alconada, Ignacio García Cepeda, Jorge López Olmedo, Alberto Moreno Regidor and David Pescador Hernández A Multidisciplinary Approach to Management, Dr. Giulio A. Santoro

[64] Borobio León, G; García Plaza, A; García Cepeda, I; González Alconada, R.; Hernández Cosido, L. (2010). Metástasis en mano de adenocarcinoma de recto. Un caso excepcional. *Cirugía Española 2010;88:195-7.-vol. 88 núm. 03*

[65] Bonnheim, D.C; Petrelli, N.J; Herrera, L.; Walsh, D; Mittelman, A.(1986). Osseous metastases from colorectal carcinoma. *Am J Surg*, vol. 151(4), (April 1986), 457-459.

[66] Chang, H.C; Lew, K.H; Low, C.O .(2001). Metastasis of an adenocarcinoma of the stomach to the 4th metacarpal bone. *Hand Surgery 2001 December; 6(2): 239-242.*

[67] Clohisy, DR; Perkins, SL; Ramnaraine ML. Review of cellular mechanisms of tumor osteolysis (2000). *Clin Orthop 2000;3743:104-114*

[68] Desmanet, E; Amrani, M; Fievez, R; Six Ch. Les acrométastases. A propos de deux cas.(1991). *Revue de la littérature. Ann Chir Main 1991; 10, nº2: 154-157.*

[69] Flynn, CJ; Danjoux, C; Wong, J; Christakis, M; Rubenstein, J; Yee, A; et al.(2008). Two cases of acrometastasis to the hands and review of the literature. *Curr Oncol 2008 October; 15 (5): 51-58.*

[70] Galasko, CS. Diagnosis of skeletal metastases and assessment of response to treatment.(1995). *Clin Orthop 1995;312:64-75*

[71] García Plaza, A. (2003). *Aspectos terapéuticos y pronósticos del carcinoma colorrectal.* Ediciones Universidad de Salamanca. (Marzo 2003). Colección Vitor 105.

[72] Healey, J.H; Turnbull, A.D; Miedema, M; Lane, J.M.(1986). Acrometastases. A study of twenty-nine patients with osseous involvement of the hands and feet. *.J Bone Joint Surg Am. 1986; 68:743-746.*

[73] Kose, F; Sakalli, H ; Sezer, A; Mertsoylu, H; Pourbagher, A; Reyhan, M; Ozyilkan, O. (2008). Colon adenocarcinoma and solitary tibia metastasis: Rare entity. *J Gastrointest Canc*, vol.39, (February 2008), 146-148.

[74] Méndez López, JM; García Mas, R; Salvà Coll, G. (1997). Metastasis of an adenocarcinoma of the colon to the 1st metacarpal bone. *Ann Chir Main Memb Super 1997; 16(2): 134-7.*

[75] Mundy, JR & Yoneda, T. Facilitation and supresion of bone metastasis (1995). *Clin Orthop 1995;312:34-44*

[76] Nozue, M; Oshiro, Y; Kurata, M; Seino, K; Koike, N; Kawamoto, T et al (2002). Treatment and prognosis in colorectal cancer patients with bone metastasis. *Oncol Rep 2002 Jan-Feb; 9(1): 109-112.*

[77] Ross, J.R; Saunders ,Y; Edmonds, P.M; Patel, S; Wonderling, D; Normand, C. (2004). A systematic review of the role of bisphosphonates in metastatic disease. *Health Technol Assess*. vol 8. (August 2004). 1-176.

[78] Roth, E.S; Fetzer, D.T; Barron,B.J; Usha, A; Joseph, U. A; Isis, W; Gayed, I. W; Wan, D.Q. (2009). Does colon cancer ever metastasize to bone first? a temporal analysis of colorectal cancer progression. *BMC Cancer*. vol. 9, (August 2009), 274.

[79] Schlüter, K; Gassmann, P; Enns, A.(2006) Organ-Specific Metastatic Tumor Cell Adhesion and Extravasation of Colon Carcinoma Cells with Different Metastatic Potential. *The American Journal of Pathology. vol.169,* (September 2006),1064–1073.

[80] Schlüter, K; Gassmann, P; Enns, A; Korb, T; Hemping-Bovenkerk, A; Hölzen, J; Haier,J. (2006). Organ-Specific Metastatic Tumor Cell Adhesion and Extravasation of Colon Carcinoma Cells with Different Metastatic Potential. *American Journal of Pathology.* Vol 169, (September 2006), 1064-1073.

[81] Spiteri, V; Bibra, A; Ashwood, N; Cobb, J. Managing acrometastases treatment strategy with a case illustration (2008). *Ann R Coll Surg Engl 2008 October; 90(7): 8-11.*

[82] Sundermeyer, M. L; Meropol, N.J; Rogatko, A; Wang, H; Cohen, S.J. (2004). Changing patterns of colorectal cancer metastases: A 10-year retrospective review. *Journal of Clinical Oncology*, vol 22, nº 14S ,(July 15 Supplement 2004), 3548.

[83] Sundermeyer, M. L; Meropol, N.J; Rogatko, A; Wang, H; Cohen, S.J. (2005).Changing Patterns of Bone and Brain Metastases in Patients with Colorectal Cancer. Clinical Colorrectal Cancer. vol 5, nº 2 (July 2005). 108-113. www.intechopen.

Chapter 10

New Strategies to Enhance the Efficacy of Surgical Treatment for Colorectal Liver Metastasis

Teodoro Palomares, Ana Alonso-Varona,
Ignacio García-Alonso and Vicente Portugal

Additional information is available at the end of the chapter

http://dx.doi.org/10.5772/57326

1. Introduction

Colorectal cancer (CRC) is the second most common cause of cancer death worldwide [1]. The liver is the most frequent site of metastasis in CRC, both at the time of diagnosis (15-20% of cases) and after apparently radical surgery on the primary tumour (nearly 40% of cases). If patients with colorectal liver metastasis (CRC-LM) are not treated, prognosis is very poor, with a near zero five-year survival rate. At present, liver resection is the only treatment modality that has the potential to achieve long-term survival and to offer the possibility of a cure. Patients who undergo complete (R0) resection of liver metastases have a five-year survival rate of approximately 40-50% [2]. Unfortunately, however, 50% to 70% of patients develop secondary metastatic disease after R0-resection of CRC-LM [3].

In order to obtain the best results in a systemic disease such as metastatic CRC (mCRC), the optimal integration of medical treatment and surgery is essential. The introduction of several effective cytotoxic and targeting agents, in combination with surgical treatment, has extended survival [4]. In addition, promising emerging therapies –cancer stem cell (CSC)-targeted therapies, pathway inhibitors for CRC, induction of tumour cell differentiation, improving liver regeneration, and nanoparticle (NP)-guided tumour ablation, among others– may be found to be effective in achieving better control and even complete eradication of CRC-LM. If confirmed, these strategies will bring significant benefits to patients, particularly in terms of long-term survival. Further, in this era of multimodality treatment of CRC, it is critically important to identify effective biomarkers for prognosis and prediction of individual treatment responses, and these are expected to become useful tools for improving therapeutic approaches.

The present chapter aims i, to present the state of the art related to criteria for appropriate decision making for CRC-LM treatment; ii, to review the current data on the role of biomarkers used for the prediction of response to CRC-LM therapies; and iii, to outline emerging targeting agents and new therapeutic techniques to improve life expectancy and quality of life in CRC-LM patients.

2. Therapeutic approaches to colorectal liver metastases: The state of the art

More than half of patients with CRC will develop liver metastases, and nearly 80% of them are initially unresectable. Hence, optimal management of hepatic metastases often requires a multidisciplinary approach. The availability of new medical therapies, including neoadjuvant chemotherapy and targeted therapies, render a considerable percentage (up to 40%) of initially unresectable patients potentially resectable, improving the overall outcomes of patients with mCRC.

Nowadays, to optimise the integration between surgery and medical approaches in the treatment of mCRC it is necessary to consider different groups, based on current guidelines for stratification of patients according to clinical goals and treatment. In this section, we summarise the recommended therapeutic approaches for CRC-LM according to the afore-mentioned patient stratification.

2.1. Selection criteria for resection of colorectal liver metastases: Definition of resectability

Patients diagnosed with mCRC should undergo an upfront evaluation by a multidisciplinary team, including medical oncologists, surgeons, radiotherapists and radiologists, in order to assess resectability status and to achieve the best therapeutic results [5]. The target end point for assessing resectability is the potential of surgery to cure the disease when achieving RO resection of all evident disease. Incomplete resection (macroscopic or microscopic), so-called debulking surgery, has not been found to help achieve this end point [6].

Classically, surgical criteria have determined resectability [7], but over recent years several authors have questioned the relevance of many of them. Nowadays, the only surgical criteria that continue to be widely used are complete tumour resection with the preservation of two contiguous liver segments (with adequate vascular inflow and outflow) and an adequate liver remnant (at least 25% of the total liver volume considering the healthy organ) [8]. If, however, we seek a more comprehensive definition of resectability, we should also take into account prognostic evaluation and predicted response to different treatments, by including multiple clinical and molecular factors, which influence patient outcome. Some validated clinical scores are already available, while molecular factors are still under investigation (discussed in more detail below in the section entitled *Predictive biomarkers for response to treatment in colorectal cancer*. In relation to this, the study conducted by Fong *et al.* [9]at the Memorial-Sloan Kettering Cancer Center has been one of the most useful attempts to define prognosis after surgical management of CRC-LM. The score proposed integrates a range of risk factors which influence the risk of death after surgery: preoperative carcinoembryonic antigen (CEA) level > 200 ng/ml, synchronous metastases or metachronous metastases with a disease-free interval of less than twelve months, more than one metastasis, extrahepatic disease, a tumour > 5 cm in diameter and lymph node involvement associated with the primary tumour.

Over recent years, several studies, well summarised in the systematic review of Quan *et al.* [10], have investigated the validity of these various criteria. Notably, the value of the following indicators have been questioned: the number of lesions, maximum lesion dimensions, timing of metastases, absence of metastatic spread outside the liver, and margin of healthy liver tissue, as has the definition of an adequate liver remnant after resection [11].

In summary, the criteria listed in this section can be regarded as an invaluable tool for patient stratification before liver resection, but failure to meet them should not constitute an absolute contraindication to surgery.

2.2. Optimal chemotherapy timing and regimes

In the case of resectable CRC-LM, current guidelines recommend the administration of a course of an active systemic chemotherapy regimen for a total perioperative treatment time of approximately six months [12]. The preferred regimens are combination chemotherapy based on fluoropyrimidines XELOX (capecitabine plus oxaliplatin), FOLFOX (5-fluorouracil, leucovorin and oxaliplatin) and FOLFIRI (5-fluorouracil, leucovorin and irinotecan), optionally together with antiangiogenic biological agents (bevacizumab, cetuximab or panitumumab). In order to improve the selection of the regimen to be used, KRAS mutation status should be determined in all patients at the time of diagnosis of metastatic disease. If no KRAS mutations are identified, BRAF testing should be considered [13]. New targeting biological agents are emerging and they can be expected to lead to improvements in clinical effectiveness. Their effects, pathways and theoretical and practical applications will be discussed in more detail below in the section entitled *Emerging targeting agents for colorectal liver metastases*.

In patients with few metastases that are easy to surgically resect and no poor prognostic indicators, postoperative chemotherapy is usually preferred [14]. On the other hand, in other clinical situations, perioperative (neoadjuvant plus postoperative) chemotherapy can be used [15]. The optimal sequencing of chemotherapy is not clear, however, and recent studies have assessed the pros and cons of different possible timings of administration [16-17]. Potential advantages of administering chemotherapy preoperatively include earlier treatment of micrometastatic disease, evaluation of responsiveness to chemotherapy (which can be prognostic and help decision making) and avoidance of surgery in patients who progress early. On the other hand, several disadvantages have also been highlighted: the risk of missing the window of opportunity for resection, which may be due to disease progression or due to a complete response making it difficult to identify areas for resection; radiological complete response does not always mean pathological response, as viable cancer cells can remain at the original sites of metastases [18]; hepatotoxicity develops with some regimens with serious clinical implications both before and after surgery [19]; and finally, frequent radiological examinations must be undertaken to determine the appropriate timing for surgery [20]. There is now a general trend towards the use of perioperative chemotherapy for patients with resectable CRC-LM, but more studies are necessary to provide stronger evidence regarding the benefit of this approach.

It is important to note that patients diagnosed with rectal cancer and resectable synchronous liver metastases usually need a specific approach due to the risk of locoregional failure. Preoperative chemoradiotherapy in locally advanced rectal tumours (cT3/4, cN+) decreases the risk of pelvic recurrence after surgery, and postoperative chemotherapy is also mandatory [21]. Some studies suggest that pelvic radiotherapy diminishes tolerance to biological agents, but there is not enough data to guide decisions on when this approach may be suitable. After surgical resection of metastases and rectal lesions, pathological rectal disease determines adjuvant therapy. Specifically, postoperative chemoradiotherapy is advised for patients who have not received prior chemoradiation and have a higher risk of pelvic recurrence (pT3/4 or pN1/2) [22]. Patients with pT1-2pN0 tumours should receive six months of adjuvant chemotherapy without pelvic radiation.

In brief, the choices of type of chemotherapy/chemoradiotherapy regimen and its timing depend on a number of factors, namely a patient's disease history and pathological status, tumour gene expression, and previous treatment (including chemotherapy and associated drug toxicity/safety), as well as institutional preferences.

2.3. Conversion or downsizing chemotherapy

When patients present initially unresectable disease, owing to technical difficulties and/or the presence of poor prognostic factors, treatment decisions are difficult. In this clinical situation, preoperative chemotherapy is being considered in highly selected cases in an attempt to downsize CRC-LM and convert them to a resectable status. In these cases, any active metastatic chemotherapy regimen can be used, the goal being to reduce the size of the visible metastases as much as possible. Several trials have been conducted using different combinations of chemotherapy and biological agents, but they have not provided compelling evidence to favour one regimen over another [23-24].

Further, there are other factors we must keep in mind when considering this kind of treatment. Some chemotherapy regimens may cause hepatotoxicity (steatohepatitis and sinusoidal liver injury, among others) [25]with clinical implications for liver surgery, and we must measure responsiveness, so radiological and clinical reassessment should be scheduled approximately every two months after the initiation of chemotherapy. If the disease becomes resectable, surgery should be performed as soon as possible, in order to limit toxicity.

In addition, we must optimise imaging of CRC-LM choosing the most accurate methods. Radiological imaging techniques, namely computed tomography (CT), magnetic resonance imaging (MRI), and positron emission tomography-PET/CT in selected cases, are the essential tools to measure patient tumour response and resectability, while intraoperative ultrasonography (IOUS) remains mandatory in all patients undergoing surgical resection of CRC-LM. Indeed, several authors have demonstrated that IOUS can change the surgical management in up to 35% of patients [26-27].

Furthermore, it must be taken into account that sometimes a radiological complete response can be achieved in patients with one or more metastases. However, a systematic review of the literature suggests that between 17 and 51% of such patients will have residual microscopic disease [28-29]. Accordingly, all liver metastases, including those with radiological complete response after chemotherapy, should be resected when technically feasible. In addition, almost all authors recommend postoperative chemotherapy in these cases.

Overall, recent studies have reported that resectability is achieved in 10 to 40% of selected patients after chemotherapy. It remains difficult, however, to draw firm conclusions as the definition of unresectable disease, patient selection criteria, drug regimens, and outcome measures vary, and there is insufficient data from randomised controlled trials [10].

2.4. Surgical strategy

Liver resection remains the only treatment modality that can achieve long-term survival and offers a possibility of a cure [2]. Selection criteria for resection of CRC-LM are continually being refined (see the aforementioned *Definition of resectability*). In this field, advances in surgical strategy (timing, techniques, etc.) have improved results, but patient management is complex and tends to require a combination of different approaches (colorectal resection, liver resection, chemotherapy, and radiotherapy, among others).

At present, when oncology committees evaluate CRC-LM for surgical treatment, several clinical scenarios are considered: resectable synchronous metastases, resectable metachronous metastases and unresectable disease amenable to conversion chemotherapy.

2.4.1. Resectable synchronous metastases

Close to a third (15-34%) of patients have liver metastases at the time of diagnosis (synchronous metastases). Evidence-based protocols for the management of synchronous metastases are, however, poor, and few prospective studies have been published recently, such results as are available being difficult to generalise [30]. In any case, some suggestions can be made.

One of the open questions is the timing of colorectal and liver surgery (simultaneous versus staged). The traditional approach has been to perform surgery on the primary lesions (colorectal resection), followed by chemotherapy and subsequent liver surgery. Nowadays, simultaneous colorectal and liver resections are preferred when feasible [31]. This combined surgery can be safely performed whenever minor hepatectomies are planned, but there is no consensus on the best approach in cases requiring major hepatectomies. Considering the largest series, some show similar rates in simultaneous and staged resections [32], but a multicentre database analysis in the USA found increased morbidity and mortality after simultaneous major hepatectomy and colorectal resection [33]. Thus, in the absence of clear evidence, the decision to undertake more complex procedures must be made on a case-by-case basis. Even though surgery is the key treatment in patients with CRC-LM, chemotherapy (and sometimes radiotherapy) must also be administered. The sequencing of chemotherapy has been discussed above, and often influences surgical timing.

On the other hand, we should not forget that patients with synchronous metastases have a poorer prognosis [34]. Various strategies have been proposed in an attempt to improve results. One possibility, suggested by Mentha *et al.* [35], is a change in the treatment sequence, the so-called reverse approach, which consists of treatment with systemic chemotherapy followed by liver resection and subsequent primary tumour treatment (with the option of radiotherapy of the rectal tumour prior to resection). More recently, Bruquet *et al.* [36], have reported their experience at the MD Anderson Cancer Center comparing the traditional approach, combined or simultaneous resection, and a "reverse" strategy. These authors found similar oncological outcomes, morbidity and mortality with the three options. This lack of strong evidence makes us cautious, but we believe that the reverse strategy can be considered a reasonable option in patients with asymptomatic primary CRC but advanced CRC-LM.

2.4.2. Resectable metachronous metastases

Most patients with CRC-LM (2/3 of cases) develop liver metastases after initial treatment, during the course of the disease (metachronous metastases). The management of resectable metachronous disease is distinct from that of synchronous disease, though it should also include diagnostic imaging of CRC-LM, as well as evaluation of the chemotherapy and surgical history.

In this group of patients, PET/CT should be considered preoperatively to characterise the extent of metastatic disease and to identify possible sites of extrahepatic disease that could preclude surgery [37]. In addition, it is important to evaluate previous chemotherapy to guide the choice of regimen. In general, six months of perioperative (pre- and/or postoperative) chemotherapy is recommended, but in selected cases observation is also considered appropriate. In addition, previous hepatotoxicity and other side effects should be taken into account [12].

In relation to the type of surgery to be performed, previous surgery can preclude surgical treatment of metachronous metastases, especially if upfront liver resection was performed, it being necessary to assess the remnant liver and technical difficulties. Finally, recent data suggest that it is safe to adopt a surgical approach to the treatment of recurrent hepatic disease isolated to the liver, but that survival decreases with each subsequent curative surgical approach [38].

2.4.3. Unresectable disease amenable to conversion chemotherapy

In this clinical situation, preoperative chemotherapy is considered in highly selected cases, with the aim of downsizing CRC-LM [39]. After disease becomes resectable, surgery should be performed as soon as possible and all liver metastases, including those with radiographic complete response after chemotherapy, should be resected when technically feasible [10]. The treatment of the primary tumour can be postponed until the completion of adjuvant therapy [36].

2.4.4. New surgical techniques

A feasible approach has emerged for patients who would be left with an inadequate future liver remnant (FLR) if complete disease clearance were to be attempted with a single hepatectomy: this is a two-stage hepatectomy for bilobular liver metastases in combination with selected use of portal venous embolization. It offers the best chance of achieving an adequate degree of liver remnant hypertrophy, being more effective than portal venous embolization before a single hepatectomy [40].

Although the standard of care for resectable liver metastases is surgical resection, in selected patients other liver-directed therapies can be used in addition to or instead of surgical resection. These include intrahepatic arterial chemotherapy [41], radiofrequency tumour ablation [42], radioembolization [43]and stereotactic external beam radiation [44]. Some of these innovative techniques will be discussed in more depth below in the section entitled *New therapeutic techniques for colorectal liver metastases*.

3. Predictive biomarkers for response to treatment in colorectal cancer

Over the past decade, developments in CRC-LM therapy have improved the prognosis of patients. Combination chemotherapy, such as FOLFOX or FOLFIRI, has become the standard regimen for unresectable advanced or recurrent CRC, and high response rates have been reported. On the other hand, not all patients respond well to these therapies, and it has been suggested that differential responses are due to the specific molecular profile of each patient and/or tumour. To facilitate the design of personalised therapeutic strategies for CRC patients, it is therefore important to identify biomarkers which are able to accurately predict the sensitivity of patients to the potential therapies and to estimate the likely course of the illness.

Recent advances in the fields of genomics and proteomics have contributed to our understanding of CRC at the molecular level by evaluating the expression profiles of genes and proteins in tissues and body fluids. To date, some of the candidate biomarkers have yielded somewhat contradictory results. On the other hand, several studies have identified candidate molecular biomarkers that may help to predict the response to cytotoxic chemotherapy and guide treatment selection.

3.1. Molecular predictors of response to chemotherapy

5-Flurouracil (5-FU) is the main stay of all current standard CRC chemotherapy regimens, despite the fact that it causes serious side effects (grade 3 or 4) in up to 30% of patients. Several enzymes involved in 5-FU metabolism have been proposed as predictors of response to fluopyrimidine treatment: 5-FU exerts its activity by inhibiting thymidylate synthase (TS), a key enzyme of nucleotide pyrimidine metabolism that is essential for DNA synthesis and cellular proliferation. Thymidine phosphorylase (TP) is another enzyme involved in thymidine metabolism, which regulates the conversion of thymine to thymidine; this is why it is thought to limit the toxicity of high levels of thymidine and prevent replication errors during DNA synthesis. In this role, TP degrades 5-FU, limiting the activity of this chemotherapeutic agent. Dihydropyridimine dehydrogenase (DPD) is a rate-limiting hepatic enzyme involved in the catabolism of 5-FU [45]. It was found that low levels of expression of TP, DPD and TS were independently associated with improved overall survival [46]. Specifically, deficiency in DPD activity caused by mutations in the gene encoding DPD (the *DYPD* gene) can lead to severe 5-FU-related toxicities, which can be fatal. However, as mutations in the *DPYD* gene are responsible for only some of the adverse reactions to 5-FU and the association between genotype and phenotype is not clear [47], further assay development and prospective trials are needed to evaluate the clinical usefulness of these enzymes in predicting which patients are likely to develop serious, life-threatening toxicity to 5-FU [48].*Irinotecan (CPT-11),* a topoisomerase inhibitor, shows efficacy in the treatment of mCRC when used either as a single agent or in combination with radiotherapy and/or other chemotherapeutic drugs. Irinotecan acts as an inhibitor of DNA topoisomerase I (Topo I) and exerts a cytotoxic effect in replicating cells by inducing DNA strand breaks [49]. The active metabolite of irinotecan is SN-38, which is metabolised *in vivo* through conjugation by the liver enzyme uridine diphosphate glucuronosyltransferase (UGT1A1). A variant of the gene encoding this enzyme (UGTA1*28) has come to be considered the main pharmacogenetic marker for severe haematological toxicity (neutropaenia) of the drug. Nevertheless, UGT1A1*28 testing as a predictive marker of adverse effects needs to be further investigated before translation to clinical practice and the available data are not conclusive in defining a precise genotype-based dosage [50-51]. In addition, tumour expression of Topo-I has been explored as a biomarker of the efficacy of irinotecan-based therapies [52]. Although further studies are needed, it has been shown that high levels of Topo-I in tumour tissue are associated with a good response to irinotecan [53-54]; these data are consistent with the hypothesis that a larger amount of Topo I would facilitate the activity of a Topo I inhibitor [55].*Oxaliplatin* is a platinum analogue that improves response rate and survival in patients with advanced CRC. DNA kinking is the major feature of platinum-DNA adducts that block DNA replication and lead to cancer cell death. These DNA strand breaks are recognised and repaired by the nucleotide excision repair (NER) pathway, whose major components are excision repair cross-complementation group (ERCC1 and ERCC2) proteins, acting as the rate-limiting enzymes of oxaliplatin efficacy. Several studies have demonstrated that low levels of ERCC1 and/or ERCC2 gene expression correlate well with better response rates following oxaliplatin-based therapy in advanced CRC patients, leading to improved survival [56-58]. Despite these promising findings, most of the studies have been retrospective and differed significantly in design, and results have not been consistent. Further prospective trials are needed to assess the correlation between decreased expression of *ERCC1* and *ERCC2* and platinum toxicities.

3.2. Molecular predictors of response to anti-EGFR therapy

We should also consider other markers which it has been suggested may be useful for predicting patient responses to biological agents, in particular anti-epidermal growth factor receptor (EGFR) monoclonal therapy. EGFR is a member of the transmembrane tyrosine kinase receptor family ErbB, involved in tumour cell proliferation, inhibition of apoptosis, invasion, migration and angiogenesis [59-60]. When a ligand binds the EGFR homo or hetero-dimers are formed with other ErbB family members, initiating two main intracellular cascades, which are important for cell survival, proliferation and migration. On the one hand, membrane localization of the lipid kinase PIK3CA counteracts PTEN and promotes AKT1 phosphorylation and, on the other, KRAS activates BRAF, which in turn triggers the mitogen-activated protein kinases [61]. Abnormal expression of EGFR has been demonstrated in many advanced tumours, including in breast cancers, gliomas and lung cancer. In the case of mCRC, EGFR overexpression has been detected in 60-80% of cases [59]and a correlation has been reported with early tumour recurrence and extra-hepatic metastasis [62]. For these reasons, researchers started to explore therapeutic strategies to disrupt EGFR function.

Cetuximab, a chimeric IgG1 monoclonal antibody (mAb), and panitumumab, a humanised IgG2 mAb, target the EGFR and have small, but nonetheless clinically important response rates of around 10% in unselected patients with chemotherapy-refractory metastatic CRCs. However, its exact role in the CRC metastatic cascade has not yet been characterised due to controversial results obtained with anti-EGFR antibody therapy. In fact, it has been shown that the response to this therapy is independent of EGFR expression in tumour tissue [63]. In relation to this, some studies suggest that EGFR expression in the primary tumour does not necessarily correspond with the level of expression in metastatic tissue, while other studies have reported 78-100% concordance in EGFR expression in the two tissue compartments [64]. These findings prompted an effort to identify alternative predictive molecular biomarkers that could help to select patients more likely to benefit from anti-EGFR agents. Candidates that have been investigated so far include not only molecular alterations affecting the EGFR, but also molecular events downstream in the pathway, such as aberrations in the interlinked RAS-RAF-mitogen-activated protein kinase and PI3K-AKT-mTOR intracellular signalling transducers.

KRAS encodes for a cytoplasmic GTP-binding protein with low inherent GTPase activity. When the KRAS protein is bound to GTP, it relays signals of cellular proliferation and inhibition of apoptosis, acting as a typical oncogene. Activating mutations in KRAS lead to a gain in function of this gene, and hence over-expression of RAS/RAF-dependent proteins. Specifically, mutations in codons 12 and 13 of exon 2 have been demonstrated to predict low response rate to EGFR monoclonal antibodies-targeted therapy [65]. A lack of efficacy and also a possible detrimental effect on anti-EGFR–based chemotherapy in KRAS-mutated patients have been suggested by some trials using cetuximab in first-line therapy for mCRC, such as OPUS (oxaliplatin plus cetuximab) [66] and CRYSTAL (irinotecan plus cetuximab) [67]. These data indicate that KRAS mutations can be considered a highly specific biomarker to predict poor response to treatment with anti-EGFR mAbs. In addition, due to the fact that anti-EGFR agents fail to achieve either objective responses or disease stabilization in a substantial proportion of patients with wild-type KRAS tumours also, it seems necessary to investigate mutations in other genes involved in signalling pathways downstream of EGFR, including NRAS, BRAF, PIK3CA and PTEN.

Activating mutations in other members of the RAS family are less common than those found in KRAS. For instance, the reported frequency of *NRAS* mutations is 2.2 to 2.6%. Patients with tumours with these mutations had a significantly poorer response rate to anti-EGFR therapy [68], although no significant differences were seen in overall survival between patients with wild-type and mutant *NRAS.*

Mutations in *BRAF,* the major effector of *KRAS,* have also been associated with reduced sensitivity to EGFR-directed therapy. In a retrospective study, Di Nicolantino *et al.*

[69]examined tumours from patients who had received anti-EGFR therapy. They found that none of the patients carrying the BRAF V600E mutation responded and that none of the responders had a BRAF mutation. Moreover, De Roock *et al.* [68]recently conducted a large trial in which they analysed tumour specimens from CRC patients treated with the anti-EGFR agent cetuximab. They found that KRAS and BRAF mutations were mutually exclusive; the *BRAF* mutation was identified in 4.7% of cases and those carrying the mutation had a significantly lower response to anti-EGFR therapy, than those with BRAF wild-type tumours.

The phosphatidylinositol 3-kinase/Akt/mammalian target of rapamycin, *PI3K/AKT/mTOR,* pathway is another major intracellular signalling effector pathway activated by EGFR stimulation. Mutations in this pathway are present in as many as 30-40% of CRC patients. In particular, mutations in PI3KCA have been described in 15% of colon carcinomas, 20% of these being found in exon 20. Patients carrying these mutations and treated with anti-EGFR therapy have poorer clinical outcomes than wild-type PIK3CA carriers. However, because the number of patients with these mutations is very low in most studies, there is a need for controlled trials to assess whether the use of BRAF and PIK3CA mutation analysis as predictors of anti-EGFR therapy efficacy improves clinical outcomes [70].
PTEN is the only tumour suppressor gene involved in the PI3K/AKT-mTOR pathway. Loss of PTEN function, due to mutations, deletions or epigenetic silencing, leads to activation of this pathway. On the other hand, intact PTEN expression in metastatic tissue was found to be predictive of response to cetuximab, while this was not observed in patients with intact PTEN expression in primary tumour tissue [71]. These data are, however, limited and the findings need to be explored in larger confirmatory studies.

3.3. Molecular predictors of response to anti-VEGFR therapy

VEGF is overexpressed in CRC and the level of expression is directly correlated with the development of metastasis [72]. The VEGF family is made up of six growth factors (GFs) which exert their effects via binding to one of the three VEGFRs which belong to the tyrosine kinase receptor (TKR) family, mostly found in endothelial cells and angioblasts [64]. Bevacizumab is a humanised mAb which binds to VEGFA blocking the binding of this GF to VEGFR, thereby avoiding the corresponding intracellular signal transduction. Although several groups have focused their research efforts on finding a biomarker to accurately predict the clinical benefit of adding bevacizumab to therapy, no predictive molecules have yet been identified.

Several candidate predictive biomarkers similar to the KRAS mutation for cetuximab, have been proposed for bevacizumab, but they have remained elusive [73]. Specifically, it has been shown that the efficacy of bevacizumab therapy is independent of KRAS, BRAF and p53 status [74-75].

Another candidate is Ang-2, a regulator of angiogenesis that exerts context-dependent effects on endothelial cells. Although this ligand binds the endothelial-specific receptor tyrosine kinase 2 (TIE2) and acts as a negative regulator of angiogenesis, recent data from analysis of tumours indicate that, under certain conditions, Ang-2 can stimulate endothelial cells, acting as an anti-apoptotic agent in these cells [76]. In this context, serum Ang-2 has been proposed as a candidate biomarker due to the fact that patients having low pre-therapeutic Ang-2 serum levels was significantly associated with response rate after receiving bevacizumab-containing treatment, though results should be further validated [77].

Recently, the development of quantitative predictive biomarkers has led to the increased use of imaging in the evaluation of tumour angiogenesis. Dynamic contrast enhanced-MRI (DCE-MRI) is a technique that can assess tumour perfusion and microvascular vessel wall permeability. Although it is difficult to evaluate the subtle changes occurring during bevacizumab treatment, correlations between tumour grade, microvessel density and VEGF expression in clinical trials of angiogenesis inhibitors have led to DCE-MRI parameters being proposed as biomarkers of drug efficacy [73]. Lastly, some authors have investigated changes in plasma cytokines and angiogenic factors during treatment as potential markers of therapeutic response and resistance [78].

3.4. DNA microarray-based gene expression profiling

Due to the genetic heterogeneity of CRC, many authors agree that it is likely to be necessary to assemble a panel of biomarkers to obtain high enough sensitivity to use these types of biomarkers as a screening test in clinical practice [48, 52]. To date, however, a limited number of markers have been identified in CRC, and their individual use has led to conflicting results.

In this context, advances in genomic techniques, such as DNA microarrays (allowing high-throughput analysis of genes), are very important as they provide large volumes of data which increases the probability of uncovering potential biomarkers. Recently, a total of 66 genes associated with benefit from adjuvant 5-FU/leucovorin treatment were identified. Six of the so-called "chemotherapy benefit genes" were selected to create treatment score algorithms. If validated, these signatures will quantify the likelihood of differential treatment benefit from 5-FU-based therapy [79]. Further, DNA microarray-based gene expression profiling provides a strategy to search systematically for molecular markers of colon cancer. Gene expression analysis studies have already resulted in many new insights into cancer biology and mRNA expression analysis is turning out to be a very useful tool for disease outcome prediction [80-81].

4. Emerging targeting agents for colorectal liver metastasis

The current treatment recommendations for mCRC indicate that therapeutic approach should be multidisciplinary [82], as surgery plus perioperative treatment offers better survival than surgery alone in patients with resectable or potentially resectable disease. Thus, whereas primary surgery is the gold standard for individuals with a single mestatasis, it seems that for multinodular disease, neoadyuvant chemotherapy followed by surgery may be more appropriate [83]. Though in cases of unresectable aggressive disease, treatment should be decided on a case-by-case basis (adapting the strategy to the characteristics of the patient), a multidisciplinary approach should be taken to planning treatment from the outset. In fact, in select unresectable patients chemotherapy allows subsequent rescue surgery and achieves a significant increase in five-year survival rates [39]. An essential aspect of the treatment strategy for advanced CRC is the consideration of treatment as a continuum. Thus, sequential administration of conventional drug combinations based on fluoropyrimidines plus oxaliplatin or irinotecan, results in longer survival. While XELOX, FOLFOX and FOLFIRI are the schemes most commonly used, the trend has been for the standard of care chemotherapy for first-line mCRC to change from FOLFIRI to FOLFOX [84]. In order to improve the poor prognosis of patients with mCRC, treatment intensification has been also tested using the combination of the three active agents 5-FU/leucovorin, oxaliplatin and irinotecan (FOLFOXIRI), and this has achieved increase in R0 secondary resection rate and in overall survival [85]. Other schemes are currently being evaluated in randomised phase II trials as first-line chemotherapy for advanced CRC; these include TOMOX (oxaliplatin plus raltitrexed) which has been found to have a similar efficacy to FOLFOX [86].

The development of new drugs that selectively target specific molecular pathways involved in tumour progression (targeted therapy) has resulted in one of the most important advances in mCRC in the last decade, with biological agents today being a commonly used weapon in the armamentarium against mCRC, particularly in chemorefractory patients and those who are not initially suitable liver resection candidates [87]. In recent years, intense efforts have been focused on developing new molecules to inhibit targets that are critical for CRC, including new anti-angiogenesis agents, novel tyrosine kinase inhibitors (TKIs), agents to act on the PI3K/Akt signalling pathway, modulators of autophagy, and proteasome inhibitors, as well as targeted therapies against cancer stem cells, among others.

4.1. Targeting angiogenesis

GFs have been identified as important targets [88]and the development of targeting biological agents, directed to block effects of GFs on tumour cells, and their integration with cytotoxic chemotherapy regimens has resulted in significant improvements in efficacy outcomes.

One of the most important effects of some GFs is the promotion of angiogenesis, an essential mechanism for both primary tumour growth and metastasis. Due to this, novel therapeutic approaches have focused on the role of angiogenesis-targeting inhibitors. So far, three antiangiogenic biological agents have been approved for the treatment of patients with mCRC: bevacizumab, cetuximab and panitumab. The first successful targeting agent was bevacizumab; today, there is clear evidence to recommend addition of this anti-VEGF antibody to cytotoxic therapy (irrespective of the selected chemotherapy regimen) in both the first- and second-line treatment, this significantly increasing overall survival [75]. Moreover, it has been shown that bevacizumab, combined with FOLFOX or FOLFIRI, may also be active in chemorefractory and selected mCRC patients [89]. Currently, new trials (CHARTA and PERIMAX) are being conducted with bevacizumab plus FOLFIRI, designed to assess the benefits and limitations of a highly active four-drug regimen in mCRC [4]. In addition, it is also important to note that in patients with mCRC on a bevacizumab-containing regimen who show disease progression and hence need a change in the chemotherapy regimen, maintenance therapy with bevacizumab appears to be associated with significantly longer overall survival than the same regimen without bevacizumab [90]; this fact highlights the importance of bevacizumab therapy beyond disease progression in patients with mCRC, although this use is not currently recommended outside clinical trials.

The other two antiangiogenenic biological agents, cetuximab and panitumumab target the ligand-binding domain of EGFR. Signalling of this receptor appears to modulate angiogenesis via the upregulation of VEGF and other angiogenic factors [60]. The use of these EGFR inhibitors was approved for mCRC in patients with wild-type KRAS, whose tumours express EGFR. In fact, as described previously, BRAF and codon 12 KRAS mutations are predictive of adverse outcome in CRC patients receiving cetuximab, being associated with a shorter time to progression and poor survival [91]. In contrast, it has been demonstrated that the combination of chemotherapy, such as irinotecan or FOLFIRI, and cetuximab as a first line in patients with wild-type KRAS significantly improves survival [67, 92]. Cetuximab is also indicated as a monotherapy in such patients following failure of both irinotecan- and oxaliplatin-based chemotherapy [93], while panitumumab is also a valid second-line option for wild-type KRAS patients, as a monotherapy or combined with FOLFIRI [94], though the addition of this EGFR inhibitor to oxaliplatin-based chemotherapy in first-line treatment of mCRC did not improve survival or response rate [95]. In an attempt to increase anti-tumour activity by simultaneously blocking both VEGF and EGFR pathways, some randomised studies have explored the combination of cetuximab or panitumumab with bevacizumab plus chemotherapy, but no benefits were observed, and in some cases the outcome was actually poorer with a greater toxicity, so this type of combination is not recommended for mCRC [64].

In relation to toxicity, treatment with these biological agents is associated with a wide range of adverse events that sometimes require discontinuation of treatment; these include severe hypersensitivity and skin toxicities, in the case of EGFR mAbs, and hypertension, thromboembolic events, bleeding and proteinuria, with bevacizumab treatment [93].

Despite the aforementioned advances, the targeted biological agents currently available are only effective in a small subset of patients (for example, less than half of the KRAS-wild type patient population benefits from anti-EGFR strategies) [96]and their overall impact on the treatment of mCRC has been relatively modest (beneficial effects only lasting on the order of weeks to a few months). These limited results, coupled with the undesirable effects, has led to intensification of the search for novel antiangiogenic therapies to increase the anti-tumour activity in advanced CRC. There are currently several molecules in phase II and III trials for treatment of mCRC that target various members of the VEGF family (aflibercept), signalling by VEGFRs (ramucirumab and IMC-18F1) or the tyrosine kinase components of these receptors (regorafenib, brivanib alaninate, cediranib and linifanib) [93, 97].

Aflibercept is a multiple angiogenic factor trap designed to block the angiogenesis network by binding VEGF-A, VEGF-B and placental growth factor (PLGF) [98]. The recent results of a multinational phase III study (VELOUR trial: aflibercept/FOLFIRI *vs.* placebo/FOLFIRI) demonstrated significant improvements in median overall survival, supporting the use of this VEGF Trap as a second-line option for patients with prior oxaliplatin treatment [99]. Ramucirumab is a fully humanised mAb directed against the extracellular domain of VEGFR-2, which binds VEGF-A and is believed to be the key VEGFR involved in tumour angiogenesis. Like aflibercept, ramucirumab is currently being evaluated in combination with FOLFIRI in a phase III trial for the second-line treatment of mCRC patients for whom prior oxaliplatin- and bevacizumab-containing initial therapy has failed [100]. In addition, a phase II study of ramucirumab in the first-line setting in combination with FOLFOX6 therapy is also in progress [101]. Another anti-VEGFR mAb, IMC-18F1, which targets VEGFR-1 has been developed recently [102], and is also being studied in a phase II trial in mCRC.

Other candidate molecules represent new approaches to intracellular signal blockade of the VEGF and fibroblast growth factor (FGF) signalling pathways, via TKIs. In a recent phase III study (CORRECT trial), regorafenib has been found to improve survival in mCRC patients who progressed after all standard therapies, making it the first small-molecule multikinase inhibitor to have demonstrated survival benefits in such patients [103]. Brivanib alaninate is an oral TKI that specifically inhibits the VEGFR-1 and FGFR. This FGF signalling blockade may represent an important advantage, since it has been suggested that resistance to bevacizumab is associated with increased expression of FGF [78], and hence brivanib could have antiangiogenic activity in bevacizumab-resistant patients. In addition, a phase III trial combining brivanib and cetuximab in second/third line therapy in patients with advanced wild-type *KRAS* mCRC found improved progression free survival with no impact in overall survival [97]. Cediranib is an inhibitor of VEGFRs, platelet-derived growth factor-(PDGF) receptor beta and FGF receptor, whose activity has been compared with that of bevacizumab as a first-line treatment in combination with FOLFOX (HORIZON phase III trial) for mCRC patients; although cediranib activity was comparable to that of bevacizumab, the patient-reported outcomes were significantly less favourable [104]. Similarly, linifanib (a TKI that targets both VEGFRs and PDGFRs), in combination with FOLFOX, did not offer any advantages (over bevacizumab) in a randomised phase II trial as a second-line treatment for mCRC [105].

4.2. Targeting PI3K/Akt/mTOR pathway

The PI3K/Akt/mTOR pathway, an essential regulator of protein translation and cell proliferation, is another important target being investigated for mCRC in phase II and III trials. The PI3K/AKT/mTOR signalling cascade is constitutively active in many types of cancer and, in particular, it plays a critical role in the growth and progression of CRC. In addition, it has been demonstrated that this pathway may be upregulated after blockade of both VEGF- and EGFR-mediated signalling [101].

These aforementioned data provide the rationale for targeting this pathway therapeutically in CRC patients. Perifosine is an oral alkylphospholipid that targets both AKT and nuclear transcription factor-kappa B (NF-κB) pathways. This novel molecule appears to enhance the cytotoxic effects of 5-FU: it has produced promising results in a phase II randomised trial of capecitabine ± perifosine in previously treated patients with mCRC and, hence, is currently in phase III clinical development in combination with this 5-FU prodrug [106].

Activation of the PI3K/AKT cascade promotes mTOR, a serine-threonine kinase whose activation results in cell cycle progression and protein synthesis, and is involved in the CRC metastatic process. The mTOR inhibitors are analogues of rapamycin, including everolimus and temsirolimus, which are being investigated in clinical trials in combination with irinotecan, cetuximab, FOLFOX, bevacizumab or panatimumab in patients with mCRC progressing on prior chemotherapy [101]. Current expert opinion suggests that mTOR inhibitors may represent an attractive anti-tumour target in combination with strategies to target other pathways that may overcome resistance [107]. In relation to this, it has been demonstrated that addition of the multikinase inhibitor, sorafenib, enhances the therapeutic effect of rapamycin on induction of apoptosis and inhibition of cell-cycle progression, migration and invasion of CRCs [108]. In addition, it has been suggested that mTOR inhibition by metformin (an antidiabetic drug), via activation of the AMP-activated protein kinase (AMPK) pathway, which functions as a sensor for cellular nutrient and energy levels, could be a new option for CRC [109].

4.3. Autophagy modulators and proteasome inhibitors

Autophagy is a multistep process of sequestration and subsequent elimination of cytosolic proteins, damaged organelles and protein aggregates in autophagosomes [110]. This self-degradation, via the lysosome, is responsible for the maintenance of intracellular homeostasis and enables cell survival under stress conditions. In the cancer cell, autophagy can be used as a strategy of self-adaption to generate nutrients and energy during tumour progression and in periods of hypoxia and stress, such as induced by chemotherapy, leading to development of drug resistance. The role of autophagy after chemotherapy remains controversial, it having been suggested that autophagy induction may increase efficacy of other anti-tumour agents, while most evidence suggests that the inhibition of autophagy is what can increase the effectiveness of these agents. As autophagy inhibitor, an analogue of chloroquine, hydroxy-chloroquine (HCQ), is currently involved in two different phase II studies for advanced CRC in combination with FOLFOX/bevacizumab or capecitabine/oxaliplatin/bevacizumab [111]. Given that HCQ induces ocular toxicities, such as retinopathy, novel autophagy inducers, such as Lys05, are currently being investigated in CRC [112].

In relation to autophagy inducers, since the PI3K/Akt/mTOR pathway is a key regulator of autophagy [113], mTOR inhibitors have been also used to modulate this mechanism, proving to be effective in many models for CRCs, but their clinical use has been less successful [114]. Proteasome inhibitors have also been described as autophagy inducers. It has been shown that proteasome inhibition generates a stress response through alteration of the protein milieu, which, in turn, induces endoplasmic reticulum stress; this causes an accumulation of misfolded proteins in the endoplasmic reticulum lumen and, consequently, induction of cellular stress responses, such as the unfolded protein response and autophagy to maintain endoplasmic reticulum homeostasis [110]. Bortezomib, the main proteasome inhibitor, was shown to induce autophagy in CRC cells [115]. However, in a randomised phase II study in relapsed or refractory CRC, bortezomib alone or in combination with irinotecan was not effective [116]. There are current trials examining combinations of bortezomib with other chemotherapies, such as oxaliplatin, 5-FU and leucovorin, in patients with advanced CRC [117]. In view of the limited results with autophagy inducers, some authors have suggested that optimal anti-tumour efficacy might be achieved by the combination of proteasome inhibitors and autophagy inhibitors [118].

4.4. Targeting cancer stem cells, Wnt pathway inhibitors, and tumour cell differentiation inducers

Cancer stem cells (CSCs) are a subpopulation of tumour cells that possess the capacity to self-renew and to give rise to the heterogeneous lineages of cancer cells that comprise the tumour, and it is believed that they could be crucial in controlling and curing cancer [119]. Specifically, there is increasing evidence that CSCs play an important role in the occurrence, growth, and progression of tumours, as well as possibly in the initiation of distant metastases. In addition, CSCs are also involved in resistance to conventional chemotherapeutic drugs, novel tumour-targeted drugs, and radiation therapy [120].

CSCs have been identified not only in leukaemias, but also in solid tumours, including CRC. In fact, it has been suggested that CRC stem cells are responsible for tumour relapse, because conventional drugs fail to eliminate the CSC reservoir [121]. Due to this important clinical feature, CRC stem cells have recently been identified as a rational therapeutic target. Several CSC-targeted therapies have been proposed, including microbial- and plant-derived biomolecules; therapies directed at CSC-specific surface markers; some classical drugs, such as tranilast, curcumin and thioridazine; and reversal of their resistance to anti-tumour agents; so far, however, the toxicity of some of these approaches in normal stem cells and treatment resistance remain important limitations [122].

Various signalling pathways, such as Wingless/Int (Wnt), Hedgehog and Notch, are involved in maintaining the stemness of CSCs. Among these, Wnt, stands out for being particularly active in the majority of CRCs, and hence is the first being investigated for therapeutic targeting in CRC. A primary consequence of Wnt signalling activation is the stabilization of β-catenin in the cytoplasm, resulting in an increased translocation of β-catenin to the nucleus and, in turn, activation of Wnt target gene expression. Misregulation of the canonical Wnt/β-catenin pathway and aberrant activation of Wnt signalling target genes are common in CRC and contribute to cancer progression [123]. Despite the importance of this pathway, few compounds have progressed beyond preclinical development. Efforts have been made to investigate the inhibition of a number Wnt genes, including the matrix metalloproteinases (MMPs), which play an important role in the degradation of extracellular matrix component, crucial for invasion and metastasis. Some studies have shown that increased expression of various MMPs (MMP-1, MMP-2 and MMP-9) favours CRC progression and could predict liver metastasis. Further, several therapeutic MMP inhibitors have been developed, but so far they have failed to produce a survival benefit and, in addition, they have been associated with adverse effects, such as musculoskeletal syndrome. The development of more selective MMP inhibitors is seen as a possible way forward [124].

Another novel compound is salinomycin, a polyether ionophore antibiotic that has been shown to kill CSCs in various types of human cancer, including CRC cells, mostly by interfering with ABC drug transporters and the Wnt/β-catenin signalling pathway. Salinomycin inhibits the migratory and invasive capacity, and reduces the proportion of CD133 CSCs in HT29 and SW480 CRC cells [125]. The results from preclinical trials and its ability to kill therapy-resistant cancer cells make salinomycin a promising anticancer drug [126].

In recent years, other agents have been shown to suppress the self-renewal of CSCs *in vitro* and *in vivo*; these include metformin, DECA-14, rapamycin, oncostatin M, some natural compounds, oncolytic viruses, microRNAs, TNF-related apoptosis inducing ligand, telomerase inhibitors, mAbs and all-*trans* retinoic acid (ATRA). It has been suggested that combina-

http://dx.doi.org/10.5772/57326

tions of these agents and conventional therapy could significantly reduce tumour growth, metastasis and recurrence [127].

CSCs are characterised by two main properties of normal stem cells, self-renewal and differentiation. Given this, the induction of differentiation using retinoids would be a plausible therapeutic strategy. ATRA, a potent differentiating agent, has been demonstrated to induce CSC growth inhibition, and this has been associated with down-regulation of Wnt/β-catenin signalling [128]. In a CRC tumour model of liver metastasis, we have demonstrated the anti-tumour effects of ATRA. This pro-differentiating agent hindered or completely abolished the pro-tumour stimulus produced by serum obtained from hepatectomised rats, and by a wide variety of GFs (HGF, VEGF, PDGF, EGF, and bFGF). In addition, in combination with 5-FU, an additive effect was observed in *in vitro* studies [129]. In *in vivo* experiments, ATRA also reduced tumour progression, though it failed to increase survival, both alone and in combination with 5-FU (unpublished data).

5. New therapeutic techniques for colorectal liver metastasis

Although surgical excision of tumour tissue remains the only potentially curative treatment for CRC-LM, several other techniques are now being developed to be used when surgery is not feasible or to improve surgical results.

The list of possible new therapeutic techniques for CRC-LM seems likely to increase over the next five years, including:

- Surgical approaches focused on increasing the size of the liver lobes (staged surgery or portal branch ligatures), as the percentage of remnant liver after hepatectomy is a limiting factor in many patients
- Techniques for percutaneous tumour ablation, which can reduce CRC-LM volume and allow surgery or at least delay the progression of the illness
- Nanoparticles (NPs) to selectively deliver drugs to tumour cells or induce local hyperthermia.

First, let us consider patients who could benefit from surgical excision of their liver metastases, but in whom the FLR would be less than 25%, which is currently considered the threshold of what can be tolerated. Initially, strategies for such cases were focused on selectively increasing the liver mass of liver lobes free of tumour. Some clinical trials have found that portal vein embolization (PVE) of the lobes bearing metastases induces regeneration of the other lobes, and this has been found to result in a 20-45% increase in their relative volume in two to eight weeks [130]. However, the clinical benefit of this procedure is not clear and, as there were also reports of tumour progression due to hepatectomy, it has not been widely adopted.

In patients who have inadequate FLR to undergo disease clearance with a single hepatectomy, two-stage hepatectomy for bilobar liver metastases in combination with selected use of portal venous embolization is feasible. It offers the best chance of achieving adequate FLR hypertrophy, better than a strategy involving PVE before a single hepatectomy. In addition, rates of macroscopic surgical clearance greater than 65% have been reported [131].

Surgical strategies must be individualised after careful assessment of disease distribution and its relationship to key underlying vascular and biliary structures. Thus, the majority of authors perform the first surgical stage focused on the minor hepatectomy and concurrent procedures as required. When necessary, ligature or embolization of the portal vein is carried out, to enhance the hepatic regeneration response induced by hepatectomy [132]. Nowadays, embolization is preferred to avoid surgical manipulation of the porta hepatis prior to major hepatectomies, and to achieve segment IV total portal inflow occlusion if a right hepatectomy is planned. Hypertrophy after PVE is maximal in the first three weeks, and tends to plateau after this period [133]. The time interval between hepatectomies must be long enough for adequate recovery from the first hepatectomy and liver hypertrophy, but not so long as to enable disease progression, since tumour volume may still increase within the occluded liver [134]. This interval is not well defined but is believed to be around eight to sixteen weeks. In the second-stage operation, the liver surgery usually is complex, often involving other procedures such as radiofrequency ablation. Consequently, postoperative morbidity is significant (50-60%) after this second surgery, particularly due to transient or permanent liver insufficiency. Nevertheless, when performed in referral centres for hepatic surgery the mortality rate is low (2.6-5%). Further, reported three-year survival rates after two-staged hepatectomy range from 30 to 58% [135], and in all series were significantly higher than in those patients treated with best palliative chemotherapy. Given this survival benefit and the feasibility of the surgery, this two-stage approach can be justified in suitably selected patients.

More recently, *in situ* liver transection with portal vein ligation has been proposed as a useful alternative for patients who have some segments of the left liver free of tumour, but an FLR that is too small [136]. In a first surgical intervention, arterial vessels and veins draining the lobes containing metastases are dissected and marked with vessel loops; then, the portal branches to those lobes are severed (most commonly, all right portal branches and segment I and IV branches). Some clinical trials have found that a 40-80% increase in FLR is achieved after three to eight days, and the patient can be re-operated on to remove the previously prepared lobes [137]. The results so far reported (daily increases of FRL up to 22%) are promising, but further clinical trials need to be carried out before this procedure can be generally recommended.

A quite different approach is percutaneous tumour ablation, an old design that is continuously being refined and improved with new technical developments. Initially, ablation of liver metastases was achieved by alcoholisation (ethanol injection), this being used as a downstaging procedure prior to surgery, then came radiofrequency thermoablation [42], and this was soon followed by microwave thermoablation. These procedures proved to be useful tools to reduce tumour volume, but only provided a transient effect when applied to CRC-LM. More recently, laser tumour ablation and cryoablation have gone through experimental trials in animals and are now being tested in patients, but still limited to primary liver tumours. As with previous treatments, if and when they prove to be useful in hepatocarcinomas, they will be tried in CRC-LM [138]

A different, perhaps more subtle, approach is embolization of the arterial vessels supplying the tumour. Transarterial embolisation with 300- to 500-µm microspheres has been widely used either as a downstaging procedure or as a palliative treatment. This classic technique was improved by adding selective transarterial chemotherapy prior to embolisation, which allowed higher doses of chemotherapy with fewer side effects [139].

One of the problems in treating CRC-LM is the low tolerance of the liver parenchyma to radiation [140]. An elegant solution to overcome this limitation is known as *selective internal radiation therapy* and consists in the administration of ^{90}Y-resin microspheres through the arterial branches supplying the tumour. First applied to non-resectable hepatocarcinoma patients, achieving a reduction in tumour burden, relief of symptoms and increase in survival, it is now being tested in CLR-LM with promising results. However, the type of radiolabelled microspheres, indications and dosing schedules have to be better defined [141].

A novel approach has been the use of precharged particles to chemoembolise liver tumours. Smaller (50- to 100-µm) electrically-activated microspheres are exposed to a chemotherapeutic agent which binds to them by electrostatic forces. These spheres are delivered to the vascular tumour bed where they are widely and uniformly seeded; then the drug is released and exerts its effect specifically on the tumour tissue, while the spheres block further blood supply. Preliminary reports have been quite promising, and may lead to the procedure being applied in CRC-LM [142].

All these techniques can, however, only be applied to selected macroscopic liver metastases, leaving untreated residual microfoci responsible for tumour recurrence. We need therapeutic tools to attack individual cancer cells seeded throughout the whole liver parenchyma from the primary colorectal tumour. Currently, one of the most promising avenues is radioimmunotherapy, with ongoing preclinical and clinical studies in CRC. This type of therapy involves the administration of radiolabeled mAbs that are directed specifically against tumour-associated antigens or against the tumour microenvironment. Some phase II trials have suggested that radioiodinated antibodies against CEA, as an adjuvant treatment after R0-resection of CRC-LM, improve overall survival [143]. More recently, new studies are being undertaken to assess the safety and efficacy of combining anti-CEA-RIT and kinase inhibitors, such as imatinib, to increase antibody distribution in CRC tumours [144].

On the other hand, the new field of nanosystems for cancer diagnostics and treatment is highly promising [145]. NPs, which easily escape detection and destruction by our immune system, are being used to deliver drugs directly to the tumour bed and selectively destroy cancer cells. It has been suggested that this strategy may be able to overcome tumour resistance and reduce toxicity in healthy organs. Tumour tissue tends to retain NPs, probably due to its particular characteristics (abnormally leaky endothelium and underdeveloped lymphatic drainage) [146], and this could explain the tendency of NPs to accumulate in liver metastases more than in normal liver parenchyma when administered through the hepatic artery, as we have recently shown [147]. Further, in order to decrease the severe dose-limiting toxicity of 5-FU and to enhance the concentration of this agent in the tumour mass, some researchers are investigating the use of 5-FU-loaded biodegradable NPs, and have already shown a significant improvement in the anticancer activity of the drug in an *in vitro* CRC model [148]. Finally, magnetic NPs are being investigated in combination with high-frequency magnetic fields to induce local hyperthermia in the tumour, promising results having been obtained in experimental settings (CRC-LM in rats) [149].

6. Conclusion

Liver metastases are a common undesirable development in CRC and represent the leading cause of death in this high-prevalence disease. The management of CRC-LM has significantly changed over the past two decades, with dramatic improvements in patient outcomes. This has been made possible by the application of several key concepts when implementing different therapeutic approaches for subsets of patients with mCRC. Firstly, there is a clear consensus that the best management is achieved with a multimodality approach, including surgery, perioperative chemotherapy, biological agents and/or radiotherapy. Secondly, the therapeutic option with the best potential for cure in patients with CRC-LM remains complete resection of the metastases. Strategies to facilitate liver resection are allowing significantly increases in overall survival in this complex disease. In relation to this, the use of optimal first-line chemotherapy doublet (FOLFOX, FOLFIRI, XELOX) or triplet regimens (FOLFOXIRI) in combination with targeted therapy is now recognised as a good therapeutic approach in potentially resectable patients. In particular, the development of new biological molecules for targeted therapy (bevacizumab, cetuximab, and panatimumab) has been a key factor in the most important advances in mCRC treatment.

Nevertheless, much remains to be done. The fact that these current targeted biological agents are only effective in small subsets of patients with mCRC, and that their overall impact in the management of the disease is still relatively modest, has encouraged researchers to search for novel molecules that selectively target specific molecular pathways. This has resulted in a plethora of new antiangiogenic agents (aflibercept, ramucirumab, regorafenib, etc.) and novel molecules directed against new biological targets (such as, autophagy or CSCs) or various different signalling pathways (Wnt and PI3K/AKT/mTOR, among others); these are currently being tested in preclinical studies or in phase II and III trials.

Additionally, new therapeutic techniques, such as surgical approaches focused on increasing the size of the liver lobes, SIRT, radiofrequency ablations and, more recently, NPs to selectively deliver drugs or to induce local hyperthermia in the tumour bed, promise to increase overall outcome in patients with advanced mCRC, in particular, in those with special characteristics that complicate treatment of their disease (inadequate FLR and others).

Finally, it is important not to forget the need to continue the search for new biomarkers to enable better patient stratification for each treatment option. Based on a better understanding of the process involved in the development and progression of CRC, biomarker panels will be developed and this will greatly facilitate the design of personalized medicine for CRC patients.

http://dx.doi.org/10.5772/57326

Acknowledgements

Our ongoing research effort in this field is supported by research grants from the University of the Basque Country (Project GIU 10/16) and the Gangoiti Barrera Foundation.

Author details

Teodoro Palomares[1*], Ana Alonso-Varona[2], Ignacio García-Alonso[1] and Vicente Portugal[3]

*Address all correspondence to: teodoro.palomares@ehu.es

1 Dpt. of Surgery and Radiology and Physical Medicine, Faculty of Medicine and Dentistry, University of the Basque Country, Leioa, Spain

2 Dpt. of Biology and Histology, Faculty of Medicine and Dentistry, University of the Basque Country, Leioa, Spain

3 Unit of Colorectal Surgery, Hospital Galdakao-Usansolo, Galdakao, Spain

References

[1] Jemal A, Bray F, Center MM, Ferlay J, Ward E, Forman D. Global cancer statistics. CA Cancer J Clin 2011;61(2): 69-90.

[2] Kanas GP, Taylor A, Primrose JN, Langeberg WJ, Kelsh MA, Mowat FS, et al. Survival after liver resection in metastatic colorectal cancer: review and meta-analysis of prognostic factors. Clin Epidemiol 2012;4: 283-301.

[3] Lopez P, Marzano E, Piardi T, Pessaux P. Repeat hepatectomy for liver metastases from colorectal primary cancer: a review of the literature. J Visc Surg 2012;149(2): e97-e103.

[4] Stein A, Glockzin G, Wienke A, Arnold D, Edelmann T, Hildebrandt B, et al. Treatment with bevacizumab and FOLFOXIRI in patients with advanced colorectal cancer: presentation of two novel trials (CHARTA and PERIMAX) and review of the literature. BioMed Central Cancer 2012;12: 356. doi: 10.1186/1471-2407-12-356.

[5] Masi G, Fornaro L, Caparello C, Falcone A. Liver Metastases from Colorectal Cancer. How to Best Complement Medical Treatment With Surgical Approaches. Future Oncol 2011;7(11): 1299-1323.

[6] Yoo PS, Lopez-Soler RI, Longo WE, Cha CH. Liver resection for metastatic colorectal cancer in the age of neoadjuvant chemotherapy and bevacizumab. Clin Colorectal Canc 2006;6(3): 202-207

[7] Steele G Jr, Ravikumar TS. Resection of hepatic metastases from colorectal cancer. Biologic perspective. Ann Surg 1989;210: 127–138.

[8] Pawlik TM, Schulick RD, Choti MA. Expanding criteria for resectability of colorectal liver metastases. The Oncologist. 2008;13(1): 51-64.

[9] Fong Y, Fortner JG, Sun RL, Brennan MF, Blumgart LH. Clinical score for predicting recurrence after hepatic resection for metastatic colorectal cancer: analysis of 1001 consecutive cases. Ann Surg 1999;230(3): 309-18.

[10] Quan D, Gallinger S, Nhan C, Auer RA, Biagi JJ, Fletcher GG, et al. The role of liver resection for colorectal cancer metastases in an era of multimodality treatment: a systematic review. Surgery 2012;151(6): 860-870.

[11] Pulitanò C, Bodingbauer M, Aldrighetti L, de Jong MC, Castillo F, Schulick RD, et al. Liver resection for colorectal metastases in presence of extrahepatic disease: results from an international multi-institutional analysis. Ann Surg Oncol 2011;18(5): 1380-1388.

[12] Ciliberto D, Prati U, Roveda L, Barbieri V, Staropoli N, Abbruzzese A, et al. Role of systemic chemotherapy in the management of resected or resectable colorectal liver metastases: a systematic review and meta-analysis of randomized controlled trials. Oncol Rep 2012;27(6):1849-1856.

[13] Santini D, Spoto C, Loupakis F, Vincenzi B, Silvestris N, Cremolini C, et al. High concordance of BRAF status between primary colorectal tumours and related metastatic sites: implications for clinical practice. Ann Oncol 2010;21(7): 1565.

[14] Simmonds PC, Primrose JN, Colquitt JL, Garden OJ, Poston GJ, Rees M. Surgical resection of hepatic metastases from colorectal cancer: a systematic review of published studies. Brit J Cancer 2006;94(7): 982-999.

[15] Neumann UP, Thelen A, Rocken C, Seehofer D, Bahra M, Riess H, et al. Non-response to pre-operative chemotherapy does not preclude long-term survival after liver resection in patients with colorectal liver metastases. Surgery 2009;146(1): 52-59.

[16] Nordlinger B, Sorbye H, Glimelius B, et al. Perioperative chemotherapy with FOLFOX4 and surgery versus surgery alone for resectable liver metastases from colorectal cancer (EORTC Intergroup trial 40983): a randomised controlled trial. Lancet 2008;371(9617): 1007-1016.

[17] Nordlinger B, Sorbye H, Glimelius B, Poston GJ, Schlag PM, Rougier P, et al. EORTC liver metastases intergroup randomized phase III study 40983: Long-term survival results. J Clin Oncol 2012;30(15s): 3508.

[18] van Vledder MG, de Jong MC, Pawlik TM, Schulick RD, Diaz LA, Choti MA. Disappearing colorectal liver metastases after chemotherapy: should we be concerned? J Gastrointest Surg 2010;14(11): 1691-1700.

[19] Brouquet A, Benoist S, Julie C, Penna C, Beauchet A, Rougier P, et al. Risk factors for chemotherapy-associated liver injuries: a multivariate analysis of a group of 146 patients with colorectal metastases. Surgery 2009;145(4): 362-371.

[20] van Kessel CS, Buckens CF, van den Bosch MA, van Leeuwen MS, van Hillegersberg R, Verkooijen HM. Preoperative Imaging of Colorectal Liver Metastases After Neoadjuvant Chemotherapy: A Meta-Analysis Ann Surg Oncol 2012;19(9): 2805-2813.

[21] Rödel C, Liersch T, Becker H, Fietkau R, Hohenberger W, Hothorn T, et al (German Rectal Cancer Study Group). Preoperative chemoradiotherapy and postoperative chemotherapy with fluorouracil and oxaliplatin versus fluorouracil alone in locally advanced rectal cancer: initial results of the German CAO/ARO/AIO-04 randomised phase 3 trial. Lancet Oncol 2012;13(7): 679-687.

[22] Smalley SR, Benedetti JK, Williamson SK, Robertson JM, Estes NC, Maher T, et al. Phase III trial of fluorouracil-based chemotherapy regimens plus radiotherapy in postoperative adjuvant rectal cancer: GI INT 0144. J Clin Oncol 2006;24(22): 3542-3547.

[23] Folprecht G, Gruenberger T, Bechstein WO, Raab HR, Lordick F, Hartmann JT, et al. Tumour response and secondary resectability of colorectal liver metastases following neoadjuvant chemotherapy with cetuximab: the CELIM randomised phase 2 trial. Lancet Oncol 2010;11(1): 38-47.

[24] Masi G, Vasile E, Loupakis F, Cupini S, Fornaro L, Baldi G, et al. Randomized trial of two induction chemotherapy regimens in metastatic colorectal cancer: an updated analysis. J Natl Cancer I 2011;103(1): 21-30.

[25] Choti MA. Chemotherapy-associated hepatotoxicity: do we need to be concerned? Ann Surg Oncol 2009;16(9): 2391-2394.

[26] Wildi SM, Gubler C, Hany T, Petrowsky H, Clavien PA, Jochum W, et al. Intraoperative sonography in patients with colorectal cancer and resectable liver metastases on preoperative FDG-PET-CT. J Clin Ultrasound 2008;36(1): 20–26.

[27] Sahani DV, Kalva SP, Tanabe KK, Tanabe KK, Hayat SM, O'Neill MJ, et al. Intraoperative US in patients undergoing surgery for liver neoplasms: comparison with MR imaging. Radiology 2004;232(3): 810–814.

[28] Elias D, Goere D, Boige V, Kohneh-Sharhi N, Malka D, Tomasic G, et al. Outcome of post-hepatectomy-missing colorectal liver metastases after complete response to chemotherapy : impact of adjuvant intra-arterial hepatic oxaliplatin. Ann Surg Oncol 2007;14(11): 3188-3194

[29] Tanaka K, Takakura H, Takeda K, Matsuo K, Nagano Y, Endo I. Importance of complete pathologic response to prehepatectomy chemotherapy in treating colorectal cancer metastases. Ann Surg 2009;250(6): 935-942.

[30] Slesser AA, Simillis C, Goldin R, Brown G, Mudan S, Tekkis PP. A meta-analysis comparing simultaneous versus delayed resections in patients with synchronous colorectal liver metastases. Surg Oncol 2013;22(1): 36-47.

[31] Chen J, Li Q, Wang C, Zhu H, Shi Y, Zhao G. Simultaneous versus staged resection for synchronous colorectal liver metastases: a meta-analysis. Int J Colorectal Dis 2011;26(2): 191–199.

[32] Viganó L. Treatment strategy for colorectal cancer with resectable synchronous liver metastases: Is any evidence-based strategy possible? World J Hepatol 2012;4(8): 237–241.

[33] Reddy SK, Pawlik TM, Zorzi D, Gleisner AL, Ribero D, Assumpcao L, et al. Simultaneous resections of colorectal cancer and synchronous liver metastases: a multi-institutional analysis. Ann Surg Oncol 2007;14(12): 3481–3491.

[34] Tsai MS, Su YH, Ho MC, Liang JT, Chen TP, Lai HS, et al. Clinicopathological features and prognosis in resectable synchronous and metachronous colorectal liver metastasis. Ann Surg Oncol 2007;14(2): 786-794.

[35] Mentha G, Majno PE, Andres A, Rubbia-Brandt L, Morel P, Roth AD. Neoadjuvant chemotherapy and resection of advanced synchronous liver metastases before treatment of the colorectal primary. Brit J Surg 2006;93(7): 872-878.

[36] Brouquet A, Mortenson M, Vauthey JN, Rodriguez-Bigas M, Overman MJ, Chang GJ, et al. Surgical strategies for synchronous colorectal liver metastases in 156 consecutive patients:classic, combined or reversed strategy? J Am Coll Surgeons 2010;210(6): 934-941.

[37] Briggs RH, Chowdhury FU, Lodge JP, Scarsbrook AF. Clinical impact of FDG PET-CT in patients with potentially operable metastatic colorectal cancer. Clin Radiol 2011;66(12): 1167-1174.

[38] Andreou A, Brouquet A, Abdalla EK, Aloia TA, Curley SA, Vauthey JN. Repeat hepatectomy for recurrent colorectal liver metastases is associated with a high survival rate. HPB (Oxford) 2011;13(11): 774-782.

[39] Adam R, Wicherts DA, de Haas RJ, Ciacio O, Lévi F, Paule B, et al. Patients with initially unresectable colorectal liver metastases: is there a possibility of cure? J Clin Oncol 2009;27(11): 1829-1835.

[40] Tanaka K, Kumamoto T, Nojiri K, Takeda K, Ichikawa Y, Endo I. Timing of Two-stage Liver Resection during Chemotherapy for Otherwise Unresectable Colorectal Metastases World J Surg 2012;36(8): 1832–1841.

[41] Fiorentini G, Aliberti C, Tilli M, Mulazzani L, Graziano F, Giordani P, et al. Intra-arterial infusion of irinotecan-loaded drug-eluting beads (DEBIRI) versus intravenous therapy (FOLFIRI) for hepatic metastases from colorectal cancer: final results of a phase III study. Anticancer Res 2012;32(4): 1387-1395.

[42] Ansari D, Andersson R. Radiofrequency ablation or percutaneous ethanol injection for the treatment of liver tumors. World J Gastroenterol 2012;18(10): 1003-1008.

[43] Kosmider S, Tan TH, Yip D, Dowling R, Lichtenstein M, Gibbs P. Radioembolization in combination with systemic chemotherapy as first-line therapy for liver metastases from colorectal cancer. J Vasc Interv Radiol 2011;22(6): 780-786.

[44] Kress MS, Collins BT, Collins SP, Dritschilo A, Gagnon G, Unger K. Stereotactic body radiation therapy for liver metastases from colorectal cancer: analysis of safety, feasibility, and early outcomes. Frontiers in Oncology 2012;2: 8. doi: 10.3389/fonc. 2012.00008.

[45] Meinsma R, Fernandez-Salguero P, Van Kuilenburg AB, Van Gennip AH, Gonzalez FJ. Human polymorphism in drug metabolism: mutation in the dihydropyrimidine dehydrogenase gene results in exon skipping and thymineuracilurea. DNA and Cell Biology 1995;14(1): 1-6.

[46] Gustavsson B, Christopher K, Carlsson G, Wettergren Y, Odin E, Lindskog EB, et al. Molecular determinants of efficacy for 5-FU-based treatments in advanced colorectal cancer: mRNA expression for 18 chemotherapy-related genes. Int J Cancer 2009;124(5): 1220-1226.

[47] Yen JL, McLeod HL. Should DPD analysis be required prior to prescribing fluoropyrimidines? Eur J Cancer 2007;43(6): 1011-1016.

[48] Newton KF, Newman W, Hill J. Review of biomarkers in colorectal cancer. Colorectal Dis 2012;14(1): 3-17.

[49] Alagoz M, Gilbert DC, El-Khamisy S, Chalmers AJ. DNA Repair and Resistance to Topoisomerase I Inhibitors: Mechanisms, Biomarkers and Therapeutic Targets. Curr Med Chem 2012;19(23): 3874-3885.

[50] Cecchin E, Innocenti F, D'Andrea M, Corona G, De Mattia E, Biason P, et al. Predictive role of the UGT1A1, UGT1A7, and UGT1A9 genetic variants and their haplotypes on the outcome of metastatic colorectal cancer patients treated with fluorouracil, leucovorin, and irinotecan. J Clin Oncol 2009;27(15): 2457-2465.

[51] Palomaki GE, Bradley LA, Douglas MP, Kolor K, Dotson WD. Can UGT1A1 genotyping reduce morbidity and mortality in patients with metastatic colorectal cancer treated with irinotecan? An evidence-based review. Genetic Medicine 2009;11(1): 21-34.

[52] Dienstmann R, Vilar E, Tabernero J. Molecular Predictors of Response to Chemotherapy in Colorectal Cancer. Cancer J 2011;17(2): 114-12 6.

[53] Braun MS, Richman SD, Quirke P, Daly C, Adlard JW, Elliott F, et al. Predictive biomarkers of chemotherapy efficacy in colorectal cancer: results from the UK MRC FOCUS trial. J Clin Oncol 2008;26(16): 2690-2698.

[54] Ikeguchi M, Arai Y, Maeta Y, Ashida K, Katano K, Wakatsuki T. Topoisomerase I expression in tumors as a biological marker for CPT-11 chemosensitivity in patients with colorectal cancer. Surg Today 2011;41(9): 1196-1199.

[55] Rasheed ZA, Rubin EH. Mechanisms of resistance to topoisomerase I-targeting drugs. Oncogene 2003;22(47): 7296–7304.

[56] Lenz HJ, Zhang W, Shi MM, Jacques C, Barrett JC, Danenberg KD, et al. ERCC-1 gene expression levels and outcome to FOLFOX chemotherapy in patients enrolled in CONFIRM1 and CONFIRM2. J Clin Oncol 2008;26(suppl): abstract 4131.

[57] Yin M, Yan J, Martinez-Balibrea E, Graziano F, Lenz HJ, Kim HJ. ERCC1 and ERCC2 Polymorphisms Predict Clinical Outcomes of Oxaliplatin-based Chemotherapies in Gastric and Colorectal Cancer: A Systemic Review and Meta-analysis. Clin Cancer Res 2011;17(6): 1632-1640.

[58] Lin YL, Liau, JY, Yu SC, Ou DL, Lin LI, Tseng LH, Chang YL, et al. KRAS Mutation Is a Predictor of Oxaliplatin Sensitivity in Colon Cancer Cells. PLOS ONE 2012;7(11) e50701. doi: 10.1371/journal.pone.0050701.

[59] LeGolvan MP, Resnick M. Pathobiology of colorectal cancer hepatic metastases with an emphasis on prognostic factors. Journal of Surg Oncol 2010;102(8): 898-908.

[60] Wanebo HJ, Berz D. The neoadjuvant therapy of colorectal hepatic metastases and the role of biologic sensitizing and resistance factors. J Surg Oncol 2010;102(8): 891-897.

[61] Olayioye MA, Neve RM, Lane HA, Hynes NE. The ErbB signaling network: receptor heterodimerization in development and cancer. EMBO J 2000;19(13): 3159-3167.

[62] Christophi C, Harun N, Fifis T. Liver regeneration and tumor stimulation-A review of Cytokine and angiogenic factors. J Gastrointest Surg 2008;12(5): 966-980.

[63] Chung KY, Shia J, Kemeny NE, Shah M, Schwartz GK, Tse A, et al. Cetuximab shows activity in colorectal cancer patients with tumors that do not express the epidermal growth factor receptor by immunohistochemistry. J Clin Oncol 2005;23(9): 1803-1810.

[64] Tol J, Punt CJA. Monoclonal antibodies in the treatment of metastatic colorectal cancer: a review. Clin Ther 2010;32(3): 437-453.

[65] De Roock W, Piessevaux H, De Schutter J, Janssens M, De Hertogh G, Personeni N, et al. KRAS wild-type state predicts survival and is associated to early radiological response in metastatic colorectal cancer treated with cetuximab. Ann Oncol 2008;19(3): 508-515.

[66] Bokemeyer C, Bondarenko I, Makhson A, Hartmann JT, Aparicio J, de Braud F, et al. Fluorouracil, leucovorin, and oxaliplatin with and without cetuximab in the first-line treatment of metastatic colorectal cancer. J Clin Oncol 2009;27(5): 663-671.

[67] Van Cutsem E, Köhne CH, Láng I, Folprecht G, Nowacki MP, Cascinu S, et al. Cetuximab plus irinotecan, fluorouracil, and leucovorin as first-line treatment for metastatic colorectal cancer: updated analysis of overall survival according to tumor KRAS and BRAF mutation status. J Clin Oncol 2011;29(15): 2011-2019.

[68] De Roock W, Claes B, Bernasconi D, De Schutter J, Biesmans B, Fountzilas G. Effects of KRAS, BRAF, NRAS, and PIK3CA mutations on the efficacy of cetuximab plus chemotherapy in chemotherapy-refractory metastatic colorectal cancer: a retrospective consortium analysis. Lancet Oncol 2010;11(8) 753-762.

[69] Di Nicolantonio F, Martini M, Molinari F, Sartore-Bianchi A, Arena S, Saletti P, et al. Wild-type BRAF is required for response to panitumumab or cetuximab in metastatic colorectal cancer. J Clin Oncol 2008;26(35): 5705-5712.

[70] George B, Scott K. Predictive and Prognostic Markers in Colorectal Cancer. Current Oncol Rep 2011;13(3): 206-215.

[71] Loupakis F, Pollina L, Stasi I, Ruzzo A, Scartozzi M, Santini D, et al. PTEN expression and KRAS mutations on primary tumors and metastases in the prediction of benefit from cetuximab plus irinotecan for patients with metastatic colorectal cancer. J Clin Oncol 2009;27(16): 2622-26299.

[72] Ellis LM, Takahashi Y, Liu W, Shaheen RM. Vascular endothelial growth factor in human colon cancer: biology and therapeutic implications. Oncologist 2000;5(s1): 11-15.

[73] Hirashima Y, Yamada Y, Tateishi U, Kato K, Miyake M, Horita Y, et al. Pharmacokinetic parameters from 3-Tesla DCE-MRI as surrogate biomarkers of antitumor effects of bevacizumab plus FOLFIRI in colorectal cancer with liver metastasis. Int J Cancer 2012;130(10): 2359-2365.

[74] Ince WL, Jubb AM, Holden SN, Holmgren EB, Tobin P, Sridhar M, et al. Association of k-ras, b-raf and p-53 status with the treatment effect of bevacizumab. J Natl Cancer I 2005;97(13): 981-989.

[75] Zoratto F, Rossi L, Zullo A, Papa A, Zaccarelli E, Tomao L, et al. Critical appraisal of bevacizumab in the treatment of metastatic colorectal cancer. OncoTargets Ther 2012;5: 199-211.

[76] Felcht M, Luck R, Schering A, Seidel P, Srivastava K, Hu J. Angiopoietin-2 differentially regulates angiogenesis through TIE2 and integrin signalling. J Clin Invest 2012;122 (6): 1991-2005.

[77] Goede V, Coutelle O, Neuneier J, Reinacher-Schick A, Schnell R, Koslowsky TC, et al. Identification of serum angiopoietin-2 as a biomarker for clinical outcome of colorec-

tal cancer patients treated with bevacizumab-containing therapy. Brit J Cancer 2010;103(9): 1407-1414.

[78] Kopetz S, Hoff PM, Morris JS, Wolff RA, Eng C, Glover KY, et al. Phase II trial of infusional fluorouracil, irinotecan, and bevacizumab for metastatic colorectal cancer: efficacy and circulating angiogenic biomarkers associated with therapeutic resistance. J Clin Oncol 2010;28(3): 453-459.

[79] Tabernero J, Baselga J. Multigene assays to improve assessment of recurrence risk and benefit from chemotherapy in early-stage colon cancer: has the time finally arrived, or are we still stage locked? J Clin Oncol 2010;28(25): 3904-3907.

[80] Sikaroodi M, Galachiantz Y, Baranova A. Tumor markers: the potential of "omics" approach. Curr Mol Med 2010;10(2): 249-257.

[81] García-Bilbao A, Armañanzas R, Ispizua Z, Calvo B, Alonso-Varona A, Inza I, et al. Identification of a biomarker panel for colorectal cancer diagnosis. BioMed Central Cancer 2012;12: 43.

[82] Schwarz RE, Berlin JD, Lenz HJ, Nordlinger B, Rubbia-Brandt L, Choti MA. Systemic cytotoxic and biological therapies of colorectal liver metastases: expert consensus statement. HPB 2013;15(2): 106-115.

[83] Aranda E, Abad A, Carrato A, Cervantes A, García-Foncillas J, García-Alfonso P, et al. Treatment recommendations for metastatic colorectal cancer. Clin Translat Oncol 2011;13(3): 162-178.

[84] Song X, Zhao Z, Barber B, Gregory C, Wang PF, Long SR. Treatment patterns and metastasectomy among mCRC patients receiving chemotherapy and biologics. Curr Med Res Opin 2011;27(1): 123-130.

[85] Fornaro L, Vasile E, Masi G, Loupakis F, Baldi GG, Allegrini G, et al. Outcome of Second-Line Treatment After First-Line Chemotherapy with the GONO FOLFOXIRI Regimen. Clin Colorectal Cancer 2012;11(1): 71-76.

[86] Gravalos C, Salut A,García-Girón C, García-Carbonero R, León AI, Sevilla I, et al. A randomized phase II study to compare oxaliplatin plus 5-fluorouracil and leucovorin (FOLFOX4) versus oxaliplatin plus raltitrexed(TOMOX) as first-line chemotherapy for advanced colorectal cáncer. Clin Translat Oncol 2012;14(8): 606-612.

[87] Nordlinger B, Adam R, Arnold D, Zalcberg JR, Gruenberger T. The role of biological agents in the resection of colorectal liver metastases. Clin Oncol-UK 2012;24(6): 432-442.

[88] Palomares T, Caramés M, García-Alonso I, Alonso-Varona A. Growth Factors and the Redox State as New Therapeutic Targets for Colorectal Cancer. In: Ettarh R. (ed.) Colorectal Cancer Biology. From genes to tumor. Rijeka: InTech;2012. p189-216.

[89] Geva R, Vecchione L, Tejpar S,Piessevaux H, Cutsem EV, Prenen H. Bevacizumab plus chemotherapy as salvage treatment in chemorefractory patients with metastatic colorectal cancer. Oncotargets Ther 2013;6: 53-58.

[90] Grothey A, Sugrue MM, Purdie DM, Dong W, Sargent D, Hedrick E, et al. Bevacizumab beyond first progression is associated with prolonged overall survival in metastatic colorectal cancer: results from a large observational cohort study (BRiTE). J Clin Oncol 2008;26(33): 5326-5334.

[91] Pentheroudakis G, Kotoula V, De Roock W, Kouvatseas G, Papakostas P, Makatsoris T, et al. Biomarkers of benefit from cetuximab-based therapy in metastatic colorectal cancer: interaction of EGFR ligand expression with RAS/RAF, PIK3CA genotypes. BioMed Central Cancer 2013;13(1): 49-63.

[92] García-Foncillas J, Díaz-Rubio E. Progress in metastatic colorectal cancer: growing role of cetuximab to optimize clinical outcome. Clin Translat Oncol 2010;12(8): 533-542.

[93] Fuloria J. Safety profiles of current antiangiogenic therapies for metastatic colorectal cancer. Oncotargets Ther 2012;5: 133-142.

[94] Ballestrero A, Garuti A, Cirmena G, Rocco I, Palermo C, Nencioni A, et al. Patient-tailored treatments with anti-EGFR monoclonal antibodies in advanced colorectal cancer: KRAS and beyond. Curr Cancer Drug Tar 2012;12(4): 316-328.

[95] Zhou SW, Huang YY, Wei Y, Jiang ZM, Zhang YD, Yang Q, Xie DR. No survival benefit from adding cetuximab or panitumumab to oxaliplatin-based chemotherapy in the first-line treatment of metastatic colorectal cancer in KRAS wild type patients: a meta-analysis. PLOS One 2012;7(11). e50925. doi: 10.1371/journal.pone.0050925.

[96] Saridaki Z, Georgoulias V, Souglakos J. Mechanisms of resistance to anti-EGFR mAb treatment in metastatic colorectal cancer. World J Gastroenterol 2010;16(10): 1177-1187.

[97] Grothey A, Allegra C. Antiangiogenesis therapy in the treatment of metastatic colorectal cancer. Ther Adv Med Oncol 2012;4(6): 301-319.

[98] Holash J, Davis S, Papadopoulos N, Croll SD, Ho L, Russell M, et al. VEGF-Trap: a VEGF blocker with potent antitumor effects. PNAS-USA 2002;99(17): 11393-11398.

[99] Van Cutsem E, Tabernero J, Lakomy R, Prenen H, Prausová J, Macarulla T, et al. Addition of aflibercept to fluorouracil, leucovorin, and irinotecan improves survival in a phase III randomized trial in patients with metastatic colorectal cancer previously treated with an oxaliplatin-based regimen. J Clin Oncol 2012;30(28): 3499-3506.

[100] Spratlin J. Ramucirumab (IMC-1121B): MAb inhibition of vascular endothelial growth factor receptor-2. Curr Oncol Rep 2011;13(2): 97-102.

[101] Chu E. An update on the current and emerging targeted agents in metastatic colorectal cancer. Clin Colorectal Canc 2012;11(1): 1-13.

[102] Schwartz JD, Rowinsky EK, Youssoufian H, Pytowski B, Wu Y. Vascular endothelial growth factor receptor-1 in human cancer: concise review and rationale for development of IMC-18F1 (human antibody targeting vascular endothelial growth factor receptor-1). Cancer 2010;116(4s): 1027-1032.

[103] Grothey A, Van Cutsem E, Sobrero A, Siena S, Falcone A, Ychou M, et al. CORRECT Study Group. Regorafenib monotherapy for previously treated metastatic colorectal cancer (CORRECT): an international, multicentre, randomised, placebo-controlled, phase 3 trial. Lancet 2013;381(9863): 303-312.

[104] Schmoll HJ, Cunningham D, Sobrero A, Karapetis CS, Rougier P, Koski SL, et al. Cediranib with mFOLFOX6 versus bevacizumab with mFOLFOX6 as first-line treatment for patients with advanced colorectal cancer: a double-blind, randomized phase III study (HORIZON III). J Clin Oncol 2012;30(29): 3588-3595.

[105] O'Neil BH, Cainap C, Van Cutsem E, Gorbunova VA, Karapetis CS, Berlin J, et al. Randomized phase II open-label study of mFOLFOX6 in combination with linifanib or bevacizumab for metastatic colorectal cancer. J Clin Oncol 2012;30(15s): 3532.

[106] Richardson PG, Eng C, Kolesar J, Hideshima T, Anderson KC. Perifosine, an oral, anti-cancer agent and inhibitor of the Akt pathway: mechanistic actions, pharmacodynamics, pharmacokinetics, and clinical activity. Expert Opin Drug Met 2012;8(5): 623-633.

[107] Kim DD, Eng C.The promise of mTOR inhibitors in the treatment of colorectal cancer. Expert Opin Inv Drugs 2012;21(12): 1775-1788.

[108] Gulhati P, Zaytseva YY, Valentino JD, Stevens PD, Kim JT, Sasazuki T, et al. Sorafenib enhances the therapeutic efficacy of rapamycin in colorectal cancers harboring oncogenic KRAS and PIK3CA. Carcinogenesis 2012;33(9): 1782-1790.

[109] Feng YH, Wu CL, Shiau AL, Lee JC, Chang JG, Lu PJ, et al. MicroRNA-21-mediated regulation of Sprouty2 protein expression enhances the cytotoxic effect of 5-fluorouracil and metformin in colon cancer cells. Int J Mol Med 2012;29(5): 133-142.

[110] Suh DH, Kim MK, Kim HS, Chung HH, Song YS. Unfolded protein response to autophagy as a promising druggable target for anticancer therapy. Ann N.Y. Acad Sci 2012;1271: 20-32.

[111] Carew JS, Kelly KR, Nawrocki ST. Autophagy as a target for cancer therapy: new developments. Cancer Manag Res 2012;4: 357-365.

[112] McAfee Q, Zhang Z, Samanta A, Levi SM, Ma XH, Piao S, et al. Autophagy inhibitor Lys05 has single-agent antitumor activity and reproduces the phenotype of a genetic autophagy deficiency. PNAS-USA 2012;109(21): 8253-8258.

[113] Jegga AG, Schneider L, Ouyang X, Zhang J. Systems biology of the autophagy-lysosomal pathway. Autophagy 2011;7(5): 477-489.

[114] García-Mauriño S, Alcaide A, Domínguez C. Pharmacological control of autophagy: therapeutic perspectives in inflammatory bowel disease and colorectal cancer. Curr Pharm Design 2012;18(26): 3853-3873.

[115] Hong YS, Hong SW, Kim SM, Jin DH, Shin JS, Yoon DH, et al. Bortezomib induces G2-M arrest in human colon cancer cells through ROS-inducible phosphorylation of ATM-CHK1. Int J Oncol 2012;41(1): 76-82.

[116] Kozuch PS, Rocha-Lima CM, Dragovich T, Hochster H, O'Neil BH, Atiq OT, et al. Bortezomib with or without irinotecan in relapsed or refractory colorectal cancer: results from a randomized phase II study. J CLin Oncol 2008;26(14): 2320-2326.

[117] Caponigro F, Lacombe D, Twelves C, Bauer J, Govaerts AS, Marréaud S, et al. An EORTC phase I study of Bortezomib in combination with oxaliplatin, leucovorin and 5-fluorouracil in patients with advanced colorectal cancer. Eur J Cancer 2009;45(1): 48-55.

[118] Benbrook DM, Long A. Integration of autophagy, proteasomal degradation, unfolded protein response and apoptosis. Exp Oncol 2012;34(3): 286-297.

[119] Fábián A, Barok M, Vereb G, Szöllosi J. Die hard: are cancer stem cells the Bruce Willises of tumor biology? Cytometry Part A 2009;75(51): 67-74.

[120] Moitra K, Lou H, Dean M. Multidrug efflux pumps and cancer stem cells: insights into multidrug resistance and therapeutic development. Clin Pharm Ther 2011;89(4): 491–502.

[121] Vaiopoulos AG, Kostakis ID, Koutsilieris M, Papavassiliou AG. Colorectal cancer stem cells. Stem cells 2012;30(3): 363-371.

[122] Prud'homme GJ. Cancer stem cells and novel targets for antitumor strategies. Current Pharmaceutical Design 2012;18(19): 2838-2849.

[123] McDonald SL, Silver AR. On target? Strategies and progress in the development of therapies for colorectal cancer targeted against WNT signalling. Colorectal Dis 2011;13(4): 360-369.

[124] Herszényi L, Hritz I, Lakatos G, Varga MZ, Tulassay Z. The behavior of matrix metalloproteinases and their inhibitors in colorectal cancer. Int J Mol Sci 2012;13(10): 13240-13263.

[125] Dong TT, Zhou HM, Wang LL, Feng B, Lv B, Zheng MH. Salinomycin selectively targets 'CD133+' cell subpopulations and decreases malignant traits in colorectal cancer lines. Ann Surg Oncol 2011;18(6): 1797-1804.

[126] Naujokat C, Steinhart R.Salinomycin as a drug for targeting human cancer stem cells. J Biomed Biotechnol 2012;2012: 1-17.

[127] Ning X, Du Y, Ben Q, Shu J, Li Z. Therapeutic strategies targeting cancer stem cells. Cancer Biol Ther 2013;14(4): 1-9.

[128] Lim YC, Kang HJ, Kim YS, Choi EC. All-trans-retinoic acid inhibits growth of head and neck cancer stem cells by suppression of Wnt/β-catenin pathway. Eur J Cancer 2012;48,(17): 3310-3318.

[129] García-Alonso I, Palomares T, Alonso-Varona A, Díaz-Sanz I, Miró B, Méndez J. All-Trans Retinoic Acid blocks the proliferative effect of growth factors on rat colocarcinoma cells. Brit J Surg 2010;97(S4): 15.

[130] van Gulik TM, van den Esschert JW, de Graaf W, van Lienden KP, Busch OR, Heger M, et al. Controversies in the use of portal vein embolization. Digest Surg 2008;25(6): 436-444.

[131] Bowers KA, O'Reilly D, Bond-Smith GE, Hutchins RR. Feasibility study of two-stage hepatectomy for bilobar liver metastases. Am J Surg 2012;203(6): 691-697.

[132] Abulkhir A, Limongelli P, Healey AJ, Damrah O, Tait P, Jackson J, et al. Preoperative portal vein embolization for major liver resection: a meta-analysis. Ann Surg 2008;247(1): 49-57.

[133] Ribero D, Abdalla EK, Madoff DC, Donadon M, Loyer EM, Vauthey JN. Portal vein embolization before major hepatectomy and its effects on regeneration, resectability and outcome. Brit J Surg 2007;94(11):1386-1394.

[134] Barbaro B, Di Stasi C, Nuzzo G, Vellone M, Giuliante F, Marano P. Preoperative right portal vein embolization in patients with metastatic liver disease. Metastatic liver volumes after RPVE. Acta Radiol 2003;44(1): 98-102.

[135] Wicherts DA, Miller R, de Haas RJ, Bitsakou G, Vibert E, Veilhan LA, et al. Long-term results of two-stage hepatectomy for irresectable colorectal cancer liver metastases. Ann Surg 2008;248(6): 994-1005.

[136] Knoefel WT, Gabor I, Rehders A, Alexander A, Krausch M, Schulte am Esch J, et al. In situ liver transection with portal vein ligation for rapid growth of the future liver remnant in two-stage liver resection. Brit J Surg 2012;100(3): 388-394.

[137] Schnitzbauer AA, Lang SA, Goessmann H, Nadalin S, Baumgart J, Farkas SA, et al. Right portal vein ligation combined with in situ splitting induces rapid left lateral liver lobe hypertrophy enabling 2-staged extended right hepatic resection in small-for-size settings. Ann Surg 2012;255(3): 405-414.

[138] Sindram D, Lau KN, Martinie JB, Lamnitti DA. Hepatic tumor ablation. Surg Clin N Am 2010;90(4): 863-876.

[139] Hoffmann RT, Paprottka P, Jakobs TF, Trumm CG, Reiser MF. Arterial therapies of non-colorectal cancer metastases to the liver (from chemoembolization to radioembolization). Abdom Imagin 2011;36(6): 671-676.

[140] Malik U, Mohiuddin M. External-beam radiotherapy in the management of liver metastases. Sem Oncol 2002;29(2): 196-201.

[141] Van de Wiele C, Maes A, Brugman E, D'Asseler Y, De Spiegeleer B, Mees G, et al. SIRT of liver metastases: physiological and pathophysiological considerations. Eur J Nucl Mol I 2012;39(10): 1646-1655.

[142] Namur J, Citron SJ, Sellers MT, Dupuis MH, Wassef M, Manfait M, et al. Embolization of hepatocellular carcinoma with drug-eluting beads: doxorubicin tissue concentration and distribution in patient liver explants. J Hepatol 2011;55(6): 1332-1338.

[143] Liersch T, Meller J, Kulle B, Behr TM, Markus P, Langer C, et al. Phase II Trial of Carcinoembryonic Antigen Radioimmunotherapy With 131I-Labetuzumab After Salvage Resection of Colorectal Metastases in the Liver: Five-Year Safety and Efficacy Results. J Clin Oncol 2005;23(27): 6763-6770.

[144] Rajkumar VS, Boxer G, Robson M, Muddle J, Papastavrou Y, et al. A comparative study of PDGFR inhibition with imatinib on radiolabeled antibody targeting and clearance in two pathologically distinct models of colon adenocarcinoma. Tumor Biol 2012;33(6): 2019-2029.

[145] Gonçalves AS, Macedo AS, Souto EB. Therapeutic nanosystems for oncology nanomedicine. Clin Translat Oncol 2012;14(12): 883-890.

[146] Garcia-Bennett A, Nees M, Fadeel B. In search of the Holy Grail: folate-targeted nanoparticles for cancer therapy. Biochemical Pharmacology 2011;81(8): 976-984.

[147] Echevarria-Uraga JJ, García-Alonso I, Plazaola F, Insausti M, Etxebarria N, Saiz-López A, et al. Study of the intra-arterial distribution of Fe3O4 nanoparticles in a model of colorectal neoplasm induced in rat liver by MRI and Spectrometry. Int J Nanomed 2012;7: 2399-2410.

[148] Ortiz R, Prados J, Melguizo C, Arias JL, Ruiz MA, Alvarez PJ, et al. 5-Fluorouracil-loaded poly(epsilon-caprolactone) nanoparticles combined with phage E gene therapy as a new strategy against colon cancer. Int J Nanomed 2012;7: 95-107.

[149] Echevarria-Uraga JJ, García-Alonso I, Herrero B, Marin H, Insausti M, Plazaola F, et al. Liver hyperthermia induced by different iron magnetic nanoparticles ''ex vivo'' and correlation to pathological damage in the tissue. Brit J Surgery 2013;100(S1): 12.

Chapter 11

Rare Tumors of the Colon and Rectum

Goran Stanojević and Zoran Krivokapić

Additional information is available at the end of the chapter

http://dx.doi.org/10.5772/56937

1. Introduction

Malignant tumors of the colon and rectum represent a separate entity, due to their early clinical manifestation, specific methods of examination and, particularly, due to treatment, which is predominantly based on the need for conservation of the sphincter mechanism, without disturbing the oncological principles of surgical treatment and the necessary radicalism. In spite of introduction of the new surgical procedures, and the significant improvements in radio, i.e. chemotherapy, the prognosis of these tumors remains serious.

With regard to the histological structure, tumors can be:

1. Adenocarcinomas,
2. Carcinoids,
3. Lymphomas,
4. Gastrointestinal stromal tumors (GISTs),
5. Squamous cell carcinoma
6. Melanomas
7. Other (extremely rare forms of malignant tumors)

Adenocarcinomas account for 95-97% of all malignant tumors, while the remaining 3-5% belongs to, so called, rare tumors of colon and rectum. The annual percent change in incidence for each rare tumor increased significantly during the 10 years (range: 3.1–9.4%, $p<0.05$), except squamous cell carcinoma (5.9%, $p>0.05$) [1]. With regard to the incidence, all rare tumors of the large bowel can be divided into 2 groups:

1. tumors with the incidence 0,1-2% and
2. rare tumors with the incidence <0,1%.

In the first group the most common ones are: carcinoids 1,8%, primary lymphomas 0,1-1%, GISTs 0,9%, melanomas 0,5-1%, and squamous cell carcinoma 0,1% (without the anal canal). The second group or extremely rare forms of malignant tumors consist of: teratoma, plasmocytoma, schwannomas, metastatic tumor. Literature data are limited and mostly concern series of operated patients of some institutions or several published national studies, but there are no randomized studies or meta-analyses which have higher degree of scientific verification because these tumours are very rare [2].

The aims of studying the rare tumors of the colon and rectum are:

– determination of the incidence among population,

– determination of the clinical characteristics

– comparative analysis of the treatment outcome in different parts of the gastrointestinal tract and

– overall and five-year survival of patients.

2. Carcinoids

Carcinoid tumors represents rare, slow growing tumors and they occur in 1,8% of all malignant tumors of the large bowel. There is no clear predominance related to sex and, in the most of cases, the patients are in their sixties or seventies. They originate from the enterochromaffin (argentafil, Kulchitsky) cells, as a part of the diffuse endocrine system and they belong to the group of neuroendocrine tumors, so called well-differentiated "NET's". They are also called APUDomas, which is an abbreviation for "amine precursor uptake and decarboxylation", due to their ability to take over and decarboxylase amines, originally described by Pearse in 1969 [3]. They can occur in all parts of gastrointestinal tract as well as outside of the tract. Therefore with regard to the place of occurrence and according to the division of the primitive intestine during the embryological development, carcinoids are divided into:

1. foregut carcinoid tumors start in the lungs, bronchi, or stomach;
2. midgut carcinoid tumors start in the small intestine, appendix,or proximal large bowel;
3. hindgut carcinoid tumors start in the distal colon or rectum.

Data from literature indicate that the incidence of carcinoids in certain locations is different, although it is considered to be most often localized on the appendix vermiformis, in about 40% of cases, on ileum about 25%, on rectum 15-20% and on respiratory system around 10%. On the other hand, the Japanese National Study has identified, in 90 057 operated patients during the period of 15 years, 345 cases of carcinoids on the small and large bowel, out of which 0,9% was localized on the ileum, 2,3% on the appendix, 8,2% on the colon and 88,6% on the rectum

http://dx.doi.org/10.5772/56937

[1]. Their secretion is active and secrete around 30 vasoactive substances, the most important of which are serotonin, histamine and substance P. In 1867, Langhans [1] first described a gut carcinoid tumor, but the first detailed description of the tumor, similar to carcinoid, was given by Lubrasch 1888, after performing the autopsy on two persons, previously treated due to having multiple tumors of ileum. A German pathologist Oberndorfer first mentioned the term "carcinoid" in 1907, while Siburg published the first data about the rectum carcinoid in 1929 [4-5]. The term "carcinoid" indicates that the tumor, according to some histological characteristics, is similar to carcinoma, but it behaves in a more benign way and less aggressive. They have often been discovered accidently, during the colonoscopy, or by examination of the clinical symptoms, such as rectoragia or diarrhea. During the primary diagnosing, 60-90% of carcinoids are less than 1 cm of size.These tumors have a variable malignant potential, which depends on: size, localization, depth of invasion and way of growth of the tumor itself.

According to the data from literature, the colon and rectum carcinoids less than 1 cm of size have metastases in about 5,5% of cases. The bigger sized tumors, 1-1.9 cm, have metastasis within the range of 4 to 30%, while those above 2 cm, within the range of 70-80%. With regard to localization, the rectum carcinoids have metastasis in 18% on average, unlike the colon ones in 60%, jejunoileal localization in 34%, stomach in 23% and lungs in 21% [2]. The depth of invasion, particularly the tumors, which are less than 2 cm in size, represents a very important predictive factor in the method and outcome of treatment. Invasion of muscularis propria and lymphovascular, i.e. perineural invasion, anaplastic reaction, positive Ki-67 mutations and frequent mitosis increase the risk of metastasis of tumors, which are less than 2 cm in size. Macroscopically, these are small tumors in the nodular form, covered with the normal mucosa, with intensive fibrosis of the intestine wall. Ulcerous forms with a tendency of bleeding, have metastasis in larger percent and represent a significant risk factor. Histologically, the tumor cells look similar, rounded or polygonal with expressed nucleus and acidophilic cytoplasmic granules. Immunohistochemically, they show focal or diffuse existence of chromaganin A and/ or neuron-specific enolase, synaptophysina, CD 56 and pancreatic polypeptide. There is no clear histological difference between benign and malignant large bowel carcinoids, except the size of the tumor itself and invasion of muscularis proprie.

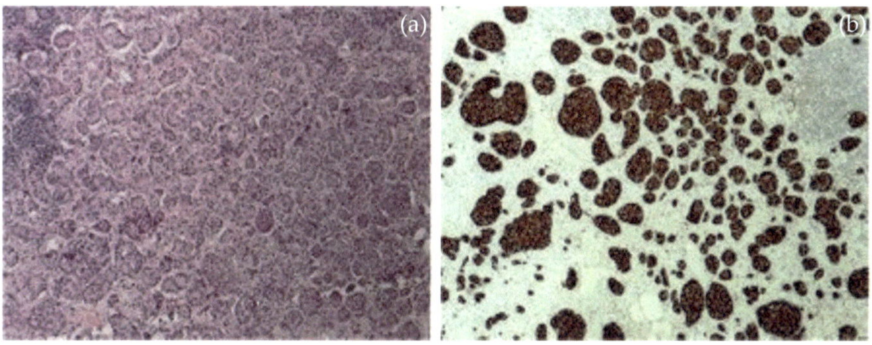

Figure 1. a) colon carcinoid (H&E 10x); b) colon carcinoid (chromogranin A 10x)

2.1. Clinical presentation and diagnosis

The clinical presentation is characterized by the existence of symptoms resulting from the secretion of different biochemical substances and growth of the tumor itself. Occasional abdominal pains, followed by facial flushing, diarrhea, bronchospasm, arrhythmia, hyperthermia, - blood pressure variations and vasomotor collapse, which, based on the intensity can lead to a life dangerous condition, or so called "carcinoid crisis". Various daily activities and psychological conditions, such as alcohol drinking, emotional stress, increased body temperature and difficult defecation potentiate the intensity of symptoms.

The diagnosis of the large bowell carcinoids was usually made by detailed anamnesis and clinical examination of the abdomen and digital rectal examination. Very often, it is an unclear finding, due to the intact mucosa, so it is necessary to take biopsy from the part of the tumor surface, as well as, from the deeper structures. It is also necessary to include a colonoscopy in clinical examination, due to the possible existence of the synchronous lesion, and magnetic resonance imaging or endoluminal ultrasound of the small pelvis, because of the pre-operative staging. The examination of the liver metastatsis, should be completed with an ultra-sound and CT scan. The modern diagnostics of carcinoids understands also the, so called, functional or biochemical examinations based on taking over of the certain substances by the tumor cells, which makes them different from the normal tissue. The biochemical properties of carcinoid tumors reflect the presence of neurosecretory granules. They are classified as biochemically typical or atypical based on the presence of high levels of serotonin in so-called typical tumors. The best known metabolite of serotonin in carcinoid tumors is 5-HIAA(hydroxyl indole acetic acid). In a 24-hour sample, the urinary level of 5-HIAA is the test most commonly used in the endocrine work-up of carcinoid tumors. Despite its popularity, it lacks the sensitivity and specificity for the diagnosis of carcinoid tumors because 5-HIAA may not be elevated in atypical carcinoids and can be elevated in other conditions such as tropical sprue, celiac disease, Whipple's disease, and small bowel obstruction, and can be caused by ingestion of food high in serotonin, or certain medications.

Although a number of other tumor markers have been investigated for carcinoid tumor overproduction, serum analysis of chromogranin A, a glycoprotein that is secreted with other hormones by neuroendocrine tumors, appears to be the most promising, with specificity approaching 95% and sensitivity for carcinoid tumors approaching 80 percent. A 40 percent false-positive rate has been seen in patients with multiple myeloma[6].

For this purpose, the scintigraphy of the somatostin receptors on the surface of tumor cells is applied, or SRS and PET scan, which uses a metabolic taking over of FDG Fluorin- 18 fluorodeoxyglucose, by the tumor cells. The results of the research indicate that, Octreoscan is the most optimal for identification of the primary tumor and existence of the positive lymph nodes, while in the case of distant metastasis, it is CT or NMR. Within the frame of the biochemical analyses, in case of doubt that there is a carcinoid present, it is necessary to determine the level of 5 hydroxy-indole acetic acid in urine.

http://dx.doi.org/10.5772/56937

2.2. Treatment

The treatment of the colon carcinoid can be divided into two groups:

a. minimally invasive procedure

b. laparatomy

c. Minimally invasive procedure includes several types of interventions:

   – endoscopic mucosectomy or submucosectomy

   – transanal tumor extirpation

   – TEM (transanal endoscopic microsurgery)

   – laparoscopic resections of colon and rectum

Endoscopic mucosectomy or submucosectomy represent one of the possible methods in the conditions of the initial stadium of disease, without penetration into muscularis mucosae, and up to 1 cm of size. The literature data show that endoscopic mucosetomy or submucosetomy are performed in 54% of patients suffering from rectum carcinoid, transanal extirpation of tumor /TEM in 27% of the operated patients, on one hand, as well as in 6% of patients treated by the invasive procedure, on the other [7-9].

The results of the treatment indicate that, in patients treated by the endoscopic methods, in 83% of cases, it was about the positive limits (R1 status), in 16% it was the residual tumor (R2 status) with 2% of acute complications in terms of the occurrence of post-operative bleeding. In 12 patients (14%), a sub-mucosectomy was done, with 42% of the positive margins present.

The advantage of the endoscopic approach is a minimally invasive procedure, faster recovery of a patient and smaller operative trauma, but there are also disadvantages in terms of the high percent of R1 or R2 procedure, (positive margins or residual tumor).

Transanal exstirpation/TEM is indicated in the conditions of rectal carcinoid invasion to the submucose and muscularis proprie. They are mainly performed after the unsuccessful, previously done mucosectomy i.e. sub-mucosectomy. The results of treatment indicate that in 43% of the operated patients, RO resection was done, while in 52% of cases R1, i.e. R2 resection was done. The post-operative complications occurred in about 9% of patients. The disadvantage of the procedure is still a high percentage of R1 and R2 operations.

Laparoscopic resections of colon and rectum represent a trend in the modern colorectal surgery, with all characteristics of the minimally invasive procedure. It is indicated in tumors, which spread to the structures deeper than lamina muscularis mucosa (T2 stadium), most often to the upper third of rectum, but the other parts of rectum as well, where performing the endoscopic procedure would lead to a high percent of R1 and R2 operations.

2.2.1. Laparatomy

– resection of colon (according to the type of segmental or right/left hemicolectomies)

– (resections of rectum with different forms of reconstructions T-T anastomosis, L-T anastomosis, colonic J pouch, etc.)

– incontinence operations (abdominoperineal amputation of rectum, etc.)

– in case of inoperability of tumor, the performance of colostomy.

Laparotomy is indicated in carcinoids of greater median size, so-called bulky tumors, with infiltration to the surrounding organs, as well as, with the potential risk of the colon obstruction. In relation to the outcome of treatment, the resection procedures are loaded with a higher percent of the local recurrence rate, which is explained by the existence of the more invasive and bigger tumors, treated in this way [10-13].

Systemic therapy in carcinoid treatment has two aims

– to reduce intensity of the systemic effects of disease and

– treatment of metastasis.

Reducing intensity of the systemic effects means the use of various medicaments, such as: H2 blockers, Phenothiazin, corticosteroids, serotonin blockers serotonin, bronchodilators etc. The analogues of Somatostatin have a significant effect that, by blocking the receptors reduce the production and systemic effects, primarily the intensity of flushing and diarrhea, in 80% of patients.

Staging system	Colon carcinoids		Rectal carcinoids	
	% patien.	5-year surv.%	% patient.	5-year surv.%
I	13	97	83	97
II	32	69	6,5	84
III	12	21	2,8	27
IV	43	17	7,4	20
N 0	52		96	
1	48		4	
M 0	76		97,6	
1	24		2,4	

Table 1. Staging system and 5- year survival rate [14-16]

In treatment of metastasis, the effect of chemotherapy application (5-fluorouracil, strreptozotocin, doxorubicin,, etoposide, cisplatin, carboplatin, etc.) is insignificant, with a clinical response (Response Rate- RR) from 0 to 30%. In some cases, Interferon is used, in duration of up to 2,5 years, but due the numerous unfavorable effects, its use is limited [6].

The prognosis of the disease, depending on TNM stadium. A search of 15,983 patients with carcinoid tumors from the National Cancer Institute's SEER (Surveillance Epidemiology and

End Results) database identified 2459 with colon tumors and 4701 patients with rectal carcinoid tumors from 1973 to 2004. Patients were analyzed according to various clinicopathologic factors and a tumor (T1, T2, T3), lymph node (N0, N1), and metastasis (M0, M1) staging system was created according to these parameters. Results is shown in Table 1.

3. Primary non-Hodgkin lymphomas

Lymphomas of colon and rectum are the rare tumors that make 1,4% of human lymphomas, 10-20% of gastrointestinal lymphomas, 0,2-0,6% of all malignant tumors of colon, that is, 0,1-1% of all tumors of the large bowel. According to the incidence in the gastrointestinal system in adults, they take a third place, following the stomach and small intestine, unlike with the age of up to seventeen, where the intestinal localization is predominant. In relation to the incidence of all malignant colon and rectum diseases, they take a third place, following adenocarcinoma and carcinoids [17,18]. The predilection places of occurrence are cecum and rectum, due to large amount of lymph tissue in these regions of the large bowel.

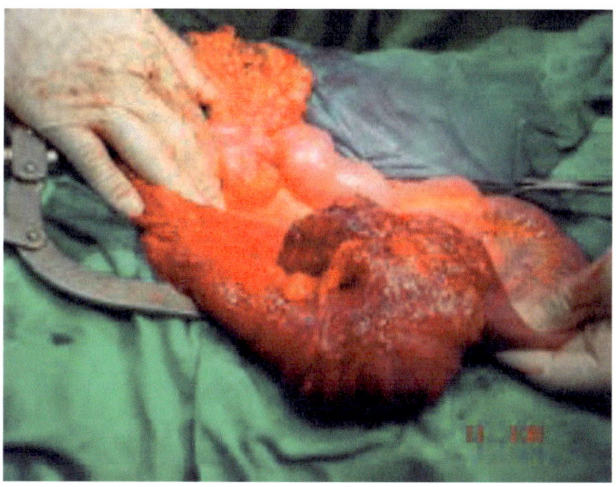

Figure 2. Primary non-Hodgkin lymphoma of the cekum

It occurs more often in male patients, older than 50. With regard to the degree of spreading, diseases can be: primary (localized) and secondary (diffuse form). The primary lymphomas of the large bowel are characterized by the existence of the so-called Dawson's criteria [19]:

1. no palpable, superficial lymph nodes at presentation;l
2. no enlarged mediastinal lymph nodes on chest x-ray;
3. normal range for white blood cell count including total and differential
4. at surgery, only the regional lymph nodes are involved;

5. the liver and spleen are without disease

Primary lymphoma of the colon is a predominantly extranodal form of non-Hodgkin lymphoma, while Hodgkin type is much rarer, present in less than 5% of all patients autopsied due to this disease [20-22]. Devin and his coworkers from the Mayo Clinic, published the largest study of patients with rectum lymphomas,which shows that, out of 61 patients treated in the period of 27 years, 49 of them had a diffuse form and only 12 had a localized disease [23]. The tumors usually have a form of polypoid and ulceriform mass, and sometimes, they form excrescent on mucosa, similar to multiple adenomatous polyposis.

Etiological factors in formation of the large bowel lymphoma are unknown, as well as for the other types of malignant diseases. However, the higher incidence was noticed in the conditions of immunosuppression, such as the inflammatory disease – ulcerative colitis, HIV virus infections and conditions after organ transplantations, although there are no clear scientific proofs about the connections among these diseases.

More than two-thirds of intestinal lymphomas are supposed to be of B cell lineage, while T cell intestinal lymphomas are rather infrequent and often multifocal and most frequently localized in the small bowel. In relation to the histological type of B cell, non-Hodgkin lymphomas can be: diffuse B cell type, MALT lymphoma, mantle type, Burkitt type and follicular lymphoma. The incidence of some histopathological forms differs from study to study, so Anderson and his associates presented the data of the, so-called, International Study Group about Lymphomas, which included 1378 patients from 8 different cities from 4 continents. Out of the total number of the histopathological findings, in 80% of cases B-cell lymphoma was diagnosed, where the most common form was the one with the large cells, while the other forms, such as mantle, Burkitt and MALT types were significantly rare. In relation to the histological grades, in 75% of tumors, a moderate and intermediately type of diffuse lymphoma of the large cells was established [24-27].

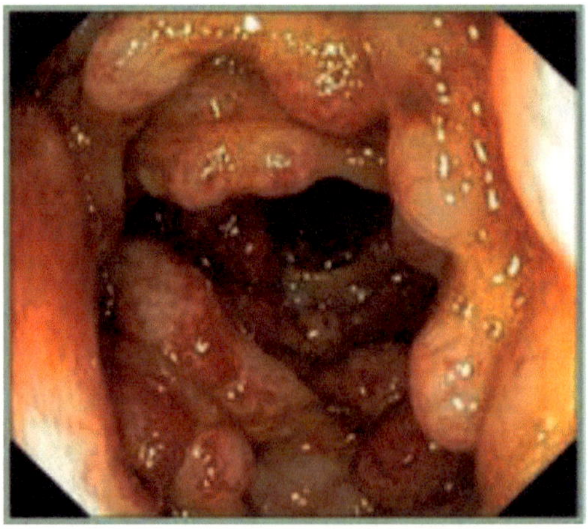

Figure 3. Mantle type of primary non-Hodgkin lymphoma

The degree of disease spreading to the surrounding structures was the best presented by the, so-called, Ann-Arbor staging, modification according to Musshoffu [28,29]. The aim of the successful treatment is the early detection of the disease in IE or IIE stage where still there is a possibility of curative resection. The data from literature are significantly different in relation to the stage of a disease in treated patients, which is a consequence of the various criteria according to which the patients were included into the study, different methodologies of performance and the level of health culture among the tested population.

Stage	Characteristics
IE	Limited to the colonic/rectal wall
IIE 1	Involvement of paracolic lymph nodes
IIE 2	Involvement of intermedial lymph nodes.
III	Involvement of the large bowel and lymph nodes on both sides of diaphragm
IV	Involvement of distant organs (large bowel and one or more extralymphatic organs or tissue)

Table 2. Ann-Arbor staging- Musshoff modifications of primary colorectal lymphoma[29].

3.1. Clinical presentation and diagnosis

The clinical presentation is characterized by the existence of rectoragia and the changed bowel habits. By analyzing the symptoms of the disease, Cho and his associates, presented the study data, which showed that, out of 23 patients, 56% had a non-specific symptoms, abdominal pain and weight loss or anorexia, that is, 35% the of tested patients were operated in the advanced stage of the disease [30]. The data from the research made by Fan and associates, showed that, out of 37 tested patients, 59% had only abdominal pain and 75,7% were operated in the stage of the disease where positive lymphoma nodes were present in the mesenterium of colon and mesorectum. The specific symptoms, such as bleeding per rectum, were present in only 12,5% of patients [17]. Non-specificity of symptoms often postpones timely visit to a doctor and timely diagnosing, which leads to a much higher incidence of the advanced stages of the disease. A special problem is primary colorectal lymphomas - present as surgical emergency, caused by tumors of the IIIE and IVE stages[31]. Surgical emergencies, caused by the obstruction of the large bowel, or perforation, initiate a need for urgent surgical intervention, which leads to significantly higher rate of mortality of 58% and more frequent disease recurrence [32-36]. The diagnosis can be made - by taking the anamnestic data and clinical examination including digito rectal examination and colonoscopy with biopsy. There are data from literature, which show that it is not always possible to establish the diagnosis by endoscopic procedures, due to inadequately made biopsy of the tumor, as well as the need for timely performance of an adequate immunohistochemical staining during histopathological examination, which is done by a pathologist. It very often leads to inability to give correct interpretation of the pathologic finding [37].

3.2. Treatment

Modern treatment of the primary lymphoma of colon and rectum implies a multi-modal approach, that is, a surgical intervention, chemotherapy and radiotherapy in selected cases. Beside the doubtless improvements achieved in surgical technique, as well as in anesthesiology and chemotherapy, during the last three decades, there is still a low level of the five-year survival among the operated patients, which is 42% [29, 37]. The treatment of the large bowel Non-Hodgkin lymphoma is characterized by the existence of different attitudes about it, from applying only chemo and radiotherapy on one side, to the performance of surgical procedures, on the other. Bilsel and his associates published a review of the case from 2005, which gave a complete clinical response of the primary rectal lymphoma, after the treatment with chemo and radiotherapy [24]. The other authors also presented similar data [38,39]. Pricolo and his associates, in their analysis of the case presentation from 2002, describe the treatment of rectum lymphoma using the resection procedures and then chemo and radio therapy, while Shimono from Japan recommends a pre-operative radiotherapy first, and then a surgical intervention [40,41]. Regarding the type of operation, there are recommendations that, with small dimension primary rectal lymphoma and low malignant potential – MALT or mantle type lymphoma, it is enough to perform a limited resection or transanal extirpation of tumor [42,43]. The differences in attitude are the consequence of the results achieved based on the presentations of cases or studies about a small number of patients and a heterogeneous groups of the treated tumors, in various stages of the disease, with different histopathological diagnosis etc. Nevertheless, based on the modest experience of the authors, the resection of the large bowel is recommended whenever possible, together with neo or adjuvant therapy [44, 45].

4. GISTs

Gastrointestinal stromal tumors or, shortly GISTs, are the most common mesenchymal tumors, which are characterized by positive c-KIT, that is, CD117, CD 34 antigens, and they make 0,1-1% of all gastrointestinal tract tumors. They occur most commonly in the stomach 60-70% and small intestine 20-25%, while they are the least present in the large bowel, around 5%, and 0,9% of all tumors in the rectum. In relation to the incidence of occurrence only in the large bowel, they occur in 80% of all patients in the rectum, while in 20% of cases it is in the colon. They occur in middle-aged persons between 40-60 and between both sexes equally, with the incidence of 6,8 / 1 000 000 [46].

At the beginning of XXth century, Theodor Bilroth provided the first descriptions of the stromal tumors. However, the term “stromal tumor” was introduced bay Mazur and Clark only in 1983, following the development of immunohistochemistry. One year later, in 1984, Henry Appelman introduced the term "GIST-gastrointestinal stromal tumors" for the first time, while Kindblom and his associates proved that GISTs originate from the interstitial Cajal cells, which represent the so called, pace maker cells of the gastrointestinal tract. Due to the similar structural and immunohistochemical characteristics of GISTs and Cajal cells, many authors are of the opinion that they originate from the same mesenchimal cell [45]. Invasiveness, or the metastasis risk assessment of the GISTs on various locations, determined by the size of tumor and mitotic index, as shown in table 4 [47].

Mitotic count	Size	Gastric GIST	Duodenal GIST	Jejunal & ileal GIST	Rectal GIST
≤5/50	<2 cm	0%	0%	0%	0%
	>2 ≤5	1.9%	8.3%	4.3%	8.5%
	>5 ≤10	3.6%	34%	24%	57%
	>10	12%		52%	
>5/50	≤2	0%	N/A	50%	54%
	>2 ≤5	16%	50%	73%	52%
	>5 ≤10	55%	86%	85%	71%
	>10	86%		90%	

Table 3. Metastasis risk assessment of GISTs in different parts of GI tract [48].

4.1. Clinical presentation and diagnosis

GISTs are symptomatic in about 70%, - in about 10% asymptomatic and in 20% they are discovered during the autopsy, which shows that 1/3 of the large bowel stromal tumors are clinically completely silent. The symptomatology is very similar to the other colon tumors, and is characterized by hematochezia, abdominal or rectal pain, occurrence of complete rectum prolapse etc.[49]. Depending on the tumor size, it is possible to get the clinical presentation of the obstruction or ileus, caused by the growth of GISTs. The diagnosis - can be made by taking the anamnestic data, clinical examination including a digital rectal exam, which should be completed with rectoscopy, colonoscopy, endorectal ultrasound and NMR. It is necessary to do a biopsy of tumor with immunohistochemical analysis, for definite confirmation of the GIST existence in the large bowel. In the case of any doubt that there is metastasis in the liver, it is also necessary to perform the ultrasound and CT scan, within the complete staging of tumor. PET scan is indicated in the operated patients in order to follow up.

4.2. Treatment

Surgical intervention is a method of choice in treatment of large bowel GISTs, and is applied in the following cases:

1. Primary disease;
2. Metastatic diseases
3. Recurrence

The main aims of surgical treatment of the primary disease are the complete resection, so-called R0 resection and preservation of the tumor pseudocapsule, without wide resection margins and lymphadenectomy. This is very important in treatment of the rectum GISTs, due to the aims of sphincter saving procedure and improve the patient's quality of life. With regard to the size and localization of the large bowel stromal tumors, it is possible to use various surgical procedures: segmental resection, local excision, anterior and abdominoperineal resection. The performance of the anterior resection (high or low), means the observance of the partial or total mesorectal excision principles, in order to prevent sacral nerves injury, bleeding or local recurrence.

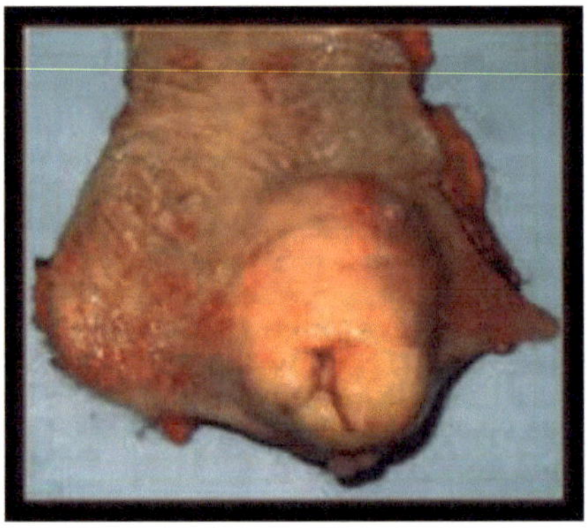

Figure 4. Rectal GIST

When GIST adheres to contiguous organs, consideration should be given to an en bloc resection. The modern aspects of the GISTs treatment also mean the use of Imatinib, a medicament, which revolutionary contributed to the significantly better results in treatment in GISTs. Joensuua, Heinrick van Oosterona and Tuveson made the first reports about the use of Imatinib in 2001. An immediate cause for the invention of this medicament was the discovery of Hirot about the existence of the abnormal activation of KIT oncoprotein or transmembrane receptor tyrosine kinase and the following mutation of C-kit gene, with exceptional cellular proliferation. Imatinib selectively inhibits the receptors of the transmembrane tyrosin kinese, thus blocking the abnormal growth of tumor. Van Oosteron and his associates published the results from 70% of clinical responses in KIT-positive metastatic GISTs [50,51]. Primary unresectable GISTs of the large bowel are initially treated with Imatinib, with an aim to reduce the size of a tumor – "downsizing". In the case of the existence of a metastatic disease, a non-adjuvant use of Imanitib is indicated, in order to secure good clinical response, meaning a disease without progression, with the possibility of performing R0 resection [52]. When there is a small volume metastasis in liver, some authors recommend the simultaneous resection of the large bowel and liver, and then the application of Imatinib[53]. Distant metastasis occur on the liver in over 50%, and they are treated with the initial application of Imatinib, followed by the various resection procedures.

The treatment of GISTs using chemotherapy has a minimum effect, RR<10%, and has no significance for the overall survival, as well as the application of radiotherapy, since the tumor is radio resistant.

4.3. Treatment outcomes

The outcome of the large bowel GISTs treatment is troubled with a high percentage of local and distant recurrences, so after the R0 resection, it occurs in 45-50% of cases, 20-25 months after the surgical intervention. The average five-year survival rate is 50%, 73% after the R0 and in 26% after R1 and R2 resections. In the case of the advanced disease with local recurrence and metastatic disease, a five-year survival rate is 28-35% [54].

5. Squamous cell carcinoma

Squamous cell Carcinoma of the large bowel is a very rare disease, unlike its localizations on the esophagus and the anal canal. The data from literature are based on the reviews of the clinical cases and series with a small number of patients. Schmidtmann first described the squamous cell carcinoma of the large bowel, actually cecum in 1919, and Reiford described the same disease on the rectum in 1933. Currently, there are about 100 cases of the squamous cell carcinoma of the large bowel described in literature, and the incidence of the disease is 0,1-0,25 on 1000 patients suffering from the colorectal carcinoma [55].

Due to a very rare occurrence of the tumor, there is a lack of prospective studies, or meta analyses, which would offer data about the demographic characteristics of the patients, risk factors, the nature of the disease behavior, as well as the optimal treatment.It mainly occurs in patients of the average age of 60, more often among women 66% than among men 34% [56].Etiology of the occurrence of colorectal squamous cell carcinoma is still unknown, as well as of the other kinds of malignant diseases, although there are several theories trying to explain the formation of this neoplasm:

– The influence of differentiation of stem cells,

– Squamous metaplasia at the place of existence of colorectal adenoma,

– Proliferation of uncommitted mucosal basal cells into squamous cells which subsequently undergo a malignant transformation

– Oncogenic influence of the chronicle kidney insufficiency, as well as, the application of the immunosuppressive therapy in terms of development of some cancerous viruses or oncogenic differentiation of the stem cells,

– Special influences of irradiation, colocutaneous fistula, ulcerous colitis, Entamoeba histolityca colitis, homosexuality, immunosuppression, schistosomiasis, and still unclear influence of HIV (human papilloma viruses types 16, 18, 31, 33) [57- 59].

5.1. Clinical presentation and diagnosis

The symptoms of the disease are very similar to the symptoms of colon carcinoma, such as bleeding, abdominal pain, change in bowel habits with the episodes of diarrhea and obstipation and weight loss.The diagnosis is established by taking the anamnestic data, clinical examination including digital rectal exam, which should be completed with rectoscopy, colonoscopy, MSCT, endorectal ultrasound andd NMR.Williams and his associates published the following criteria for diagnosing the squamous cell carcinoma of the large bowel, in 1979:

1. non-existence of the squamous cell carcinoma and its metastasis on the other locations (particularly the skin),
2. careful anoscopy and rectoscopy in order to exclude the existence proximal extension of anal squamous cell carcinoma,
3. non-existence of a fistulous tract lined by squamous cells [55, 58].

These criteria should be completed with the excision biopsy of tumor, as well as, the PH, or immunohistochemical confirmation (presence of cytokeratin CAM 5.2, AE1/AE3 i 34B12. CAM 5.2). Sub-mucous localizations of the squamous cell carcinoma represent a separate problem, due to difficult identification during standard examinations, so, in these cases, it is recommended to use endoluminal ultrasound guided needle biopsy of tumor. Determination of values of the tumor markers represents one of the possible auxiliary diagnostic procedures for determination of the disease, under the condition that the marker is specific for a particular tumor. In the case of the squamous cell carcinoma of the colon and rectum, there are no specific tumor markers, so those, usually used for the anal squamous cell carcinoma or for the so called layer plate cells of carcinoma antigen (Squamous cell carcinoma antigen "-SCC Ag)", are used. According to the opinions of some authors, SCC Ag is not specific for the initial diagnosis, but for the follow up of the occurance of local and distant recurrence after treatment [60].

5.2. Treatment

Surgical intervention is a method of choice in treatment of the squamous cell carcinoma of the large bowel. The type of surgical intervention depends on the size of tumor, its localization, depth of invasion into the colon wall, presence of local and distant metastasis, BMI (Body Mass Index), general condition of the patient and presence of comorbidity. The types of surgical intervention are similar to those used with the colon carcinoma: endoscopic mucosa/submucosa resection, segmental or hemi colectomy, local excision, resection procedures on the rectum, as well as abdominoperineal amputation of the rectum. Endoscopic mucosa/submucosa resection is applied based on the experience acquired in treatment of adenocarcinoma, and is indicated in patients with superficial tumors – T1 stage and with an expressed comorbidity. Endoscopic mucosa/sub-mucosa resection, local excision (trans-anal or trans-anal endoscopic microsurgery-TEM) is a method of choice with T1 stage of the disease, which means a tumor spreading to mucosa/sub-mucosa. There are some dilemmas about the type of treatment in T2 stage (spreading to muscularis proprie), because after application of the local excision, a recurrence rate is present in 20% of the operated patients. In these cases, it is necessary to make a good pre-operative staging of tumor in relation to the existence of the positive lymph nodes and the range of spreading to the large bowel wall.In the cases of the transmural spreading to the wall, up to the pericolic/rectal fat tissue – T3 stage, as well as the infiltration into the surrounding organs T4-stage, there are dilemmas whether it is better to do a surgical intervention first, and then the chemotherapy, or vice versa. The researches, which

http://dx.doi.org/10.5772/56937

were made based on the application of the identical treatment protocol in anal squamous cell carcinoma - (combination of the chemo and radio therapy 5-FU +mitomycin-C and radio 45 Gy), did not give the expected results in localization of the proximal parts of the rectum and colon. There are data in literature, which recommend only application of the chemo and radio therapy, as well as, the simultaneous chemo-radiation. However, the majority of authors agree that, for the time being and based on the experiences acquired in treatment of a small number of patients, the optimal therapy means surgical intervention and the adjuvant chemo radiation [52]. Surgical treatment of the advanced disease means the application of the resection procedures (colectomy, high and low resection of rectum) and abdominoperineal amputations of rectum. The resections of rectum, as a sphincter preserving operation, enable better quality of life of the patient on one hand, and compliance with the oncological principles on the other. Regardless of the advantages of the resection procedures in relation to the amputation surgery of rectum, the data from literature show that Miles's operation has been performed twice as much in treatment of the squamous cell carcinoma of rectum, which has been explained by a large number of advanced tumors at the time of diagnosing [61].

The disease prognosis is based on determination of the TNM stage, the most important prognostic factor, identical to the one in anal squamous cell carcinoma. The TNM stage is shown in Table 4.

Stadium	T	N	M
0	Tis	N0	M0
I	T1	N0	M0
	T2	N0	M0
IIA	T3	N0	M0
IIB	T4	N0	M0
IIIA	T1-T2	N1	M0
IIIB	T3-T4	N1	M0
IIIC	Any T	N2	M0
IV	Any T	Any N	M1

Table 4. TNM staging system of squamous cell carcinoma of the large bowel [56].

By comparing the disease prognosis from adenocarcinoma of the colon and rectum of the same stage, it has been established that stages of the disease I and II have a similar prognosis, unlike the advanced ones (stages III and IV), where squamous cell carcinoma has worse prognosis. The average five-year survival is 32%, with variations, which are related to the certain stages: Dukes B 50%, Dukes C 33% & Dukes D 0%. Application of the adjuvant therapy improves the overall survival of a patient, on one hand, while the pre-operative radiotherapy increases the percent of the sphincter preserving operation, on the other [58,59].

6. Melanoma

Melanoma of the gastrointestinal tract is a rare mucosal melanoma with a particularly aggressive biology compared with cutaneous one of equal stage. They most often occur as a metastatic tumor, while the primary localization is rare and possible in esophagus, stomach, small intestine and anorectum, that is, at the places where melanocyte normally exist. The colon melanoma is an extremely rare tumor with regard to the fact that, embryologically, melanocytes do not exist in this part of colon and that, up to now, only 12 cases have been describes in the English literature. There are several theories, which describe the formation of the colon melanoma: relation to neural crest cells, model of tumor regression and ectodermal differentiation, but none of them has been completely proved so far. Localization in the anorectum takes the third place regarding the incidence of localization, behind the rest of skin and eyes surfaces and it makes 1-1,5% of all melanomas in the human body, and 3-15% of all tumors of the colon and rectum [62,63]. Moore described it for the first time in 1857 and, until now, the total of 500 cases was described in the literature. The most often it occurs on the skin, under the dental line, and rarely at the level of cuboidal epithelium of the transition zone and mucosae of the distal rectum. It is more common in women (twice as much than in men), between 60 and 70 years of age [64]. The melanoma represents a disease of the neuroectodermal origin, which the most often originates from melanocytes and nevus cells of the basal layer of epidermis, and significantly less from mucosa. It has an extremely worse long-term prognosis, because of the disease discovery in the advanced stage, mainly with metastasis in the inguinal nodes. Beside the lymhogenous dissemination, spreading is possible by the local ingrowth and in hematogenous way. The local spread is according to the radial (horizontal) and vertical growth. Radial growth means circular spreading around the primary tumor, through the epithelium of mucosa and the superficial layers of sub-mucosa, without tendency of metastasizing. Vertical growth means penetration into the deeper layers of the colon wall, with simultaneous metastasizing. Determination of level of the vertical tumor growth, i.e. involvement of the colon and rectum wall layers, is essential for the choice of surgical intervention. The most important roles here have the MSCT (multi-slice scanner), NMR (magnetic resonance) and endoluminal ultrasound. Hematogenous dissemination occurs by penetration of the melanoma cells into the blood vessels, with further spreading to the whole body. About 30% of patients, at the moment of diagnosing, are considered to have a disseminated process, while only 17% of the operated ones have a five-year survival. [65,66]. It differs from skin melanoma in the way that 25% of tumors do not contain a pigment of the so called "coloured" tumor, and because ultraviolet radiation is a factor of protection, not a risk. In case of existence of the pigment tumor of the rectum, the macroscopic appearance is very similar to thrombosed external and prolapsing internal hemorrhoids (see figure 5), which can mislead a doctor in setting a diagnosis[67,68].

The symptoms of the disease are different, but the most common ones are the abdominal pain, weight loss and bleeding.The diagnosis of the disease implies to detailed anamnesis, physical examination with special reference to inspection of all parts of skin and eyes, as the most common primary localizations, as well as, taking biochemical laboratory analyses, digito rectal examination, colonoscopy, barium enema, multi-slice scanner (MSCT), magnetic resonance

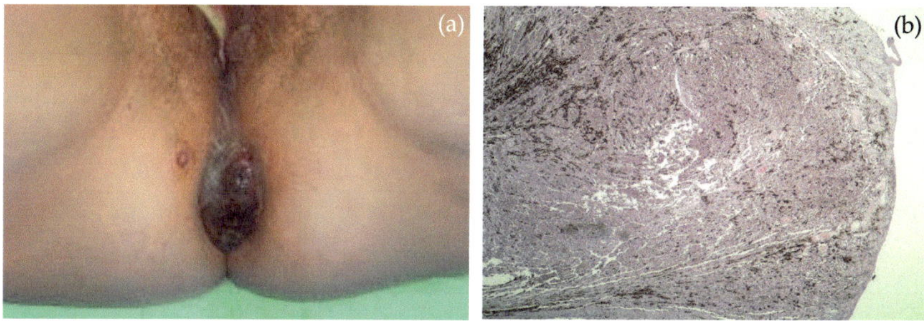

Figure 5. a). Prolapsed melanoma recti; b). Histopathological finding of melanoma recti (H&E 40x)

(NMR), endoluminal ultrasound and tumor biopsy with pathohistological and immunohistochemical processing. Special attention should be paid to the examination of certain groups of lymph nodes, depending on the primary tumor localization. Taking into account the results made by Kalid and his associates, the most often localization of the primary colon melanoma is cekum ascedens and transversum, while with the metastatic melanoma these are the ascendant and descendant parts of colon [62]. Curative treatment of the large bowel melanoma is exclusively surgical. The main aim of the treatment is to achieve a compromise between the necessity to apply a radical oncological treatment and a need to preserve the patient's quality of living. The contemporary approach to treatment of the primary colon and rectum melanoma implies to the performance of surgical interventions, such as:

a. colectomy with wide excisional margins (partial, hemi-colectomy, subtotal and total)

b. trans-anal wide local excision with preservation of the anal sphincter (in the case of the initial stage of the rectum tumor)

c. extensive surgeries according to the type of the rectum resection or abdominoperineal amputation.

There are numerous dilemmas about which type of surgical intervention to be applied in certain stages of the disease. The supporters of radical treatment recommend the resection or rectum abdominoperineal amputation, depending on the localization, with dissection of both inguinal regions, stating the following advantages:

– possibility of the detailed exploration of the abdomen and the eventual discovery of distant metastasis;

– lower percent of the local recurrence rate [69].

On the other hand, some authors recommend a wide local excision of tumor with preservation of the sphincter mechanism, for the following reasons:

– absence of definitive stoma,

– similar five-year survival [70,71].

The authors from MD Anderson Cancer Center present 20-year experience with treatment of 54 patients with localized anorectal melanoma, demonstrating that combined surgical wide local excision and adjuvant radotherapy provides good local disease control with acceptable side effects [72].The existence of such different attitudes in literature is a consequence of, primarily, uneven criteria of the researches made, comparison of different localizations of the anorectal melanoma and stage of the disease. The most significant parameter, based on which a decision about the type of surgical intervention is made, is the thickness of tumor. According to Weynadt and his associates, indication for a wide local excision are melanomas up to 4 mm thick, with the limits of excision up to 2 cm from the primary tumor, without involvement of sphincter, while the extensive surgeries on the rectum are recommended for the melanomas over 4 mm thick [73].In relation to the adjuvant therapy, melanomas are considered hemi resistant tumors, so certain cytostatic medicaments have an effect in 10-25% of the treated ones. The most often used are: dacarbazin, temozolamid, cisplatin, carboplatin, nitrosoureas.The latest research showed that determination of biological markers RAS/RAF/MEK/ERK, represent a significant indicator of the cell growth intensity degree, as well as, the invasion and survival [62]. The adjuvant therapy of anorectum melanoma is not very much successful because all these tumors are radio resistant and scarcely responsive to chemotherapy[74,75].

6. Extremely rare tumors

Other tumors include an extremely rare malignant diseases of the large bowel: primary teratomas, extramedullary plasmacytomas, schwannomas and metastasis of distant tumors.

Primary teratomas of the large bowel are very rare diseases and, there are only about 50 cases published in literature until now, mainly the ones in the rectum and in the form of clinical presentation. It occurs more often in women at the average age of 42,5. They are considered to originate as consequence of the ectopic development of the so-called "captured" ectodermal tissue although, in their composition, some structures of mesodermal endodermal origin are possible. Histologically, it is composed of the stratified squamous epithelia, fat cells, hair follicle, cartilage and, partially glandular tissue. They are usually benign tumors, however some malignant transformations are also possible, which create a need for the total elimination of tumor, due to compliance with the oncological principles. Data from literature indicate that teratomas usually occur in the ovary, testicles, mediastinum and the middle lines such as sacrococcygeal region, while they occur less frequently in the gastrointestinal tract (rectum, sigmoid part of colon, appendix and terminal ileum) [76]. The rectal teratomas usually have a polypoid cystic form, with protrusion into the lumen area. The solitary cysts are mainly present, filled in with sebaceous whitish liquid into which the sebaceous glands, hair follicles and teeth are immersed. Beside the cystic form, the existence of the solid tumors is possible, which indicates a mature form of the teratoma.

The clinical presentation is characterized by the presence of pain during defecation, bleeding and change in bowel habits. The diagnosis is established by the anamnesis and digital rectal examination, which confirms the existence of the polypoid tumor mass of mainly smooth edges and a pedicle. The cases of rupture of the ovarian teratoma into the rectal lumen are described, with the similar difficulties. The additional diagnostic procedures, such as the endoluminal ultrasound, multi-slice scanner and NMR give the additional information about the extensity of the tumor itself, as well as, the estimation of operability. Some malignant transformations of teratomas with a tendency of creating squamous cell carcinoma are possible, and due to this, it is not advisable to perform the transanal punctuation because of the danger of malignant cells spreading, on one hand, and the potential infection, on the other. The method of choice in the treatment is the complete elimination of the cystic tumor.

The most frequent form of plasma cell neoplasm is a multiple myeloma. Out of the total number of all multiple myeloma, only 2% are the so-called extramedullary plasmacytoma. More the 75% of extramedullary plasmacytoma occur in the upper part of the respiratory system, while the most common places of occurence in the gastrointestinal tract are the stomach and small intestine. Until now, 22 cases of the occurence of extramedulllary plasmacytoma in the colon, have been reported, where the average age of patients was around 52,3. The most frequent localization on the large bowel are the cecum with 36,4% and rectum with 22,7%. It is essential to make a differential diagnosis differentiation between the primary and secondary plasmacytoma, that is, the metastasis of the multiple myeloma. It is achieved by determination of the Bence-Jones proteins in urine, by serum electrophoresis, as well as, the immunohistochemical finding of the collections of monoclonal plasma cells.

The treatment involves the application of:

– surgical intervention in 81,8% of cases,

– radio-therapy in 9% of cases,

– combined application of surgical intervention and radio-therapy in 4,5% of cases [77,78].

Schwannomas originate from Schwann cells, which form neural sheath and belong to the group of stromal tumors. In the gastrointestinal tract, they most frequently appear in the stomach, while the primary Schwannomas of the large bowel are extremely rare and, until to now, only 39 clinical cases have been reported. They mainly occur in older patients around 65 years of age, of both sexes equally. They grow slowly and there is a large number of patients who do not have any symptoms at the moment of diagnosing. The symptoms occur depending on the size and localization of tumor, but vague pain in the abdomen, bleeding and change of bowel habitus mainly manifest them. The pre-operative diagnosing, using the standard procedures such as anamnesis, physical examination, colonoscopy MSCT, NMR and endoluminal ultrasound, is possible in determination of the tumor mass, but not the type and kind of tumor because it resembles to the GIST tumors of the colon. The most accurate diagnosis implies the elimination of tumor as a whole, with pathohistologic and immunohistochemical analyisis. It is also difficult to differentiate it from GISTs in respect of immunohistochemical analyisis and some authors classify it the sub-group of GISTs, such as GANT tumors, i.e. gastrointestinal autonomous nerve tumors [79].

7. Metastases in the colon and rectum from the distant tumors

The metastasis of distant primary tumors rarely spread to the large bowel, and it is usually related to the carcinoma of the surrounding organs (stomach, pancreas, ovarian etc.) which, due to their growth and size, spread to the surrounding parts of colon, or "fall" on the intraperitoneal rectum with secondary infiltration. The degree of the tumor spreading depends on the length of the primary tumor existence and the histologic type, although the literature data indicate that serosa is infiltrated in 28%, muscles' layer in 31% and mucosa in 14% of patients. The expansion of the prostate cancer is possible, with perforation to Denonvilliers fascia and the secondary spreading to the rectum, according to the type of circumferential, i.e. annular stenosis, without spreading to mucosa in men, as well as the carcinoma portie vaginalis uteri, in women [80,81]. The pouch of Douglas, as the lowest point in the abdomen and in the close vicinity of the rectum, is a place of intraperitoneal spreading of carcinoma of any intra-abdominal or retroperitoneal organ, with predomination of the stomach and ovarium. Carcinoma metastasis of retroperitoneal and extra-abdominal organs, pancreas, kidneys and breast, are described in literature [82,83]. The clinical presentation is similar to those of the other colon tumors (bleeding, change in the bowel habitus, pain in the region of anus), supplemented with symptomatology of the primary localization of the malignant process. The diagnosis implicates anamnesis, digital rectal examination, colonoscopy, endoanal ultrasound, multi-slice scanner, NMR, as well as, the biopsy with pathohisiological confirmation.

The strategy of treatment depends on:

– localization of the primary malignant process,

– advancement of the disease,

– histological type of the primary tumor

If the primary tumor localization is in the immediate vicinity of the colon and rectum (pancreas, sigma, prostate, cervix and vagina), it is recommended to use the so called en block resections, with an aim to achieve the oncological principle of radicalism or R0 procedure [84]. Sometimes, it is necessary to perform a non-adjuvant therapy in order to reduce the volume of tumor, so called "downsizing", and the biological aggressiveness of tumor, "down-staging", on one hand, or to supplement the surgical intervention with the adjuvant therapy, on the other. In the case of extra abdominal localization of the primary tumor, it is necessary to assess the effect of successfulness of the surgical intervention in achieving a R0 resection, or the application of the neoadjuvant therapy.

8. Conclusion

Rare tumors of the colon and rectum represent an important group of neoplasms, due to their specific prognosis secondary to late diagnosis, and resistance to conventional cancer therapy. Over the last 20 years, their overall incidence has increased, due to advent of novel imaging techniques, especially the development of more sophisticated diagnostic tools including high resolution CT and MRI, capsule endoscopy and somatostatin scintigraphy for NETs. Although the development of specific targeted therapies such as tyrosine kinase inhibitors for GISTs and somatostatin analogs for NETs have improved prognosis, early detection remains the critical variable in determining outcome. Similarly, promising therapeutic data in some subgroups are encouraging although the majority is still diagnosed late and targeted effective therapy is lacking. Difference in survival is the consequence of the difference in biological aggressiveness of tumor, way of the disease spreading and tendency towards metastasis on one hand, and the frequency of appearance and symptomatology on the other. Carcinoid was an indolent tumor with the best prognosis, both non-Hodgkin lymphoma and squamous cell carcinoma of the large bowel showed significantly worse overall survival rate, as compared to adenocarcinoma, while melanoma has the shortest time of survival. The aim of this chapter is to draw our attention to the rare tumors in everyday clinical practice.

Acknowledgements

We would like to express our gratitude to Mrs. Gorjana Djordjevic, for meticulous proofreading and assistance with the English text.

Author details

Goran Stanojević[1,2] and Zoran Krivokapić[3,4]

*Address all correspondence to: stgoran1964@gmail.com

1 Department of Surgery of the Medical Faculty – University of Niš, Niš, Serbia

2 Clinic for General Surgery, Clinical Center Niš, Niš, Serbia

3 Medical Faculty –University of Belgrade, Department of Surgery, Belgrade, Serbia

4 First Surgery Clinic, Clinical Center Serbia, Belgrade, Serbia

References

[1] Kang H, O'Connell JB, Leonardi MJ, Maggard MA, McGory ML, Ko CY. Rare tumors of the colon and rectum: a national review. Int J Colorectal Dis 2007; 22(2):183-189.

[2] Gordon Ph. Malignant neoplasms of the Colon. In: Gordon Ph, Nivatvongs S, (eds) Principles and Practice of the Surgery for the Colon Rectum and Anus. New York, London: Informa Healthcare; 2007. p 489-645

[3] Vilallonga R, Espín Basany E, López Cano M, Landolfi S, Armengol Carrasco. Neuroendocrine carcinomas of the colon and rectum. A unit's experience over six years Rev Esp Enferm Dig 2008;100(1):11-16.

[4] Gustafsson BI, Siddique L, Chan A, Dong M, Drozdov I, Kidd M, Modlin IM. Uncommon cancers of the small intestine, appendix and colon: an analysis of SEER 1973-2004, and current diagnosis and therapy. Int J Oncol. 2008;33:1121-1131.

[5] Yoon SN, Sik CY, Shin US. Clinicopathological characteristics of rectal carcinoids. Int J Colorectal Dis 2010; 25:1087–1092

[6] Robertson R G, Geiger W, Davis N. Carcinoid Tumors. Am Fam Physician. 2006;74(3):429-434.

[7] Devine R, Brand M. Miscellaneous Neoplasms. In: Wolff B, Fleshman J, Beck D, Pemberton J, Wexner S, (eds) The ASCRS Textbook of Colon and Rectal Surgery. Springer; 2007.p 515-524.

[8] Gibbs NM. The histogenesis of carcinoid tumours of the rectum.J Clin Pathol 1963; 22: 206-214.

[9] Kwann MR, Goldberg JE, Bleday R. Rectal carcinoid tumors: review of results after endoscopic and surgical therapy. Arch Surg. 2008;143(5):471-475.

[10] Soga J. Carcinoids of the rectum: an evaluation of 1271 reported cases. Surg Today 1997;27(2):112-119

[11] Jetmore AB, Ray JE, Gathright JB Jr, McMullen KM, Hicks TC, Timmcke AE. Rectal carcinoids: the most frequent carcinoid tumor. Dis Colon Rectum 1992;35(8):717-725

[12] Koura AN, Giacco GG, Curley SA, Skibber JM, Feig BW, Ellis LM. Carcinoid tumors of the rectum: effect of size, histopathology, and surgical treatment on metastasis free survival. Cancer 1997;79(7):1294-1298

[13] Neary P, Redmond PH, Houghton T, Watson GRK, Bouchier-Hayes D. Carcinoid disease: Review of the literature. Dis Colon Rectum 1997; 40 (3):349-362

[14] Landry CS, Brock G, Scoggins CR, McMasters KM, Martin RC. Proposed staging system for colon carcinoid tumors based on an analysis of 2,459 patients. J Am Coll Surg. 2008;207(6):874-881

[15] Landry CS, Brock G, Scoggins CR, McMasters KM, Martin RC. Proposed staging system for rectal carcinoid tumors based on an analysis of 4701 patients. Surgery. 2008;144(3):460-466.

[16] Schindl M, Niederle B, Häfner M; et al. Stage-dependent therapy of rectal carcinoid tumors. World J Surg 1998;22(6):628-634.

[17] Fan CW, Changchien Cr, Wang JY, Chen JS, Hsu KC, Tang R, et al. Primary colorectal lymphoma. Dis Colon Rectum 2005; 43: 1277-1282

[18] N. Doolabh, T. Anthony, C. Simmang, S. Bieligk, E. Lee, P. Huber, R. Hughes, et al. Primary colonic lymphoma. J Surg Oncol 2000; 74: 257-262.

[19] Dawson IM, Cornes JS, Morson BC. Primary malignant lymphoid tumours of the gastrointestinal tract. Br J Surg 1961; 49:80-9.

[20] Keighley MRB, Williams NS. Rare tumours of the colon and the rectum. In: Keighley MRB, Williams NS, (eds) Surgery of The Anus Rectum & Colon. WB Saunders, London-Toronto; 2001.p 1329-1347.

[21] Pandey M, Kothari KC, Wadhawa MK, Patel HP, Patel SM, Patel DD. Primary malignant large bowel lymphoma. Am Surg 2002; 68:121-126

[22] Koch P, del Valle F, Berdel WE, Willich NA, Reers B, HiddemannW, et al. Primary gastrointestinal Non-Hodgkin's lymphoma: I. Anatomic and histologic distribution, clinical features, and survival data of 371 patients registered in the German multicenter study GIT NHL 01/92. J Clin Oncol 2001; 19:3861-3873

[23] Devine RM, Beat RW Jr, Wolf BG. Malignant lymphoma of the rectum. Dis Colon Rectum 1986; 29: 812-814

[24] Jezersek Novakovic,B, Novakovic S, Frkovic-Grazio S. A single-center report on clinical features and treatment response in patients with intestinal T cell non-Hodgkin's lymphomas. ONCOLOGY REPORTS 2006; 16: 191-195.

[25] Harris ML, Jaffe ES, Diebold J, Flandrin G, Konrad MH, Vardiman J, et al. The World Health Organization classification of hematological malignancies. Report of the Clinical Advisory Committee meeting, Airline House, Virginia, November 1997. Mod Pathol 2000;13: 193-199.

[26] Bairey O, Ruchlemer R, Shpilberg O.Non-Hodgkin's lymphomas of the colon. Isr Med Assoc J 2006; 8:832-835

[27] Anderson JR, Armitage JO, Weisenburger DD. Epidemiology of the non-Hodgkin's lymphomas: distributions of the major subtypes differ by geographic locations. Non-Hodgkin's Lymphoma Classification Project. Ann Oncol 1998; 9: 717-720.

[28] Musshoff K. Klinische stadieneinteilung der nicht-Hodgkin lymphoma. stranlentherapie; 1977;153:218-221.

[29] National Cancer Institute. Summary and description of a working formulation for clinical usage. The Non-Hodgkin's Lymphoma Pathologic Clasisification Project 1982; 49:2112-2135.

[30] Cho MJ, Ha CS, Allen PK, Fuller LM, Cabanillas F, Cox J. Primary Non-Hodgkin Lymphoma of the Large Bowel. Therapeutic Radiology 1997; 205:535-539

[31] Gonzalez QH, Heslin MJ, Dávila-Cervantes A, Alvarez-Tostado J, de los Monteros AE, Shore G, Vickers SM. Primary colonic lymphoma. Am Surg 2008; 74: 214-216

[32] Cai S, Cannizzo F Jr, Bullard Dunn KM, Gibbs JF, Czuczman M, Rajput A.The role of surgical intervention in non-Hodgkin's lymphoma of the colon and rectum. Am J Surg 2007; 93:409-412

[33] Wang MH, Wong JM, Lien HC, Lin CW, Wang CY. Colonoscopic manifestations of primary colorectal lymphoma. Endoscopy 2001; 33:605-609.

[34] Jinnai D, Iwasa Z, Watanuki T. Malignant lymphoma of the large intestine-operative results in Japan. Surg Today 1983;13: 331-336.

[35] Contrery K, Nance FC, Becker WF. Primary lymphoma of the gastrointestinal tract. Ann Surg 1980;191:593-598.

[36] Busch E, Rodriguez-Bigas M, Mamounas E, Barcos M, Petrelli NJ. Primary colorectal non-Hodgkin's lymphoma.Ann Surg Oncol 1994;1: 222-228

[37] MTC Wong and KW Eu. Primary colorectal lymphomas. Colorectal Dis 2006;8:586-591.

[38] Devine R., Brand M. Miscellaneous Neoplasms. In: Wolff B, Fleshman J, Beck D, Pemberton J, Wexner S, (eds) The ASCRS Textbook of Colon and Rectal Surgery. Springer; 2007.p 515-524.

[39] Teare JP, Greenfield SM, Slater S. Rectal lymphoma after colectomy for ulcerative colitis. Gut 1992;33:138-139

[40] Ahmed M, El-Ghani M, Shafiey M, Fawzy M, Ismail H, Monir M. Clinico-Pathological Features and Outcome of Management of Pediatric Gastrointestinal Lymphoma J Egypt Nat Canc Inst 2005;17: 251-259.

[41] Pricolo R, Parziale A, Filosa M, Voltolini F, Zangrandi A. Primary lymphoma of the rectum: a case report and review of the literature.Chir Ital 2002; 54 (4): 549-554.

[42] Shimono R, Mori M, Kido A, Adachi Y, Sugimachi K. Malignant lymphoma of the rectum treated preoperatively with hyperthermia and radiation. Eur J Surg Oncol 1995; 21(1): 83-84

[43] Terauchi S, Yamamoto K, Fujii H, Koyama F, Sugimori S, Enomoto H, Yamanouchi M, Nakano H. Mantle cell lymphoma of the rectum at an early stage: a case report. Hepatogastroenterology 2001; 48: 675-677.

[44] G Stanojević, M Stojanović, M Jovanović, M Stojanović, M Jeremić, B Branković, N Ignjatović, V Katić. Primarni kolorektalni limfomi. Vojnosan preg 2009; 66:295-302

[45] Goran Stanojevic, Milica Nestorovic, Branko Brankovic, Miroslav Stojanovic, Milan Jovanovic, Milan Radojkovic. Primary colorectal lymphoma: An overview. World J Gastrointest Oncol 2011: 3(1): 14-18

[46] Grassi N, Cipolla C, Torcivia A, Mandala S, Graceffa G, Bottino A, Latteri F. Gastrointestinal stromal tumour of the rectum: report of a case and review of literature. World J Gastroenterol. 2008 28;14(8):1302-1304.

[47] Miettinen M, Sobin LH, Sarlomo-Rikala M. Immunohisto-chemical spectrum of GISTs at different sites and their differential diagnosis with a reference to CD117 (KIT) Mod Pathol. 2000;13:1134–1142.

[48] Miettinen M, Lasota J. Gastrointestinal stromal tumors: pathology and prognosis at different sites. Semin Diagn Pathol. 2006;23(2):70-83

[49] DeMatteo RP, Lewis JJ, Leung D, Mudan SS, Woodruff JM, Brennan MF. Two hundred gastrointestinal stromal tumors: recurrence patterns and prognostic factors for survival. Ann Surg. 2000;231:51–58.

[50] Manouras A, Pappas A, Katergiannakis V, Filis K, Chrysikos J, Pattas M, Genetzakis M, Tsekouras D, Lagoudianakis E. Gastrointestinal stromal tumors of the rectum: report of five cases. Acta Gastroenterol Belg 2009;72(2):257-261.

[51] van Oosterom AT, Judson I, Verweij J, Stroobants S, Donato di Paola E, Dimitrijevic S, Martens M, Webb A, Sciot R, Van Glabbeke M, Silberman S, Nielsen OS. European Organisation for Research and Treatment of Cancer Soft Tissue and Bone Sarcoma Group. Safety and efficacy of imatinib (STI571) in metastatic qgastrointestinal stromal tumours: a phase I study. Lancet 2001;358:1421-1423.

[52] van der Zwan SM, DeMatteo RP Gastrointestinal stromal tumor: 5 years later Cancer. 2005 ;104(9):1781-1788.

[53] Verweij J, Casali PG, Zalcberg J, LeCesne A, Reichardt P, Blay JY, Issels R, van Oosterom A, Hogendoorn PC, Van Glabbeke M, Bertulli R, Judson I. Progression-free survival in gastrointestinal stromal tumours with high-dose imatinib: randomised trial. Lancet 2004;364:1127-1134.

[54] Marc Everett M, Gutman H.· Surgical management of gastrointestinal stromal tumors: Analysis of outcome with respect to surgical margins and technique. J Surg Oncol 2008; 98:588-593

[55] M. Najeeb Al Hallak MN,Hage-Nassar G, Mouchli A. Primary Submucosal Squamous Cell Carcinoma of the Rectum Diagnosed by Endoscopic Ultrasound: Case Report and Literature Review. Case Rep Gastroenterol. 2010; 4(2): 243–249

[56] Dyson T & Draganov P. Squamous cell cancer of the rectum. World J Gastroenterol. 2009; 15(35): 4380–4386

[57] Yurdakul G, de Reijke TM, Blank LE, Rauws EA. Rectal squamous cell carcinoma 11 years after brachytherapy for carcinoma of the prostate. J Urol. 2003;169:280.

[58] Williams GT, Blackshaw AJ, Morson BC. Squamous carcinoma of the colorectum and its genesis. J Pathol. 1979;129:139–147

[59] Leung KK, Heitzman J, Madan A. Squamous cell carcinoma of the rectum 21 years after radiotherapy for cervical carcinoma. Saudi J Gastroenterol. 2009;15:196–198

[60] Audeau A, Han HW, Johnston MJ, Whitehead MW, Frizelle FA. Does human papilloma virus have a role in squamous cell carcinoma of the colon and upper rectum? Eur J Surg Oncol. 2002;28:657–660.

[61] Nahas CS, Shia J, Joseph R, Schrag D, Minsky BD, Weiser MR, Guillem JG, Paty PB, Klimstra DS, Tang LH, et al. Squamous-cell carcinoma of the rectum: a rare but curable tumor. Dis Colon Rectum. 2007;50:1393–1400

[62] Khalid U, Saleem T, Imam AM, Khan MR. Pathogenesis, diagnosis and management of primary melanoma of the colon. World J Surg Oncol 2011; 9: 1-9.

[63] Lens M, Bataille V, Krivokapic Z. Melanoma of the small intestine. Lancet Oncol. 2009;10:516-521.

[64] Keighley MRB, Williams NS Malignant Tumours of The Anal Canal and Anus. In: Keighley MRB, Williams NS, eds. Surgery of The Anus Rectum & Colon. London-Toronto:WB Saunders, 2001. p 1303-1328.

[65] Malik A, Hull TL, Milsom J. Long-term survivor of anorectal melanoma: report of a case. Dis Colon Rectum 2002 ; 45:1412-1415.

[66] Thibault C, Sagar P, Nivatvongs S. Anorectal melanoma: an incurable disease?Dis Colon Rectum 1997; 40: 661-667.

[67] Brady MS, Kavolius JP, Quan SH. Anorectal melanoma. A 64 –year experience at Memorial Sloan-Kettering Cancer Center. Dis Colon Rectum 1995; 38: 146-151

[68] Fripp VT, Esquivel J, Cerruto CA. Perianal melanoma disguised as hemorrhoids: case report and discussion. J Natl Med Assoc 2005; 97 :726-31.

[69] G Stanojević., Z Krivokapić., M Kontić., G Barišić., M Stojanović., M Jeremić Hirurgija rektuma i anusa. In: Jeremić M (ed) Abdominalna hirurgija II, Mediciniski fakultet Niš; 2009. p771-847.

[70] Roumen RMH. Anorectal melanoma in The Netherlands:a report of 63 patients. Eur J Surg Oncol 1996; 22: 598-601.

[71] Malik A, Hull TL, Floruta C. What is the best surgical treatment for anorectal melanoma ? Int J Colorectal Dis 2004 ; 19:121-123.

[72] Kelly P, Zagars GK, Cormier JN, Ross MI, Guadagnolo AB.Sphincter-Sparing Local Excision and Hypofractionated Radiation Therapy for Anorectal Melanoma. Cancer 2011;117:4747–4755

[73] Weyandt GH, Egget AO, Houf M, Raulf F, Brocker EB, Becker JC. Anorectal melanoma: surgical management guidelines according to tumour thickness. Br J Cancer 2003; 89 :2019-2022.

[74] G Stanojevic, Z Rancic, M, Jovanovic, M Stojanovic, D Mihailovic, B Brankovic. Melanoma of the anal canal. Acta Chir Yugoslavica 2006; (3): 83-85.

[75] Longo WE, Vernava AM, Wade TP, Coplin MA, Virgo KS, Johnson FE. Rare anal canal cancers in the U.S. veteran: patterns of disease and results of treatment. Am Surg 1995; 61:495-500.

[76] Gordon Ph.Malignant neoplasms of the Rectum. In: Gordon Ph, Nivatvongs S, (eds) Principles and Practice of the Surgery for the Colon Rectum and Anus. Informa Healthcare, New York, London; 2007. p 645-742.

[77] Singh O, Gupta SS, Mathur RK. A rare case of primary solid intrarectal dermoid.Saudi J Gastroenterol. 2011; 17(1):74-76.

[78] G Stanojević, Z Krivokapić, B Branković, M Nestorović. Retki tumori rektuma. In: Krivokapić Z (ed) Karcinom rektuma. Zavod za udžbenike, Beograd; 2012. p 513-528.

[79] Braumann C, Guenther N, Charalambos M, Junghans T. Schwannoma of the colon mimicking carcinoma: a case report and literature review. Int J Colorectal Dis 2007; 22:1547–1548.

[80] Laser A. Adenocarcinoma of the prostate involving the rectum. Dis Colon Rectum 1978; 21:23-25

[81] Christodoulopoulus JB, Papaionnou AN, Drakopoulou EP, et al. Carcinoma of the cervix presenting with the rectal symptomatology: Report of three cases. Dis Colon Rectum 1972; 15: 373-376

[82] Cervi G, Vettoretto N, Vinco A, et al. Rectal localizatition of the metastatic lobular breast cancer: report of a case. Dis Colon Rectum 2001; 44:453-455.

[83] Rosito MA, Damin DC, Lazzaron AR, et al. Metastatic renal cell carcinoma involving the rectum. Int J Colorectal Dis 2002; 17:359-361.

[84] Stojanovic MP, Radojkovic M, Jeremic LM, Zlatic AV, Stanojevic GZ, Jovanovic MA, Kostov MS, Katic VP. Malignant schwannoma of the pancreas involving transversal colon treated with en-bloc resection. World J Gastroenterol 2010;16:119-122.

Section 4

Adjuvant Therapy

Chapter 12

Current State-of-the-Science Adjuvant and Neoadjuvant Therapy in Surgically Resected Colorectal Cancer

I.H. Sahin and C.R. Garrett

Additional information is available at the end of the chapter

http://dx.doi.org/10.5772/57481

1. Introduction

Colorectal cancer represents the third most prevalent cancer in the United States, and the third most common cause of cancer-related mortality [1]. Due to the widespread introduction of screening of asymptomatic patients age 50 and above, the incidence of colorectal cancer has been declining [2]. Unfortunately the incidence of colorectal cancer in those under the age of 50 is increasing [3]. In its earliest stages colorectal cancer is highly treatable and curable. Cures in patients with advanced disease are uncommon, but with improved systemic therapies and oncologic surgery, is increasing over time. However, despite modern therapeutic advances, less than 20% of patients with distant metastatic disease will be alive and disease free for five years following the diagnosis [4].

Management of colorectal cancer highlights the importance of oncologic multidisciplinary care. Surgical adjuvant chemotherapy and chemoradiation therapy have led to improved outcomes for patients with colon cancer and rectal cancer, respectively. This is one of the factors associated with a decrease in colorectal cancer mortality over the last decade. Adherence to treatment guidelines has been shown to be associated with improved patient outcomes [5].Further refinements in adjuvant therapy will involve molecular risk adaption and improved selection of patients for chemotherapy and adjuvant chemoradiation therapy, incorporation of molecularly targeted agents into the treatment paradigm, and studies to define more clearly the optimal time and duration of adjuvant therapy following colorectal surgery.

2. Staging of colon cancer

The pathologic stage of colon cancer is currently based on the seventh version of the American Joint Commission of Cancer Staging [6]; a simplified version is reproduced in Table 1.

Pathologic stage is currently the most accurate predictor of those at greatest risk of relapse, and those most likely to benefit from additional adjuvant therapy. As greater than 80% of patients with stage I disease are cured with surgery alone additional adjuvant therapy has not been shown to improve the already favorable prognosis. Patients with stage II and III are at high risk of systemic relapse and in stage III patients the benefit of adjuvant chemotherapy has clearly been demonstrated and the data supporting it will be reviewed in section 3. Systemic therapy for patients with resected stage II disease remains highly controversial and will be addressed in section 4.

Stage	Description	5-year survival
I	T1,2, N0	85-95%
II	T3,4 N0	60-80%
III	Any T, N 1,2, M0	30-60%
IV	M1	< 20%

Table 1. Simplified AJCC Staging Classification and Estimated 5-year Survival

3. Treatment of stage III colon cancer

5-Flurouracil -based Adjuvant Chemotherapy

The prodrug 5-flurouracil was synthesized and patented in 1957 [7] and had shown modest efficacy in the treatment of patients with metastatic colorectal cancer, increasing the median survival from 6-9 months without therapy to an average of 12-14 months. Initial studies evaluating its efficacy, combined with the immune modulatory agent levamisole, were conducted by the North Central Cancer Treatment Group (NCCTG) in the 1980s. In a large, randomized, prospective trial, involving multiple sites across the United States, patients treated with 5-flurouracil and levamisole for 12 months were noted to have a 40% reduction in the relative risk of recurrence, and a 33% reduction in the relative risk of mortality [8]. Long term follow up data from this study confirms the increased cure rate in association with the use of adjuvant chemotherapy, not merely the representation of a lead-time bias [9]. Thus 5-flurouracil became, and remains, the backbone of surgical adjuvant therapy for resected stage III colon cancer. Levamisole was associated with significant toxicity however, and subsequent clinical trials demonstrated that 5-flurouracil, modulated by leucovorin, was also associated with a survival benefit [10] but with less neurological toxicity.

Adjuvant 5-flurouracil -based chemotherapy for colon cancer has been refined over time. Weekly 5-flurouracil has been administered (Roswell Park regimen) and in a randomized clinical trial, was demonstrated to be superior to the combination of 5-FU, semustine, and vincristine [10]. Studies comparing 5-flurouracil combined with leucovorin versus levamisole demonstrated that 6 months treatment of 5-flurouracil + leucovorin was equivalent to 12 months 5-flurouracil levamisole; 6 months of 5-flurouracil plus levamisole was determined to be less effective, in terms of 5-year disease free survival. Thus, six months of therapy is determined to be the optimal. As will be reviewed the optimal duration of chemotherapy is currently under active investigation.

It had been noted that in the metastatic setting, meta-analysis of randomized phase II trials suggested that infusional 5-flurouracil is more active when compared to bolus intravenous 5-flurouracil [11]. 5-flurouracil has a different mechanism of action when given continuously, with a greater inhibition of messenger ribonucleic acid (RNA), when compared to bolus 5-flurouracil, where the action is more directed at targeting DNA synthesis through inhibition of thymidylate synthetase. Reduced folate (leucovorin) increases the binding of 5-flurouracil to thymidylate synthase, thereby increasing the efficacy of 5-flurouracil in inhibiting DNA synthesis (see Figure 1). Although no large, randomized studies comparing bolus 5-flurouracil compared to infusional 5-flurouracil have been performed, the superior toxicity profile of infusional 5-flurouracil (less diarrhea, mucositis, and myelosuppression), and the potential for additive benefit of infusional 5-flurouracil (given its different mechanism of action) have led to infusional 5-flurouracil combined with bolus 5-flurouracil being used more commonly in 5-flurouracil adjuvant chemotherapy combined with other novel agents.

Oral Fluropyrimidines

Capecitabine is an oral pro-drug which is converted to thymidine phosphorylase into 5-flurouracil. It has been demonstrated that tumor cells have higher levels of thymidine phosphorylase and therefore at least theoretically there could be preferential accumulation of 5-FU in tumor cells. In a large phase III study (the X-ACT) trial was found to be non-inferior to bolus 5-flurouracil/leucovorin (Mayo Clinic regimen) [12]. Therefore capecitabine is currently approved for patients who are deemed to be suitable candidates for monotherapy, and is an alternative to bolus or infusional 5- flurouracil. Other oral fluropyrimidines have been examined for efficacy; UFT is a combination of uracil (a dihydropyrimidine dehydryogenase inhibitor (DPD), the enzyme responsible for metabolizing 5-FU, and tegafur (a 5-FU prodrug). When evaluated in a randomized phase III study of stage II and III patients, and compared to bolus flurouracil modulated with leucovorin (Roswell Park regimen) it was found to be equal in efficacy [13]. UFT was approved for use in much Europe and Asia but has not been approved for use in the United States.

CapeOx is currently recommended as one of the chemotherapy regimens in the latest version of the National Comprehensive Cancer Network (NCCN) Clinical Practice Guidelines in Oncology (version 1.2011) for the adjuvant treatment of stage III colon cancer. The NO16968 (XELOXA) trial, a large randomized phase III study of CapeOx versus bolus 5-flurouracil (Roswell Park) was performed in more than 1,800 stage III colon cancer patients. It showed a significantly superior three-year disease free survival with CapeOx when compared to the control arm (71% versus 67%, P = 0.0045) [14]. CapeOx was associated with less febrile neutropenia and stomatitis than 5FU/LV, although as expected peripheral neuropathy were more frequent; peripheral neuropathy was observed in a similar proportion of patients receiving FOLFOX or CapeOx.

As a consequence of the efficacy of oxaliplatin, demonstrated in the metastatic setting, a large randomized trial compared the efficacy of infusional 5-FU plus oxaliplatin, and infusional 5-FU combined with bolus 5-FU (the Multi-center International Study of Oxaliplatin, 5-FU, and Leucovorin, in the Adjuvant Treatment of Colon Cancer, or MOSAIC Study). Initial data reported a 23% risk reduction of disease recurrence at three years [15]. Updated 6-year disease-free survival data demonstrated a 6% improvement in disease-free survival, confirming the initial positive results [16]. Since 2003 FOLFOX has been the standard-of-care for patients with resected stage III disease with no contraindications to adjuvant chemotherapy.

Due to the young age of participants in the MOSIAC trial the efficacy of FOLFOX chemotherapy has been questioned in elderly patients, given its increased toxicity, primarily peripheral neuropathy. Pooled analysis of four randomized trials, involving 3,742 patients (of whom 614 were greater or equal to 70 years old) demonstrated that the benefit of FOLFOX chemotherapy did not differ by age, nor did dose intensity [17]. Thus in patients over the age of 70 who are deemed appropriate candidates may still benefit from the addition of oxaliplatin, although very few patients over 80 were included in these studies, thus the data for octogenarians and nonagenarians is limited.

Oxaliplatin was also evaluated in combination with bolus 5-FU (FLOX); in the National Surgical Adjuvant Breast **Project (NSABP)** randomized 2,407 patients with stage II or III colon cancer to either the Roswell Park regiment (bolus 5-FU modulated with leucovorin) or the Roswell Park regimen combined with fortnightly oxaliplatin. There was a superior 5-year disease-free survival with FLOX but not a difference in 5-year overall survival [18].

Adjuvant Irinotecan

Other combination cytotoxic regimens have been subjected to randomized phase III clinical trial evaluation in the stage III setting. Given the trend to evaluate agents with efficacy in the metastatic setting, and assume at least the potential for benefit in the adjuvant setting, irinotecan has been studied in combination with 5-FU. Prior metastatic studies confirmed the superiority of combination bolus 5-FU plus irinotecan when compared to bolus 5-Flurouracil monotherapy alone [19], as well as when combined with infusional 5-FU (FOLFIRI) (Douillard JY, et al. 2000). Thus irinotecan was evaluated in the surgical adjuvant setting for high risk patients, both combined with bolus 5-FU (IFL) [21] or as FOLFIRI compared to infusional and bolus 5-flurouracil (LV5-FU2), the **PETACC-3 study** [22]; neither of these studies demonstrated a benefit to the addition of irinotecan. Therefore at this time irinotecan is not indicated in the adjuvant treatment of colon cancer.

Efficacy of Anti-Epidermal Growth Factor Monoclonal Antibodies in the Adjuvant Therapy of Colon Cancer

Given the efficacy of the anti-epidermal growth factor antibodies cetuximab [23] and panitumumab [24] in the metastatic setting, it seemed reasonable to explore the efficacy of these antibodies in the adjuvant setting. A large prospective randomized study evaluated the efficacy of FOLFOX with or without cetuximab chemotherapy. During the course of the trial studies demonstrated that the benefit to cetuximab therapy was limited to those patients with KRAS wild type tumors [25]; thus protocol entry to limited to those patients whose tumors harbored a KRAS mutation (see Figure 2). Despite this selection of therapy there was no improvement in the disease-free survival in the cetuximab treated arm [26].

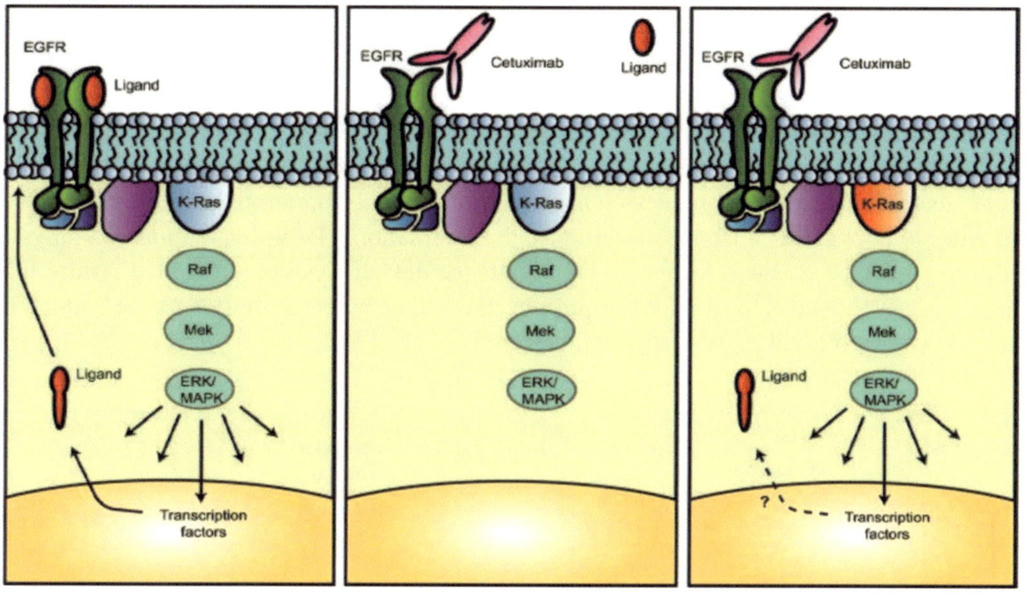

Figure 1. Possible Explanation for Lack of Efficacy of Anti-Epidermal Growth Factor Antibodies in KRAS Mutant Colorectal Cancer

Efficacy of Anti-Epidermal Growth Factor Monoclonal Antibodies in the Adjuvant Therapy of Colon Cancer

Colorectal cancer is the first tumor for which anti-angiogenesis therapies have proven to be effective. The addition of irinotecan plus 5-FU plus the fully humanized anti-vascular endothelial antibody bevacizumab was associated with a 5 month prolongation in overall survival when compared to chemotherapy alone in patients with metastatic disease. This suggested a potential role for this novel targeted agent in the adjuvant therapy of stage III colon cancer. However two studies, the C08 [27] and the AVANT trial [28], both failed to demonstrate a disease free survival benefit to the addition of bevacizumab to standard chemotherapy.

Future Cytotoxic Approaches to Adjuvant Colon Therapy

Although irinotecan did not add to the efficacy of adjuvant chemotherapy there is a suggestion that certain patients with molecular subtypes of colon cancer may benefit from it, possibly patients with microsatellite instable disease [29] Recent randomized phase III clinical trials suggests superior efficacy of the three agents (5-FU, oxaliplatin, and irinotecan, or FOLFOXIRI) when compared to two agents FOLFIRI [30-33]. The efficacy of FOLFOXIRI is under consideration for testing in a prospective randomized clinical trial compared to FOLFOX chemotherapy.

Duration of Adjuvant Therapy in Colon Cancer

As discussed previously, the standard duration of adjuvant chemotherapy was initially 12 months when adjuvant therapy was first approved for colon cancer in 1990. As noted previously subsequent studies determined that 6 months adjuvant duration was determined to be equally effective. A prospective randomized trial comparing 3 months of LV5-FU2 when compared to 6 months 5-flurouracil modulated with leucovorin (Mayo regimen) did not demonstrate a statistically significant difference in overall survival ($P>0.05$Given as the trial was not powered as a non-inferiority study, there are four ongoing studies comparing 3 versus 6 months adjuvant chemotherapy (see table 2). Although there are some differences in the study design, close to 18,000 patients will be entered on these four studies during this decade. In order to pool the data from these studies, the International Drug Evaluation of Adjuvant Chemotherapy (IDEA) was formed to coordinate the data analysis of the pooled results. It is hoped that by the end of the decade the question of whether or not the shorter course (3 months) is equally effective will be satisfactorily answered.

Clinical Trial	Stage Evaluated	Start Date	Target Accrual	Treatment Plan
SCOT*	III	3/27/2008	9,500	CapeOx/FOLFOX 6 months vs. CapeOx/ FOLFOX 3 months
TOSCA	II, III	6/20/2007	3,450	FOLFOX 6 vs. 3 months (plus optional bevacizumab randomization for stage IIIc)
GERCOR	III	5/2/2009	2,500	FOLFOX 6 vs. 3 months
CALGB/SWOG C80702	III	7/1/2010	2,500	FOLFOX 6 vs. 3 ± celecoxib/placebo

*Short Course Oncology Therapy

Table 2. Planned Randomized Phase III Studies Evaluating the Duration of Adjuvant Chemotherapy

4. Adjuvant radiation therapy for colon cancer

No prospective data to date has suggested a survival benefit with the addition of radiation therapy as adjuvant following surgery. Retrospective data suggests that patients with high risk features for recurrence may receive benefit from radiation, including those who had T4 disease (involving another organ), a positive margin (microscopic residual disease, not true adjuvant), and clinical perforation had a better disease-free survival with the addition of adjuvant chemoradiation [34]. One large prospective randomized study evaluating the efficacy of radiation in colon cancers (non-transverse colon) was inconclusive due to the failure to meet accrual. The study was underpowered but was not able to demonstrate a benefit of the addition of radiation to chemotherapy [35]. Treatment decisions have to be made based upon the

http://dx.doi.org/10.5772/57481

patient's specific risk factors for local recurrence. At this time the use of radiation as adjuvant for resected stage III colon cancer is mainly limited to those patients with microscopic residual disease (positive pathologic margin).

5. Adjuvant treatment of stage II colon cancer

Due to the significantly better prognosis, with the majority of patients being cured with surgery alone, it is more difficult to demonstrate a significant survival benefit with the use of adjuvant chemotherapy. The initial adjuvant NCCTG adjuvant study of 5-flurouracil and levamisole was unable to demonstrate a survival benefit for the chemotherapy arm; this may in part be due to the higher number of non-cancer-related deaths in the 5-flurouracil treated group [8]. A large randomized, prospective trial of 3,239 patients with resected stage II disease demonstrated a 3.6% 5-year improvement in survival following 6 months adjuvant 5-fluorouracil and leucovorin (Mayo regimen) when compared to observation alone [35]. All agree that if a benefit exists it is relatively small and that the routine use of chemotherapy is not indicated. Of note, in the MOSIAC trial, there was no difference in outcome between stage II patients treated with FOLFOX when compared to infusional and bolus 5-flurouracil chemotherapy. Different pathologic characteristics may indicate those patients at slightly higher risk of relapse [see table 3]. Tumor microsatellite instability analysis has been associated with a more favorable prognosis, as well as a lack of benefit from adjuvant 5-flurouracil chemotherapy in resected stage II and stage III tumors; in stage II tumors those patients with mismatch repair tumors had an inferior outcome with the use of 5-fluoruracil adjuvant chemotherapy when compared to observation [39]. Tumor molecular genotyping is being utilized in order to predict those stage II tumors most likely to relapse. To date, these genomic tests have not been sufficiently predictive of those most likely to relapse and are of limited clinical utility [40-41].

Pathologic Feature	Reference
Less than 12 Lymph Nodes Analyzed	36, 37
Poorly differentiated	38
Clinical Perforation	38

Table 3. Pathologic Features Associated with a Relatively Adverse Prognosis in Stage II Disease

6. Adjuvant and neoadjuvant approaches in rectal cancer

Rectal adenocarcinomas present a unique challenge given its anatomic location in the pelvis and the fact that part of the rectum is intraperitoneal and part is extraperitoneal. The vast majority of rectal malignancies are adenocarcinomas; less common pathologies are gastrointestinal stromal tumor (GIST), carcinoid, squamous, adenosquamous tumors and melanoma. For the purposes of this chapter we will limit our discussed to rectal adenocarcinomas.

Compared the large bowel the close proximity of rectum to other local organs such as urogenital system requires different surgical techniques and significantly increases the likelihood of local relapse after surgery when compared to colon cancer [42]. For this reason, in addition to total mesorectal excision combination therapeutic options have arisen to decrease local recurrence. Subsequently, these multimodality therapy approaches have become standard-of-care in locally advanced rectal cancer. In this book chapter, we aimed to summarize scientific progression in the field of treatment of locally advanced rectal cancer.

Development of Adjuvant Therapy

The standard care of rectal cancer remains surgery with a total mesorectal excision. However locally advanced disease were relapsing significantly higher than early stage disease after surgery-only approach [43]. Rectal cancer transmurally invades the rectal wall directly and can spread through the lymphatic system to regional lymph nodes. These characteristics of locally advanced disease put the patients at higher risk of local and distant recurrence which is associated worse overall survival. Given the high rate of the recurrent disease, combination treatment approaches have evolved in locally advance rectal cancer over the last two decades. First, adjuvant radiotherapy and then combined modality therapy (chemotherapy concurrently with radiation therapy) was integrated in standard care to enhance survival outcomes of locally advanced rectal cancer.

An early prospectively randomized clinical trial was conducted to assess the question of the adjuvant benefit roles of radiation, chemotherapy, or combined modality therapy (chemoradiation) in the treatment of locally advance rectal cancer by the Gastrointestinal Tumor Study Group (GTSG) in 1985 [44]. In this study, patients after having curative surgery (202 in total), were enrolled and randomized into four different groups including; patients received no adjuvant treatment, patients treated with adjuvant radiotherapy either at dose of 40 or 48 Gray, patients received adjuvant chemotherapy with semustine and 5-fluorouracil, and a final group treated with combination of chemotherapy and radiotherapy. All patients were followed up to for 80 months. Although there was no significant difference for OS in four groups, authors found significantly better disease-free survival in combination therapy arm compared to resection-alone [44]. In same study, recurrence rate was highest in resection-alone with 55%, while the lowest relapse was observed in combination therapy group (33%). The follow-up results of this study confirmed a significantly improved overall survival reported in combination treatment group compared to surgery alone group [45]. By the end of the 10 year follow up, 10-year survival rates were 26% vs. 45% in control group vs. combination treatment group and was showing the superiority of combination treatment group. Independently, The National Surgical Adjuvant and Breast and Bowel Project (NSABP) released the result of R-01 that comparing adjuvant radiation or chemotherapy to surgery alone and provided superior overall and disease-free survival in chemo group respect to the surgery alone ($P = 0.03$, $P = 0.006$ respectively) [46]. No significant survival benefit observed in radiation alone group.

The North Central Cancer Treatment Group (NCCTG) reported a trial comparing the adjuvant radiation versus the combined chemoradiation. In this study, total 209 patients randomized in two arms. The combined modality arm was found to have 34% reduced overall recurrence compared to the radiation alone. ($P < 0.003$) [47]. Decreased recurrence incidence was observed in both local (25% versus 13% $P < 0.02$) and distant relapse (43% versus 29.5% $P < 0.003$). After this study National Surgical Adjuvant Breast Program (NSABP) examined the impact of the adjuvant chemotherapy alone versus chemoradiotherapy on overall survival and disease free survival in protocol R-02. In this study, all female patients received 5-flurouracil and leucovorin whereas male patients either received MOF regimen including 5-flurouracil, semustine, vincristine or 5-flurouracil combined with leucovorin. Radiotherapy was given in 25 fractions at a daily 18 Gray dose. Although there was a significant decrease in cumulative local relapse incidence after 5-year follow-up (13% versus 8%, $P = 0.02$), they observed no overall or disease-free survival differences in between these two groups.

Neoadjuvant Radiotherapy

Absence of clinical evidence to use radiotherapy in adjuvant settings urged the researchers to test the efficacy of radiotherapy in preoperative settings. Swedish investigators conducted a phase III clinical trial to understand the possible role of neoadjuvant radiotherapy (i.e. pre-operative radiation therapy) [48]. They enrolled 1,168 patients and randomly assigned to receive either conventional surgery alone or surgery with preceded neoadjuvant radiotherapy designed as a total dose of 25 Gy in five fractions. After five years follow up, recurrence rate was found 11% in neoadjuvant radiotherapy group, whereas it was observed as high as 27% in patients with surgery alone ($P < 0.001$). Additionally, the authors reported significantly better five year-survival in radiotherapy arm (58% compared to 48%, $P = 0.004$). Since conventional surgery was performed in this study, the additive role of the radiation in TME was still not clear. In 2007, this question was addressed by Dutch Colorectal Cancer Group. They conducted a randomized clinical trial enrolled the patients into TME alone and 5 fractions radiotherapy with total 25 Gray dose plus total mesorectal excision [49]. After a median 6.1 years follow- up, no significant overall survival difference was demonstrated. Moreover, there was no significant difference in distal recurrence incidence. On the other hand, they found a significant decrease in local recurrence rate (5.6 % vs 10.9%, $P < 0.001$).

Currently, two different preoperative radiotherapy protocols are commonly preferred in locally advanced rectal cancer treatment including conventional (50.4 Gray administered in 28 fractions) and short-term treatment (25 Gray in 5 fractions). Although both models have been shown to decrease local recurrence, there are debates on prolonged side effect in short-term radiotherapy modality [50]. While short-term neoadjuvant radiation treatment is commonly used in European countries, conventional radiation is standard-of-care of locally advance rectal cancer in USA.

Neoadjuvant Chemoradiation Therapy (Combined Modality Therapy)

Better outcomes observed in chemoradiation in adjuvant settings raised the question of possible neoadjuvant chemoradiation for treatment of patients with locally advanced rectal cancer. In 2004, German Rectal Cancer Study Group (GRCSG) examined the role preoperative chemoradiation in rectal cancer patients with T3 or T4 stages or node positivity [51]. They randomized 823 patients in two groups; the neoadjuvant arm received a total 50.4 Gray dose radiation in 28 fractions and 5-flurouracil 120-hour continuous infusion during the first and fifth weeks of radiation at a dose of 1,000 mg per square meter of body surface then followed by surgery after completing the chemoradiation. Patients also received four cycles of 5-flurouracil (500 mg per square meter body surface) which was designed as five time weekly during the four weeks. The adjuvant group also received the same treatment except additional a boost of 5.4 Gray radiation after total mesorectal excision. No significant difference was reported for five year-survival in between neoadjuvant and adjuvant group (74% vs 76% respectively, $P = 0.80$). Interestingly, five years cumulative incidence of local recurrence was significantly lower in neoadjuvant group than the adjuvant. (6% versus 13% respectively, $P = 0.006$). Moreover they observed less acute and long term toxicity in neoadjuvant arm of the study compared the adjuvant arm ($P = 0.001$ versus $P = 0.01$).

In another study, European Organization for Research and Treatment of Cancer (EORTC) randomized 1,011 patients with locally advanced rectal cancer into four different groups: a) preoperative radiotherapy designed as 45 Gy in five weeks, b) preoperative radiotherapy plus two course of 5-flurouracil and leucovorin (350 mg/m^2/day and 20 mg/m^2/day), c) preoperative radiotherapy plus postoperative four course of 5-flurouracil and leucovorin, and d) preoperative radiotherapy and two course of bolus 5-flurouracil and leucovorin, plus postoperative four course of postoperative 5-flurouracil and leucovorin. In early preliminary results of the study, authors reported a significant benefit towards preoperative chemoradiotherapy groups for tumor size, lymph node involvement, pathological complete response ($P < 0.0001$, $P = 0.046$, $P < 0.001$). [52]. Later in follow up results, no significant difference was observed in OS between neoadjuvant chemoradiotherapy and neoadjuvant radiotherapy (P=0.085). On the other hand, local recurrence was significantly lower in preoperative chemoradiation groups ($P = 0.002$) [53]. Chemotherapy protocol which was given in this study was an uncommon protocol possibly is a contributing factor for absence of survival difference in between chemoradiation and radiation alone group in preoperative settings.

To better understand the additive role of neoadjuvant chemoradiation for patients with locally advanced rectal cancer, NSABP R-03 trial was conducted. Two hundreds and sixty-seven patients enrolled in two arms; patients who received neoadjuvant or adjuvant chemoradiation. Neoadjuvant group received a bolus of 5-flurouracil with leucovorin for six weeks followed by radiation given as a total 45 Gray dose in 25 fractions with an additional 5.4 Gray boost. Then, patients were resected and postoperatively received 24 more weeks of weekly 5-FU and LV. Patients in adjuvant arm also received same courses of treatment in the same order except initial surgical resection. The most striking finding of this study was superior 5-year disease-free survival observed in neoadjuvant arm (64.7% vs 53.4%, P=0.011). Although there was not a significant difference in OS (P = 0.65), There was trend for observed five-year overall survival as 74.7% vs 65.6% in the neoadjuvant and adjuvant arms respectively [54]. Overall, all these clinical trials support the use neoadjuvuvant chemotheradiation as standart-care-of locally advance colorectal cancer. Although there is no clear result proving as an evidence for the superior OS compared to adjuvant chemoradiation, decreased local recurrence incidence with neoadjuvant treatment promises better local disease control. Moreover decreased acute and prolonged treatment related toxicities and improved sphincter preservation observed in preoperative treatment also favor the neoadjuvant chemoradiation modality [54].

Current Drugs for Neoadjuvant Therapy of Rectal Cancer

5-Fluorouracil

5-flurouracil has become the recommended first-line chemotherapy in locally advanced rectal cancer patients based on the GTSG and NCCTG data [44,47].The most commonly preferred administration mode of 5-flurouracil is continuous intravenous infusion(225-300mg/m^2 daily). To compare the bolus administration with continuous intravenous infusion, the NCCTG randomized 660 patients in two arms. Both arms received concurrent radiotherapy. First group received bolus 5-flurouracil on three consecutive days as s rapid infusion of 500 mg/m^2 while the other group received as protracted infusion (225 mg/m^2/day). Four-year relapse free survival was 63% in continuous infusion group while it was 53% in the bolus arm ($P = 0.01$). Significant difference for 4-year overall survival was also observed in the same study. Four-year overall survival was 70% as compared to 60% in continuous infusion and bolus group respectively ($P = 0.005$). Interestingly, no benefit was observed for local relapse in continuous infusion group ($P = 0.110$). While leukopenia was more common in bolus group, diarrhea incidence was found higher in continuous infusion group.

Capecitabine

Since superior outcomes observed in continuous intravenous administration of 5-flurouracil in chemoradiation regimens, an equivalent fluropyrimidine, capecitabine was studied for locally advanced rectal cancer treatment. Oral administration of capecitabine which has very similar pharmacokinetics to continuous intravenous 5-flurouracil provided more convenient treatment for patients if they are able to tolerate oral administration. In a phase I clinical study, the recommended dose of the capecitabine was determined as 1800 mg/m2 daily given orally in two divided doses combined with 50.4 Gray preoperative radiation [56]. A prospectively randomized study of 1,987 patients was enrolled into two groups; a) patients who received capecitabine orally, b) patients who were administered bolus 5-flurouracil modulated with leucovorin [58]. In the results of this study, non-inferior disease-free survival was observed in capecitabine group. The capecitabine improved relapse-free survival ($P = 0.04$). Moreover, fewer adverse effects were seen with capecitabine treatment compared to bolus 5-flurouracil plus leucovorin arm ($P < 0.001$) [58].

The NSABP R-04 trial compared the use of capecitabine to continuous infusion 5-flurouracil with or without oxaliplatin during combined modality therapy in locally advance rectal cancer. 5-fluorouracil was given as a 225 mg/m^2 daily protracted venous infusion during radiation and capecitabine was given at 1650 mg/m^2 orally in two divided doses daily on the days of radiation only. There was no significant different regarding pathologic complete response, surgical downstaging or sphincter-saving surgery. Local recurrence and overall survival have yet to be reported [59].

More recently, in a randomized phase III study, German researchers compared the efficacy of capecitabine with 5-flurouracil as neoadjuvant radiosensitizing agent [60]. In this study, 392 patients were randomized into two groups. Patients in capecitabine arm were enrolled to receive two cycles of capecitabine (2,500 mg/m^2 days 1-14, repeated day 22), then followed by chemoradiotherapy (50 4 Gray plus capecitabine 1650 mg/m^2 days 1-38 and additionally three cycles of capecitabine). Two cycles of bolus 5-flurouracil (500 mg/m^2 days 1-5, repeated day 29), followed by chemoradiotherapy (50 4 Gray plus infusional 5-flurouracil 225 mg/m^2 daily), finally two cycles of bolus 5-FU were administered patients in 5-flurouracil arm. Results were promising for non-inferiority with significantly better 5-year OS in capecitabine group (76% as compared to 67%, *P* = 0.05). Similarly disease-free survival was also higher in capecitabine group (75% versus 67%, *P* = 0.07).

Oxaliplatin

Given the promising results of oxaliplatin treatment of colon cancer in adjuvant setting [15] and metastatic disease [61] its possible additive effect to the neoadjuvant treatment of rectal cancer has been investigated. In a phase II clinical trial, oxaliplatin (at 50 mg/m2 on days 1, 8, 22, and 29) plus capecitabine (1,650 mg/m^2 on days 1 to 14 and 22 to 35) with radiotherapy (50.4 Gray in 28 fraction) was tested both for activity and safety [62]. Pathologic complete response was achieved in 17% patients whereas 53/103 patients showed more than 50% tumor regression. Although results were not superior to standard 5-FU treatment phase III trials were warranted. The randomized phase III Studio Terapia Adiuvante Retto (STAR)-01 trial has tested to outcomes of addition of oxaliplatin (60 mg/m2) to chemoradiation (225 mg/m^2/day plus 50.4 Gray in 28 daily fractions) comparing with standard chemoradiation [62]. Addition of oxaliplation did not increase pathologic complete response rate (16% versus 16%) but rather increased grade 3 to 4 adverse events in oxaliplatin arms (*P* < 0.001).

Recently published German CAO/ARO/AIO-04 randomised phase III trial also investigated the role of oxaliplatin in neoadjuvant chemoradiation [63]. In the study control group was treated with standard 5-flurouracil-based combined modality treatment, consisting of preoperative radiotherapy of 50.4 Gray plus infusional 5-flurouracil (1000 mg/m^2 days 1-5 and 29-33), followed by surgery and four cycles of bolus fluorouracil (500 mg/m^2 days 1-5 and 29). Oxaliplatin arm received preoperative radiotherapy of 50.4 Gray plus infusional 5-flurouracil (250 mg/m^2 days 1-14 and 22-35) and oxaliplatin (50 mg/m^2 days 1, 8, 22, and 29), followed by surgery and eight cycles of adjuvant chemotherapy with oxaliplatin (100 mg/m^2 days 1 and 15), leucovorin (400 mg/m2 days 1 and 15), and again infusional 5-flurouracil. Authors reported better pathologic complete response outcomes in oxaliplatin treatment arm compared to standard group (17% vs 13% respectively, *P* = 0.038). Controversially, ACCORD 12/0405-PRODIGE 2 trial reported no benefit with additional oxaliplatin [64]. In this study control patients were assigned to receive 5 weeks of treatment with radiotherapy 45 Gy/25 fractions with concurrent capecitabine 800 mg/m^2 twice daily (5 days per week). The experimental arm of the study received 50 Gray in 25 fractions radiation with capecitabine 800 mg/m^2 twice daily (5 days per week) and oxaliplatin 50 mg/m^2 (once weekly). Although there was trend toward oxaliplatin plus group for pCR it was not significant (19.2% s 13.9% P=0.09). Preoperative grade 3 and 4 toxicities were observed significantly higher in oxalipatin plus arm (*P* < 0.001). Since there is no consensus in clinical trials for benefit with additional oxaliplatin it is not currently standard-of-care of locally advanced rectal cancer.

Targeted Therapies

Monoclonal antibodies targeting the critical survival signaling pathways such as epidermal growth factor receptor (EGFR) and vascular endothelial growth factor receptor (VEGFR) are currently under the investigation to determine their role in neoadjuvant chemoradiaton treatment in rectal cancers. The potential role of cetuximab and bevacizumab in the treatment of locally advanced rectal cancer has been tested in phase I and phase II clinical trials.

In a phase I/II clinical study the safety and potential benefit of cetuximab in neoadjuvant chemoradiation investigated in locally advanced rectal cancer patients. Forty patients enrolled to receive initial intravenous dose of 400 mg/m^2 cetuximab which was given 1 week before the initiation of radiation followed by 250 mg/m^2/week for 5 weeks and capecitabine during the radiotherapy 650 mg/m^2 orally twice daily and 825 mg/m^2 twice daily, as a second dose level [65]. Observed pathologic complete response was only in two patients (5%), while diarrhea was seen in 65% of the patients. Grade 3 diarrhea was detected in 15% of cases. In one patient three grade 4 toxic effect was reported by authors; one myocardial infarction, one pulmonary embolism, and one pulmonary infection with sepsis.

In the EXPERT-C trial, combination of cetuximab and capecitabine plus oxaliplatin was studied in neoadjuvant settings. One hundred sixty-five patients enrolled in two arms to receive four cycles of capecitabine/oxaliplatin and then capecitabine chemoradiotherapy, surgery, and adjuvant CAPOX (four cycles) or the same regimen plus weekly cetuximab [66]. In this study the most striking finding was significantly improved OS in cetuximab plus group ($P = 0.034$). Additionally, a better radiologic response was determined in cetuximab group. On the other hand there was no difference either in pathologic complete response rate or progression-free survival ($P = 1.0$, $P = 0.363$ respectively)

Another fully humanized monoclonal antibody, that binds circulating anti-vascular epithelial growth factor, bevacizumab, has also been investigated in combination neoadjuvant treatment of rectal cancer. In a phase I/II study, bevacizumab combined with preoperative 5-FU and radiotherapy in 32 locally advanced rectal cancer patients [67]. Patients were administered four cycles of bevacizumab infusion (5 or 10 mg/kg) on day 1 of each cycle; 5-FU (225 mg/m^2/24 hours) during cycles 2 to 4; radiotherapy in 28 fractions with a total dose of 50.4 Gy over 5.5 weeks. Surgery was performed 7 to 10 weeks after completion of all therapies. No grade4 toxicity was detected and the most frequent toxicity was diarrhea. Pathologic complete response was achieved in 5 out of 32 patients. In another phase II study, bevacizumab was explored in a combination treatment of capecitabine and radiotherapy [68]. Twenty-five rectal cancer patients received neoadjuvant therapy with radiotherapy (50.4 Gy in 28 fractions over 5.5 weeks), bevacizumab every 2 weeks (3 doses of 5 mg/kg), and capecitabine (900 mg/m^2 orally twice daily during the radiation). Surgical resection was performed a median of 7.3 weeks later initial treatment. An encouraging pathologic complete response rate was reported in 8 of 25 patients (32%). Six of 24 patients showed less than 10% viable tumor cells in final pathological specimens. No patient was reported with grade 3 gastrointestinal toxicity or significant hematologic toxicity.

In a recent study, bevacizumab was tested in a combined treatment including the oxaliplatin, 5-FU, and radiotherapy in 26 patients [69]. Patients were initially treated with 1 month of induction bevacizumab and FOLFOX6, then received 50.4 Gy of radiation and concurrent bevacizumab (5 mg/kg on Days 1, 15, and 29), oxaliplatin (50 mg/m^2/week for 6 weeks), and continuous infusion 5-FU (200 mg/m(2)/day). This trial was terminated early because of high incidence of significant grade 3 toxicity. Authors reported 19 (75%) of 25 patients experienced grade 3 toxicities. Five (20%) out of 25 patients had pathologic response. The effect of bevacuzimab was also studied with erlotinib, a small molecule epidermal growth factor receptor tyrosine kinase inhibitor in a combination treatment of 5-flurouracil and external beam radiation in 21 patients [70]. Seven (47%) of 15 patients who completed the therapy and had surgery achieved pathologic complete response. Reported toxicities were including lymphopenia 6 (40%), diarrhea 4 (24%), rash 2 (12%), cardiac ischemia 1(6%), transaminitis (6%) and mucositis (6%).

Obtained promising pathologic response and observed safety results by the addition of monoclonal antibodies in neoadjuvant chemoradiation encourages to further explore the role of these drugs in treatment of locally advanced rectal cancer. On the other hand these targeting agents are yet to be standard-care-of rectal cancer in neoadjuvant settings.

7. Conclusions

The clinical advances over the last two decades have led to demonstrable improvements in the outcomes of patients with colorectal cancer and are a testament to the success of multidisciplinary cancer care. Continued development of novel therapeutics in the metastatic setting will undoubtedly lead to changes in our surgical adjuvant treatments. Refinement in predictive and prognostic studies will allow us greater ability to tailor the appropriate therapy for patients, and allow for greater patient's participation in the shared decision process.

Author details

I.H. Sahin and C.R. Garrett

University of Texas MD Anderson Cancer Center Houston, Texas, USA

References

[1] Siegel R, DeSantis C, Virgo K, Stein K, Mariotto A, Smith T, et al. Cancer treatment and survivorship statistics, 2012. CA: a cancer journal for clinicians. 2012 Jul-Aug; 62(4):220-41. PubMed PMID: 22700443.

[2] Printz C. American Cancer Society reports progress in reducing cancer deaths. Cancer. 2011;117(20):4573-4.

[3] Siegel RL, Jemal A, Ward EM. Increase in incidence of colorectal cancer among young men and women in the United States. Cancer Epidemiology Biomarkers & Prevention. 2009;18(6):1695-8.

[4] Kopetz S, Chang GJ, Overman MJ, Eng C, Sargent DJ, Larson DW, et al. Improved survival in metastatic colorectal cancer is associated with adoption of hepatic resection and improved chemotherapy. Journal of Clinical Oncology. 2009;27(22):3677-83.

[5] Chagpar R, Xing Y, Chiang YJ, Feig BW, Chang GJ, You YN, et al. Adherence to Stage-Specific Treatment Guidelines for Patients With Colon Cancer. Journal of Clinical Oncology. 2012;30(9):972-9.

[6] Compton CC, Byrd DR, Garcia-Aguilar J, Kurtzman S, Olawaiye A, Washington MK. AJCC Cancer Staging Atlas: Springer; 2012.

[7] Chu E. Ode to 5-Fluorouracil. Clinical colorectal cancer. 2007;6(9).

[8] Moertel CG, Fleming TR, Macdonald JS, Haller DG, Laurie JA, Goodman PJ, et al. Levamisole and fluorouracil for adjuvant therapy of resected colon carcinoma. New England Journal of Medicine. 1990;322(6):352-8.

[9] Moertel CG, Fleming TR, Macdonald JS, Haller DG, Laurie JA, Tangen CM, et al. Fluorouracil plus levamisole as effective adjuvant therapy after resection of stage III colon carcinoma: a final report. Annals of internal medicine. 1995;122(5):321.

[10] Wolmark N, Rockette H, Fisher B, Wickerham DL, Redmond C, Fisher ER, et al. The benefit of leucovorin-modulated fluorouracil as postoperative adjuvant therapy for primary colon cancer: results from National Surgical Adjuvant Breast and Bowel Project protocol C-03. Journal of Clinical Oncology. 1993;11(10):1879-87.

[11] Efficacy of intravenous continuous infusion of fluorouracil compared with bolus administration in advanced colorectal cancer. Meta-analysis Group In Cancer. Journal of clinical oncology : official journal of the American Society of Clinical Oncology. 1998 Jan;16(1):301-8. PubMed PMID: 9440757.

[12] Twelves C, Wong A, Nowacki MP, Abt M, Burris III H, Carrato A, et al. Capecitabine as adjuvant treatment for stage III colon cancer. New England Journal of Medicine. 2005;352(26):2696-704.

[13] Lembersky BC, Wieand HS, Petrelli NJ, O'Connell MJ, Colangelo LH, Smith RE, et al. Oral uracil and tegafur plus leucovorin compared with intravenous fluorouracil and leucovorin in stage II and III carcinoma of the colon: results from National Surgical Adjuvant Breast and Bowel Project Protocol C-06. Journal of Clinical Oncology. 2006;24(13):2059-64.

[14] Haller D, Tabernero J, Maroun J, De Braud F, Price T, Van Cutsem E, et al. 5LBA First efficacy findings from a randomized phase III trial of capecitabine+ oxaliplatin vs.

bolus 5-FU/LV for stage III colon cancer (NO16968/XELOXA study). EJC Supplements. 2009;7(3):4-.

[15] André T, Boni C, Mounedji-Boudiaf L, Navarro M, Tabernero J, Hickish T, et al. Oxaliplatin, fluorouracil, and leucovorin as adjuvant treatment for colon cancer. New England Journal of Medicine. 2004;350(23):2343-51.

[16] De Gramont A, Boni C, Navarro M, Tabernero J, Hickish T, Topham C, et al., editors. Oxaliplatin/5FU/LV in adjuvant colon cancer: Updated efficacy results of the MOSAIC trial, including survival, with a median follow-up of six years. ASCO Annual Meeting Proceedings J Clin Oncol; 2007.

[17] Goldberg RM, Tabah-Fisch I, Bleiberg H, de Gramont A, Tournigand C, Andre T, et al. Pooled analysis of safety and efficacy of oxaliplatin plus fluorouracil/leucovorin administered bimonthly in elderly patients with colorectal cancer. Journal of Clinical Oncology. 2006;24(25):4085-91.

[18] Kuebler JP, Wieand HS, O'Connell MJ, Smith RE, Colangelo LH, Yothers G, et al. Oxaliplatin combined with weekly bolus fluorouracil and leucovorin as surgical adjuvant chemotherapy for stage II and III colon cancer: results from NSABP C-07. Journal of clinical oncology. 2007;25(16):2198-204.

[19] Saltz LB, Cox JV, Blanke C, Rosen LS, Fehrenbacher L, Moore MJ, et al. Irinotecan plus fluorouracil and leucovorin for metastatic colorectal cancer. New England Journal of Medicine. 2000;343(13):905-14.

[20] Douillard JY, Cunningham D, Roth A, Navarro M, James R, Karasek P, et al. Irinotecan combined with fluorouracil compared with fluorouracil alone as first-line treatment for metastatic colorectal cancer: a multicentre randomised trial. The Lancet. 2000;355(9209):1041-7.

[21] Saltz LB, Niedzwiecki D, Hollis D, Goldberg RM, Hantel A, Thomas JP, et al. Irinotecan fluorouracil plus leucovorin is not superior to fluorouracil plus leucovorin alone as adjuvant treatment for stage III colon cancer: results of CALGB 89803. Journal of Clinical Oncology. 2007;25(23):3456-61.

[22] Van Cutsem E, Labianca R, Bodoky G, Barone C, Aranda E, Nordlinger B, et al. Randomized phase III trial comparing biweekly infusional fluorouracil/leucovorin alone or with irinotecan in the adjuvant treatment of stage III colon cancer: PETACC-3. Journal of Clinical Oncology. 2009;27(19):3117-25.

[23] Garrett CR, Eng C. Cetuximab in the treatment of patients with colorectal cancer. Expert opinion on biological therapy. 2011;11(7):937-49.

[24] Hoda D, Simon GR, Garrett CR. Targeting colorectal cancer with anti-epidermal growth factor receptor antibodies: focus on panitumumab. Therapeutics and clinical risk management. 2008;4(6):1221.

[25] Khambata-Ford S, Garrett CR, Meropol NJ, Basik M, Harbison CT, Wu S, et al. Expression of epiregulin and amphiregulin and K-ras mutation status predict disease

control in metastatic colorectal cancer patients treated with cetuximab. Journal of Clinical Oncology. 2007;25(22):3230-7.

[26] Alberts SR, Sargent DJ, Nair S, Mahoney MR, Mooney M, Thibodeau SN, et al. Effect of Oxaliplatin, Fluorouracil, and Leucovorin With or Without Cetuximab on Survival Among Patients With Resected Stage III Colon Cancer A Randomized Trial. JAMA: the journal of the American Medical Association. 2012;307(13):1383-93.

[27] Allegra CJ, Yothers G, O'Connell MJ, Sharif S, Petrelli NJ, Lopa SH, et al. Bevacizumab in Stage II-III Colon Cancer: 5-Year Update of the National Surgical Adjuvant Breast and Bowel Project C-08 Trial. Journal of clinical oncology : official journal of the American Society of Clinical Oncology. 2012 Dec 10. PubMed PMID: 23233715.

[28] de Gramont A, Van Cutsem E, Schmoll HJ, Tabernero J, Clarke S, Moore MJ, et al. Bevacizumab plus oxaliplatin-based chemotherapy as adjuvant treatment for colon cancer (AVANT): a phase 3 randomised controlled trial. Lancet Oncol. 2012 Dec; 13(12):1225-33. PubMed PMID: 23168362.

[29] Bertagnolli MM, Niedzwiecki D, Compton CC, Hahn HP, Hall M, Damas B, et al. Microsatellite instability predicts improved response to adjuvant therapy with irinotecan, fluorouracil, and leucovorin in stage III colon cancer: Cancer and Leukemia Group B Protocol 89803. Journal of clinical Oncology. 2009;27(11):1814-21.

[30] Falcone A, Ricci S, Brunetti I, Pfanner E, Allegrini G, Barbara C, et al. Phase III trial of infusional fluorouracil, leucovorin, oxaliplatin, and irinotecan (FOLFOXIRI) compared with infusional fluorouracil, leucovorin, and irinotecan (FOLFIRI) as first-line treatment for metastatic colorectal cancer: the Gruppo Oncologico Nord Ovest. Journal of Clinical Oncology. 2007;25(13):1670-6.

[31] Souglakos J, Androulakis N, Syrigos K, Polyzos A, Ziras N, Athanasiadis A, et al. FOLFOXIRI (folinic acid, 5-fluorouracil, oxaliplatin and irinotecan) vs FOLFIRI (folinic acid, 5-fluorouracil and irinotecan) as first-line treatment in metastatic colorectal cancer (MCC): a multicentre randomised phase III trial from the Hellenic Oncology Research Group (HORG). British journal of cancer. 2006;94(6):798-805.

[32] Masi G, Loupakis F, Pollina L, Vasile E, Cupini S, Ricci S, et al. Long-term outcome of initially unresectable metastatic colorectal cancer patients treated with 5-fluorouracil/ leucovorin, oxaliplatin, and irinotecan (FOLFOXIRI) followed by radical surgery of metastases. Annals of surgery. 2009;249(3):420-5.

[33] Willett CG, Fung CY, Kaufman DS, Efird J, Shellito PC. Postoperative radiation therapy for high-risk colon carcinoma. Journal of clinical oncology. 1993;11(6):1112-7.

[34] Martenson Jr JA, Willett CG, Sargent DJ, Mailliard JA, Donohue JH, Gunderson LL, et al. Phase III study of adjuvant chemotherapy and radiation therapy compared with chemotherapy alone in the surgical adjuvant treatment of colon cancer: results of intergroup protocol 0130. Journal of clinical oncology. 2004;22(16):3277-83.

[35] Gray R, Barnwell J, McConkey C, Hills RK, Williams NS, Kerr DJ. Adjuvant chemotherapy versus observation in patients with colorectal cancer: a randomised study. Lancet. 2007;370(9604):2020.

[36] Swanson RS, Compton CC, Stewart AK, Bland KI. The prognosis of T3N0 colon cancer is dependent on the number of lymph nodes examined. Annals of surgical oncology. 2003;10(1):65-71.

[37] Le Voyer T, Sigurdson E, Hanlon A, Mayer R, Macdonald J, Catalano P, et al. Colon cancer survival is associated with increasing number of lymph nodes analyzed: a secondary survey of intergroup trial INT-0089. Journal of Clinical Oncology. 2003;21(15):2912-9.

[38] Sargent DJ, Goldberg RM, Jacobson SD, Macdonald JS, Labianca R, Haller DG, et al. A pooled analysis of adjuvant chemotherapy for resected colon cancer in elderly patients. New England Journal of Medicine. 2001;345(15):1091-7.

[39] Sargent DJ, Marsoni S, Monges G, Thibodeau SN, Labianca R, Hamilton SR, et al. Defective mismatch repair as a predictive marker for lack of efficacy of fluorouracil-based adjuvant therapy in colon cancer. Journal of Clinical Oncology. 2010;28(20): 3219-26.

[40] O'Connell M, Lavery I, Gray R, Quirke P, Kerr D, Lopatin M, et al., editors. Comparison of molecular and pathologic features of stage II and stage III colon cancer in four large studies conducted for development of the 12-gene colon cancer recurrence score. J Clin Oncol (Meeting Abstracts); 2010.

[41] Rosenberg R, Maak M, Nitsche U, Schuster T, Kuenzli B, Simon I, et al., editors. Independent validation of a prognostic genomic profile (ColoPrint) for stage II colon cancer (CC) patients. J Clin Oncol (Meeting Abstracts); 2010.

[42] Enríquez-Navascués JM, Borda N, Lizerazu A, Placer C, Elosegui JL, Ciria JP, et al. Patterns of local recurrence in rectal cancer after a multidisciplinary approach. World journal of gastroenterology: WJG. 2011;17(13):1674.

[43] Rosen L, Veidenheimer MC, Coller JA, Corman ML. Mortality, morbidity, and patterns of recurrence after abdominoperineal resection for cancer of the rectum. Diseases of the Colon & Rectum. 1982;25(3):202-8.

[44] Prolongation of the disease-free interval in surgically treated rectal carcinoma. Gastrointestinal Tumor Study Group. The New England journal of medicine. 1985 Jun 6;312(23):1465-72. PubMed PMID: 2859523. Epub 1985/06/06. eng.

[45] Douglass Jr HO, Moertel CG, Mayer RJ, Thomas PRM, Lindblad AS, Mittleman A, et al. Survival after postoperative combination treatment of rectal cancer. New England Journal of Medicine. 1986;315(20):1294-5.

[46] Fisher B, Wolmark N, Rockette H, Redmond C, Deutsch M, Wickerham DL, et al. Postoperative Adjuvant Chemotherapy or Radiation Therapy for Rectal Cancer: Re-

sults From NSABP Protocol R-011. Journal of the National Cancer Institute. 1988;80(1):21-9.

[47] Krook JE, Moertel C, Wieand HS. Radiation vs sequential chemotherapy-radiation-chemotherapy. A study of North Central Cancer Treatment Group, Duke University and Mayo Clinic. Proceedings of the American Society of Clinical Oncology. 1988;5(82).

[48] Improved survival with preoperative radiotherapy in resectable rectal cancer. Swedish Rectal Cancer Trial. The New England journal of medicine. 1997 Apr 3;336(14): 980-7. PubMed PMID: 9091798. Epub 1997/04/03. eng.

[49] Peeters KCMJ, Marijnen CAM, Nagtegaal ID, Kranenbarg EK, Putter H, Wiggers T, et al. The TME trial after a median follow-up of 6 years: increased local control but no survival benefit in irradiated patients with resectable rectal carcinoma. Annals of surgery. 2007;246(5):693-701.

[50] Stephens RJ, Thompson LC, Quirke P, Steele R, Grieve R, Couture J, et al. Impact of short-course preoperative radiotherapy for rectal cancer on patients' quality of life: data from the Medical Research Council CR07/National Cancer Institute of Canada Clinical Trials Group C016 randomized clinical trial. Journal of Clinical Oncology. 2010;28(27):4233-9.

[51] Sauer R, Becker H, Hohenberger W, Rödel C, Wittekind C, Fietkau R, et al. Preoperative versus postoperative chemoradiotherapy for rectal cancer. New England Journal of Medicine. 2004;351(17):1731-40.

[52] Bosset JF, Calais G, Mineur L, Maingon P, Radosevic-Jelic L, Daban A, et al. Enhanced tumorocidal effect of chemotherapy with preoperative radiotherapy for rectal cancer: preliminary results--EORTC 22921. Journal of clinical oncology : official journal of the American Society of Clinical Oncology. 2005 Aug 20;23(24):5620-7. PubMed PMID: 16009958. Epub 2005/07/13. eng.

[53] Bosset JF, Collette L, Calais G, Mineur L, Maingon P, Radosevic-Jelic L, et al. Chemotherapy with preoperative radiotherapy in rectal cancer. The New England journal of medicine. 2006 Sep 14;355(11):1114-23. PubMed PMID: 16971718. Epub 2006/09/15. eng.

[54] Roh MS, Colangelo LH, O'Connell MJ, Yothers G, Deutsch M, Allegra CJ, et al. Preoperative multimodality therapy improves disease-free survival in patients with carcinoma of the rectum: NSABP R-03. Journal of clinical oncology : official journal of the American Society of Clinical Oncology. 2009 Nov 1;27(31):5124-30. PubMed PMID: 19770376. Pubmed Central PMCID: 2773471. Epub 2009/09/23. eng.

[55] O'Connell MJ, Martenson JA, Wieand HS, Krook JE, Macdonald JS, Haller DG, et al. Improving adjuvant therapy for rectal cancer by combining protracted-infusion fluorouracil with radiation therapy after curative surgery. The New England journal of medicine. 1994 Aug 25;331(8):502-7. PubMed PMID: 8041415. Epub 1994/08/25. eng.

[56] Ngan SY, Michael M, Mackay J, McKendrick J, Leong T, Lim Joon D, et al. A phase I trial of preoperative radiotherapy and capecitabine for locally advanced, potentially resectable rectal cancer. British journal of cancer. 2004 Sep 13;91(6):1019-24. PubMed PMID: 15305186. Pubmed Central PMCID: 2747703. Epub 2004/08/12. eng.

[57] Kim JC, Kim TW, Kim JH, Yu CS, Kim HC, Chang HM, et al. Preoperative concurrent radiotherapy with capecitabine before total mesorectal excision in locally advanced rectal cancer. International journal of radiation oncology, biology, physics. 2005 Oct 1;63(2):346-53. PubMed PMID: 15913913. Epub 2005/05/26. eng.

[58] Hofheinz RD, Wenz F, Post S, Matzdorff A, Laechelt S, Hartmann JT, et al. Chemoradiotherapy with capecitabine versus fluorouracil for locally advanced rectal cancer: a randomised, multicentre, non-inferiority, phase 3 trial. The lancet oncology. 2012 Jun; 13(6):579-88. PubMed PMID: 22503032. Epub 2012/04/17. eng.

[59] Roh MS, Yothers GA, O'Connell MJ, Beart W, Pitot HC, Shields AF, et al. The impact of capecitabine and oxaliplatin in the preoperative multimodality treatment in patients with carcinoma of the rectum: NSABP R-04. J Clin Oncol 29: 2011 (suppl; abstr 3503) 2011.

[60] Rodel C, Liersch T, Hermann RM, Arnold D, Reese T, Hipp M, et al. Multicenter phase II trial of chemoradiation with oxaliplatin for rectal cancer. Journal of clinical oncology : official journal of the American Society of Clinical Oncology. 2007 Jan 1;25(1):110-7. PubMed PMID: 17194912. Epub 2006/12/30. eng.

[61] Goldberg RM, Sargent DJ, Morton RF, Fuchs CS, Ramanathan RK, Williamson SK, et al. A randomized controlled trial of fluorouracil plus leucovorin, irinotecan, and oxaliplatin combinations in patients with previously untreated metastatic colorectal cancer. Journal of clinical oncology : official journal of the American Society of Clinical Oncology. 2004 Jan 1;22(1):23-30. PubMed PMID: 14665611. Epub 2003/12/11. eng.

[62] Aschele C, Cionini L, Lonardi S, Pinto C, Cordio S, Rosati G, et al. Primary tumor response to preoperative chemoradiation with or without oxaliplatin in locally advanced rectal cancer: pathologic results of the STAR-01 randomized phase III trial. Journal of clinical oncology : official journal of the American Society of Clinical Oncology. 2011 Jul 10;29(20):2773-80. PubMed PMID: 21606427. Epub 2011/05/25. eng.

[63] Rodel C, Liersch T, Becker H, Fietkau R, Hohenberger W, Hothorn T, et al. Preoperative chemoradiotherapy and postoperative chemotherapy with fluorouracil and oxaliplatin versus fluorouracil alone in locally advanced rectal cancer: initial results of the German CAO/ARO/AIO-04 randomised phase 3 trial. The lancet oncology. 2012 Jul;13(7):679-87. PubMed PMID: 22627104. Epub 2012/05/26. eng.

[64] Gerard JP, Azria D, Gourgou-Bourgade S, Martel-Laffay I, Hennequin C, Etienne PL, et al. Comparison of two neoadjuvant chemoradiotherapy regimens for locally advanced rectal cancer: results of the phase III trial ACCORD 12/0405-Prodige 2. Journal of clinical oncology : official journal of the American Society of Clinical

Oncology. 2010 Apr 1;28(10):1638-44. PubMed PMID: 20194850. Epub 2010/03/03. eng.

[65] Machiels JP, Sempoux C, Scalliet P, Coche JC, Humblet Y, Van Cutsem E, et al. Phase I/II study of preoperative cetuximab, capecitabine, and external beam radiotherapy in patients with rectal cancer. Annals of oncology : official journal of the European Society for Medical Oncology / ESMO. 2007 Apr;18(4):738-44. PubMed PMID: 17208931. Epub 2007/01/09. eng.

[66] Dewdney A, Cunningham D, Tabernero J, Capdevila J, Glimelius B, Cervantes A, et al. Multicenter randomized phase II clinical trial comparing neoadjuvant oxaliplatin, capecitabine, and preoperative radiotherapy with or without cetuximab followed by total mesorectal excision in patients with high-risk rectal cancer (EXPERT-C). Journal of clinical oncology : official journal of the American Society of Clinical Oncology. 2012 May 10;30(14):1620-7. PubMed PMID: 22473163. Epub 2012/04/05. eng.

[67] Willett CG, Duda DG, di Tomaso E, Boucher Y, Ancukiewicz M, Sahani DV, et al. Efficacy, safety, and biomarkers of neoadjuvant bevacizumab, radiation therapy, and fluorouracil in rectal cancer: a multidisciplinary phase II study. Journal of clinical oncology : official journal of the American Society of Clinical Oncology. 2009 Jun 20;27(18):3020-6. PubMed PMID: 19470921. Pubmed Central PMCID: 2702234. Epub 2009/05/28. eng.

[68] Crane CH, Eng C, Feig BW, Das P, Skibber JM, Chang GJ, et al. Phase II trial of neoadjuvant bevacizumab, capecitabine, and radiotherapy for locally advanced rectal cancer. International journal of radiation oncology, biology, physics. 2010 Mar 1;76(3):824-30. PubMed PMID: 19464823. Epub 2009/05/26. eng.

[69] Dipetrillo T, Pricolo V, Lagares-Garcia J, Vrees M, Klipfel A, Cataldo T, et al. Neoadjuvant bevacizumab, oxaliplatin, 5-fluorouracil, and radiation for rectal cancer. International journal of radiation oncology, biology, physics. 2012 Jan 1;82(1):124-9. PubMed PMID: 20947267. Epub 2010/10/16. eng.

[70] Blaszkowsky LS, Hong TS, Zhu AX, Kwak EL, Mamon HJ, Shellito PC, et al. A phase I/II study of bevacizumab (beva), erlotinib (erl), and 5-fluorouracil (5-FU) with concurrent external beam radiation therapy (RT) in locally advanced rectal cancer (LARC). Journal of Clinical Oncology. 2009;suppl: abstract 4106.

Chapter 13

Adjuvant Treatment in Colorectal Cancer

Krassimir Ivanov, Nikola Kolev, Ivan Shterev,
Anton Tonev, Valentin Ignatov, Vasil Bojkov and
Tanya Kirilova

Additional information is available at the end of the chapter

http://dx.doi.org/10.5772/56914

1. Introduction

Worldwide, more than 1 million people develop colorectal cancer (CRC) annually [1]. CRC is a major health problem in the Western world and the second most common cause of cancer mortality [2]. To improve performance, the role of chemotherapy for CRC has increased dramatically over the last decade. Of course surgery remains the cornerstone of treatment, the vast majority of CRC patients now receive chemotherapy with multiple agents that are currently approved for the treatment in the appropriate setting. However, it is a complex process to select the optimal chemotherapy for each patient and practice evidence gap is still a problem. We found large differences in patterns of institution, region and country. The results suggest that the lack of evidence for CRC chemotherapy practice still exists around the world. [3] Recently, standardization of cancer treatment, including chemotherapy, has become of particular importance for the quality of cancer therapy. It is important to know whether the overhaul performed normalization of CRC chemotherapy. Measures and quality indicators are needed and several studies on indicators of quality of cancer care have been reported. However, measures to assess the standardization of cancer therapy are not well established. In this study, we evaluated the usefulness of the oncology market research to assess the evidence gap in practice CRC chemotherapy. We also discuss the role of the method to measure the effect of normalization of CRC chemotherapy. [4, 5]

Although surgery remains the cornerstone of treatment, the vast majority of CRC patients now receive chemotherapy to reduce the risk of metastatic spread by eradicating microscopic tumor foci that are distant from the primary tumor and undetectable in perioperative assessment of tumor extension. [5] Five-year survival of patients are mainly determined by the histological stage of the tumor at the time of resection. The most important prognostic factor for survival in patients without visceral metastases is the stage of the tumor determined by the depth of penetration of the tumor in the bowel wall and the number of lymph nodes [4] (lymph nodes >12 examined). Result of the meta - analysis of over 10 studies showed that each - two-month delay of adjuvant chemotherapy resulted in a 14% decrease in overall survival, suggesting that adjuvant chemotherapy should be administered as soon as possible [5].

The introduction of new cytotoxic agents such as oral fluoropyrimidines, oxaliplatin and irinotecan in chemotherapy (CT) regimens have improved the response rate, disease-free survival (DFS) and overall survival (OS) in patients with metastatic colorectal cancer. [6, 7] This has encouraged the trials in the adjuvant treatment of non-metastatic disease, especially in patients with stage III tumors. Table 1 shows the most common regimens used for the CT adjuvant. Surgery alone is usually curative for colon cancer stage II, but about 20% to 30% of these patients develop recurrence and die of metastatic disease. [8] This underpins the need for prognostic factors such as microsatellite instability (MSI), which are potentially predictive of tumor response to cytotoxic agents. [7] Prognostic factors are particularly useful in the context of stage II colorectal cancer, where the benefits of cytotoxic adjuvant therapy are more controversial than in stage III disease. The identification of accurate and validated predictive and prognostic markers help clinicians in choosing appropriate use of adjuvant chemotherapy in patients with stage II CRC.

MSI is a change in the length of microsatellite DNA due to the insertion or deletion of repeating units – from 1to 5 nucleotides caused by defects in mismatch repair genes or methylation of their promoters. [9] Tumors with MSI are more often proximal, poorly differentiated, mucinous, and show a significant lymphocytic infiltration. [9] Colon cancers with high-frequency MSI have clinical and pathological features that distinguish them from microsatellite stable tumors and MSI is a marker of favorable outcome and a predictor for the benefit decreased from fluorouracil - based adjuvant chemotherapy in patients with stage II or colon cancer stage III with microsatellite stable tumors or tumors with low-frequency microsatellite instability. [10] Silence or mutation of mismatch repair (MMR) genes can lead to protein deficiency MMR and MSI 10. This is observed in patients with Lynch syndrome, and it is a rare cause of hereditary colon cancer 2 to 4% of the 11 cases. Somatic mutation is reported in 19% of CRC [12], while silencing of MMR genes can be observed in up to 52% of sporadic colon cancers [13].

In sporadic CRC, three tumor phenotypes were defined: microsatellite stable (MSS), low-frequency MSI (MSI-L) and high frequency MSI (MSI-H). It has been reported that MSI-H are more frequently found in stage II disease than in stage III disease 14. This may partly explain the benefit decreased from 5 - fluorouracil adjuvant chemotherapy (5FU) in patients with stage II. Tente identify patients who might benefit from adjuvant chemotherapy led to the development of multigene tests as several Oncotype DX etc. Unfortunately, there is no evidence that any of them can predict the potential benefit of adjuvant chemotherapy. [13]

2. Treatment guidelines for CRC

Some guidelines for the treatment of CRC have been developed to promote the standardization of CRC treatment. Only two drugs, panitumumab and cetuximab first line were still causing discord. Bevacizumab or capecitabine combined with oxaliplatin is used for the treatment of advanced and recurrent CRC, while the FOLFOX regimen is used in patients with a high risk of recurrence in the adjuvant chemotherapy. In this major revision, current controversies are treated as clinical issues with many references.

Adjuvant 5-FU chemotherapy is the standard treatment used in patients with stage III (Dukes C) and high-risk stage II (Dukes B) tumors. Capecitabine and bolus 5FU regimes have proven efficacy and are associated with a low risk of severe toxicity. The addition of oxaliplatin to 5FU improves patient outcomes in the adjuvant setting. Mosaic of randomized trials in 2246 patients with stage 2 or 3 of the CRC to receive LV5FU2 or FOLFOX-4 chemotherapy. The operating system after 6 years of follow-up for all patients was 78.5% for FOLFOX-4 against 76% for LV5FU2. Subgroup analysis showed stage-specific 6-year OS rate of 72.9% against 68.7% in patients with stage 3 of the CRC and 86.9% compared with 86.8% in patients with stage 2 CRC for FOLFOX-4 and LV5FU2, respectively. The NSABP C-07 trial had a similar design, the addition of oxaliplatin to 5FU adjuvant chemotherapy, but used a different calendar 5FU and oxaliplatin doses delivered also less than in the MOSAIC study (nine against twelve). The first results showed a similar improvement in disease-free survival (DFS) than that observed in the MOSAIC trial. A recently presented the final results confirm improved DFS, but showed shorter survival time after recurrence in the oxaliplatin arm and an improvement in overall survival has not been seen. A significant interaction between age and survival of certain parameters were observed. Patients less than 70 years appeared to benefit from the addition of oxaliplatin while patients over 70 years, no benefit was observed consistently. The analysis of the ACCENT database, including 10, 449 patients less than 70 years and 2170 patients over 70 years from six randomized trials have demonstrated a significant interaction between age and treatment effect. No differences in results were noted between experimental (combination) chemotherapy and chemotherapy in patients with fluoropyrimidine control over 70 years. Adding oxaliplatin to 5FU increases the overall incidence of grade 3 toxicity and is associated with the occurrence of peripheral sensory neuropathy. Over 90% of patients experience temporary symptoms typically induced cold, with a minority of patients with persistent symptoms affecting activities of daily living (grade 2 and 3 toxicity). In the MOSAIC study, grade 3 peripheral sensory neuropathy was noted in 12.5% of patients treated with oxaliplatin for the treatment. After 48 months of follow-up, rates of toxicity were grade 11.9% 1, % [22] 8 degree and 0.7% grade 3, respectively. Similar data were presented for the NSABP C-07 study.

Decisions regarding the use of adjuvant chemotherapy combinations are more complex. The incidence of approximately 3% of significant long-term peripheral neuropathy and MS MT Seymour Braun could interfere with the activities of the daily life of the patient influences decision-making in relation to the small additional benefit accrued to receive the oxaliplatin. MOSAIC and NSABP the C-07 trials delivered a total dose of oxaliplatin different, but both studies noted similar improvements in DFS. International trials evaluating shorter periods of oxaliplatin-based chemotherapy in the adjuvant setting (12 versus 24 weeks of chemotherapy oxaliplatin/5FU ISRCTN 59757862) in order to assess the non-inferiority of short periods of treatment, as well as consideration of the evaluation criteria of quality of life. The relative benefit of chemotherapy is also a key factor in the choice of treatment for patients in the adjuvant setting. Patients with stage 3 are a heterogeneous group and decisions based on age, the relative risk of recurrence (N1 N2 against disease), and the additional benefit that can be achieved by adding oxaliplatin need to be carefully considered. Given the new data in patients over 70 years, it seems likely that chemotherapy oxaliplatin are used less frequently in this group. Patients with disease stage 2 have an excellent prognosis with or without chemotherapy 5FU-based and high-risk patients functions are selected for processing. Both C-07 and MOSAIC are powered to assess the benefit of adding oxaliplatin to 5-FU in patients with stage 2 disease, but a trend towards improved DFS was noted. However, no OS benefit is probably very low in absolute terms (<2%) and difficult to justify given the excellent overall performance (> 80% at 5 years of operation) and the risk of neurotoxicity. [23]

3. 5FU

In 1990, Moertel and colleagues first reported the value of adjuvant chemotherapy in patients with stage III colon cancer (Dukes C, Tx N + M0). [15] This study showed an increase in overall survival and progression-free survival in patients receiving 5FU/ Levamisole - based chemotherapy for 1 year against levamisole alone or without chemotherapy. With a median follow - up of 6.5 years, patients treated with 5-FU / levamisole showed a 40% reduction in recidivism and an estimated reduction of 33% of overall mortality [16]. 5-FU is a pyrimidine analogue, which inhibits thymidylate synthase (TS) (involved in the de novo synthesis of thymidine) and is involved in incorporation into RNA and DNA with the inhibition of DNA synthesis and function [17]. With 5FU bolus injection maximum concentration is reached in the plasma and bone marrow 100-1000 times higher than with continuous infusion. More than 85% of the administered drug is inactivated by dihydropyrimidine dehydrogenase (DPD), expressed mainly in the liver. Some mutation in DPD in about 2% in the general population can lead to serious life-threatening toxicity [17]. Leucovorin (LV) or folinic acid enhance the antitumor activity of 5FU. Today, there is a lack of LV in the United States, despite the absence of specific data confirming this statement. The QUASAR study investigators demonstrated that patients treated with 175 mg of LV similar survival and 3 - year recurrence rate of LV 25 mg when administered as a bolus 5-FU as adjuvant therapy for CRC 7. Similar results have been reported in the parameters in metastatic CRC patients - there was no difference in survival or response rate in patients receiving 5FU bolus high - dose or low-dose LV [18]. Therefore, when LV is not available without LV treatment is reasonable. Comparison of monthly bolus FU / LV regimen (5FU bolus followed by LV 15 minutes) with double - monthly infusion LV5FU2 (LV for 2 hours, followed by bolus 5-FU, followed by a continuous infusion of 5-FU over 2 days) in 905 patients with stage II (43%) or III (57%) colon cancer showed that the regime was less toxic LV5FU2, especially regarding hematological and gastrointestinal events (P <0.001) [19]. No significant difference in DFS and OS was observed in one of two regi mens median follow-up 6 years. Two other studies have shown that the two ways of 5FU bolus administration combined with LV with or without levamisole and a continuous infusion of 5-FU are equivalent. Saini and colleagues conducted a multicenter randomized trial comparing the efficacy and toxicity of 12 weeks of 5FU delivered by continuous intravenous infusion against the standard bolus 5-FU and LV for 6 months as adjuvant treatment in colorectal cancer. The two schemes are equivalent, but the plan 12 weeks was less toxic [20]. The analysis of data from several trials in which patients were randomly resection of the tumor or tumor resection followed by adjuvant 5-FU/LV showed that the benefit of adjuvant chemotherapy was observed in patients with stage III [21, 22], which suggests that because of nodal status of these patients are at higher risk. Both studies showed that the addition of oxaliplatin to 5-FU/LV as adjuvant therapy in stage II and elderly patients showed no significant DFS or OS [23, 24] benefits even in patients with characteristics high risk - T4 tumors, intestinal obstruction, venous invasion, etc. This suggests that, despite the failure of our definition of high-risk patients with stage II, 5-FU/LV regimen may be preferable. QUASAR investigators reported their analysis of 3238 patients, the majority of them were in stage II colon cancer. Patients were randomized to receive 5-FU/LV or observation. The relative risk of death from all causes in the 5-FU/LV arm versus observation was 0.82 (95% CI, 0.70 to 0.95, p = 0.008). The relative risk of recurrence was 0.78 (95% CI, 0.67-0, 91, p = 0.001) [7]. The investigators did not separate patients into individuals high or low risk. Risk factors are obstruction or bowel perforation, elevated preoperative CEA, poorly differentiated tumors, removal of CDC patients and MSI-S. The impact of adjuvant chemotherapy and the potential benefit of this new could not be clearly demonstrated in this study of patients with stage II.

4. Oral fluoropyrimidines

Two oral prodrugs of 5FU - capecetabine and uracil / tegafur (UFT), has demonstrated efficacy in metastatic disease, which is comparable with bolus 5-FU/LV regimens [25, 26]. After oral administration, capecitabine is rapidly absorbed with plasma concentrations peaking after 1.5 hours [27]. Pharmacokinetics is largely dose - dependent. The pharmacology of capecitabine is not significantly influenced by gender, race, performance status, body surface area, albumin or hepatic dysfunction [28]. The half-life of capecitabine is between 0.49 and 0.89 hours, whereas the half-life of the metabolite (5-FU) extends from 0.67 to 1.15 hours [29]. Regarding renal excretion primarily (more than 70% of metabolites), capecitabine is against - in patients with severe renal impairment (creatinine clearance less than 30 mL / min).

Therapy	Mechanism of Action	Indications	Potential Common Toxicities
5- Fluorouracil (5FU)	Blocks the enzyme thymidylate synthase (TS), which is essential for DNA synthesis	Multiple uses in combination with other agents, both in the adjuvant (postop) and palliative setting	Gastrointestinal (nausea, diarrhea) Myelosuppression Fatigue
Capecitabine	Blocks thymidylate synthase (orally administered prodrug converted to 5FU)	Multiple uses in combination with other agents, both in the adjuvant (postop) and metastatic setting	Gastrointestinal (nausea, diarrhea) Myelosuppression Fatigue Palmar-plantar syndrome (hand-foot syndrome)
Oxaliplatin	Inhibits DNA replication and transcription by forming inter- and intra-strand DNA adducts/cross-links	Used in combination with 5FU, leucovorin (LV) (FOLFOX) in the adjuvant (postop) and metastatic setting	Peripheral neuropathy Gastrointestinal (nausea, diarrhea) Fatigue Myelosuppression Hypersensitivity
Irinotecan	Inhibits topoisomerase I, an enzyme that facilitates the uncoiling and recoiling of DNA during replication	Used alone or in combination with 5FU, LV (FOLFIRI) in the metastatic setting	Cholinergic (acute diarrhea) Gastrointestinal (nausea, late diarrhea) Fatigue Myelosuppression Alopecia
Bevacizumab	Monoclonal antibody which binds to VEGF ligand	Used in combination with either FOLFOX or FOLFIRI in the metastatic setting	Hypertension Arterial thrombotic events Impaired wound healing Gastrointestinal perforation
Cetuximab	Monoclonal antibody to EGFR (chimeric) that blocks the ligand-binding site	Used with irinotecan or as a single agent in the metastatic setting	Acneform rash Hypersensitivity Hypomagnesemia Fatigue
Panitumumab	Monoclonal antibody to EGFR (fully humanized) that blocks the ligand-binding site	Used as a single agent in the metastatic setting	Acneform rash Hypomagnesemia Fatigue

VEGF, vascular endothelial growth factor; EGFR, epidermal growth factor receptor.

Table 1. Types of therapeutical agents and their mechanism of action

The X-ACT (Xeloda (capecitabine) in adjuvant therapy of colon cancer) Phase III trial in patients (N = 1.987) compared capecitabine (2500 mg / m 2 / day, 14 to 21 days) for bolus 5-FU/

LV. After a median follow-up of 6.9 years, both treatments showed similar efficacy in terms of DFS and OS [30]. The HR for DFS of capecitabine compared 5-FU/LV was 0.88 (95% CI, 0.77 to 1.01), the upper limit of the 95% is well below the predefined non-inferiority margin of 1.20 ($p < 0.0001$) [30]. The 5-year DFS rate for capecitabine and 5-FU/LV were 60.8% and 56.7%, respectively. These monitoring data confirm that, as adjunctive therapy for patients with colon cancer resected stage III oral capecitabine is at least equivalent to iv bolus treatment of 5-FU/LV in terms of 5 - year DFS, the primary endpoint of X-ACT study. Infusional 5-FU regimens are now often favored because they offer similar efficacy or improved slightly bolus 5-FU/LV regimes and are generally better tolerated [31]. However, the plasma concentration profile of capecitabine is administered twice daily for 14 days, closer to that of a continuous infusion of 5-FU bolus injections as daily or weekly 5FU.La capecitabine Profile improved safety compared to bolus 5-FU/LV in terms of significantly lower rates of diarrhea, stomatitis, neutropenia, nausea, alopecia, febrile neutropenia [30].

UFT and oral LV was evaluated in the adjuvant setting in the NSABP C-06 trial. More than 1000 patients with colon cancer were randomized to receive either oral or intravenous UFT with LV 5FU with LV. 47% of patients had colon cancer stage II, and 53% had colon cancer stage III. Median follow-up was 62.3 months time. There was no significant difference in disease-free survival - or overall showing that the UFT is an acceptable alternative to parenteral 5-FU/LV [32]. No difference in toxicity profiles of the two regimens has been reported.

5. Adjuvant therapy combination

The hypothesis that the antitumor activity of the combination agent, including oxaliplatin, irinotecan, bevacizumab, cetuximab in metastatic cure rates would result in increased adjuvant proved to be often wrong. Oxaliplatin is a platinum compound and third generation of the safe administration of evidence of clinical activity has been reported 33. Platinum compounds exert their effect through the development of covalent adducts with cellular DNA, which is not portable - specific cycle [34]. Platinum derivative oxaliplatin is described as having a "tri-exponential" reason for removing the half - life being successively 0.28 hours, 16.3 hours and 273 hours [35]. The fact that the third half-life of oxaliplatin hundreds of hours, the accumulation of the drug in the tissues can reasonably be expected. In this regard, one study examined the long - term retention of platinum 8-75 months after treatment with cisplatin and oxaliplatin [36]. Narrow therapeutic index of oxaliplatin and adverse reactions are mainly reported in the hematopoietic system, peripheral nerves, and gastrointestinal tract [35]. The addition of oxaliplatin to 5FU improves patient outcomes in the adjuvant setting. Mosaic of randomized 2246 patients with stage II or III CRC will LV5FU2 or FOLFOX-4 (which is LV5FU2 chemotherapy plus oxaliplatin on day 1]. The 5-year DFS rate of Phase II and III patients were 73.3% and 67.4% in the FOLFOX-4 groups and LV5FU2, respectively (RR 0.80, 95% CI, 0.68-0, 93, $p = 0.003$) [37]. Subgroup analysis showed stage - specific 6 years OS rate of 72.9% against 68.7% in patients with stage III CRC (HR 0.80, 95% CI, 0.65-0, 97, $P = 0.023$) and 85.0% against 83.3% in patients with stage II CRC ($P = 0.65$] in the FOLFOX-4 and LV5FU2, respectively [38]. As expected, the toxicity of the regimen FOLFOX-4 was higher than that observed in the LV5FU2 arm. All - cause mortality in the first 60 days was the same in both arms.The NSABP C-07 trial had a similar design, the addition of oxaliplatin to 5-FU adjuvant chemotherapy, but using a different calendar 5FU and also provide fewer doses of oxaliplatin in the MOSAIC study (nine against twelve). FLOX regimen in this trial was studied - oxaliplatin was given on weeks 1, 3, and 5 more per week 5-FU/LV bolus of 1-6 weeks, repeated at 8 week cycle, depending on the standard weekly 5-FU/LV treatment. Over 2000 patients were randomized to receive 5-FU/LV and FLOX treatment. Stage II patients were 29% and stage III patients was 71%. The median duration of follow up was 34 months. The hazard ratio of FLOX against 5-FU/LV was 0.79 (95% CI, 0.67 to 0.93], with a risk reduction of 21% in favor of FLOX [39]. As expected, treatment toxicity FLOX was higher than that observed in the 5-FU/LV arm. 15 deaths were recorded in the treatment with FLOX and 14 deaths 5-FU/LV. Update this study showed that the benefit of FLOX in DFS was observed in 7 - year median follow - but there was no significant difference in overall survival when the two arms were compared 24 (HR, 0.88, 95% CI, 0.74 to 1.05, P = 0.1428). A significant interaction between age and survival of certain parameters were observed. Patients less than 70 years appeared to benefit from the addition of oxaliplatin while in patients over 70 years, no benefit was observed consistently. MOSAIC and NSABP the C-07 trials delivered a total dose of oxaliplatin different, but both studies noted similar improvements in DFS. International trials evaluating shorter periods of oxaliplatin - based chemotherapy in the adjuvant setting (12 versus 24 weeks of chemotherapy oxaliplatin/5FU ISRCTN 59757862) in order to assess the non-inferiority of short periods treatment.Both NSABP C-07 and MOSAIC are powered to assess the benefit of adding oxaliplatin to 5-FU in patients with stage II disease, but a trend towards improved DFS was noted.However, no OS benefit is probably very low in absolute terms (<2%) and difficult to justify given the excellent overall performance (> 80% at 5 years of operation) and the risk of neurotoxicity. Analysis of a phase III trial comparing capecitabine plus oxaliplatin (XELOX) with bolus 5-FU/LV as adjuvant treatment for colon cancer stage III showed that XELOX was an improvement of 3 years compared to 5-FU/LV DFS rate [40, 41]. Patients receiving XELOX had less adverse reactions such as diarrhea, alopecia, and more neurosensory toxicity, vomiting and hand-foot syndrome than patients receiving FU / LV. All these studies suggest that FOLFOX, XELOX FLOX and can be used interchangeably in contexts adjuvant. Irinotecan is a semisynthetic analogue of camptothecin, originally isolated from the China / Tibet ornamental tree Camptotheca acuminata.It is a chemotherapy agent that causes destruction of cells in S phase-specific topoisomerase I poison in the cell [42]. CALGB 89803 trial by Saltz and colleagues randomized 1264 patients to receive standard weekly bolus 5-FU / LV bolus regimen or weekly irinotecan and 5-FU bolus / LV. The primary endpoints of the study were overall survival and disease-free survival. Surprisingly, they found no difference in either DFS (0.84] or OS (P = 0.74] between the two treatment arms with lethal and non-lethal toxicity increased by the addition of irinotecan to standard 5FU / LV pattern 43.This trial showed the need for randomized controlled trials adjuvant because advances in the treatment of metastatic disease does not necessarily translate into advances in adjuvant therapy. Phase III trial was conducted by large investigators PETACC-3. They investigated whether the addition of irinotecan to LV5FU2 would improve disease-free survival in patients with colon cancer. After surgery, patients with stage II and III colon cancer were randomized to receive surgery LV5FU2 (LV 200 mg / m 2 infused over 2 hours, followed by 5-FU as a 400 mg / m 2 bolus and then one of 600 mg / m 2 by continuous infusion over 22 hours on days 1 and 2 every 2 weeks for 12 cycles) with or without irinotecan (180 mg / m 2 infused over 30 to 90 minutes, day 1, every 2 weeks) [44]. After a median follow-up of 66.3 months, the rate at 5 years was 56.7% with DFS irinotecan/ LV5FU2 and 54.3% for LV5FU2 alone (p = 0.106). They observed that the addition of irinotecan to LV5FU2 was associated with an increased incidence of adverse reactions and neutropenia. They concluded that irinotecan added to LV5FU2 as adjuvant therapy does not confer a statistically significant improvement in overall survival or DFS in patients with colon cancer stage III versus LV5FU2 alone. For the moment, there are no data supporting the use of irinotecan-containing regimens in adjuvant stage II and III patients. Analysis PETACC-3 trial could not confirm the expected benefit of adding irinotecan in MSI-H patients. Bevacizumab is a recombinant humanized monoclonal antibody directed against the vascular endothelial growth factor (VEGF) which is used to inhibit the function of VEGF in vascular endothelial cells and thereby inhibit tumor angiogenesis-dependent solid tumors for growth and metastasis [45]. Bevacizumab has demonstrated clinical activity to increase in the standard CT metastatic settings.This led to the consideration of this agent in the adjuvant chemotherapy in the NSABP C-08 trial. More than 2500 patients, most of whom had stage III were randomized to receive FOLFOX6 modified 6 months, alone or with bevacizumab [46]. In the bevacizumab arm, bevacizumab was administered for more than 6 months, for a total of 1 year of bevacizumab.The primary endpoint of the study was 3 years DFS. The relative risk of FOLFOX plus bevacizumab versus FOLFOX alone was 0.89 (95% CI, 0.76 to 1.04, p = 0.15). This study did not demonstrate the benefits of the use of bevacizumab in the adjuvant treatment of stage II and III CRC and for this reason the use of bevacizumab cannot be recommended for use in the adjuvant treatment of patients with colon cancer. Cetuximab is a monoclonal antibody capable of inhibiting the degradation and transmembrane receptor EGFR epidermal growth factor 47.Inhibition of EGFR is of major importance because EGFR control many important activities of tumor cells, including tumor growth and neo - angiogenesis, inhibition of the apoptotic response to chemotherapy and radiotherapy. In a Phase III, randomized, Alberts and colleagues evaluated the potential benefit of cetuximab added to the sixth amended plan FOLFOX.Ils randomized over 2500 patients to receive 12 cycles of FOLFOX every two weeks with or without cetuximab. The mutational status of the KRAS gene was decided at the central level. The median follow-up of 28 months. Three-year disease-free survival for FOLFOX alone was 74.6% against 71.5% with the addition of cetuximab (HR, 1.21, 95% CI, 0.98 to 1.49, P = 0 08) in patients with wild-type KRAS, and 67.1% against 65.0% (HR 1.12, 95% CI, 0.86 to 1.46, p = 0.38) in patients with mutated KRAS 48.The trial did not demonstrate any benefit when adding cetuximab to FOLFOX regimen. More patients with grade 3 or higher adverse events (72.5% versus 52.3%, odds ratio (OR) 2.4, 95% CI, 2.1 to 2.8, p <.001) and failure to carry Good 12 cycles (33% versus 23%, OR 1.6, 95% CI, 1.4 to 1.9, p <0, 001) were significantly higher with cetuximab.Increased toxicity was observed in patients aged 70 years or older. Therefore, the role of cetuximab in the adjuvant treatment is insignificant for the moment.

6. Chemotherapy in elderly

Colon cancer usually occurs in the elderly with a median age at diagnosis> 70 years in the USA. Given the increasing life expectancy, patients aged >75 years will be an important component of oncology practice in the future. Despite this fact, very few patients >75 years participate in clinical trials. There is disagreement in the administration of standard adjuvant therapy between young and elderly patients, despite a significant survival benefit for most patients [49]. The pooled analyzes of safety and efficacy of adjuvant chemotherapy in the elderly showed comparable rates of toxicity and similar survival benefits compared to younger patients [50].The majority of data for adjuvant therapy in elderly patients is not the incorporation of new therapeutic agents such as oxaliplatin. Subsequent population-based studies have suggested that older people (eg the elderly category <75 years versus> 75 years [51] were less likely to have received adjuvant therapy, but experienced similar survival rates compared younger patients [52]. Finally, although the majority of recommendations to reduce colorectal cancer screening for persons aged <75 years, the study results indicate that [53] patients aged >75 years account for almost 20% of cases of colon cancer lymph nodes.In this large population-based study, investigators found that age was associated with significantly lower rates of adjuvant chemotherapy administration, whereas the survival benefits of such treatment are comparable to those of younger patients with stage III in [53] colon cancer.Although chronological age alone should not be an exclusion criterion, more work is needed to establish an optimal strategy and effective way to understand who would benefit most from adjuvant therapy after surgical resection.

7. Efectivness

Patients with metastatic CRC being treated with chemotherapy are followed closely to monitor efficacy. There are standardized efficacy measures, such as the RECIST (response evaluation criteria in solid tumors) criteria, used as endpoints for large clinical trials. A partial response is defined as a 30% decrease in the longest dimension of each measurable tumor deposit, using unidimentional, or RECIST criteria [54-56]. A complete response is complete disappearance of all clinically detectable disease. The response rate (RR) is the percentage of patients who meet either a partial or complete response. Measures used to determine the duration of treatment benefit include:

1. progression-free survival (PFS), which is the time from the start of treatment to the date the disease, worsens;

2. disease-free survival (DFS), which is the length of time patients are free of disease after completion of curative treatment; and

3. overall survival (OS), which is the length of time patients are alive after diagnosis or initiation of treatment for metastatic disease.

8. Postoperative management

Postoperative, or "adjuvant" systemic therapy has become standard for stage III colon cancer. Adjuvant therapy should also be strongly considered in stage II patients. It is generally recommended for any medically fit patient with stage II cancer with unfavorable factors, including colonic perforation, poorly differentiated histology, colonic obstruction, lympho vascular invasion, or inadequately sampled lymph nodes [61]. The optimal choice of adjuvant chemotherapy has recently changed from a 6-month course of 5FU-based chemotherapy alone to a 6-month course of infusional 5FU plus LV and oxaliplatin (FOLFOX) based on a large trial of adjuvant systemic therapy for resected stage II or III colon cancer [62].This trial demonstrated an increase in disease-free survival at 3 years from 72.9 to 78.2% ($p = 0.002$) with addition of oxaliplatin to FU/LV. Five-year disease-free survival remained significant (HR: 0.80; $p = 0.003$) and at 6 years there was an overall survival benefit for stage III patients (68.3% versus 72.9%) [64].Toxicities were comparable between the two groups, with the exception that oxaliplatin is associated with a much higher rate of paresthesia: 12.4% versus 0.2% grade 3 (serious) toxicity. This neurotoxicity persisted at a grade 3 level in 1.1% of treated patients at one-year of follow-up.

Many advances have occurred recently in the treatment of metastatic CRC. Active agents, in addition to the original 5FU, that have been approved by the Food & Drug Administration (FDA) for mCRC include irinotecan, capecitabine, oxaliplatin, bevacizumab, cetuximab, and panitumumab. The goals of systemic therapy of mCRC include palliation of symptoms, prolongation of life, and in selected cases of liver-only metastases, tumor regression to facilitate surgical resection of these metastases. The median survival of a patient with mCRC has improved during the last decade from less than 1 year, with only 5FU-based therapy, to ~2 years, with multiagent systemic therapy.

5FU, often modified by LV, has been clinically used for half a century as a standard agent for mCRC [64]. This was the only available agent until 1996, when irinotecan was approved. Over the last decade, chemotherapies such as oxaliplatin and capecitabine and targeted agents such as bevacizumab, cetuximab, and panitumumab have been approved. 5FU blocks the enzyme thymidylate synthase (TS), which is essential for DNA synthesis. Leucovorin (LV), also known as folinic acid, enhances the antineoplastic effects of 5FU. Both LV (FOL = folinic acid) and 5FU (F = fluorouracil) can be combined with irinotecan (IRI) or oxaliplatin (OX) with the treatment acronyms FOLFIRI or FOLFOX, respectively. These alternative treatments consist of administration of a bolus of 5FU, LV, and either oxaliplatin or irinotecan. The patient is then sent home with a 2-day infusion of low-dose 5FU, administered by a small, lightweight, portable pump, usually worn on a belt or shoulder strap, infused through a centrally placed catheter. The patient or health care provider can simply disconnect the catheter after the 2-day infusion. Capecitabine is an oral fluoropyrimidine with a similar mechanism of action and similar efficacy as 5FU.

Irinotecan is a derivative of camptothecin, found in *Camptotheca acuminata,* a plant native to China. It potently inhibits topoisomerase I, an enzyme that facilitates the uncoiling and recoiling of DNA during replication by cleaving one strand and subsequently reattaching that strand. Oxaliplatin is a platinum chemotherapy that inhibits DNA replication and transcription by forming inter- and intrastrand DNA adducts/cross-links.

In patients with mCRC, optimal chemotherapy consists of initial administration of a fluoropyrimidine and oxaliplatin or irinotecan (e.g., FOLFOX or FOLFIRI). Tournigand et al [65] and Colucci et al [66] performed randomized trials where patients received either FOLFIRI followed by FOLFOX, or vice versa. In the Tournigand et al study, FOLIRI was found to have a response rate (RR) of 56% and a 8.5-month median progression free survival (mPFS), whereas FOLFOX had a RR of 54% and a mPFS of 8 months. Colucci et al found that FOLFIRI had a RR of 31% and FOLFOX had a RR of 34%. Both regimens had a mPFS of 7 months. Both investigators concluded that both regimens had similar efficacy when used as first-line therapy. Therefore, either FOLFOX or FOLFIRI can be considered standard options for first-line treatment of mCRC. These regimens are typically given with bevacizumab.

Bevacizumab is a monoclonal antibody that binds to vascular endothelial growth factor (VEGF) ligand to inhibit angiogenesis. Its antineoplastic effect is ascribed to regression of microvascular density, inhibition of neovascularization, and "normalization" of grossly abnormal tumor vasculature that permits more effective chemotherapy delivery to the tumor. The FDA recently approved bevacizumab in combination with 5FU-based chemotherapy for mCRC based on findings that addition of bevacizumab to irinotecan, 5FU, and LV for mCRC improved PFS from 6.2 months to 10.6 months, improved the response rate from 35 to 45 [67] and improved overall survival from 15.6 to 20.3 months. Saltz et al found that the addition of bevacizumab to oxaliplatin-based chemotherapy significantly improved PFS from 8.0 to 9.3 months without an improvement in response rate [68]. The finding of improved PFS without improved RR is common in trials of targeted therapy because the metastatic lesions can cavitate or has necrosis rather than regress. Recently, XELOX chemotherapy with or without bevacuzimab was found to be noninferior to FOLFOX with or without bevacuzimab [69]. XELOX chemotherapy includes a combination of oral 5FU known as capecitabine or xeloda (XEL) plus oxaliplatin (OX). XELOX can be used as an alternative in patients who cannot tolerate FOLFOX side effects.

In 2004, the FDA approved cetuximab, the chimeric (human/mouse) monoclonal antibody targeting epidermal growth factor receptor (EGFR), for treatment of mCRC with irinotecan, and as a single agent for patients intolerant of irinotecan-based therapy. Early randomized trials showed benefit of cetuximab in previously treated mCRC patients. When cetuximab was combined with irinotecan in patients refractory to irinotecan-based chemotherapy, the response rate was 22.9% versus 10.8% for irinotecan alone [70]. Among patients who failed previous lines of treatment, monotherapy with cetuximab was found to improve overall survival, PFS, and quality of life compared with best support care alone [71]. Cetuximab causes an acneform rash on the face and upper body in more than 80% of patients. The rash is associated with improved survival.

Although the FDA approved cetuximab for use in epidermal growth factor receptor (EGFR) expressing mCRC, there is no evidence that the presence or absence of EGFR expression influences RR, and routine testing for this is unnecessary. K-ras mutations have been shown to predict response to cetuximab. The K-ras gene encodes a GTPase protein that is involved in cell signal transduction pathways [72]. Wild-type (nonmutated) K-ras is found in normal cells. Approximately 40% of colorectal tumor cells have a mutated K-ras gene resulting in constitutively active protein and abnormal cell growth, proliferation, and differentiation. Evidence suggests there is no benefit in using cetuximab monotherapy in previously treated and untreated mCRC patients who have mutated K-ras tumors. Previously treated metastatic colorectal patients with mutated K-ras tumors did not benefit from cetuximab monotherapy, in contrast to patients with wild-type K-ras who had significantly improved overall survival and PFS [74]. FOLIFIRI and cetuximab as first-line therapy in mCRC was found to reduce the risk of disease progression; however, the benefit was limited to patients with K-ras wild-type tumors (HR 0.68, CI 0.50–0.94) [73].

In 2006, the FDA approved panitumumab, a monoclonal antibody to EGFR, which unlike cetuximab, is fully humanized (not chimeric). It is indicated for patients with mCRC who have progressed on or are following 5FU, oxaliplatin, and irinotecan-containing regimens. In a large randomized trial of panitumumab versus best supportive care for mCRC, a response rate of 10% was found [74]. Like cetuximab, panitumumab causes an acneform skin rash. As a fully human monoclonal antibody, panitumumab has a lower risk of serious infusion reactions than the 3% rate observed with cetuximab. Similar to cetuximab, panitumumab monotherapy is more efficacious in patients with wild- rather than mutant-type K-ras tumors. In a randomized clinical trial of previously treated mCRC patients, median PFS and OS was significantly improved in the wild-type K-ras group compared with the mutant group [75]. 17% of patients with wild-type K-ras responded to treatment versus 0% of patients with mutant K-ras. The relative activity of cetuximab versus panitumumab, as well as the relative activity of panitumumab when given with chemotherapy, is currently unknown.

9. Rectal cancer

Given the higher local recurrence rates and poorer overall survival of patients with rectal cancer, multimodality management is important. In the early 1990s, the standard of care following surgical resection for full thickness (T3–4) or lymph node positive rectal cancer was postoperative chemoradiotherapy as it was found to improve both local control and OS compared with surgery alone [77, 78]. Recently, preoperative chemoradiotherapy has become the treatment of choice for full thickness rectal cancers prior to total mesorectal excision based on a randomized clinical trial conducted by Sauer et al. Although this trial showed no difference in OS, improved local recurrence rates (6% versus 13%) were found for patients receiving preoperative 5FU-based chemoradiotherapy as compared with postoperative chemoradiotherapy [79]. Preoperative 5FU chemoradiotherapy as compared with preoperative radiation alone also has been shown to improve local recurrence rates (2.7% versus 14.6%) [80].

10. Liver metastases

The standard of care for patients with resectable liver metastases as their only site of cancer spread is changing from previous surgical resection alone to a combination of perioperative chemotherapy and surgery based on a trial conducted by Nordlinger et al [76]. This trial randomized patients with one to four potentially resectable liver metastases to either perioperative chemotherapy (six cycles of FOLFOX chemotherapy both pre- and postresection) or surgery alone. The authors concluded that perioperative chemotherapy reduced the risk of events such as progressive or recurrent disease and death by 25% in eligible and resected patients without increased severe, life-threatening toxicity. The results of this trial are controversial because when all randomized patients were included in the analysis only a trend and not significance in PFS favoring the chemotherapy arm was found.

11. Targeted therapy

Although new drug development takes years, targeted drug use can occur more quickly with advanced tests and will be a focus of future work. In addition, efforts will focus on identifying biomarkers that predict response to systemic therapy so that tailored therapy can be initiated.

With regards to the future of adjuvant systemic chemotherapy, microsatellite-instability (MSI) testing of tumor DNA may be used to identify which patients will benefit from additional therapy (i.e., predictive biomarker) [81, 82]. Approximately 15% of colon cancers exhibit MSI commonly caused by loss of DNA mismatch-repair pathways. Tumors display short repeated nucleotide sequences called microsatellites secondary to frame-shift mutations and base-pair substitutions. Recent retrospective evidence demonstrated that adjuvant 5FU-based chemotherapy improved OS among patients with microsatellite-stable tumors. However, there was no benefit to those patients with high MSI [83-90]. Ongoing trials are attempting to replicate these findings in a prospective manner. The clinical benefit of cetuximab, a monoclonal antibody against EGFR, varies greatly depending on tumor biology: the greatest benefit is among patients with wild-type (nonmutated) K-ras tumors. In the metastatic setting, potential predictive biomarkers of interest include K-ras, epiregulin, B-raf, PTEN, and Pi3K. Jonker et al found that mCRC patients with both high epiregulin (ligand for EGFR) gene expression and K-ras wild-type status had greater benefit from cetuximab therapy (HR for overall survival 0.43, p = 0.001) [94]. In addition, loss of the tumor-suppressor gene PTEN [95] and having mutated protein kinase B-raf may [96]predict for resistance to EGFR therapy such as cetuximab.

12. Discussion

Over the past decade, the prevention and treatment of colorectal cancer has rapidly evolved. To implement evidence-based care a multidisciplinary team is required including surgeons, radiation and medical oncologists, as well as gastroenterologists, radiologists, pathologists, and primary care physicians. Unfortunately, despite improvements in surgical techniques and systemic therapy CRC still remains the number two cause of cancer mortality in North America. This study evaluated the usefulness of oncology assess the standardization of CRC chemotherapy and the results at the rate of recurrence and survival. The methodology has enabled the understanding of patterns used for CRC chemotherapy around the world. The results showed significant differences in patterns between countries, regions and institutions. In addition, the actual use of CRC chemotherapy may depend on the health policies of the respective governments. Schemes used are in line with the recommendations of the new guidelines, with the exception of hospital characteristics depended specialization. In first-line chemotherapy for stage IV CRC, general hospitals still favored the use of oral fluoropyrimidines, such as UFT / LV and S-1. However, the differences between general hospitals, cancer centers and university hospitals has decreased after the revision of the guidelines. In adjuvant chemotherapy for stage III CRC, cancer centers and general hospitals used similar patterns, but those that are used in different hospitals. Measures and indicators are greatly needed to evaluate and improve the quality of cancer treatment. Using market research to develop indicators for the standardization of care against cancer is a new methodology. Data not only showed evidence practice gap, but also the growing standardization of CRC affected by chemotherapy treatment guidelines. Methodology indicates a lack of standardization in the care of CRC. Oncology market research also has the potential for cost-effectiveness analyzes, such as sales data for each agent can be evaluated using the analysis system of oncology. Efforts to improve screening utilization by the general population are required to improve mortality and morbidity from CRC. Research advances in medical oncology will result in better understanding of tumor genetics and biology of the host. This will allow systemic therapy to be tailored to specific tumor molecular targets, while sparing toxicity to normal tissue. With these improvements in CRC care, the disease will be treatable with tailored medical treatments that are effective with low toxicity.

13. Recommendations

13.1. Stage II colorectal cancer

- The routine use of adjuvant chemotherapy for all patients with stage II colon cancer is not recommended. However, the subset of patients with high-risk stage II disease who should be considered for adjuvant therapy includes patients with inadequately sampled nodes, T4 lesions, perforation, or poorly differentiated histology.
- The ultimate clinical decision should be based on discussions with the patient about the nature of the evidence supporting treatment, the anticipated morbidity of treatment, the presence of high-risk prognostic features on individual prognosis, and patient preferences.
- When treated with adjuvant therapy, high-risk stage II patients should receive similar regimens to those recommended for stage III patients. The enrolment of resected high-risk

stage II patients in clinical trials is encouraged. Additional trials comparing adjuvant therapy with observation are needed and are ethically acceptable in stage II colon cancer.

13.2. Stage III colorectal cancer

It could be recommended that patients with completely resected stage III colon cancer should be offered adjuvant chemotherapy and that this treatment should start within eight weeks of surgery. Treatment should depend on factors such as patient suitability and preference, and patients and clinicians must work together to determine the optimal course of treatment. The recommended treatment option is:

- 5-FU given intravenously in combination with leucovorin (LV) and oxaliplatin in the regimens known as FOLFOX or FLOX. These 5-FU/LV/oxaliplatin regimens have demonstrated superior DFS when compared with 5-FU plus LV and are the recommended regimens. Oxaliplatin administration is associated with a 1% risk of persistent grade 3 neuropathy that needs to be considered in conjunction with expected benefits of therapy.
- Some patients would not be considered appropriate for oxaliplatin regimens. Examples include patients with underlying neurologic conditions or at increased risk of neuropathy, patients at increased risk for infections, and patients likely to poorly tolerate infections as a result of chemotherapy. For these patients, the treatment options are:
- Oral capecitabine administered for six months, which has equivalent efficacy to intravenous 5-FU/LV. Capecitabine results in significantly less diarrhea, stomatitis, neutropenia, nausea/vomiting, and alopecia but significantly more hand-foot syndrome when compared with 5-FU/LV.
- 5-FU in combination with LV administered for six months using either the weekly or monthly schedule.

Suitable patients should be offered entry into clinical trials testing new adjuvant treatments for resected stage III colon cancer.

Author details

Krassimir Ivanov[1], Nikola Kolev[1], Ivan Shterev[2], Anton Tonev[1], Valentin Ignatov[1], Vasil Bojkov[4] and Tanya Kirilova[3]

1 Department of General and Operative Surgery, University Hospital "St. Marina", Varna, Bulgaria

2 Department of Medical Oncology, University Hospital "St. Marina", Varna, Bulgaria

3 Department of Gastroenterology, University Hospital "St. Marina", Varna, Bulgaria

4 Department of Surgery, University Hospital "St. Marina", Varna, Bulgaria

References

[1] Parkin DM, Bray F, Ferlay J, Pisani P. Global cancer statistics, 2002. *CA: a cancer journal for clinicians* 2005;55(2):74-108.

[2] Ries LA, Wingo PA, Miller DS, Howe HL, Weir HK, Rosenberg HM, et al. The annual report to the nation on the status of cancer, 1973-1997, with a special section on colorectal cancer. *Cancer* 2000;88(10):2398-424.

[3] Siegel R, Ward E, Brawley O, Jemal A. Cancer statistics, 2011: the impact of eliminating socioeconomic and racial disparities on premature cancer deaths. *CA: a cancer journal for clinicians* 2011;61(4):212-36.

[4] Meyerhardt JA, Mayer RJ. Systemic therapy for colorectal cancer. *The New England journal of medicine* 2005;352(5):476-87.

[5] Biagi JJ, Raphael MJ, Mackillop WJ, Kong W, King WD, Booth CM. Association between time to initiation of adjuvant chemotherapy and survival in colorectal cancer: a systematic review and meta-analysis. *JAMA : the journal of the American Medical Association* 2011;305(22):2335-42.

[6] Goldberg RM, Sargent DJ, Morton RF, Fuchs CS, Ramanathan RK, Williamson SK, et al. A randomized controlled trial of fluorouracil plus leucovorin, irinotecan, and oxaliplatin combinations in patients with previously untreated metastatic colorectal cancer. *Journal of clinical oncology : official journal of the American Society of Clinical Oncology* 2004;22(1):23-30.

[7] Andre T, Afchain P, Barrier A, Blanchard P, Larsen AK, Tournigand C, et al. Current status of adjuvant therapy for colon cancer. *Gastrointestinal cancer research : GCR* 2007;1(3):90-7.

[8] Benson AB, 3rd, Schrag D, Somerfield MR, Cohen AM, Figueredo AT, Flynn PJ, et al. American Society of Clinical Oncology recommendations on adjuvant chemotherapy for stage II colon cancer. *Journal of clinical oncology : official journal of the American Society of Clinical Oncology* 2004;22(16):3408-19.

[9] Chun P, Wainberg ZA. Adjuvant Chemotherapy for Stage II Colon Cancer: The Role of Molecular Markers in Choosing Therapy. *Gastrointestinal cancer research : GCR* 2009;3(5):191-6.

[10] Ribic CM, Sargent DJ, Moore MJ, Thibodeau SN, French AJ, Goldberg RM, et al. Tumor microsatellite-instability status as a predictor of benefit from fluorouracil-based adjuvant chemotherapy for colon cancer. *The New England journal of medicine* 2003;349(3):247-57.

[11] Lynch HT, de la Chapelle A. Hereditary colorectal cancer. *The New England journal of medicine* 2003;348(10):919-32.

[12] Halvarsson B, Anderson H, Domanska K, Lindmark G, Nilbert M. Clinicopathologic factors identify sporadic mismatch repair-defective colon cancers. *American journal of clinical pathology* 2008;129(2):238-44.

[13] Cunningham JM, Christensen ER, Tester DJ, Kim CY, Roche PC, Burgart LJ, et al. Hypermethylation of the hMLH1 promoter in colon cancer with microsatellite instability. *Cancer research* 1998;58(15):3455-60.

[14] Roth AD, Tejpar S, Delorenzi M, Yan P, Fiocca R, Klingbiel D, et al. Prognostic role of KRAS and BRAF in stage II and III resected colon cancer: results of the translational study on the PETACC-3, EORTC 40993, SAKK 60-00 trial. *Journal of clinical oncology : official journal of the American Society of Clinical Oncology* 2010;28(3):466-74.

[15] Moertel CG, Fleming TR, Macdonald JS, Haller DG, Laurie JA, Goodman PJ, et al. Levamisole and fluorouracil for adjuvant therapy of resected colon carcinoma. *The New England journal of medicine* 1990;322(6):352-8.

[16] Moertel CG, Fleming TR, Macdonald JS, Haller DG, Laurie JA, Tangen CM, et al. Fluorouracil plus levamisole as effective adjuvant therapy after resection of stage III colon carcinoma: a final report. *Annals of internal medicine* 1995;122(5):321-6.

[17] Ackland SP, Beale P, Peters GJ. Thymidylate synthase inhibitors. *Cancer chemotherapy and biological response modifiers* 2003;21:1-28.

[18] Jager E, Heike M, Bernhard H, Klein O, Bernhard G, Lautz D, et al. Weekly high-dose leucovorin versus low-dose leucovorin combined with fluorouracil in advanced colorectal cancer: results of a randomized multicenter trial. Study Group for Palliative Treatment of Metastatic Colorectal Cancer Study Protocol 1. *Journal of clinical oncology : official journal of the American Society of Clinical Oncology* 1996;14(8):2274-9.

[19] Andre T, Colin P, Louvet C, Gamelin E, Bouche O, Achille E, et al. Semimonthly versus monthly regimen of fluorouracil and leucovorin administered for 24 or 36 weeks as adjuvant therapy in stage II and III colon cancer: results of a randomized trial. *Journal of clinical oncology : official journal of the American Society of Clinical Oncology* 2003;21(15):2896-903.

[20] Saini A, Norman AR, Cunningham D, Chau I, Hill M, Tait D, et al. Twelve weeks of protracted venous infusion of fluorouracil (5-FU) is as effective as 6 months of bolus 5-FU and folinic acid as adjuvant treatment in colorectal cancer. *British journal of cancer* 2003;88(12):1859-65.

[21] Efficacy of adjuvant fluorouracil and folinic acid in B2 colon cancer. International Multicentre Pooled Analysis of B2 Colon Cancer Trials (IMPACT B2) Investigators. *Journal of clinical oncology : official journal of the American Society of Clinical Oncology* 1999;17(5):1356-63.

[22] Efficacy of adjuvant fluorouracil and folinic acid in colon cancer. International Multicentre Pooled Analysis of Colon Cancer Trials (IMPACT) investigators. *Lancet* 1995;345(8955):939-44.

[23] Tournigand C, Andre T, Bonnetain F, Chibaudel B, Lledo G, Hickish T, et al. Adjuvant therapy with fluorouracil and oxaliplatin in stage II and elderly patients (between ages 70 and 75 years) with colon cancer: subgroup analyses of the Multicenter International Study of Oxaliplatin, Fluorouracil, and Leucovorin in the Adjuvant Treatment of Colon Cancer trial. *Journal of clinical oncology : official journal of the American Society of Clinical Oncology* 2012;30(27):3353-60.

[24] Yothers G, O'Connell MJ, Allegra CJ, Kuebler JP, Colangelo LH, Petrelli NJ, et al. Oxaliplatin as adjuvant therapy for colon cancer: updated results of NSABP C-07 trial, including survival and subset analyses. *Journal of clinical oncology : official journal of the American Society of Clinical Oncology* 2011;29(28):3768-74.

[25] Hoff PM, Ansari R, Batist G, Cox J, Kocha W, Kuperminc M, et al. Comparison of oral capecitabine versus intravenous fluorouracil plus leucovorin as first-line treatment in 605 patients with metastatic colorectal cancer: results of a randomized phase III study. *Journal of clinical oncology : official journal of the American Society of Clinical Oncology* 2001;19(8):2282-92.

[26] Douillard JY, Hoff PM, Skillings JR, Eisenberg P, Davidson N, Harper P, et al. Multicenter phase III study of uracil/tegafur and oral leucovorin versus fluorouracil and leucovorin in patients with previously untreated metastatic colorectal cancer. *Journal of clinical oncology : official journal of the American Society of Clinical Oncology* 2002;20(17):3605-16.

[27] Van Cutsem E, Twelves C, Cassidy J, Allman D, Bajetta E, Boyer M, et al. Oral capecitabine compared with intravenous fluorouracil plus leucovorin in patients with metastatic colorectal cancer: results of a large phase III study. *Journal of clinical oncology : official journal of the American Society of Clinical Oncology* 2001;19(21):4097-106.

[28] Pasetto LM, Monfardini S. The role of capecitabine in the treatment of colorectal cancer in the elderly. *Anticancer research* 2006;26(3B):2381-6.

[29] Reigner B, Blesch K, Weidekamm E. Clinical pharmacokinetics of capecitabine. *Clinical pharmacokinetics* 2001;40(2):85-104.

[30] Twelves C, Scheithauer W, McKendrick J, Seitz JF, Van Hazel G, Wong A, et al. Capecitabine versus 5-fluorouracil/folinic acid as adjuvant therapy for stage III colon cancer: final results from the X-ACT trial with analysis by age and preliminary evidence of a pharmacodynamic marker of efficacy. *Annals of oncology : official journal of the European Society for Medical Oncology / ESMO* 2012;23(5):1190-7.

[31] Poplin EA, Benedetti JK, Estes NC, Haller DG, Mayer RJ, Goldberg RM, et al. Phase III Southwest Oncology Group 9415/Intergroup 0153 randomized trial of fluorouracil, leucovorin, and levamisole versus fluorouracil continuous infusion and levami-

sole for adjuvant treatment of stage III and high-risk stage II colon cancer. *Journal of clinical oncology : official journal of the American Society of Clinical Oncology* 2005;23(9): 1819-25.

[32] Lembersky BC, Wieand HS, Petrelli NJ, O'Connell MJ, Colangelo LH, Smith RE, et al. Oral uracil and tegafur plus leucovorin compared with intravenous fluorouracil and leucovorin in stage II and III carcinoma of the colon: results from National Surgical Adjuvant Breast and Bowel Project Protocol C-06. *Journal of clinical oncology : official journal of the American Society of Clinical Oncology* 2006;24(13):2059-64.

[33] Raymond E, Chaney SG, Taamma A, Cvitkovic E. Oxaliplatin: a review of preclinical and clinical studies. *Annals of oncology : official journal of the European Society for Medical Oncology / ESMO* 1998;9(10):1053-71.

[34] Culy CR, Clemett D, Wiseman LR. Oxaliplatin. A review of its pharmacological properties and clinical efficacy in metastatic colorectal cancer and its potential in other malignancies. *Drugs* 2000;60(4):895-924.

[35] Alcindor T, Beauger N. Oxaliplatin: a review in the era of molecularly targeted therapy. *Curr Oncol* 2011;18(1):18-25.

[36] Brouwers EE, Huitema AD, Beijnen JH, Schellens JH. Long-term platinum retention after treatment with cisplatin and oxaliplatin. *BMC clinical pharmacology* 2008;8:7.

[37] Andre T, Boni C, Navarro M, Tabernero J, Hickish T, Topham C, et al. Improved overall survival with oxaliplatin, fluorouracil, and leucovorin as adjuvant treatment in stage II or III colon cancer in the MOSAIC trial. *Journal of clinical oncology : official journal of the American Society of Clinical Oncology* 2009;27(19):3109-16.

[38] Adjuvant chemotherapy with oxaliplatin, in combination with fluorouracil plus leucovorin prolongs disease-free survival, but causes more adverse events in people with stage II or III colon cancer Abstracted from: Andre T, Boni C, Mounedji-Boudiaf L, et al. Multicenter international study of oxaliplatin/5-fluorouracil/leucovorin in the adjuvant treatment of colon cancer (MOSAIC) investigators. Oxaliplatin, fluorouracil, and leucovorin as adjuvant treatment for colon cancer. N Engl J Med 2004;350:2343-51. *Cancer treatment reviews* 2004;30(8):711-3.

[39] Kuebler JP, Wieand HS, O'Connell MJ, Smith RE, Colangelo LH, Yothers G, et al. Oxaliplatin combined with weekly bolus fluorouracil and leucovorin as surgical adjuvant chemotherapy for stage II and III colon cancer: results from NSABP C-07. *Journal of clinical oncology : official journal of the American Society of Clinical Oncology* 2007;25(16):2198-204.

[40] Schmoll HJ, Cartwright T, Tabernero J, Nowacki MP, Figer A, Maroun J, et al. Phase III trial of capecitabine plus oxaliplatin as adjuvant therapy for stage III colon cancer: a planned safety analysis in 1, 864 patients. *Journal of clinical oncology : official journal of the American Society of Clinical Oncology* 2007;25(1):102-9.

[41] Haller DG, Tabernero J, Maroun J, de Braud F, Price T, Van Cutsem E, et al. Capecitabine plus oxaliplatin compared with fluorouracil and folinic acid as adjuvant therapy for stage III colon cancer. *Journal of clinical oncology : official journal of the American Society of Clinical Oncology* 2011;29(11):1465-71.

[42] Xu Y, Villalona-Calero MA. Irinotecan: mechanisms of tumor resistance and novel strategies for modulating its activity. *Annals of oncology : official journal of the European Society for Medical Oncology / ESMO* 2002;13(12):1841-51.

[43] Saltz LB, Niedzwiecki D, Hollis D, Goldberg RM, Hantel A, Thomas JP, et al. Irinotecan fluorouracil plus leucovorin is not superior to fluorouracil plus leucovorin alone as adjuvant treatment for stage III colon cancer: results of CALGB 89803. *Journal of clinical oncology : official journal of the American Society of Clinical Oncology* 2007;25(23): 3456-61.

[44] Van Cutsem E, Labianca R, Bodoky G, Barone C, Aranda E, Nordlinger B, et al. Randomized phase III trial comparing biweekly infusional fluorouracil/leucovorin alone or with irinotecan in the adjuvant treatment of stage III colon cancer: PETACC-3. *Journal of clinical oncology : official journal of the American Society of Clinical Oncology* 2009;27(19):3117-25.

[45] McCormack PL, Keam SJ. Bevacizumab: a review of its use in metastatic colorectal cancer. *Drugs* 2008;68(4):487-506.

[46] Allegra CJ, Yothers G, O'Connell MJ, Sharif S, Petrelli NJ, Colangelo LH, et al. Phase III trial assessing bevacizumab in stages II and III carcinoma of the colon: results of NSABP protocol C-08. *Journal of clinical oncology : official journal of the American Society of Clinical Oncology* 2011;29(1):11-6.

[47] Merlano M, Occelli M. Review of cetuximab in the treatment of squamous cell carcinoma of the head and neck. *Therapeutics and clinical risk management* 2007;3(5):871-6.

[48] Alberts SR, Sargent DJ, Nair S, Mahoney MR, Mooney M, Thibodeau SN, et al. Effect of oxaliplatin, fluorouracil, and leucovorin with or without cetuximab on survival among patients with resected stage III colon cancer: a randomized trial. *JAMA : the journal of the American Medical Association* 2012;307(13):1383-93.

[49] Ades S. Adjuvant chemotherapy for colon cancer in the elderly: moving from evidence to practice. *Oncology (Williston Park)* 2009;23(2):162-7.

[50] Gill S, Loprinzi CL, Sargent DJ, Thome SD, Alberts SR, Haller DG, et al. Pooled analysis of fluorouracil-based adjuvant therapy for stage II and III colon cancer: who benefits and by how much? *Journal of clinical oncology : official journal of the American Society of Clinical Oncology* 2004;22(10):1797-806.

[51] Kahn KL, Adams JL, Weeks JC, Chrischilles EA, Schrag D, Ayanian JZ, et al. Adjuvant chemotherapy use and adverse events among older patients with stage III colon cancer. *JAMA : the journal of the American Medical Association* 2010;303(11):1037-45.

[52] Dobie SA, Baldwin LM, Dominitz JA, Matthews B, Billingsley K, Barlow W. Completion of therapy by Medicare patients with stage III colon cancer. *Journal of the National Cancer Institute* 2006;98(9):610-9.

[53] Abraham A, Habermann EB, Rothenberger DA, Kwaan M, Weinberg AD, Parsons HM, et al. Adjuvant chemotherapy for stage III colon cancer in the oldest old: Results beyond clinical guidelines. *Cancer* 2012.

[54] Jemal A, Siegel R, Ward E, et al. Cancer statistics, 2008. CA Cancer J Clin. 2008;58(2): 71–96.

[55] Canadian Cancer Society/National Cancer Institute of Canada. Canadian Cancer Statistics. Toronto, Canada: 2008.

[56] Therasse P, Arbuck S G, Eisenhauer E A, et al. New guidelines to evaluate the response to treatment in solid tumors. European Organization for Research and Treatment of Cancer, National Cancer Institute of the United States, National Cancer Institute of Canada. J Natl Cancer Inst. 2000;92(3):205–216.

[57] Wolmark N, Fisher B, Rockette H, et al. Postoperative adjuvant chemotherapy or BCG for colon cancer: results from NSABP protocol C-01. J Natl Cancer Inst. 1988;80(1):30–36.

[58] Wolmark N, Rockette H, Fisher B, et al. The benefit of leucovorin-modulated fluorouracil as postoperative adjuvant therapy for primary colon cancer: results from National Surgical Adjuvant Breast and Bowel Project protocol C-03. J Clin Oncol. 1993;11(10):1879–1887.

[59] Scheithauer W, Rosen H, Kornek G V, Sebesta C, Depisch D. Randomised comparison of combination chemotherapy plus supportive care with supportive care alone in patients with metastatic colorectal cancer.BMJ. 1993;306(6880):752–755.

[60] Jonker D S, Maroun K J. Adjuvant Systemic Chemotherapy for Stage II and III Colon Cancer Following Complete Resection: Guideline Recommendations. Toronto: Cancer Care Ontario Evidence-Based Series#2–29; Cancer Care Ontario; 2008.

[61] André T, Boni C, Mounedji-Boudiaf L, et al. Multicenter International Study of Oxaliplatin/5-Fluorouracil/Leucovorin in the Adjuvant Treatment of Colon Cancer (MOSAIC) Investigators Oxaliplatin, fluorouracil, and leucovorin as adjuvant treatment for colon cancer. N Engl J Med. 2004;350(23):2343–2351.

[62] De Gramont A, Boni C, Navarro M, et al. Oxaliplatin/5-FU/LV in adjuvant colon cancer: Updated efficacy results of the MOSAIC trial, including survival, with a median follow-up of six years. Journal of Clinical Oncology, 2007 ASCO Annual Meeting Proceedings Part 1. 2007;25(18S) Abstract 4007.

[63] Krueger G M, Alexander L L, Whippen D A, Balch C M. Arnoldus Goudsmit, MD, PhD: chemotherapist, visionary, founder of the American Society of Clinical Oncology, 1909-2005. J Clin Oncol.2006;24(24):4033–4036.

[64] Tournigand C, André T, Achille E, et al. FOLFIRI followed by FOLFOX6 or the reverse sequence in advanced colorectal cancer: a randomized GERCOR study. J Clin Oncol. 2004;22(2):229–237.

[65] Colucci G, Gebbia V, Paoletti G, et al. Gruppo Oncologico Dell'Italia Meridionale Phase III randomized trial of FOLFIRI versus FOLFOX4 in the treatment of advanced colorectal cancer: a multicenter study of the Gruppo Oncologico Dell'Italia Meridionale. J Clin Oncol. 2005;23(22):4866–4875.

[66] Hurwitz H, Fehrenbacher L, Novotny W, et al. Bevacizumab plus irinotecan, fluorouracil, and leucovorin for metastatic colorectal cancer. N Engl J Med. 2004;350(23): 2335–2342.

[67] Saltz L, Clarke S, Diaz-Rubio E, et al. Bevacizumab (Bev) in combination with XELOX or FOLFOX4: efficacy results from XELOX-1/NO16966, a randomized phase III trial in the first-line treatment of metastatic colorectal cancer (MCRC). Orlando, FL: Paper presented at: Gastrointestinal Cancers Symposium, American Society of Clinical Oncologists; July 19–21, 2007. Abstract 238.

[68] Cassidy J, Clarke S, Díaz-Rubio E, et al. Randomized phase III study of capecitabine plus oxaliplatin compared with fluorouracil/folinic acid plus oxaliplatin as first-line therapy for metastatic colorectal cancer.J Clin Oncol. 2008;26(12):2006–2012.

[69] Cunningham D, Humblet Y, Siena S, et al. Cetuximab monotherapy and cetuximab plus irinotecan in irinotecan-refractory metastatic colorectal cancer. N Engl J Med. 2004;351(4):337–345.

[70] Jonker D J, O'Callaghan C J, Karapetis C S, et al. Cetuximab for the treatment of colorectal cancer. N Engl J Med. 2007;357(20):2040–2048.

[71] Cutsem E Van, Köhne C H, Hitre E, et al. Cetuximab and chemotherapy as initial treatment for metastatic colorectal cancer. N Engl J Med. 2009;360(14):1408–1417

[72] Karapetis C S, Khambata-Ford S, Jonker D J, et al. K-ras mutations and benefit from cetuximab in advanced colorectal cancer. N Engl J Med. 2008;359(17):1757–1765.

[73] Cutsem E Van, Peeters M, Siena S, et al. Open-label phase III trial of panitumumab plus best supportive care compared with best supportive care alone in patients with chemotherapy-refractory metastatic colorectal cancer. J Clin Oncol. 2007;25:1658–1664.

[74] Amado R G, Wolf M, Peeters M, et al. Wild-type KRAS is required for panitumumab efficacy in patients with metastatic colorectal cancer. J Clin Oncol. 2008;26(10):1626–1634.

[75] Nordlinger B, Sorbye H, Glimelius B, et al. EORTC Gastro-Intestinal Tract Cancer Group. Cancer Research UK. Arbeitsgruppe Lebermetastasen und-tumoren in der Chirurgischen Arbeitsgemeinschaft Onkologie (ALM-CAO) Australasian Gastro-Intestinal Trials Group (AGITG) Fédération Francophone de Cancérologie Digestive

(FFCD) Perioperative chemotherapy with FOLFOX4 and surgery versus surgery alone for resectable liver metastases from colorectal cancer (EORTC Intergroup trial 40983): a randomised controlled trial. Lancet. 2008;371(9617):1007–1016.

[76] Gastro-intestinal Tumor Study Group. Prolongation of the disease-free interval in surgically treated rectal carcinoma. N Engl J Med. 1985;312:1465–1472.

[77] Krook J E, Moertel C G, Gunderson L L, et al. Effective surgical adjuvant therapy for high-risk rectal carcinoma. N Engl J Med. 1991;324(11):709–715.

[78] Sauer R, Becker H, Hohenberger W, et al. German Rectal Cancer Study Group Preoperative versus postoperative chemoradiotherapy for rectal cancer. N Engl J Med. 2004;351(17):1731–1740.

[79] Gérard J P, Conroy T, Bonnetain F, et al. Preoperative radiotherapy with or without concurrent fluorouracil and leucovorin in T3-4 rectal cancers: results of FFCD 9203. J Clin Oncol. 2006;24(28):4620–4625.

[80] Gryfe R, Kim H, Hsieh E T, et al. Tumor microsatellite instability and clinical outcome in young patients with colorectal cancer. N Engl J Med. 2000;342(2):69–77.

[81] Hemminki A, Mecklin J P, Järvinen H, Aaltonen L A, Joensuu H. Microsatellite instability is a favorable prognostic indicator in patients with colorectal cancer receiving chemotherapy. Gastroenterology.2000;119(4):921–928.

[82] Ribic C M, Sargent D J, Moore M J, et al. Tumor microsatellite-instability status as a predictor of benefit from fluorouracil-based adjuvant chemotherapy for colon cancer. N Engl J Med. 2003;349(3):247–257.

[83] Jonker D J, Karpetis C, Harbison C, et al. High epiregulin (EREG) gene expression plus K-ras wild-type (WT) status as predictors of cetuximab benefit in the treatment of advanced colorectal cancer (ACRC): results from NCIC CTG CO.17- A phase III trial of cetuximab versus best supportive care (BSC) J Clin Oncol. 2009;27(15S) Abstract 4016.

[84] Loupakis F, Pollina L, Stasi I, et al. PTEN expression and KRAS mutations on primary tumors and metastases in the prediction of benefit from cetuximab plus irinotecan for patients with metastatic colorectal cancer. J Clin Oncol. 2009;27(16):2622–2629.

[85] Di Nicolantonio F, Martini M, Molinari F, et al. Wild-type BRAF is required for response to panitumumab or cetuximab in metastatic colorectal cancer. J Clin Oncol. 2008;26(35):5705–5712.

Section 5

Genomics

Chapter 14

Possible Role of Proto-Oncogenes in Colorectal Cancer — A Population Based Study

Syed Mudassar, Mosin S Khan, Nighat P. Khan, Mahboob ul- Hussain and Khurshid I. Andrabi

Additional information is available at the end of the chapter

http://dx.doi.org/10.5772/57380

1. Introduction

Cancer is not just one disease, but a generic term used to encompass a group of more than two hundred diseases sharing common characteristics. From a clinical point of view, cancer is a large group of diseases, that vary in their age of onset, rate of growth, state of cellular differentiation, diagnostic detectability, invasiveness, metastatic potential, response to treatment, and prognosis. From a molecular and cell biological point of view, however, cancer may be a relatively small number of diseases caused by similar molecular defects in cell function resulting from common types of alterations to a cell's genes. Ultimately, cancer is a disease of abnormal gene expression. There are a number of mechanisms by which this altered gene expression occurs. These mechanisms may occur via a direct insult to DNA, such as a gene mutation, translocation, amplification, deletion, loss of heterozygosity, or via a mechanism resulting from abnormal gene transcription or translation. The overall result is an imbalance of cell replication and cell death in a tumor cell population that leads to an expansion of tumor tissue. Cancers (carcinomas) are characterized by their unregulated growth and spread of cells to other parts of the body [1,2]. Treatment of an individual diagnosed with cancer is not only dependent upon which type of malignancy (cancer) they have, but also on the extent of its spread, together with its sensitivity to treatment [3].The total care of the patient will involve assessment of their physical, psychological and social needs, so that a complete care package can be developed to support them and their carer(s) throughout the whole of their patient.

1.1. Colorectal cancer

Colorectal cancer (CRC), less formally known as bowel cancer, is a cancer characterized by neoplasia in the colon, rectum, or vermiform appendix. CRC is a leading cause of cancer mortality in the Western World. In the United States, CRC is the third most commonly diagnosed cancer in men and women and the second leading cause of cancer-related mortality [4]. Because 5% of persons (1 in 20 persons) will develop colorectal cancer, this disease is an important public health issue.

1.2. Incidence of colorectal cancer

Globally, cancer of the colon and rectum is the third mostcommon cancer in males and in females with mortality paralleling incidence [5]. An estimated 141,210 cases (71,850 male and 69360 female) of CRC were expected to occur in 2011.An estimated 49, 380 deaths (25,250 male and 24,130 female)of CRC were expected to occur in 2011, accounting for about 9% of all cancer deaths (Table 1). The5-year survival is 90% when CRC is diagnosed at an early stage however, less than 40% cases are diagnosed when the cancer is still localized [6]. The frequency of CRC varies remarkably among different populations. The incidence of colorectal cancer is increasing in certain countries where risk was historically low (Japan, Puerto Rico). In high-risk countries, trends are gradually increasing (England), stabilizing (New Zealand), or declining (United States) with time. The greatest increases in the incidence of colorectal cancer are in Asia (Japan, Hong Kong, Singapore), Eastern Europe (Hungary, Poland), Israel, and Puerto Rico. In contrast to the recent decrease in rates seen in some western and northern European countries, relatively large increases have been observed in Spain. The decrease in incidence in the United States partially reflects the increase in detection and removal of precancerous lesions; the increase in several Asian and Eastern European countries may reflect changes in the prevalence of obesity and dietary patterns. Age standardized incidence of colorectal cancer around the world is depicted in graph 1.

In India, CRC does not figure amongst the 10 most common malignancies. The age-standardized rates of CRC in India have been estimated to be 4.2 and 3.2/100,000 for males and females, respectively.

Inter-regional differences in the incidence of CRC, including difference among population groups living in geographic proximity but with different life styles, suggest that environment plays a role in the development of the disease [7]. Change in the location of these tumours is seen with increasing age. The proportion of tumours beyond the reach of sigmoidoscopy increases with age [8]. Sub site distribution also may differ according to ethnicity [9]

1.3. Risk factors

Epidemiologic studies have revealed a number of risk factors for colorectal cancer including age, family history of colon cancer or inflammatory bowel disease, smoking, alcohol consumption, obesity, and diet.

http://dx.doi.org/10.5772/57380

Estimated New cases		Estimated Deaths	
Male	Female	Male	Female
Prostate 240,890 (29%)	Breast 230,480 (30%)	Lung & bronchus 85,600 (28%)	Lung & bronchus 71,340 (26%)
Lung & bronchus 115,060 (14%)	Lung & bronchus 106,070 (14%)	Prostate 33,720 (11%)	Breast 39,520 (15%)
Colon & rectum 71,850 (9%)	Colon & rectum 69,360 (9%)	Colon & rectum 25,250 (8%)	Colon & rectum 24,130 (9%)
Urinary bladder 52,020 (6%)	Uterine corpus 46,470 (6%)	Pancreas 19,360 (6%)	Pancreas 18,300 (7%)
Melanoma of the skin 40,010 (5%)	Thyroid 36,550 (5%)	Liver & intrahepatic bile duct 13,260 (4%)	Ovary 15,460 (6%)
Kidney & renal pelvis 37,120 (5%)	Non-Hodgkin lymphoma 30,300 (4%)	Leukemia 12,740 (4%)	Non-Hodgkin lymphoma 9,570 (4%)
Non-Hodgkin lymphoma 36,060 (4%)	Melanoma of the skin 30,220 (4%)	Esophagus 11,910 (4%)	Leukemia 9,040 (3%)
Oral cavity & pharynx 27,710 (3%)	Kidney & renal pelvis 23,800 (3%)	Urinary bladder 10,670 (4%)	Uterine corpus 8,120 (3%)
Leukemia 25,320 (3%)	Ovary 21,990 (3%)	Non-Hodgkin lymphoma 9,750 (3%)	Liver & intrahepatic bile duct 6,330 (2%)
Pancreas 22,050 (3%)	Pancreas 21,980 (3%)	Kidney & renal pelvis 8,270 (3%)	Brain & other nervous system 5,670 (2%)
All sites 822,300 (100%)	All sites 774,370 (100%)	All sites 300,430 (100%)	All sites 271,520 (100%)

Table 1. Leading Sites of New Cancer Cases and Deaths (2011, American Cancer Society, Inc., Surveillance) 2011.

Age

Colorectal cancer is most commonly found in those aged 50 years and over.

Sex

Men are more likely than women to develop colorectal cancer. The incidence rate of colorectal cancer between 2000 and 2004 was 69.2 per 100,000 population among men and 45.8per 100,000 populations among women [10]

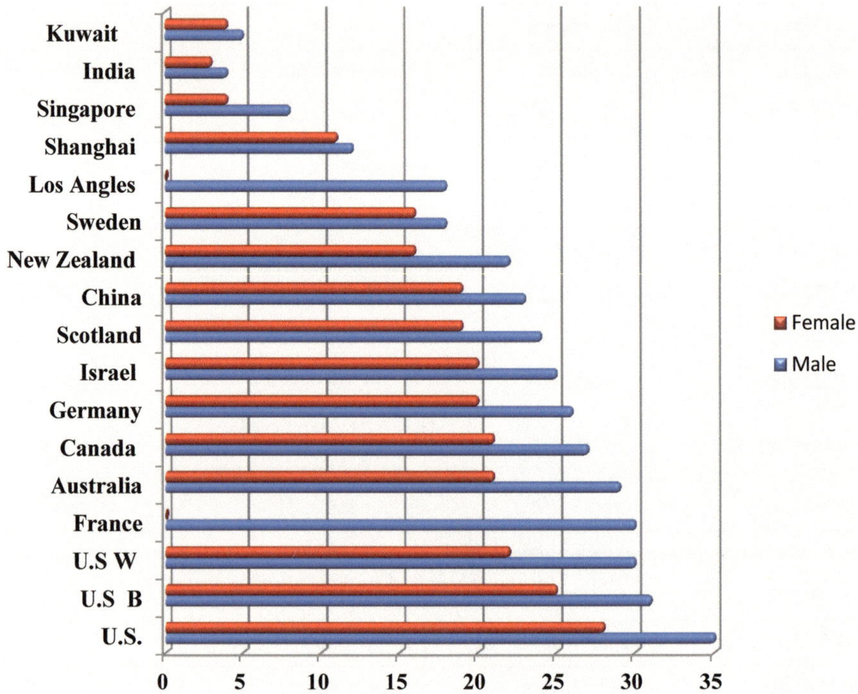

Graph 1 Family History

Graph 1: Age standardized incidence of colorectal cancer/100,000populations around the world (Arshad et al., 2011)

According to the CDC (Centre for Disease Control and Prevention), those who have a family history of colorectal cancer are at higher risk for developing colorectal cancer themselves. In addition to particular genetic pathways that are activated in the development of colon cancer, there are also known genetic mutations that can be inherited and make up approximately10% of all colorectal cancer cases [11]

Smoking

Tobacco use does not only put persons at risk for higher rates of lung, mouth, and esophageal cancers, it has also been associated with higher risk for developing colon cancer [11,12]

Diet

There have been a number of different dietary factors that have been linked to a higher risk of colorectal cancer including higher levels of red meat consumption, low levels of fruit and vegetable consumption, and diets that are low in fiber.

Obesity

Obesity is an important risk factor to consider based on the recent trends in the U.S. A number of studies have shown that being overweight is associated with increased risk of colorectal cancer. A case-control study conducted by Caan *et al* [13] found that men who had a BMI in the highest quintile were almost 2 times as likely to develop colon cancer as men with a BMI in the lowest quintile.

1.4. Classification and grade of CRC

Staging describes the extent or spread of the disease at the time of diagnosis. It is essential in determining the choice of therapy and in assessing prognosis. Stage is based on the primary tumour's size and location and whether it has spread to other areas of the body. A number of different staging systems are used to classify tumours. For CRC patients' pathologic stage represents one of the most important prognostic factors. The Dukes' system was the classic staging method for CRC, however the tumour, node, metastasis (TNM) staging system is more detailed and is most commonly used today. On occasion, Roman numerals I through IV are used in CRC staging (Table 2). These numerals correspond with Dukes' classes.TNM staging system is useful for descriptive and statistical analysis of tumour registry data. If cancer cells are present only in the layer of cells where they originated and have not penetrated the basement membrane of the tissue, the stage is in situ; otherwise it is invasive. Stage is categorized as local if cancer cells are confined to the organ of origin, regional if the cells have spread beyond their original (primary) site to nearby lymph nodes or tissues, and distant if they have spread from the primary site to distant organs or distant lymph nodes.

AJCC stage	TNM stage	TNM stage criteria for colorectal cancer
Stage 0	Tis N0 M0	Tis: Tumour confined to mucosa; cancer-in-situ
Stage I	T1 N0 M0	T1: Tumour invades submucosa
Stage I	T2 N0 M0	T2: Tumour invades muscularispropria
Stage II-A	T3 N0 M0	T3: Tumour invades subserosa or beyond (without other organs involved)
Stage II-B	T4 N0 M0	T4: Tumour invades adjacent organs or perforates the visceral peritoneum
Stage III-A	T1-2 N1 M0	N1: Metastasis to 1 to 3 regional lymph nodes. T1 or T2.
Stage III-B	T3-4 N1 M0	N1: Metastasis to 1 to 3 regional lymph nodes. T3 or T4.
Stage III-C	any T, N2 M0	N2: Metastasis to 4 or more regional lymph nodes. Any T.
Stage IV	any T, any N, M1	M1: Distant metastases present. Any T, any N.

Table 2. TNM staging for colorectal cancer

1.5. Genetics of CRC

Fifteen years ago, Fearon and Vogelstein [14] proposed a genetic model to explain the stepwise formation of CRC from normal colonic tissues. This model states that 1) CRC is the result of changes (mutations) of genes with important functions in regulating cell proliferation or repair of DNA damages, 2) mutations in more than one gene are required, and 3) the sequence of mutations is important in determining the eventual formation of CRC. The model is illustrated in (Figure 1), which also incorporated information from more recent studies.

The genes involved in the genetic paradigm leading to CRC can be broadly divided into two classes: tumour suppressor genes (TSGs) and oncogenes. TSGs encode proteins that either inhibit cell proliferation or promote apoptosis.

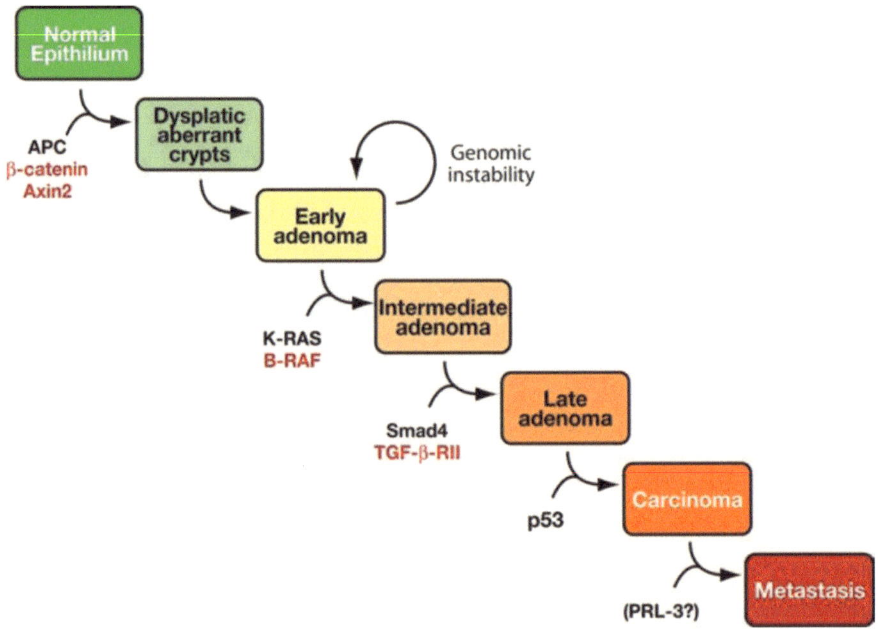

Figure 1. Correlation between CRC Progression and the accumulation of genetic alterations according to Fearon & Vogelstein (1990). The genetic alterations frequently found in CIN tumours are depicted in black; genetic alterations more common in MIN tumours are depicted in red.

TSGs are often inactivated in CRC. In contrast, oncogenes are activated versions of proto-oncogenes, which are often involved promoting cell proliferation or development. Once activated, oncogenes can lead to accelerated cell growth and contribute to tumour formation [15]. It is widely accepted that the molecular genetics of human cancers can be used to categorize colorectal carcinomas into two major types of genomic instabilities, chromosomal instability (CIN) and microsatellite instability (MSI) [16].The majority of colorectal carcinomas are categorized into the CIN pathway, which is characterized by a high frequency of allelic losses, deletions, and/or mutations of tumour suppressor genes such as APC and p53, and abnormal tumour DNA (Figure 2) [16]. Aneuploidy in CIN phenotype tumours had been demonstrated in colorectal cancer cell lines and tumour tissues. Although CIN is a common finding in colorectal carcinomas, the mechanism of CIN has not been clearly elucidated. Defects in DNA replication check point genes and many other genes increase the rate of genome rearrangement and it is suggested to be associated with CIN [17].

The other pathway, namely the MSI pathway, begins with the inactivation of one of a group of genes responsible for DNA nucleotide mismatch repair, which leads to extensive mutations in both repetitive and non-repetitive DNA sequences with low frequencies of allelic losses and rare alterations of tumour DNA content [18]. The mechanism of tumorigenesis in high-microsatellite instability (MSI-H) tumours is thought to involve frame shift mutations of microsatellite repeats within coding regions of the affected target genes, and the inactivation of these target genes is believed to directly contribute to tumour development and progression. Although these two distinct major genetic pathways of genetic instabilities are widely accepted, some tumours reveal different genetic pathways i.e., some tumours show both types of genomic instabilities and some tumours do not show any of these two instabilities. Further evidence for alternative pathways come from studies which show that mutations in *APC, KRAS* as well as *p53* do not occur in all tumours and some tumours may only contain a mutation in one of these genes. Another novel pathway has been described termed the CpG island methylator phenotype (CIMP) [17]. Two groups of tumours were identified. CIMP-positive tumours show a high degree of CpG island methylation in genes such as *p16* and *hMLH1* and are accompanied by mutations in *KRAS* and *TGF RII.* CIMP-negative tumours, which by definition do not contain a high degree of methylation, are characterized by *p53* mutations. CIMP-positive tumours may show a degree of correlation with the MSI pathway. Finally, colorectal cancers, arising from ulcerative colitis, do not develop from adenomas suggesting that they follow yet another different pathway 9 (Figure 2) [19]

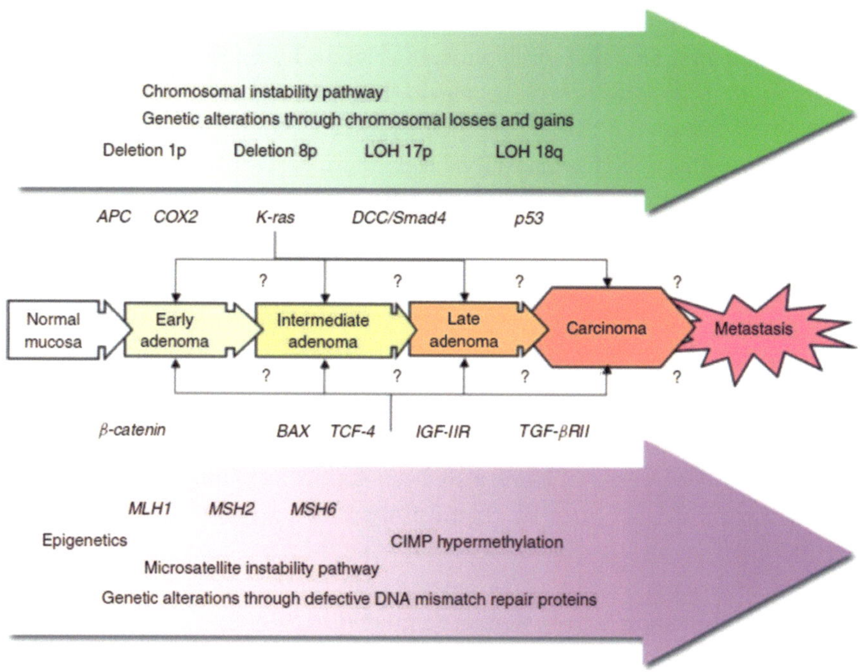

Figure 2. Characteristics of the two major pathways in CRC.

1.6. Axin

Axin1 (also simply called Axin), which encodes isoformaand b, and *Axin2* (also called Axil or Conductin) have 45%identity at the nucleotide level and the proteins they encode appear to be functionally similar. However, whereas *Axin1* is expressed ubiquitously during mouse embryogenesis, *Axin2* is expressed in a restricted pattern [20]. *Axin1* is the constitutively expressed component of the degradation complex and is essential for the maintenance of low Wnt signalling activity in the basal state. In contrast, *Axin2* is upregulated in response to increased β-catenin concentrations and thus serves to limit the duration and intensity of the Wnt signal [21]. *Axin* is downregulated in a Wnt dependent manner and is dephosphorylated after Wnt stimulation, which leads to *Axin1* destabilisation over time. Cells that receive Wnt ligand signals have low concentrations of *Axin*. Biochemical studies show that the intracellular concentrations of *Axin* are approximately 1000 times lower than other destruction complex components, suggesting that *Axin* is the limiting factor in this pathway [22]

1.6.1. Role of Axin in signaling pathways

Axin has emerged as a major scaffold protein for regulating a variety of signaling pathways and biological functions (Figure 3). In Wnt signalling, *Axin* binds to many components in the pathway, including the Wnt co-receptor LRP (low-density lipoprotein-related protein receptor) [23] Dishevelled or Dvl [24], tumour suppressor adenomatous polyposis coli (APC), GSK-3β, β-catenin [25], Casein kinases [26], protein phosphatase 2A (PP2A) [27], Diversin [28] *Ccd1* [29], and *Axam* [30].Interestingly, *Axin* itself is regulated with its stability being modulated by Wnt receptors, Dvl [31], and phosphorylation by GSK-3β. Inaddition, *Axin* also interacts with proteins that have no close relevance to Wnt signalling, including MAP kinase kinase (MEKK) [32, 33], I-MFA [34], DCAP [35], SH2/3 adaptor protein Grb4 [36], and Smad3. Interaction of *Axin* with MEKK leads to JNK activation, proceeding through a cascade from Axin, MEKK, and MKK to JNK[37].The most intriguing aspect of JNK activation by Axin is that multiple seemingly concrete structural elements of Axin are required [38]. Axin interacts with Smad3 and affects TGF-β signalling pathway.

1.6.2. Mutation of Axin in colorectal cancers

Alterations in both *Axin1* and *Axin2* have been detected in several different tumours. Mutations are found in most *Axin* domains including the APC (RGS) and β-catenin-binding domains. *Axin* sequence variants have also been found in colon, ovarian, endometrioid, adenocarcinoma, and HCC cell lines. Biochemical and functional studies have shown that these mutations interfere with the binding of GSK3 and that they also alter the interaction between *Axin* and two upstream activators of TCF-dependent transcription, Frat1, and DVL. Many components of the Wnt signalling system are mutated in colorectal cancer. Germ line loss of function mutations in the APC gene are associated with an inherited form of colorectal cancer —familial adenomatous polyposis— with 90–95% penetrance. Somatic APC mutations are also found in most sporadic colorectal cancers [39]. Alterations in other components of Wnt

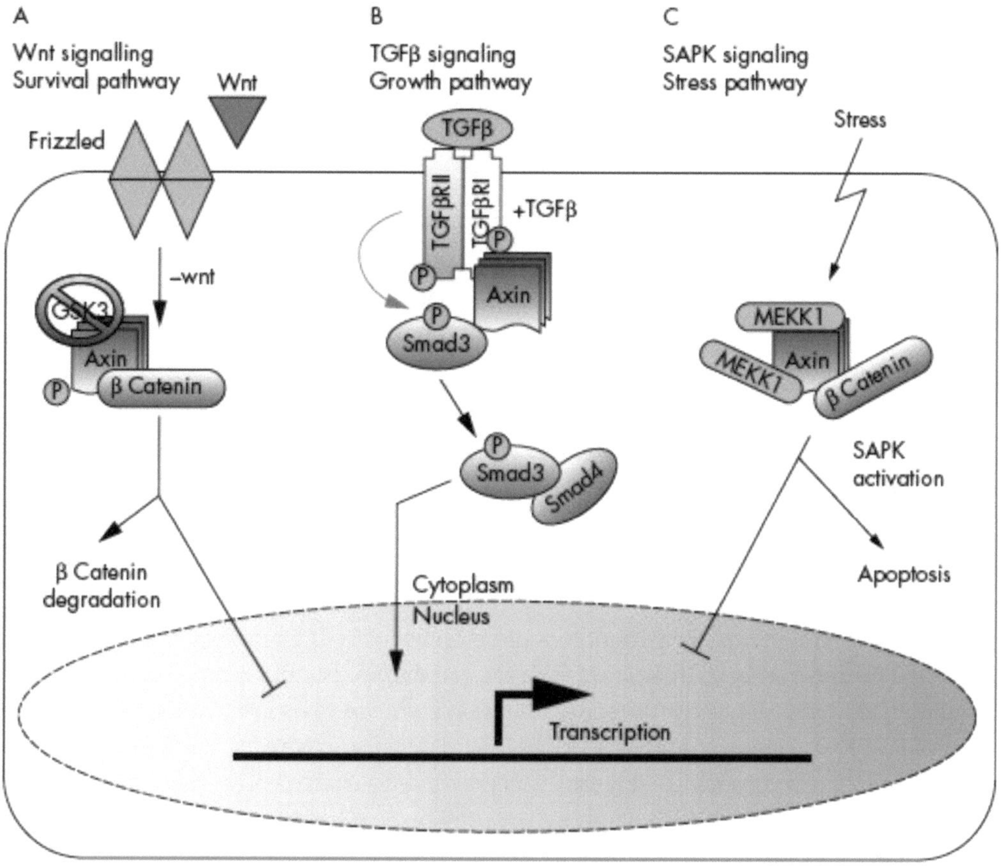

Figure 3. Regulation of three signalling pathways by Axin (1) Axin in the absence of Wnt ligand stimulates β-catenin degradation by proteosome complex and halts its transcriptional activity (2) The presence of transforming growth factor receptor signals Axin and stimulates Smad phosphorylation by TGF-β receptor I & II. The activated Smads then translocate into nucleus and stimulates transcription of downstream target gene. (3) Cells subjected to stress Axin bind to mitogenactivated protein and stimulate stress-activated protein kinase (SAPK/Jun) mediated apoptosis. (courtesy. S Salahshor et al. 2004)

signalling, including β-catenin, TCF, *Axin1*, and *Axin2*, found in colorectal cancer indicate the important role that this pathway plays in the etiology of this disease [40]. Most *Axin1* mutations in colorectal cancer occur between exon 1 and 5, where the APC, GSK3, and β-catenin-binding domains are located. Mutations in *Axin2* have been found in approximately 20% of mismatch repair deficient colorectal tumours [41]. In most cases, one base deletion or insertion occurs in the mononucleotide repeat sequences located in exon 7, leading to a frame shift and premature protein truncation [42]. These mutations lead to elimination of the DIX domain, where DVL binds and negatively regulates *Axin* activity. This domain is also essential for homo-oligomerization of *Axin*. The mutant form of *Axin2* appears to be more stable than the wild-type protein. Transfection of normal fibroblasts with *Axin2* mutants led to the accumulation of β-catenin in the nuclei. Li-Hua Jin *et al*.2003analysed 54 colorectal tumour tissues for *Axin1* mutation and reported 11% missense mutation suggesting *Axin* mutation may contribute to the onset of colorectal tumourigenesis. Webster *et al* [43] screened *Axin* gene in a range of human tumour cell lines including colon cancer cell lines. They identified two sequence variants carrying a substitution in four colon cancer cell lines. Biochemical and functional studies carried out by them showed that the L 396M change interfered with Axin'sability to bind GSK-3. Interestingly, this mutation and a neighboring L392M change differentially altered Axin'sability to interfere with two upstream activators of TCF dependent transcription factor Frat-1 and Dishevelled. Suraweera *et al* [44] reported heterozygous frame shift mutation and an in frame deletion in exon 7 of *Axin2*. They also reported 8% mutation of *Axin* in colon cancer cell lines. These studies indicates role of *Axin* gene in colorectal carcinogenesis.

1.7. Deleted in colorectal cancers (DCC) gene

The development of human cancer has been proposed to be a multistep process [45]. Vogelstein et al., 1988 showed that colonic tumorigenesis provides the systematic course to the multistep hypothesis at the molecular level. Several genes have been identified that alter during tumour progression. Frequent and consistent loss of heterozygosity (LOH) of specific chromosomes in human cancers has been associated with the presence of tumour suppressor genes [46]. In particular, the long arm of chromosome 18 has been shown to be lost in about 75% of colonic cancers [47].The tumour-suppressor gene *DCC* (deleted in colorectal carcinoma),located on the long arm of chromosome 18 (Figure 2) encodes a cell surface protein containing homology with N-CAM [14].*DCC* a putative tumour suppressor gene has been mapped on the long arm of 18th chromosome (18q). In normal conditions, *DCC* induced apoptosis limits cellular lifespan in the intestinal crypt and thereby inhibits the initiation of malignant transformation. Transfection of *DCC* cDNA into a human cell line lacking *DCC* expression suppresses tumour growth and results in apoptosis and cell cycle arrest [48].

1.7.1. Loss of heterozygosity of DCC gene

Human cancers arise by a combination of discrete mutations and chromosomal alterations. Loss of heterozygosity (LOH) of chromosomal regions bearing mutated tumour suppressor genes is a key event in the evolution of epithelial and mesenchymal tumours. The term Loss of heterozygosityv (LOH), refers to a technique widely used in cancer research.LOH relies upon an individual processing two non-identical alleles for specific genetic marker, which can be distinguished from each other. These individuals are referred to as heterozygote with respect to this allele. Distinguishing between alleles can be done by the presence of a restriction site on one allele or through polymorphic microsatellite repeats (also referred to as microsatellite markers).In the latter the alleles differ from one another based on their size. Using LOH, a comparison is made between the DNA extracted from normal and tumour tissue. If an allele is present in the normal DNA but missing in the tumour than we can suggest that this region of DNA has been lost or deleted through mutation. Therefore the tumour cells have lost an allele as only one is detected, hence loss of heterozygosity. Most commonly the deletion of DNA will not be isolated to just this marker but will more than likely also involve the loss of gene surrounding that region. This is important if the surrounding region contains one or more tumour suppressor genes. In fact LOH studies are often used to examine neoplasms to locate frequent chromosomal regions that are lost and hence may harbor putative tumour suppressor genes pivotal in the development of cancer. The greater the degree of LOH, the more genetically unstable the tumour type and more aggressive it is likely to be.

Global patterns of LOH can be understood through allele typing of tumours with polymorphic genetic markers. Simple sequence length polymorphisms (SSLPs or microsatellites) are reliable genetic markers for studying LOH. Microsatellites are short repetitive sequences of DNA that are scattered throughout the genome and are stably inherited, unique to each individual and have low inherent mutation rate [49]. Several studies have shown that alterations due to mutations in the simple repeat sequences or microsatellites are a feature in a number of cancers [50].Researchers working on colon cancers found the length of microsatellite DNA in tumour tissue vary from matching normal tissue. This variation in length of microsatellite represents a mutational process of insertion or deletion within tumour DNA [51].Loss of heterozygosity (LOH) i.e., loss of one allele at a constitutional heterozygous locus indicates the probability of loss of a tumour suppressor gene, which might promote neoplastic progression [52].

2. Aim and objectives

India is heavily burdened with CRC. Most of the genes implicated in CRC (like *APC, KRAS, SMAD* etc) have been studied in CRC patients of this population. Results therein have depicted either some semblance or little discrepancies in CRC in comparison to other studies conducted in other ethnic groups. The important genes like *Axin 1, Axin 2* and *DCC* have been reported to be involved in etio-pathology of CRC, but their role is yet to be elucidated in CRC patients of North India. Keeping in view of this, we carried out this study with following objectives

- To analyse the mutations, if any, in the coding exons (1a,1b,1c,2,4,6 and 10) of *Axin*1 gene
- To analyse the mutations, if any, in exon 7 of *Axin2* gene.
- To establish the correlation of *Axin1* and *Axin2* gene mutation with clinicopathological variables of CRC patients
- To analyse expression of *Axin* in CRC patients using western blotting technique andto correlate the altered expression of *Axin* with clinico -pathological characteristics of CRC patients.
- To analyse Loss of Heterozygosity of *DCC* gene at VNTR and D18S8-M2 markers in CRC patients and to correlate LOH of *DCC* gene with clinicopathological variables.
- Polymorphic studies of SNPs at codon 399 of *XRCC1* genes.

The main goals of this work are based on the hypothesis to understand

- What is the role of *Axin* 1 and *Axin* 2 gene aberrations in CRC?
- To understand the pattern of Axin expression in CRC tumours with respect to normal samples?
- What is the role of *DCC* gene aberrations in CRC?
- What is the role of Arg399Gln SNP of *XRCC1* gene in CRC?

3. Methodology and results

3.1. Mutational analysis of *Axin 1* and *Axin* 2 gene

Characteristics of the study subjects

A total of fifty (n=50) tissue samples of colorectal carcinoma and their adjacent normal samples were used for mutational analysis of *Axin1* and *Axin2* gene. Same samples were used for analysis of Axin protein expression. Tumour and adjacent normal tissue samples were collected in the General Surgery Department (SKIMS) after surgical resection. All the resected tissue specimens were histologically confirmed to be colorectal carcinomas by a panel of 2 expert pathologists. Median age at the time of diagnosis was 52 years (range 30-75); and male: female ratio was 1:1. Clinico-pathological characteristics of patients are given in table 3.On the basis of age, the patients were grouped into two categories, less than 50 years (<50) and greater than or equal to 50 years of age (≥50). The number of cases in the age group of ≥50 were 62 % (31/50) and less than <50 years were 38 % (19/50).In this study 29(58%) patients had cancer in the colon while as cancer of rectum accounted for 21(42%) of CRC cases. 33(61%) cases of CRC were well differentiated and 17(34%) were poorly/moderately differentiated. 31(62%) of CRC patients belonged to rural area and 19 (38%) to urban area. Based on the smoking status, 21(42%) patients were non-smokers and 29 (58%) were smokers. Almost all the patients with left colon carcinoma had attended the hospital with a clinical presentation of bleeding per rectum.

3.2. Molecular analysis of *Axin* 1 and *Axin* 2 gene

High molecular weight genomic DNA isolated from the samples (tumour tissues and corresponding normal tissues) (Figure 4) were subjected to PCR to amplify the exon 1a, 1b, 1c, 2, 4, 6 and 10 of *Axin1* and exon 7 of *Axin2*.The representative gel pictures of each amplified exon of *Axin1* and *Axin2* genes are given in figure 5. PCR products were purified manually and then purified samples were subjected to DNA sequence analysis. To identify the sequence variations, the electrophoregram obtained after sequencing of the PCR products were compared manually with the reference sequence of the *Axin1* and *Axin2* gene deposited in the NCBI Gene Bank database (Accession No.NC 000016 & NC 000017).

Clinico-epidemiological Parameters	Subgroup	Cases (n=50)
Grade/Differentiation	WD	33 (66%)
	MD/PD	17 (34%)
Stage	I/II	28(56%)
	III/IV	22(44%)
Location	Colon	29 (58%)
	Rectum	21 (42%)
Dwelling	Rural	31(62%)
	Urban	19 (38%)
Age	<50	19 (38%)
	≥50	31 (62%)
Sex	Male	24 (48%)
	Female	26 (52%)
Smoking status	Never	21(42%)
	Ever	29(58%)

WD: well differentiated; MD: moderately differentiated, PD: poorly differentiated

Table 3. Clinico-epidemiological characteristics of the CRC patients

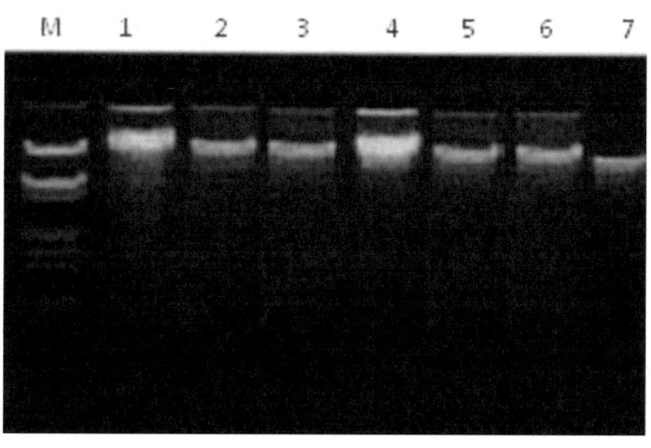

Lane M: 100bp DNA ladder; Lane 1: DNA derived from blood of CRC patients; Lane 2: DNA derived from blood of a normal healthy control; Lane 3 and 4: DNA derived from Tumour Tissue; Lane 5, 6 and 7: DNA derived from adjacent Normal Tissue

Figure 4. Agarose gel electrophoresis of DNA isolated from blood, tumour tissue, and adjacent normal tissue of CRC patients.

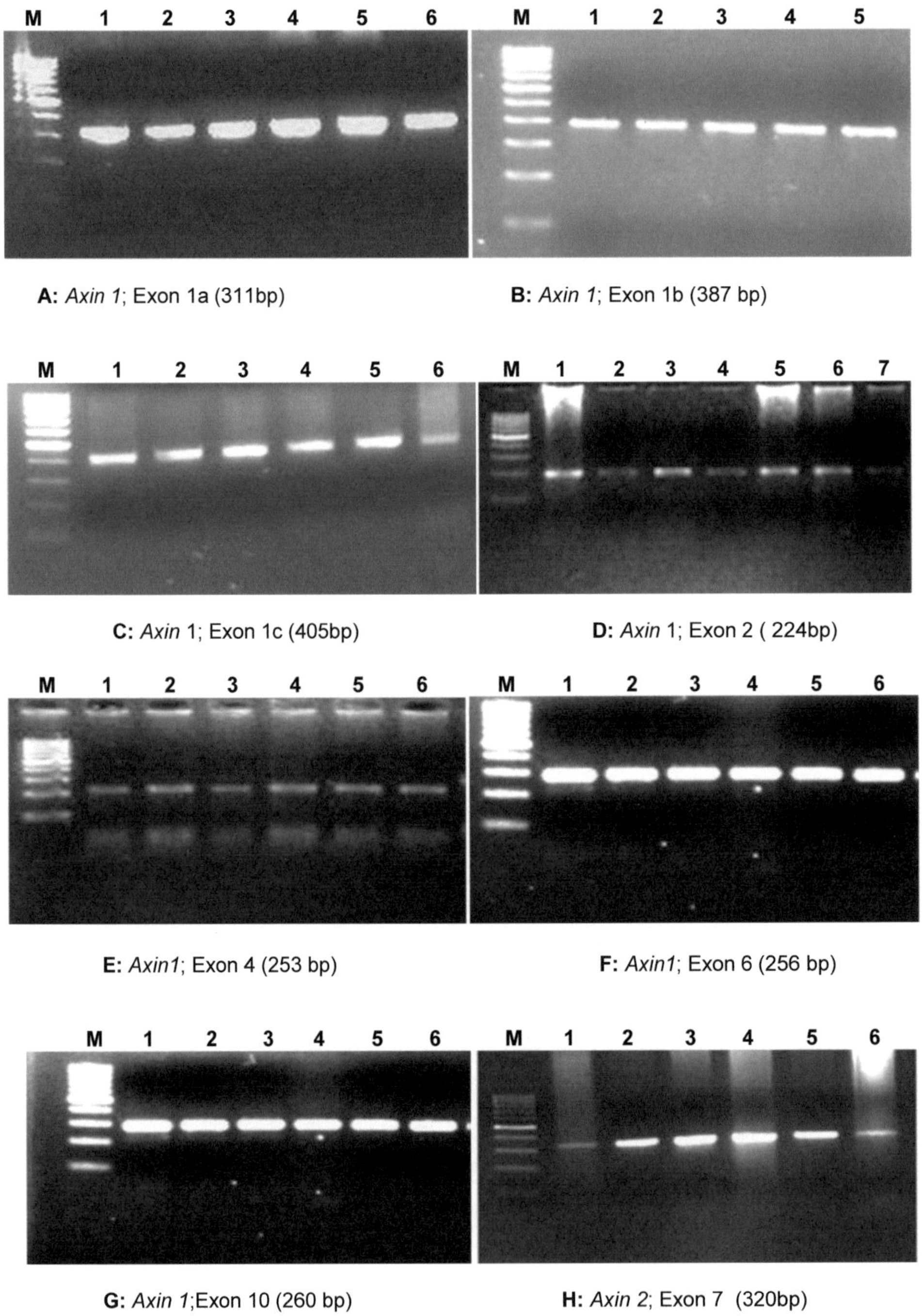

Lane M Molecular size marker 100bp; Lane 1-5, 6 and 7 Amplified product of DNA.

Figure 5. PCR amplification of different exons of Axin1 and Axin2 genes

3.3. Mutational spectrum of *Axin* 1 and *Axin* 2 gene

In this study DNA sequencing was used to analyze the exon 1a, 1b, 1c, 2, 4, 6 and 10 of *Axin1* and exon 7 of *Axin2* in a series of 50 CRC patients. No previously reported mutations were detected in any of the analysed exons of *Axin1* and *Axin2* genes in CRC patients except two SNPs mentioned below. However, an interesting finding of this study was that we detected a novel mutation of G>T (GCT>TCT) transversion in exon 7 of *Axin2* gene at codon G695T (p.alanine>serine) which has not been reported before this study [53] This G695T novel mutation was further confirmed by reverse sequence of the same samples. This novel mutation was found at a frequency of 6% (3/50). Among these three patients two were chronic smokers with mean age of fifty seven years. All the three patients had well differentiated adenocarcinoma. Clinico-pathological characteristics of patients having novel mutation are given in *Table 4*. In the same exon of *Axin2* gene a single nucleotide polymorphism (SNP) (rs 35415678) of C>T transition was detected in codon L688L (CCT>CTT) at a frequency of 18/50(36%). In exon1c of Axin1 we detected a SNP of T>C transition at codon D726D (GAT>GAC) at a frequency of 31/50 (62.5%) (Table 5.). This SNP is synonymous and does not lead to any change of amino acid (Figures 6, 7 & 8). Table 4.3 shows the changes in nucleotides of *Axin1* and *Axin2* genes observed in our study. No significant association of these SNPs was found in this report with any clinico-epidemiological characteristics (Table 6 & 7).

3.4. Analysis of protein expression of Axin

In the present study, 50 colorectal cancer tissues and their adjacent normal samples previously studied for mutation spectrum were analysed for the protein expression of the *Axin*. The clinicopathological characteristics of the studied subjects are given in Table 3. The representative picture of the proteins extracted that were run on SDS page is shown in the figure 9. Out of 50 cases of CRC, 26% (13/50) showed reduced expression of *Axin* (Figure 10) and the rest 74% (37/50) of the cases showed normal protein (*Axin*) expression. Among 13 cases of CRC with reduced expression,27% (9/33) were of well differentiated grade and 24% (4/17) of moderately/poorly differentiated grade. Reduced expression of Axin was found to be 25% (7/28) and 27% (6/22) of cases of stage I/II and III/IV respectively. Reduced expression of Axin was found to be in 4/21 (19%) of never smokers and 9/29 (31%) of ever smokers. Reduced expression of Axin in males was observed as 5/24 (21%) and in females as 8/26 (31%). 24% (7/29) of the CRC cases with colon carcinoma and 29% (6/21) cases of rectal carcinoma showed reduced expression of *Axin*. Association of reduced expression of Axin with clinicopathological characteristics is shown in Graph 2. No significant association of reduced expression of Axin with any of the clinicopathological characteristic was found (p>0.05) (Table 8).

3.5. Loss of heterozygosity (LOH) of *DCC* gene

Loss of heterozygosity of *DCC* gene was determined by PCR-LOH assay in eighty samples of colorectal carcinoma and corresponding adjacent normal tissue. Mean age at the time of diagnosis was 52 years (range 30-80) with male: female ratio of 1:1.All the tumour samples included in this study were histopathologically confirmed cases of CRC. Histopathological findings of the CRC cases revealed 51 of 80 (64%) as well differentiated grade and 29 of 80

(36%) as moderately/poorly differentiated grade. In order to analyse LOH of *DCC* gene at two markers both the markers were amplified the amplified PCR products for D18S8-M2 (396bp) was digested by *Msp*I restriction enzyme and analyzed on 8% polyacrylamide gel whereas amplified product of VNTR region was directly run on 8% PAGE (Figure 12) and photographed under ultraviolet light.

S. code	Age	Gender	S. Status	Dwelling	Location	HPG	C.change	A.Achange	N. change
CRC 29	50	Male	C.smoker	Urban	A. Colon	WD	GCT→TCT	Alanine →serine	2397 G→T
CRC 32	65	Male	C.smoker	Urban	Rectum	WD	GCT→TCT	Alanine →serine	2397 G→T
CRC 38	57	Female	N.smoker	Rural	Colon	WD	GCT→TCT	Alanine →serine	2397 G→T

Abbrevations: S.code=sample code;S.Status=Smaoking status; C.smoker=chronic smoker;

N.smoker=non-smoker HP G = Histopathological grade;WD=well differentiated; A.A change=Amino acid change;

N.N change =nucleotide change C.Change=codon change; A. Colon= ascending colon.

Table 4. Clinico-epidemiological characteristics of the patients with novel mutation in Axin 2 gene

Gene/Exon	Nucleotide change	Codon change	Amino Acid change	Frequency
Axin1 Exon 1c	1134 T→C	GAT→GAC	Asp→ Asp	31/50(62.5%)
Axin2 Exon 7	2376 C→T	CCT→CTT	Leu→ Leu	18/50(36%)

(Transcript ID of Axin1 gene ENSG00000103126, NCBI Reference Sequence NC_000016.9) (Transcript ID of Axin2 gene ENSG00000168646, NCBI Reference Sequence: NC_000017.10)

Table 5. Single nucleotide changes in Axin1 & Axin2 genes in CRC patients.

In this study only informative cases were included (cases in which normal samples were heterozygous at M2-D18S8 marker), whereas uninformative cases (cases in which normal sample showed no heterozygosity) (Figure 11) were excluded from the study. Digested product of D18S8-M2 region yielded products of size 396, 257 and 139bp. LOH was considered positive for samples with absence of 396 bp bands and presence of 257 and139 bp (Figure 11). PCR product of VNTR when run directly on 8% PAGE generated a spectrum of alleles ranging

Variables	**Cases (n=50)**	**Wild allele 19(38%)**	**Variant allele 31(62%)**	**OR(95%CI)**	***P-Value***
Grade					
WD	33(66%)	13(39%)	20(61%)	Reference	0.77
MD/PD	17(34%)	06(35%)	11(65%)	1.2(0.3-4.7)	
Age Group					
<50	19(38%)	08(42%)	11(58%)	Reference	0.63
≥50	31(62%)	11(35%)	20(65%)	1.3(0.4-4.1)	
Gender					
Male	24(48%)	10(42%)	14(58%)	Reference	0.63
Female	26(52%)	09(35%)	17(65%)	1.3(0.4-4.1)	
Smoking					
Never	21(42%)	09(43%)	12(57%)	Reference	0.62
Ever	29(58%)	10(34%)	19(66%)	1.4(0.4-4.0)	
Residence					
Rural	31(62%)	12(39%)	19(61%)	Reference	0.33
Urban	19 (38%)	10(53%)	09(47%)	0.5(0.09-2.9)	
Tumor site					
Colon	29(58%)	10(34%)	19(66%)	Reference	0.54
Rectum	21 (42%)	09(43%)	12(57%)	0.7(0.2-2.2)	

WD=Well Differentiated; MD= Moderately differentiated

Table 6. Single nucleotide changes in Axin1 & Axin2 genes in CRC patients.

in size from 150 to 210bp (Figure 12) depending on insertion or deletion. LOH at both D18S8-M2 and VNTR markers was observed as 39% (20/51) in samples with well differentiated grade and 86% (25/29) in moderately/poorly differentiated samples. 47 of 80 (59%) cases of CRC were of stage I-II and 33 of 80 (41%) of stage III-IV. LOH was found 47% (22/47) and 70% (23/33) at both the markers in stage I-II and III-IV respectively. The overall combined frequency of LOH at two markers (D18S8-M2 and VNTR) in CRC cases was reported to be 56.25 % (45/80) (Table 10; see Graph 3 also). LOH of DCC was found to be highly frequent in patients with higher stage/grade of CRC and this association was found to be significant ($p<0.05$). However no association of LOH was observed with any of the etiological parameter as depicted in Table 9.

Variables	Cases (n=50)	Wild allele 32(64%)	Variant allele 18(36%)	OR(95%CI)	*P*-value
Grade					
WD	33(66%)	19(58%)	14(42%)	Reference	0.19
MD/PD	17(34%)	13(76%)	04(24%)	0.4(0.2-1.5)	
AgeGroup					
<50	19(38%)	13(68%)	06(32%)	Reference	0.10
≥50	31 (62%)	19(61%)	12(39%)	1.3(0.4-4.8)	
Gender					
Male	24(48%)	16(67%)	08(33%)	Reference	0.7
Female	26 (52%)	16(62%)	10(38%)	1.3(0.3-4.2)	
Smoking					
Never	21(42%)	13(62%)	08(38%)	Reference	0.79
Ever	29(58%)	19(66%)	10(34%)	0.8(0.24-2.6)	
Residence					
Rural	31(62%)	20(65%)	11(35%)	Reference	0.9
Urban	19 (38%)	12(63%)	07(37%)	1(0.3-3.2)	
Tumorsite					
Colon	29(58%)	18(62%)	11(38%)	Reference	0.7
Rectum	21 (42%)	14(67%)	07(33%)	0.8(0.24-3.0)	

Table 7. Clinico-epidemiological Characteristics of the CRC Patients with single nucleotide polymorphism at codon 688 CCT>CTT Axin2 gene.

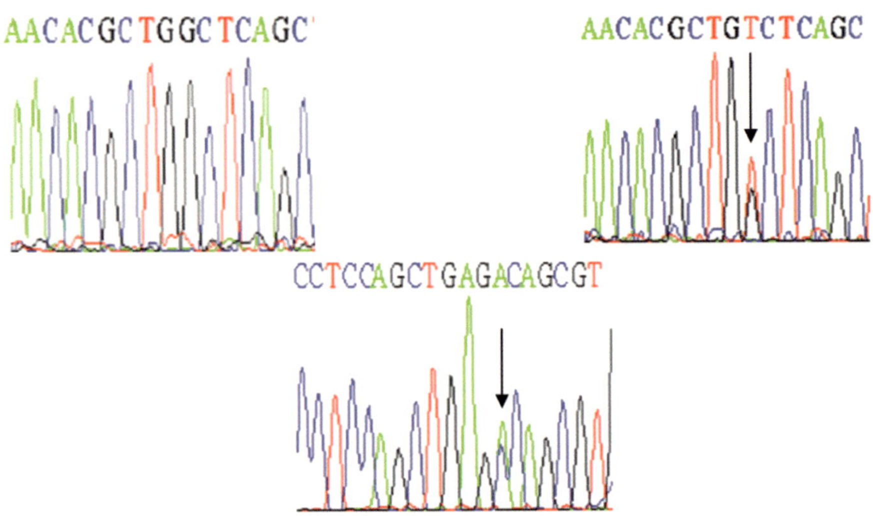

Figure 6. Partial nucleotide sequences in Exon 7 of normal (left) and of the mutants in (right) of the Axin 2 gene codon (GCT>TCT) Partial reverse sequence of the same mutation (below). Arrow points toward base change in mutants with respect to normal sequence.

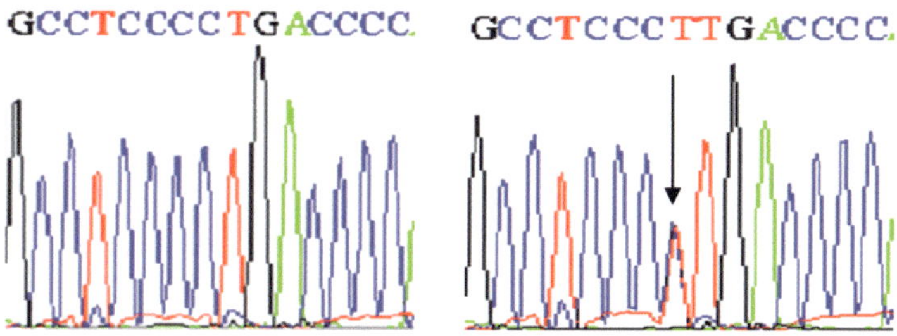

Figure 7. Partial nucleotide sequences in Exon 7 of the normal (left) and mutants in exon 7 of the Axin2 gene codon (CCT→CTT). Red arrow points toward base change in mutants with respect to normal sequence.

		Normal expression N (%)	Reduced expression N (%)	OR(95%CI)	P-Value
Clinico pathological variables	Overall results Case (n=50)	37(74%)	13(26%)	-	-
Age				Reference	0.3
<50	19(38%)	15(79%)	4(21%)	1.9(0.57-7)	
>50	31(62%)	22(71%)	9(29%)		
Sex				Reference	0.4
Male	24(48%)	19(79%)	5(21%)	1.68(1.0-2.3)	
Female	26(52%)	18(69%)	8(31%)		
Dwelling				Reference	0.2
Rural	31(62%)	21(68%)	10(32%)	0.39(0.09-1.6)	
Urban	19(38%)	16(84%)	03(16%)		
Smoking				Reference	0.3
Never	21(42%)	17(81%)	4(19%)	1.9(0.57-7.2)	
Ever	29(58%)	20(69%)	9(31%)		
Grade				Reference	0.77
WD	33(66%)	24(73%)	9(27%)	0.8(0.2-3.0)	
MD/PD	17(34%)	13(76%)	4(24%)		
Stage				Reference	0.8
I/II	28(56%)	21(75%)	7(25%)	1.1(0.3-3.8)	
III/IV	22(44%)	16(73%)	6(27%)		
Location				Reference	0.7
Colon	29(58%)	22(76%)	7(24%)	1.25(0.35-4.3)	
Rectum	21(42%)	15(71%)	6(29%)		

χ^2 was used to calculate the p-value of the variables. *P-Value <0.05 was considered statistically significant

Table 8. Association of Clinic pathological characteristics with reduced expression of Axin

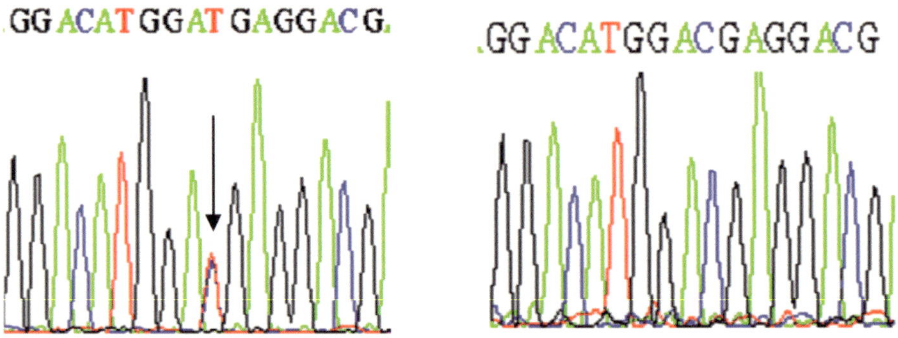

Figure 8. Partial nucleotide sequences in Exon1c of the normal (left) and mutants in exon 1c of the Axin1 gene codon (GAT →GAC).Arrow points toward base change in mutants with respect to normal sequence.

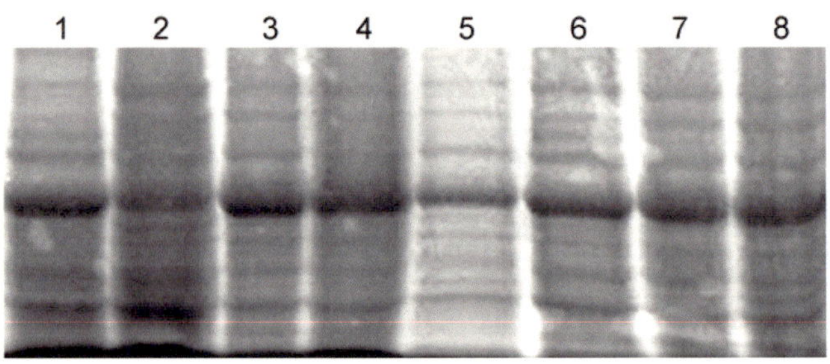

Figure 9. Representative gel picture of 10% SDS-PAGE. In each case 25 μl of the crude protein extract from tumor as well as normal tissue was loaded.

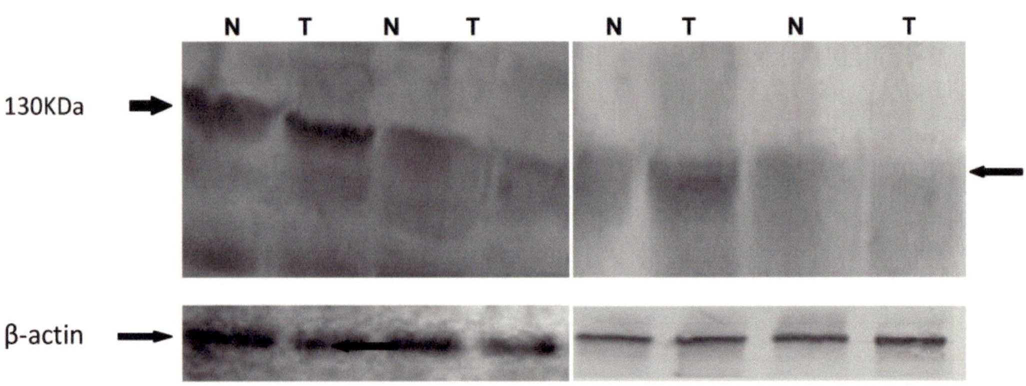

Lanes N: Protein extracted from Normal tissues; Lanes T: Protein extracted from Tumour tissue; Membrane was probed with a polyclonal antibody specific for Axin

Figure 10. Western blot analysis of Axin protein in colorectal tumour and adjacent normal tissues. Figure A-D Representative immunoblot showing the expression of Axin in Colorectal carcinoma as compared to their adjacent normals. Extract from samples was separately run for β-actin protein expression as loading control.

Variables	Cases n=80	LOH–ve [%]	LOH+ve [%]	P-value
Grade(differentiation)				
Well differentiated	51(64%)	31(61%)	20 (39%)	0.00019*
Mod/Poorly differentiated	29(36%)	4(14%)	25 (86%)	
Clinical staging				
Stages I-II	47(59%)	25(53%)	22(47%)	0.044*
Stages III-IV	33(41%)	10(30%)	23(70%)	
Location				
Colon	42(52.5%)	15 (36%)	27 (64%)	0.12
Rectum	38(47.5%)	20 (53%)	18 (47%)	
Dwelling				
Rural	46(57.5%)	22 (48%)	24 (52%)	0.393
Urban	34(42.5%)	13 (38%)	21 (62%)	
Age				
<50	33(41.25%)	14 (42%)	19 (58%)	0.8412
≥50	47(58.75%)	21 (45%)	26 (55%)	
Sex				
Male	43(53.75%)	21(49%)	22(51%)	0.323
Female	37(46.25%)	14(38%)	23(62%)	

χ^2 was used to calculate the p-value of the variables. *p-Value<0.05 was considered statistically significant

Table 9. Relation of clinico-pathological variables with LOH of DCC gene

Markers(n=80)	LOH-ve	LOH+ve	p-value
D18S8M2	61(76%)	19(24%)	0.21
VNTR	54(67.50%)	26(32.50%)	

χ^2 was used to calculate the P-value of the variables

Table 10. Percentage of Cases with and without Loss of Heterozygosity at two different markers

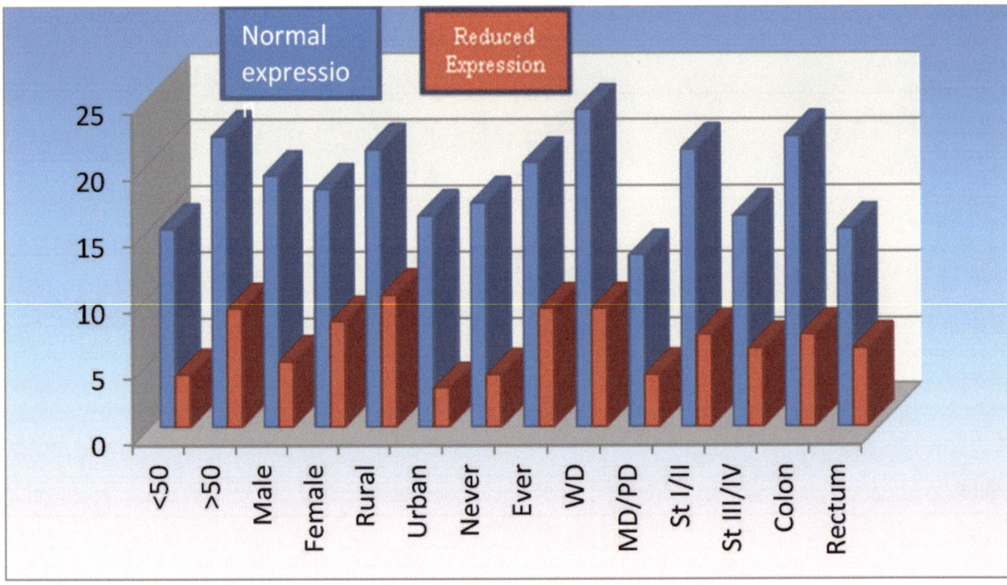

Graph 2. Association of reduced expression of Axin with clinic-pathological characteristics

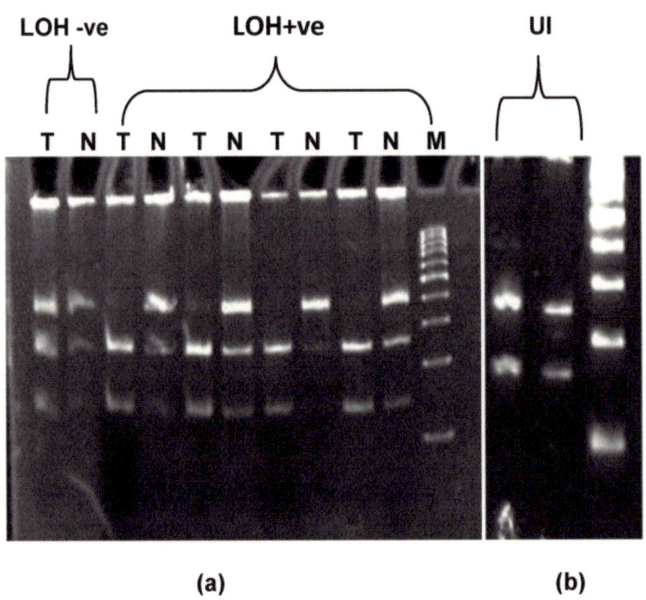

Lane M: 100bp DNA ladder,N=Normal; T=tumour. Normal samples showed three bands (band size 396,257 &139). LOH^{+ve} Informative cases. LOH -ve samples showed no loss of heterozygosity.

Figure 11. (a): LOH of DCC gene at D18S8-M2 region, (b): Uninformative cases (UI) were excluded from the study.

http://dx.doi.org/10.5772/57380

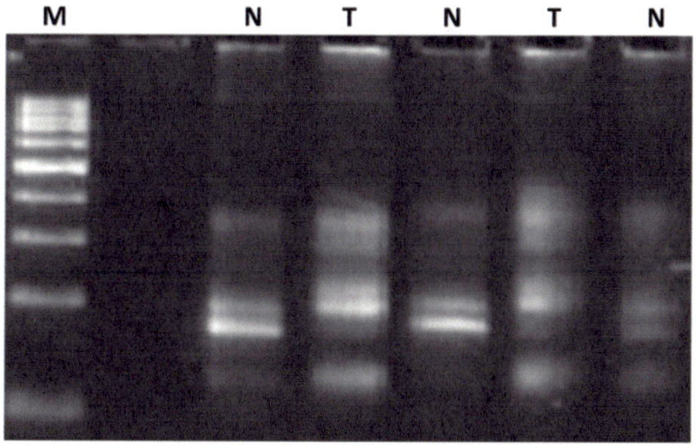

Figure 12. LOH of DCC gene at VNTR region. Lane M: 100bp DNA ladder, N: normal DNA, T: tumor DNA. Strong allelic imbalance is seen in tumor showing range of bands (150-200bp) not in adjacent normal tissues, with dominance of the larger 200-base pair allele.

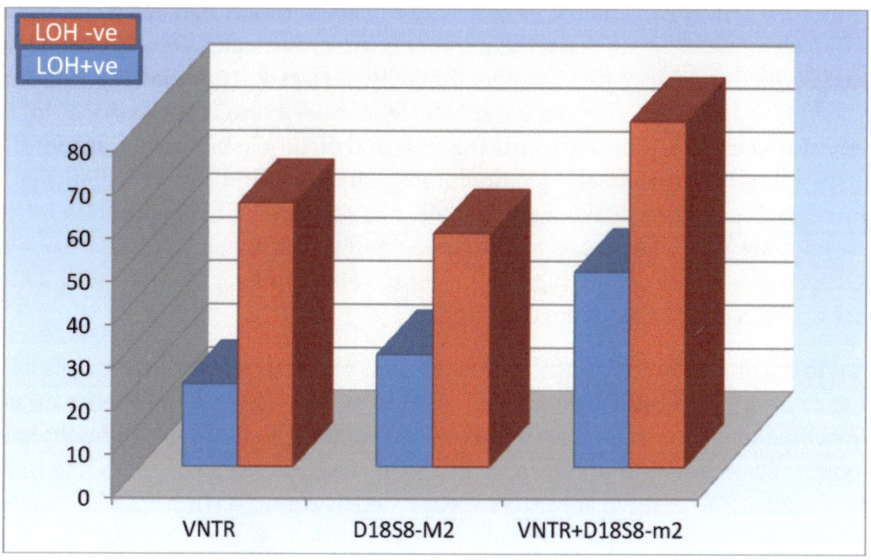

Graph 3. Frequency of distribution of LOH at two markers D18S8-M2 & VNTR of DCC gene

4. Summary and conclusion

Colorectal cancer (CRC) is a leading cause of death in the western world. [54]. The frequency of CRC varies remarkably among different populations. In India, CRC does not figure amongst the 10 most common malignancies [55]. In Kashmir incidence of cancer is showing an increasing trend and sites among the top ten common cancers [56]

Multiple factors contribute to the development of CRC, dietary and life style factors on one hand and genetic factors on the other [57]. Colon cancer is a common disease in both men and women. Because 5% of persons (1 in 20 persons) will develop colorectal cancer, this disease is an important public health issue. Colon cancer is usually observed in one of three specific patterns: sporadic, inherited or familial. Sporadic disease, with no familial or inherited predisposition, accounts for approximately 70% of colorectal cancer in the population. Sporadic colon cancer is common in persons older than 50 years of age, probably as a result of dietary and environmental factors as well as normal aging. Fewer than 10% of patients have an inherited predisposition to colon cancer. The inherited syndromes include those in which colonic polyps are a major manifestation of disease and those in which they are not. The polyposis syndromes are subdivided into familial adenomatous polyposis and the hamartomatous polyposis syndromes. The non-polyposis predominant syndromes include hereditary non-polyposis colorectal cancer (HNPCC) (Lynch syndrome I) and the cancer family syndrome (Lynch syndrome II). Although uncommon, these syndromes provide insight into the biology of all types of colorectal cancer. The third and least understood pattern of colon cancer development is known as familial colon cancer. In affected families, colon cancer develops too frequently to be considered sporadic colon cancer but not in a pattern consistent with an inherited syndrome. Up to 25% of all cases of colon cancer may fall into this category. CRC is more common in North America, parts of Europe, Australia, New Zeeland and Japan than in eastern Asia and Africa [58] This together with the fact that populations migrating from a low-incidence to a high-incidence geographical area show a similar incidence as those living in the high-incidence area, points towards life style and dietary habits being causative [59] The exact causes are still controversial but epidemiological studies indicate that diets that include low fruit, vegetable or fiber intake, high red meat or saturated fat consumption increase the risk of developing CRC. Exposure to caffeine, cigarette smoke and alcohol has also been suggested to increase risk. Diets high in calcium, folate and regular physical activity are associated with a reduced risk of developing CRC [60]

According to the model developed by Vogelstein and coworkers, colorectal neoplasia evolves through a series of genetic alterations that includes the activation of oncogenes by mutation and the inactivation of tumor suppressor genes by mutation, loss of gene, or methylation [61]. As per their multistage model of colorectal carcinogenesis alteration of genes like Axin, APC, β-Catenin, Smads, TGF-β, B-Raf are early events whereas alteration of p53,DCC are late events in the development of CRC. In our population genes like APC, β-catenin and Smads have been previously studied in relation to the development of colorectal cancer. As per one of the study carried out on Kashmiri population by Sameer et al., 2010 the mutational aberrations of APC and β-catenin were reported to be low in CRC cases in Kashmiri populations however, frequency of the epigenetic silencing of the APC gene was reported to be high. SMAD4 gene aberrations were reported to be the common event in CRC development [62].

We studied genetic alterations of *Axin* 1, *Axin* 2 and *DCC* genes in CRC patients of Kashmiri population. Following are the major findings of our study

- In the present study we studied fifty CRC and adjacent normal samples, we found a novel mutation in exon 7 of *Axin2* gene at codon 695.This G>T transversion leads to the change of codon GCT>TCT.

- The frequency of this novel mutation was found to be 6 % (3/50).
- This novel mutation leads to the change of amino acid alanine to serine.
- A SNP (rs 35415678) of C>T was found in exon 7 of *Axin2* gene at a frequency of 32% (18/50).This SNP was found at codon L688L resulting in the change of codon CCT>CTT. However this SNP was synonymous and hence does not lead to the change of amino acid.
- A SNP (rs 1805105) of T>C was found in exon 1c of *Axin1* gene at a frequency of 62.5% (31/50).This SNP was found at codon D726D leading to the change of codon GAT>GAC. This SNP was also found to be synonymous and hence does not lead to the change of amino acid
- No other sequence variation in any other analysed exons of *Axin* gene was found
- We did not find any significant association of any of the clinical epidemiological characteristic with the development of CRC.
- Protein expression of *Axin* gene in fifty tumour specimens with respect to their adjacent normal samples was studied. The samples which were studied for protein expression were same studied for mutational analysis.
- 26% (13/50) CRC patients showed reduced expression of Axin.
- No association was found with any of the clinico-pathological characteristic of CRC with the reduced expression of Axin.
- LOH of *DCC* gene at D18S8-M2 and VNTR marker was studied in eighty CRC tumour samples with respect to adjacent normal samples.
- LOH of *DCC* gene at D18S8M2 marker was found to be 23.75 % (19/80).
- LOH of *DCC* gene at VNTR marker was found to be 32.50 % (26/80).
- Aggregate percentage of loss of heterozygosity of *DCC* gene was found to be 55.25%.
- We found a significant association of LOH of *DCC* gene with higher stage and grade ($P<0.05$)
- No significant association of any other clinical pathological parameter was found with the development of CRC.
- Arg/Arg (GG) and Arg/Gln (GA) were found to be significantly associated with higher risk of CRC.
- The frequency of the *XRCC1* allele Gln/Gln was found to be 6(5%) for cases & 34(23.3%) for controls with $P<0.05$
- The frequency of the *XRCC1* allele Arg/Gln was found to be 80(66.7%) for cases & 62(42.5%) for controls.
- No significant association of Arg399Gln SNP with any clinico-pathological parameters was found.

- We found a protective role of Gln/Gln allele against the risk of development of CRC in Kashmiri population.

In conclusion, our study demonstrates significant role of *Axin* in the development of colorectal cancer. Eventhough we did not find any of the reported mutation in *Axin1* gene but we found reduced expression of *Axin1* in majority of CRC cases which clearly suggests its possible role in the development of CRC. Thus, our study points to the fact those other possible genetic alterations other than mutation could be responsible for malfunctioning of *Axin1* gene which may be responsible for the development of CRC. In *Axin2* gene the novel mutation was found at low frequency of 6% leading to the change of amino acid from alanine to serine. The codon at which this novel mutation was found lies in the region capable of binding to various proteins and thus may somehow render *Axin* incapable of binding various other proteins involved in different pathways. This may lead to the derangement of Wnt, TGF-β, and Jun/SAPK pathways. Aberration in specific binding of these signaling molecules to *Axin* due to the mutation G695T found in our study perhaps may aid in the deregulation of pathways and hence may lead to colorectal carcinogenesis.

Our study also supports the multistep model of colorectal carcinogenesis in which alteration of DCC gene has been reported to be the late event in the development of CRC as observed in our report. In this study we found that LOH has a frequency of 56% in patients with CRC and is highly frequent in patients with higher stage/grade in CRC suggesting that LOH of DCC gene may be one of the genetic events involved in the development of colorectal cancer in Kashmiri population.

Author details

Syed Mudassar[1], Mosin S Khan[1], Nighat P. Khan[1], Mahboob ul- Hussain[2] and Khurshid I. Andrabi[2*]

*Address all correspondence to: andrabik@uok.edu.in

1 Department of Clinical Biochemistry, Sher-I-Kashmir Institute of Medical Sciences, Srinagar, India

2 Department of Biotechnology, University of Kashmir, Srinagar, India

References

[1] Corner, J. What is cancer? In: Cancer Nursing Care in Context, Blackwell Publishing, Oxford; 2011

[2] Yarbro,C., Frogge,M. and Goodman,M. Cancer Nursing:Principles and Practice, 6th edn, Jones and Bartlett Publishers, Boston, MA; 2005

[3] Gabriel, J. Cancer: Health promotion, early detection and staging. In: Oncology Nursing in Practice Whurr Publishers, London; 2001

[4] American Cancer Society. Cancer Facts & Figures;2005. http://www.cancer.org/downloads/STTCAFF2005f4PWSecured.pdf.

[5] Parkin DM, Pisani P, Ferlay J. Global cancer statistics. CA Cancer J Clin 1999; 49 33–64.

[6] Ries LA, Wingo PA, Miller DS, Howe HL, Weir HK, Rosenberg HM. The annual report to the nation on status of cancer, 1973– 1977, with a special report on colorectal cancer. Cancer 2000; 88 2398–424.

[7] Potter JD. Colorectal cancer: molecules and population. J Natl Cancer Inst 1999; 91 916–32.

[8] Cooper GS, Yuan Z, Landefeld CS, Rimin AA. A national population-based study of incidence of colorectal cancer and age; implication for screening in older Americans. Cancer; 1995; 75 775–81.

[9] Demers RY, Severson RK, Lazar L. Incidence of colorectal adenocarcinoma by anatomic subsite; an epidemiologic study of time trend and racial difference in the Detroit, Michigan area. Cancer 1997; 79 441–7.

[10] Jemal A, Siegel R, Ward E, et al. Cancer statistics, 2008. CA Cancer J Clin. 2008; 58 71-96.

[11] Heavey P M, McKenna D and Rowland I R. Colorectal cancer and the relationship between genes and the environment. Nutr Cancer 2004; 48:124-141.

[12] Giovannucci E. An updated review of the epidemiological evidence that cigarette smoking increases risk of colorectal cancer. Cancer Epidemiol Biomarkers Prev 2001; 10 725-731.

[13] Caan BJ, Coates AO, Slattery ML et al. Body size and the risk of colon cancer in a large case-control study. International Journal of Obesity 1998; 22 178-184.

[14] Fearon ER, Vogelstein B. A genetic model for colorectal tumorigenesis. Cell 1990; 61 759-67.

[15] Irfan M. Hisamuddin, MD, Vincent WY. Molecular Genetics of Colorectal Cancer: An Overview. Curr Colorectal Cancer Rep 2006; 2(2) 53–59.

[16] Lengauer C, Vogelstein B. Genetic instabilities in human cancers. Nature 1998; 396 643–649

[17] Toyota M, Ahuja N, Ohe-Toyota M, Herman JG, Baylin SB,Jean-Pierre JI. CpG island methylator phenotype in colorectal cancer. Proc Natl Acad Sci 1999; 96 8681–8686.

[18] Satya Narayan, Deodutta Roy. Role of APC and DNA mismatch repair genes in the development of colorectal cancers. Molecular Cancer 2003; 2 41-47

[19] So°reide K, Janssen EA, Soiland H, Korner H, Baak JP. Microsatellite instability in colorectal cancer. Br J Surg 2006; 93 395–406

[20] Zeng L, Fagotto F, Zhang T, Hsu W, Vasicek TJ, Perry WL, Lee JJ, Tilghman SM, Gumbiner BM, Costantini F. The mouse Fused locus encodes Axin, an inhibitor of the Wnt signaling pathway that regulates embryonic axis formation. Cell 1997; 90 181–192.

[21] Lustig B, Jerchow B, Sachs M, Weiler S, Pietsch T, Karsten U, van de Wetering M, Clevers H, Schlag PM, Birchmeier W,Behrens J. Negative feedback loop of Wnt signaling through upregulation of conductin/axin2 in colorectal and liver tumors. Mol Cell Biol 2002; 22(11) 84–93.

[22] Lee E, Salic A, Kruger R, Heinrich R, Kirschner MW. The roles of APC and Axin derived from experimental and theoretical analysis of the Wnt pathway. PLoSBiol 2003; E 1-10.

[23] Tolwinski NS, Wehrli M, Rives A, Erdeniz N, DiNardo S, Wieschaus E. Wg/Wnt signal canbe transmitted through arrow/ LRP5, 6 and Axin independently of Zw3/ GSK-3ß activity. Dev Cell 2003; 4 407–18.

[24] Li L, Yuan H, Weaver CD, Mao J, Farr GH III, et al. Axin and Frat1 interact with Dvl and GSK, bridging Dvl to GSK in Wnt-mediated regulation of LEF-1. EMBOJ 1999; 18 4233–40.

[25] Nakamura T, Hamada F, Ishidate T, Anai K, Kawahara K, Toyoshima K, Akiyama T. Axin, an inhibitor of the Wnt signaling pathway, interacts with b-catenin, GSK-3b and APC and reduces the b-catenin level. Genes Cells 1998; 3 395–403.

[26] Rubinfeld B, Tice DA, Polakis P. Axin-dependent phosphorylation of the adenomatous polyposis coli protein mediated by casein kinase A. J Biol Chem 200; 276(390) 37–45.

[27] Hsu W, Shakya R, Costantini F. Impaired mammary gland and lymphoid development caused by inducible expression of Axin in transgenic mice. J Cell Biol 2001; 155 1055–1064.

[28] Schwarz-Romond T, Asbrand C, Bakkers J. et al. The ankyrin repeat protein Diversin recruits Casein kinase Ie to the beta-catenin degradation complex and acts in both canonical Wnt and Wnt/JNK signaling. Genes Dev 2002; 16 2073–84.

[29] Shiomi K, Uchida H, Keino-Masu K, Masu M. Ccd1, a novel protein with a DIX domain, is a positive regulator in the Wnt signaling during zebrafish neural patterning. Curr Biol 2003; 13 73–7.

[30] Kadoya T, Kishida S, Fukui A, Hinoi T, Michiue T, Asashima M,Kikuchi A. Inhibition of Wnt signaling pathway by a novel Axin binding protein. J Biol Chem 2000; 275 37030–7.

[31] Cliffe A, Hamada F, Bienz M. A role of Dishevelled in relocating axin to the plasma membrane during wingless signaling. Curr Biol 2003; 13 960–6.

[32] Zhang Y, Neo SY, Wang X, Han J, Lin SC. Axin forms a complex with MEKK1 and activatesc-Jun NH (2)-terminal kinase/ stress-activated protein kinase through domains distinct from Wnt signaling. J Biol Chem 1999; 274 35247–54.

[33] Luo W, Ng WW, Jin LH, Ye Z, Han J, Lin SC. Axin utilizes distinct regions for competitive MEKK1 and MEKK4 binding and JNK activation. J Biol Chem 2003; 278 37451–8.

[34] Kusano S, Raab-Traub N. I-mfa domain proteins interact with Axin and affect its regulation of the Wnt and c-Jun N-terminal kinase signaling pathways. Mol Cell Biol 2002; 22 6393–405.

[35] Yamazaki H, Nusse R. Identification of DCAP, a Drosophila homolog of a glucose transport regulatory complex. Mech Dev 2002; 119 115–9.

[36] Cowan CA, Henkemeyer M. The SH2/SH3 adaptor Grb4 transduces B-ephrin reverse signals. Nature 2001; 413 174–9.

[37] Zhang Y, Neo SY, Han J et al. Dimerization choices control the ability of axin and dishevelled to activate c-Jun N-terminal kinase/stress-activated protein kinase. J Biol Chem 2000; 275 25008–14.

[38] Rui HL, Fan E, Zhou HM, Xu Z, Zhang Y, Lin SC. SUMO-1 modification of the C-terminal KVEKVD of Axin is required forJNK activation but has no effect on Wnt signaling. J Biol Chem 2002; 277 42981–6.

[39] Liu W, Dong X, Mai M, et al. Mutations in Axin2 cause colorectal cancer with defective mismatch repair by activating beta-catenin/TCF signalling. Nat Genet 2000; 26 146–7.

[40] Wu R, Zhai Y, Fearon ER, Cho KR. Diverse mechanisms of betacatenin deregulation in ovarian endometrioid adenocarcinomas. Cancer Res 2001; 61 8247–8255.

[41] Domingo E, Espin E, Armengol M, et al. Activated BRAF targets proximal colon tumors with mismatch repair deficiency and MLH1 inactivation. Genes Chromosomes Cancer 2004; 39 138–42.

[42] Marie-Therese W, Magdalena R, Elizabeth S, Elaine D, Matthew S, Neville Y. Sequence Variants of the Axin gene in breast, colon, and other cancers: an analysis of mutations that interfere with GSK3 binding. Chromosomes & Cancer 2000; 28 443–453.

[43] Webster MT, Rozycka M, Sara E, Davis E,Smalley M, Young N, Dale TC, Wooster R. Sequence variants of the axin gene in breast, colon, and other cancers: An analysis of mutations that interfere with GSK3 binding. Genes Chromosomes Cancer 2000; 28 443–453.

[44] Suraweera N, James R, Emmanuoil V, Thomas G, Ian T,Ian T, Andrew S. Mutations within Wnt pathway genes in sporadic colorectal cancers and cell lines. Int J Cancer 2006; 119 1837–1842.

[45] Nowell PC. Mechanisms of tumor progression. Cancer Res 1986; 46 2203-2207.

[46] Baker SJ, Fearon ER, Nigro JM, Hamilton SR, Preisinger AC, Jessup JM, VanTuinen P, Ledbetter DH, Baker DF, Nakamura Y, White R and Vogelstein B. Chromosome 17 deletions and p53 gene mutations in colorectal carcinomas. Science 1989; 244 217-221.

[47] Vogelstein B, Fearon ER, Kern SE, et al. Allelotype of colorectal carcinomas. Science 1989; 244 207-11.

[48] Klingelhutz AJ, Hedrick L, Cho KR and McDougall JK. The DCC gene suppresses the malignant phenotype of transformed human epithelial cells.Oncogene 1995; 10 1581-1586.

[49] Hearne CM, Ghosh S, Todd JA. Microsatellites for linkage analysis of genetic traits.Trends Genet 1992; 8 288-294.

[50] Sturzeneker R, Bevilacqua R, Haddad L, Simpson A, Pena S. Microsatellite instability in tumours as a model to study the process of microsatellite mutations. Hum Mol Genet 2000; 9 347–352.

[51] Brentnall T. Microsatellite instability, shifting concepts in tumourigenesis. AmJ Pathol 1995; 147 561–563.

[52] Lasko D, Cavenee W, Nordenskjold M. Loss of constitutional heterozygosity inhuman cancer. Annu Rev Genet 1991; 25 281-314.

[53] Nighat P. Khan, Arshad A. Pandith, Mahboob Ul Hussain, Adfar Yousuf, Mosin S. Khan, Khursheed A. Wani, Syed Mudassar.Novelty of Axin 2 and lack of Axin 1 gene mutation in colorectal Cancer: a study in Kashmiri population. Mol Cell Biochem 2011; 355:149–155.

[54] Ferlay J, Bray F, Pisani P, Parkin DM. GLOBOCAN: Cancer Incidence, Mortality, and Prevalence Worldwide, 2002.Lyon: IARC Press; 2004.

[55] National Cancer Registry Programme Consolidated Report of Population based cancer. Registries 2001–2004 Chapter 5–6.www.icmr.nicin.

[56] Arshad AP,Mushtaq AS. Burden of cancers in the valley of Kashmir: 5 year epidemiological study reveals a different scenario. Tumor Biol.2011;DOI 10.1007/s13277-012-0418-z.

[57] Zauber AG, O'Brien MJ, Winawer SJ. On finding flat adenomas: is the search worth the gain? Gastroenterology 2002; 122 839–40.

[58] Cancerfonden. Cancerfondsrapporten; 2008.

[59] Cardoso J, Boer J, Morreau H and Fodde R. Expression and genomic profiling of colorectal cancer. Biochim Biophys Acta 2007; 1775 103-137.

[60] Peters U, Sinha R, Chatterjee N, Subar A F, Ziegler R G, Kulldorff M, Bresalier R, Weissfeld J L, Flood A, Schatzkin A and Hayes R B. Dietary fibre and colorectal adenoma in a colorectal cancer early detection programme. Lancet 2003; 361 1491-1495.

[61] Vogelstein B, Fearon ER, Hamilton SR, Kern SE, Preisinger AC, Leppert M, Nakamura Y, White R, Smits AMM and Bos JL.Genetic alterations during colorectal-tumor development. NEngl J Med 1988; 319 525-530.

[62] Syed Sameer, Nissar A. Chowdri, Nidda Syeed, Mujeeb Z Banday, Zaffar A. Shah and Mushtaq A. Siddiqi. SMAD4 - Molecular gladiator of the TGF-β signaling is trampled upon by mutational insufficiency in Colorectal Carcinoma of Kashmiri population: An analysis with relation to KRAS proto-oncogene. BMC Cancer 2010;10 300-309.

Chapter 15

Prospects of 'Omics Based Molecular Approaches in Colorectal Cancer Diagnosis and Treatment in the Developing World: A Case Study in Cape Town, South Africa

Henry Adeola, Ryan William Goosen,
Paul Goldberg and Jonathan Blackburn

Additional information is available at the end of the chapter

http://dx.doi.org/10.5772/57485

1. Introduction

The emergence of the field of genomics, proteomics and more recently lipidomics in science has advanced diagnostic and therapeutic medicine in no small measure. These fields typically deal with the documentation of the identity, abundance and localization of DNA, RNA, protein and lipid biomolecules in a given cell, tissue or organism. An in-depth knowledge of the biologic and physiologic localization, chemistry, and methodology for isolation of these essential biomolecules is key to a successful analysis and interpretation of information retrieved in the 'omics field.

The recent rapid development of these fields can be accounted for by the concurrent development of new state of the art, high throughput technologies such as real time qualitative polymerase chain reaction (RTqPCR), microarrays, flow cytometry, mass spectrometry and sequencing. These high throughput technologies have found extensive utility in diverse areas of human biology, particularly following the completion of the human genome project (HGP) in 2003. This project, which successfully documented the full complement of genes present physiologically within the human cell, gave a scientific platform to newer experimental initiatives thereafter.

Clinical application of 'Omics based approaches have gained popularity and are believed to be the future of medicine because of its inherent ability to determine disease-associated changes in the human genome, transcriptome, proteome, lipidome and metabolome. Documentation of these changes in principle enables the identification of disease-associated biomarkers for use in diagnostic tests, as well as with identifying molecular mechanisms of disease.

Establishment of the HGP was then followed by the initiation of the Cancer Genome Atlas project to create a repertoire of genomic profiles for 20 different types of cancers. This project is designed to evaluate, across-the-board, the molecular and genomic depiction of different cancer types and to delineate the networks and maps for disease pathogenesis; the first results to be published from this project were for human glioblastomas [1], followed by ovarian carcinomas. [2]

Most recently, human colon and rectal cancers have been added to the Cancer Genome Atlas Project [3], the aim being to evaluate somatic modifications in such carcinomas using genome level methodologies to assess variation in DNA copy number, methylation patterns, micro-RNA expression, exon utilization; and acquired mutations: To date, genetic mutations have been found in 29 genes and amplifications of ERBB2 and IGF2 have also been observed. This large scale identification of novel genetic changes in human colorectal cancer (CRC) may in due course enable the identification of underlying molecular mechanisms of cancer development and new therapeutic targets, as well as the development of diagnostic and/or predictive tests for CRC.

Current knowledge of cancer cell biology shows that the complex carcinogenesis process is made up of several intricate molecular pathways and that different cancer cells express a heterogeneous array of signals. Hence individualized administration of beneficial treatment regimens to patients, rather than a 'one-size-fits-all' approach, is becoming more acceptable as a generic principle to strive towards, not least since it would be similar to the use of specific antibiotics based on microscopic culture and drug sensitivity testing instead of using a broad spectrum/empirical antibiotic approach.

According to the GLOBOCAN cancer fact sheet of the International Agency for Research on Cancer (IARC), over 12 new cancer cases and 7 million cancer deaths are reported worldwide annually. Colorectal cancer is the third most common cancer in males (663,000 new cases representing 10.0% of the total cancer cases) and the second most common cancer in females (571,000 new cases representing 9.4% of the total cancer cases). [4] Roughly 600,000 cases of colorectal cancer deaths are expected annually, accounting for almost a tenth of all cancer deaths, making it the fourth leading cause of cancer death worldwide. In trend, mortality rates are higher in males than in females except in the Caribbean regions.

Over half of the global CRC burden is occurs in developed countries and its incidence is known to be lowest in third world countries. The lowest incidence is reported in Africa; however in South Africa the incidence of CRC more closely resembles that of developed countries. Even though the mortality and incidence figures are poorly reported and cannot be harmonized reliably, reports from the currently defunct National Cancer Registry of South Africa revealed that in 1999 CRC was the sixth commonest cancer in the general population, accounting for about 2,367 cases of the total 26,606 new cancer cases reported. [5]

Whilst research and health institutions in the developed world are replete with ongoing studies and discoveries of candidate disease biomarkers, significant attendant challenges are associated with 'omics based studies in a developing world setting, *inter alia*: infrastructure, human capacity and funding. Here we provide a synoptic overview of the prospects, challenges and benefits of 'omics based approaches in the diagnosis and treatment of CRC in a developing world, using our Cape Town experience as a case example.

2. Diagnostic inaccuracies in colorectal cancer

The intricacies of CRC are due in part to its multiple implicated aetiologies and the heterogeneity of the tumour. Important aetiologic considerations include; location (right sided or left sided, surface or cryptic, colonic or rectal), whether sporadic or hereditary, de novo or sequel to adenomatous polyp; intra-tumour heterogeneity (ITH) also plays an important role in the accuracy of histopathologic and molecular diagnosis. The classical theory of 'field cancerisation' [6] presupposes that cancer develops from multifocal areas of precancerous changes; this concept is supported by latter studies which demonstrated that true cancer boundaries often exceed the physically discernible margin taken out at surgery, with histological analyses showing that these multiple abnormal tissues constituting premalignant cancer cell field changes persist and surround the tumor and may form multiple independent lesions that sometimes coalesce. The implications of such findings are profound when differentiating the cancer field recurrence from second primary tumours [6-8]. Subsequently, others have considered the concept of 'sequential carcinogenesis' which suggests that cancers develop as a progression from patchy premalignant lesions which later show evidence of mild, then moderate and then severe epithelial dysplasia. [7] These dysplastic lesions eventually progress to carcinoma-in-situ (high grade intraepithelial neoplasm), then to microinvasive carcinoma and advanced invasive carcinoma.

The literature is replete with the extensive application of the field concept of Slaughter in surgical management of head and neck cancers and is gradually becoming a major consideration in the management of cancer of other organs such as the stomach, skin, cervix, lungs, vulva, bladder, colon, breast, and ovaries. [9, 10] In addition, molecular investigations have been used to assess correlation between phenotypic stages of cancer progression and expression of cancer specific genes and mutations; these studies have demonstrated significant correlations between both [7, [11], implying that molecular markers have the potential to significantly enhance the precise diagnosis, staging and treatment monitoring of cancers.

The possibility of a physically normal tissue adjacent to the tumour area and expressing cancer specific genetic profiles has spurred interest in the origin of molecular level heterogeneity and histologic variability in the immediate field surrounding the cancer area. Some researchers have suggested that the heterogeneity in cancer growth follows a Darwinian evolutionary theory of natural selection [12], whilst others have concluded that there are two plausible origins of diversity in tumour cells expansion, described by the 'clonal evolution' theory and the 'cancer stem cell' theory. [13-15] The clonal evolution theory (cancer monoclonality) presupposes that tumour cells result from a solitary clone of mitotically unstable cell that differentiate into different offspring lineage clones that have developed additional unique genetic damage down the lineage. [13] By contrast, the cancer stem cell theory (cancer polyclonality) is premised on the possibility of cancer developing from multiple cancer stem cells that proliferate concurrently and drive the expansion of the tumour. Both theories have therapeutic implications in that only a fraction of the tumour bulk drives its expansion, hence targeted molecular therapies at these 'driver cells' could in principle be established for cancer treatment.

Phylogenetic evidence suggests that well-characterized subpopulations of tumour cells, including annotations of genetic mutations, have been derived from sequential genetic events [16] and mathematical models have been described to account for this, but to date have mostly provided a one-dimensional insight into the complexities of ITH. [17, 18] The mechanistic development of cancer is a multi- dimensional event and multiple factors have been established to govern its progression such as: the shape of the organ in which it occurs; blood supply; surgical interference; the consistency of the surface on which it occurs; tumour microenvironment; and the genetic nature of the cell. Clearly ITH is a reality that affects tumour diagnosis, classification, prognosis, and treatment; and requires further understanding.

2.1. Reliability of histopathology reports

Introduction: Histopathology is the science of utilising classical histological techniques to assess micro- and macroscopic evidence of potential disease. Classical histology routinely utilises microscopic observation of micrometer cross-sections of tissue, differential staining techniques, as well as immunohistochemical assays, to assess the tissue specimen in question. The visual evidence provided by each technique, or combination thereof, allows a pathologist to identify potential evidence of pathology, thereby providing a pathological diagnosis for a given specimen.

Classical histological techniques are inherently limited in their scope for the detection of pathology as they rely on a microscopically visible presentation of clear or strong evidence of pathology, e.g. in the case of advanced disease. Furthermore, any aberrant change at the sub-microscopic level, i.e. the molecular level, needs to have translated into morphological change at the subcellular and/or overall cellular morphological level, or to have produced a variation in the abundance of a particular protein, or set of proteins, that is detectable through immunohistochemistry.

Evidence of molecular changes that are not yet detectable at the histological level: In molecular studies of tumour biopsies and adjacent "paired" normal samples, researchers often seek to identify molecular signatures that can distinguish tumour samples compared to histologically normal samples obtained from anatomical sites distal to the primary lesion. However, recent studies have investigated the possibility of significant molecular differences between histologically normal colorectal tissue from patients with polyps, or colorectal carcinoma, versus the same tissue from healthy individuals [19], suggesting that significant aberrant molecular changes occur in apparently normal colorectal tissue, despite being apparently distinctly located from the original lesion. In turn, this suggests that classic histopathological techniques are limited in their scope to identify such clinically relevant aberrant changes in tissue that appears morphologically normal; interestingly, these molecular observations are entirely consistent with Slaughter's 'field cancerisation' theory. [6] However, whether or not such a field has a gradually tapering aberrant effect as function of distance from the tumour remains incompletely answered. For instance, it has been found that there was no significant correlation between the degree of aberrant gene expression perturbation and distance from a polyp or tumour. [20] Irrespective, of the specific characteristics of any field effect, it is interesting to note that supporting evidence of aberrant perturbations in histologically normal colorectal mucosa appeared five decades after Slaughter's original hypothesis as a direct result of modern genomic, epigenomic, and proteomic research.

In a study of normal colonic mucosa from individuals with a family history of sporadic cancer conducted by Hao et al [21], it was found that there was a significant difference in the expression of several genes in these individuals' normal mucosa relative to the same tissue from healthy controls. In particular, the gene expression levels of PPAR-gamma, SAA1, and IL-8 were found to be significantly different in the morphologically normal rectosigmoid tissue samples in the individuals with a family history of CRC. Furthermore, a follow-up study in individuals with adenomatous polyps with or without familial history of colorectal carcinoma again found that there was a difference between gene expression in normal rectosigmoid mucosa from these individuals and healthy controls, regardless of the presence of a familial history of cancer. [22]

Polley et al [19] observed significantly different proteomic signatures in morphologically normal mucosa from patients with colorectal neoplasia compared to the same tissue from healthy subjects. It therefore appears that a larger than anticipated field of tissue in the colorectum may be affected by the presence of a neoplastic lesion, implying in turn that the method used to determine clear margins estimated during surgical resection may need the support of molecular assays in the future. However, whether or not the molecularly perturbed normal mucosa will progress to disease remains to be determined.

In addition to genomic and proteomic perturbations, epigenetic changes have also been reported in CRC tissues, one example being the hypomethylation of L1 promoter sequences in colorectal tumours and in adjacent normal tissue of 6 out of 19 cancer patients, but not in colonic mucosa of 14 healthy individuals. Furthermore, genomic CpG methylation appeared to be lower in normal colorectal tissue from diseased patients, compared to healthy subjects, and significantly lower in patients with hypomethylation of the L1 promoter sequences. [23]

The above examples at the genomic, proteomic and epigenetic level provide substantial evidence of molecular aberrations in morphologically normal tissue sample adjacent to a tumour. These changes might be subtle and may not effect a microscopically visible phenotype, but could well represent significant perturbations that impart normal tissue samples with precancerous characteristics. It is therefore important that such findings are considered when assessing individual biopsies by histopathology since these samples may in fact have underlying molecular signals of disease that, if interpreted correctly, could provide insight into the disease.

Molecular Intratumour heterogeneity due to branched evolutionary clonal expansion: Intratumour heterogeneity in terms of cellular morphology and types of cells, is a well-established observation in anatomical pathology. However, it is only recently that a further layer of complexity has been introduced through the discovery of an added layer of heterogeneity at the genomic and epigenomic level. This molecular heterogeneity further complicates biopsy selection and subsequent histopathological assessment because a specific lineage of clones, with a distinct genomic profile, may occur in physical clusters on a given tumour and thus be physically separated from other clonal populations. Therefore, each biopsy taken may present a uniform or slightly variable morphological appearance but might be distinct at the molecular level with unique functional potential and characteristics. This has fundamental ramifications when it comes to assessing the severity of disease and the prognosis, as well as deciding the appropriate course of treatment. Furthermore, intra-tumour heterogeneity governs how each unique tumour lineage evolves and adapts to therapeutic interventions and should therefore ideally be understood when developing new chemo- and biological treatments.

In a landmark study by Gerlinger et al [14], multiple spatially separated biopsy samples obtained from primary renal carcinomas and associated metastatic sites showed evidence of branched evolutionally growth by unique clonal population lineages. Furthermore, the majority of all somatic mutations (63 – 69%) were not found to be present across all tumour biopsies. One clinically relevant consequence of these findings was the identification of both good and poor prognostic signatures in different biopsies of the same tumour. This study highlights the inherent complexity of utilising a single biopsy for biomarker development, prognostic or predictive measures based on molecular markers to guide treatment regimen. It is clear that future biopsy collection - for the purpose of treatment planning or for biomarker research - should ensure collection and molecular assessment of multiple biopsies from physically separate sites on the same tumour.

A recent study by Kreso et al [24] has provided supporting evidence, in the context of colorectal carcinoma, that the distinct genetic profile of each intratumoural clonal subpopulation has implications in growth potential and chemotherapy tolerance and therefore has an impact on treatment outcomes. This appears to be due to Darwinian style natural selection, with certain subpopulations becoming more dominant by leveraging their intrinsic tolerance to selective pressure such as chemotherapeutic intervention. These findings highlight the fact that different tumour subpopulations have distinct proliferative potentials and chemotherapy tolerance mechanisms; as such, treatment regimens in the future my need to target each type of cellular population individually in order to prevent disease recurrence.

Future directions for modern pathological assessments of cancer tissue samples: Given the recent developments in the field of intratumour heterogeneity, and the evidence of significant molecular aberrations in histologically normal mucosa, it is clear that classical histopathological techniques are limited in their ability to assess the underlying clinically relevant heterogeneity in tumour and normal tissue samples, suggesting that modern, validated, cost-effective molecular assays should be integrated into histopathological assessments. Amongst others, this would ensure that clinically relevant phenotypic or functional characteristics - whether dormant or active - which may directly govern a tumours response to therapeutic intervention can be identified. This enhanced approach should facilitate the development of novel treatment regimens that efficaciously target all heterogeneous subpopulations for a given tumour and, in doing so, potentially also thwart aberrant histologically normal tissue from progressing to a malignant lesion.

The possibility that distinct subpopulation of cells and/ or genetic signals exist in different areas of a particular biopsy specimen poses a major challenge in implementing personalized therapy. [25] 'Omics based research can in principle generate a more robust predictor of therapeutic benefits, but this often involve an extensive sample collection for discovery and validation, adequate funding and availability of appropriate manpower: an example of one such initiative is the 'Personalized RNA Interference to Enhance the Delivery of Individualized Cytotoxic and Targeted Therapeutics' (PREDICT) consortium [26] that aims to identify reliable biomarkers of different cancer types.

2.2. Tumour classification and staging

The earliest classification system for CRC by Dukes [27], modified by Astler [28], considered the staging of CRC severity to be based on its depth of invasion. More recently, a standardized widely accepted staging system of the American Joint Committee on Cancer (AJCC) also known as the TNM system which incorporated the tumour size, nodal involvement and presence of distant metastasis was introduced [29]: These three classifications are largely based on morphologic evidence and can be subject to inaccuracies. To minimize errors in diagnosis, these phenotypically driven systems of staging colorectal tumour could now in principle be usefully complemented with a validated molecular diagnostic method.

Newer and often more reliable molecular based assessment of tumour staging and prognosis are beginning to emerge for CRC based on new molecular cancer knowledge and 'omics based techniques and complement existing orthodox morphology based methods. One of such molecular classification is based on CpG island methylator phenotype (CIMP), as well as microsatellite instability (MSI), and is scored as type 1-5 based on different combinations of these molecular features. [11] Chromosomal instability (CIN) has also been identified as an important global molecular classifiers of CRC. [30] In addition, KRAS mutations have emerged as the most common prognostic biomarker of CRC for anti-EGFR therapy patients and many more candidate markers for prediction of therapeutic outcomes in colorectal cancer are being discovered now using 'omics based techniques, including loss of PTEN signals, PI3KCA mutation and BRAF gene mutation. [31]

Identification of cancer specific genes, proteins, lipids and metabolites is increasingly regarded as a promising route to early diagnosis, treatment and monitoring of disease progress. For instance, the following genes have been recognized as associated with the risk of developing colorectal cancer; TP53, MLH1, MSH2, MSH6, MYH, EPCAM, KIT, BLM, SMAD4, PGDFRA, BMPR1A, APC, AXIN2, and STK11. *Vogelstein et al* [32] In a recent meta-analysis of 25 different genetic expression studies of colorectal cancer, a statistically significant down-regulation of carbonic anhydrase II (CAII) and CEACAM1 was observed, while there was up-regulation of TGFβ1, IFITM1, SPARC, GDF15 and MYC genes. [33] Based on these molecular patterns, a novel staging and classification system that is devoid of errors can now potentially be evolved.

2.3. Role of surgical pathology

The rationale behind the histopathologic use of slide sections from biopsy samples has been to evaluate for diagnostic purposes a representative microcosm of disease from a routinely processed, waxed, and miniaturized specimen blocks. However this has sometimes led to mis- or under- diagnosis of tumour depending on the exact site from which the biopsy was taken from. In principle, the goal of surgical resection is to take adequate 'tumour-free' margin; however achievement of this goal in practice is at best an estimated blind procedure, since cancer specific molecular alterations in the 'apparently' tumour free regions are largely unknown. This makes it difficult to readily determine the adequacy of a surgically resected margin. Not least, pathologists have had to take multiple biopsies from different sites in a resected tumour mass, trying to maximize the chances of locating the accurate tumour areas. This blind sampling procedure is a major potential source of diagnostic inaccuracies in practice and it is therefore important to detect colorectal cancer early to improve the chances of getting an adequate 'tumour free' surgical margin. Prompt surgical intervention, coupled with accurate determination of the most beneficial adjuvant therapy for the specific patient, appears to hold the key. Surgical pathology - which is the interface between surgery and pathologic specimen processing - is thus a vital control point for the eradication of diagnostic inaccuracies. Given the current molecular evidences on intratumour and interbiopsy heterogeneity, an exclusive morphology based sampling technique is a potential minefield for diagnostic errors, even with the best mastery.

A delicate balance needs to be achieved during sampling of surgical specimens for the assessment of tumour heterogeneity. The most prominent, average pattern of expression is most likely to be identified during sampling of a large tumour biopsy sample, but this approach risks masking the less prominent but potentially equally important information about sub-populations of tumour cells in the biopsy sample. By contrast, signal-to-noise ratios have to be carefully balanced when analysing smaller biopsy samples since this approach presents a smaller sampling frame within which it may be impractical to identify all possible biomarker signals a tumour could express. [34] Surgeons and pathologists also need to bear in mind the downstream requirements and applications of 'omics based research when surgical biopsy samples are taken, especially since mining the molecular archives of formalin fixed paraffin embedded (FFPE) specimens through genomics, proteomics and lipidomics research is beginning to gain traction now. However, factors such as age of tissue, condition of storage, tissue sample size, fixation time, pH influences and buffers are known to influence the outcome of 'omics based analyses on surgical specimens. [35] In particular, RNA degrades rapidly at room temperature, whilst formalin damages nucleic acids within the specimen by forming sclerotic crosslinks of DNA and RNA *via* methylol adducts and methylene bridges. [35] Thus, immediate snap freezing of fresh sections in liquid nitrogen or dry ice is good practice, whilst use of newer alcohol-based kits [36], or of phosphate buffered formalin [37, 38], provide useful alternatives to standard formalin for rapid fixation of surgical specimens prior transport to the lab.

2.4. Patient evaluation and therapeutic loopholes

Biomarker discovery research will in principle enable accurate stratification of patients into appropriate risk categories. The orthodox clinical approach of prescribing a common therapeutic cancer regimen to all colorectal cancer patients is fast becoming a subject of evidence-based debates. Certain differences exist between patients who come from demographically, geographically and genetically divergent backgrounds. Such inter-patient variability may also present significant differences in tumour phenotype, behavior and natural histories across a population, an important observation that is referred to as single nucleotide polymorphism (SNP) noise. [39] Patient stratification based on these natural clusters can enable meaningful biomarker discovery using 'omics based techniques. For instance, in a culturally heterogeneous South African population composed of Caucasians, Indigenous African, Indian, and Mixed Ancestries, the *a priori* expectation is that different racial groups may express different biomarkers of disease. In the same light, candidate biomarkers discovered from studies on developed world patient cohorts may not necessarily be effective for the management of colorectal cancer in a developing world situation due to differing ethnicities, which has clear implications for the planning and execution of 'omics based discovery and validation of biomarkers.

In principle, it is possible to predict response to specific targeted therapies (e.g. Herceptin) using 'omics based approaches, with patients who would not respond to specific targeted therapies being identified at the outset and given alternative therapies. Patient dependent source of variation for biomarker discovery includes individual genetic make-up, metabolism, stage of disease, health, immunocompetence, nutritional factors, and environmental factors. Careful patient selection to eliminate confounders must be carried out prior to experiments and biomarkers must be validated in a standardized acceptable manner.

Genetic profiling of patients for KRAS mutation, BRAF genes, Microsatellite instability (MSI) and CpG island methylator phenotypes (CIMP) is now being increasingly carried out for colorectal cancer patients in the developed world and this has contributed significantly to treatment planning. Patients that exhibit MSI have been found to possess better overall survival than those with chromosomal instability and are less affected by p53 mutations [40], whilst CRC with p53 +, MSI + profiles are usually more aggressive than those with p53-, MSI + profiles. [41] Biomarkers such as telomerase and survivin have been used to assess the long term risk of CRC development [42] whilst morphologic biomarkers in patients include neoplastic colorectal polyposis and the presence of aberrant cryptic foci (AFC); the presence of adenomas with Intraepithelial Neoplasm in the colorectal region can also be used in surveillance as surrogate endpoint biomarkers. [43] Paradoxically, most anti-cancer agents do not have well-established single predictors of individualized response, however with the advances in 'omics based approaches it should be possible to provide such molecular predictors. For example, MSI has been documented to be an effective predictor of response to fluoropyrimidine therapy, whilst ERCC1 was found to be beneficial in patients using platinum containing anticancer regimen. [31]

'Omics based techniques relevant to colorectal cancer management

The management of CRC has to date been based on fairly invasive techniques for diagnosis and treatment. In contrast, 'omics based techniques in most instances are non- or minimally invasive, thereby improving patient compliance, eliminating surgical morbidities and ultimately reducing the burden of disease through early diagnosis and effective treatment monitoring. The potential utility of increasingly common-place 'omics based techniques in the diagnosis, surveillance, treatment, and prevention of colorectal cancer is thus discussed below.

2.5. Genomics and epigenomics

Introduction: In genomic investigations, high-throughput technologies such as microarray platforms or DNA/ RNA sequencing are now commonplace. These technologies are now routinely applied to large sample collections, with complete clinical annotations, and aim to produce profound insights into disease at the resolution of single nucleotide polymorphisms, gene expression, and the status of epigenetic regulatory mechanisms such as hypo- and hypermethylation.

Extensive bioinformatic analysis of these high-throughput, multi-level, datasets has provided in-depth insights into the mechanisms of disease and treatment resistance. These findings have been translated into biomedical research aimed at addressing the significant challenge in treating cancer of the colorectum. While it is well established that cure rate for treating TNM stage I colorectal cancer is over 90%, the clinical management of stage II CRC is more complicated. [44, 45] Furthermore, improved chemo- or biological treatment regimens are needed to address the high rates of recurrent disease observed with stage II and III CRC disease, as well as for TNM stage IV disease which is generally considered incurable at present. [46, 47]

The overall disease-free survival statistics for TNM stage II disease, treated with surgery alone, are as high as 75%. [44] However, certain sub-populations of patients experience a worse prognosis and have clinical outcomes more similar to TNM stage III disease. Therefore, much focus has been on finding genetic markers to guide treatment regimen selection in stage II and III disease, the goal being to improve overall efficacy, decrease treatment failures, reduce the incidence of recurrent disease, whilst at the same time lowering the cost of treatment by limiting costly chemotherapeutics to those patients with predicted benefit.

High-throughput genomic studies today provide a comprehensive means to analyse amongst others the expression level of every individual gene, as well as to assess chromosomal segment copy number- and DNA methylation pattern variations and to determine single nucleotide polymorphism and mutation frequencies, all in a genome-wide manner. Biomarker research can thereafter be carried out to identify and validate distinct signatures derived from integrated value measurements associated with each gene, as a prelude to translating such findings into a clinical setting, as either biomarkers or novel therapeutic targets.

3. Transcriptomics

The field of transcriptomic research, within the context of prognosis and treatment outcome prediction, has seen much attention in recent years. High-volume real-time gene expression assays, gene expression microarrays and, more recently, 'next generation sequencing' based methods have provided the necessary platforms to investigate putative prognostic and predictive genetic markers. These platforms, combined with known clinical outcomes, enable panels of genes to be significantly correlated with prognosis, or the outcome of treatment with various chemotherapeutic agents. However, genetic association studies require large datasets in order to identify putative prognostic and predictive markers with significance worthy of clinical utility. As such, there are to date a limited number of landmark publications that present such multi-gene panel lists associated with prognosis and treatment outcome prediction in TNM stage II and III colon and rectal cancers.

A study by O'Connell et al [48] involved the combined analyses of four independent studies of colorectal cancer patients. Samples were obtained from 1851 CRC patients in the United States, with stage II or III disease, who participated in the National Surgical Adjuvant Breast and Bowel Project (C-01/C-02 and Cleveland Clinic (CC); C04; C-06) and 1136 candidate genes (761 genes assessed in C-01/C-02; 375 genes in CC/C-06) were evaluated. The aim of the study was to establish a panel of markers that could be associated with the risk of disease recurrence and that could determine the likelihood of patients benefitting from adjuvant 5-fluorouracil/leucovorin adjuvant therapy. The analyses resulted in the identification of 48 genes significantly associated with the risk of disease recurrence and 66 genes significantly associated with 5-FU/LV benefit (with four genes in common between the two sets). For practical reasons a gene panel of 7 genes predictive of disease recurrence, 6 predicted of 5-FU/LV benefit, and 5 reference genes were selected. The clinical utility of this predictive panel was then independently evaluated in the Quick and Simple and Reliable (QUASAR) study. [49] The aforementioned study validated the use of this gene panel, and it's consequent recurrence score, as an independent predictor of the risk of recurrent disease in stage II colon cancer patients who had undergone surgery. This gene panel was then commercialized by Genomic Health by the production of a multi-gene panel called the Oncotype DX® Colon Cancer Assay.

In separate work, Salazar et al [50] described a gene expression signature - named ColoPrint - in early 2011 that allowed for improved prediction of prognosis in TNM stage II and III colorectal cancer. The gene signature consists of 18 genes that were identified from analysis of 188 frozen tumour samples (TNM stage I-IV; 78.7% not treated with adjuvant chemotherapy), and a cross-validated on 206 independent tumour samples (TNM stage I-III; 60.7% not treated with adjuvant chemotherapy) originating from three sites in the Netherlands. This panel showed better predictive accuracy, in comparison to the American Society of Clinical Oncology criteria for assessing the risk of cancer recurrence without prescreening for microsatellite instability (MSI), with a hazard ratio of 2.69 (95% CI, 1.41 to 5.13; P = 0.003) for patients with stage II disease. Results such as these are encouraging, and provide strong supporting evidence for the utility of molecular approaches over purely clinical markers.

In a related study, a panel of 13 genes - referred to as ColoGuideEx - was reported by Ågesen *et al* [51] to be significantly associated with predicting prognosis for stage II colorectal cancer patients. This study was conducted on an initial dataset obtained from 207 colorectal samples originating from three independent Norwegian patient series, and validated on a 108-sample gene expression dataset originating from the USA and Australia. The independent prognostic value of the panel of genes was confirmed by multivariate Cox regression analyses (p≤0.004), which included various clinicopathological variables and all three-sample series.

O'Connell et al (2010)	O'Connell et al (2010) Oncotype DX® Colon Assay	Salazar et al (2011) ColoPrint®	Ågesen et al (2012) ColoGuideEx
5FU benefit	**Disease recurrence**	**Disease recurrence**	**Disease recurrence**
ATP5E	ATP5E	CA438802	AZGP1
AXIN2	BGN	CTSC	BNIP3
BIK	C-MYC	CYFIP2	CXCL10
EFNB2	FAP	EDEM1	CXCL13
GPX1	GADD45B	HSD3B1	DSC3
HSPE1	GPX1	IL2RA	ENPP3
MAD2L1	INHBA	IL2RB	EPHA7
PGK1	Ki-67	LAMA3	KLK6
RUNX1	MYBL2	LIF	MMP3
UBB	PGK1	MCTP1	PIGR
VDAC2	UBB	PIM3	SEMA3A
	VDAC2	PLIN3	SESN1
		PPARA	TUBA1B
		PYROX D1	
		SLC6A11	
		THNSL2	
		ZBED4	
		ZNF697	

Table 1. A list of multi-gene panels that are significantly associated with disease recurrence, or benefit from adjuvant 5-fluorouracil (5-FU) and leucovorin (LV) chemotherapy, as published in three independent studies.

Table 1 illustrates the various gene panels from the four studies described above and it is noteworthy that there are no genes in common between these gene panels. Furthermore, the biological relevance the genes utilised in each panel has yet to be fully explained and may represent an opportunity to identify pathologically associated genes and pathways when molecular enrichment analyses are applied across multiple gene panel studies in the context of prognostic and predictive biomarkers used in recurrent colorectal cancer. For example, there are genes across the lists in Table 1 that share a relationship by virtue of their KEGG pathway associations: (1) *Cytokine-cytokine receptor interaction* (n=6 genes; CXCL10 and CXCL13 [Chemokines; CXC subfamily] from Ågesen et al (2012), LIF [gpl30 shared] from Salazar et al (2011), IL2RA and IL2RB [IL2RG shared] from the Hematopoietins from Salazar et al (2011), and

INHBA [TGF-ß family] O'Connell et al (2010); (2) *Axon guidance* (n=3 genes; EPHA7 from Ågesen et al (2012), EFNB2 from O'Connell et al (2010), and SEMA3A from Ågesen et al (2012); (3) *Pathways in Cancer* (n=3 genes; LAMA3 from Salazar et al (2011), AXIN2 from O'Connell et al (2010), RUNX1 from O'Connell et al (2010)); (4) *p53 signaling pathway – target genes* (n=2 genes; SESN1 from Ågesen et al (2012), and GADD45B from O'Connell et al (2010)). These KEGG pathway association mappings were adapted from outputs generated by GeneCodis. [52-54]

In a novel study that utilised eight published prognostic and predictive gene expression signatures, Shi et al [55] combined the datasets and integrated them with publically available protein-protein interaction network data in order to identify candidate molecular markers associated directly with the recurrent colorectal cancer phenotype. As a result, they were able to not only infer pathophysiological mechanisms underpinning the recurrent disease phenotype, but also used the augmented and cross-study integrated signature to identify both a prognostic signature and a multi-gene signature to predict treatment outcome. The resultant gene signature consists of 487 genes and is referred to as the NEM signature (as it integrates information from Network, Expression, and Mutation datasets).

It is clear therefore that gene expression panels are developing to the point where they are close to translation into a clinical setting and adoption into routine clinical practice. It remains to be seen though how many of the published gene panels will make it into the clinic after appropriate validation studies have been carried out to assess performance across larger and more ethnically diverse patient populations. In this context, it is important to note that such signatures might yet be inherently compromised by the likely existence of multiple, possibly opposing, signatures in the same tissue sample (*vide supra*). Therefore, testing of multiple biopsies from the same tumour may be necessary in order to generate a holistic prognosis and to provide guidance on treatment strategy. Furthermore, in developing nations where the incidence of colorectal cancer is not yet decreasing and cases consistently present at more advanced stages of disease, it remains to be seen whether the cost of such diagnostic or prognostic panels will be affordable in the public sector where there is the most need and where the greatest diversity exists.

Single nucleotide polymorphisms: Colorectal cancer has classically been treated by 5-fluorouracil (Capecitabine; Xeloda®; Hoffmann-La Roche Inc.), combined with either Oxaliplatin (Eloxatin®; Sanofi-Synthélabo Inc.) or Irinotecan (Camptosar® or CPT-11; Pfizer Pharmaceuticals Inc.). Over the past decade these regimens have been augmented by the addition of biological therapeutic agents, such as the monoclonal antibodies Cetuximab (Erbitux®; ImClone Systems Inc.), Panitumumab (Vectibix®; Amgen Inc.), and Bevacizumab (Avastin®; Genentech Inc).

Each drug has a different mechanism of action and a unique set of molecular targets, as well as distinct sets of enzymes responsible for its metabolism; furthermore, particularly in the case of biological agents, specific enzymes that are functionally important to the pathways targeted by the biologic are major determinants of response. It is well-established that polymorphic variations in enzymes involved in drug metabolism can alter drug availability, thereby causing a variation in clinical response, by altering the rate and specificity of drug metabolism. Such variant drug metabolizing enzymes are generally encoded by single nucleotide polymorphisms (SNPs) that result in changes in the amino acid composition of the relevant gene product (i.e. protein), resulting in altered enzymatic activity. As such, the biomedical community has utilised an arsenal of molecular techniques, including high-throughput genomic platforms, to identify such SNPs and to quantify their frequency in populations in order to correlate with treatment outcomes and thereby to identify biomarkers that are predictive of therapeutic response.

This area of research has been comprehensively reviewed recently by Asghar et al [56], Bandrés et al [57], Benheim et al [58], Coate et al [59], De Roock et al [60], and Ross et al [61] and forms the basis of the rich pharmacogenetic resource, PharmGKB® (http://www.pharmgkb.org) which documents each therapeutic agent together with an aggregated list of SNPs reported in the literature to be associated with treatment outcome.

4. Pharmacogenomics

4.1. Markers of treatment outcomes when treated with classical chemotherapeutics

5-Fluorouracil: 5-Fluorouracil (5-FU) was introduced more than 50 years ago by Heidelberger et al [62] and is the foundational cytotoxic agent used in the treatment of colorectal neoplasia. 5-FU can be administered in three different physical forms: either through an intravenous solution, or as an oral compound (Capecitabine, and Tegafur). The metabolism of either of these compounds results in the formation of fluoronucleotides. A subset of these molecules, fluorouridine triphosphate (FUTP) and fluorodeoxyuridine monophosphate (FdUMP) are misincorporation into DNA and RNA during their *in vivo* biosynthesis. In addition, FdUMP inhibits thymidylate, synthase thereby resulting in a nucleotide imbalance due to a depleted intracellular reserve of thymidine for DNA synthesis. The enzymes responsible for producing the active metabolites have been studied for polymorphic variation and analysed for their correlation to treatment response (as seen in Table 2).

Gene	SNP	Molecular effect	Associated treatment outcome	Reference
TP		Increased expression	Increased response	Bandrés et al (2007)
TS	TSER2R	Decreased expression	Increased response	Bandrés et al (2007)
DPD	DYPD*2A	Decreased activity	Increased response Increased toxicity	Bandrés et al (2007)
MTHFR	677T	Increased production of CH_2FH_4	Increased response	Bandrés et al (2007)

Table 2. A list of single nucleotide polymorphism (SNP) markers associated with treatment outcome, as reported by Bandrés et al (2007), when using a 5-fluorouracil-based regimen.

Oxaliplatin: Oxaliplatin is a platinum analog that results in inter- and intra-molecular DNA cross-links, resulting in the inhibition of DNA synthesis, transcription and repair processes.

This compound has been extensively utilised in combination with 5-FU and Leucovorin, a regimen referred to as FOLFOX and commonly prescribed for treatment of advanced colorectal cancer.

There are two groups of genes that are primarily responsible for altered response to Oxaliplatin, namely genes involved in DNA repair and in glutathione conjugation reactions. In the former group, a polymorphism in the X-ray repair cross-complementing group 1 enzyme (XRCC1) - which is part of the base excision repair system - has been associated with variable initiation of DNA repair. [57] In addition, a polymorphism in a component of the ubiquitous nucleotide excision repair pathway - the excision repair cross complementing group 2 (ERCC2) gene - has been significantly associated with a clinical response to platinum-based chemotherapy. [57] However, there are no known polymorphisms in the DNA mismatch repair pathway associated with variation in treatment response with Oxaliplatin. In the second group, it has been reported that platinum compounds are inactivated by glutathione conjugation and therefore the enzymes responsible for catalyzing this reaction have been investigated. In particular, SNPs in several glutathione-S-transferase (GST) genes have been implicated in conferring resistance to Oxaliplatin. [57]

Gene	SNP	Molecular effect	Associated treatment outcome	Reference
GSTP1	613G	Decreased activity	Increased response	Bandrés et al (2007)
GSTT1	Deletion	Decreased activity	Increased response	Bandrés et al (2007)
GSTM1	Deletion	Decreased activity	Increased response	Bandrés et al (2007)
XRCC1	388Gln	Decreased activity	Increased response	Bandrés et al (2007)
ERCC2	751Gln	Decreased activity	Increased response	Bandrés et al (2007)

Table 3. A list of single nucleotide polymorphism (SNP) markers associated with treatment outcome, as reported by Bandrés et al (2007), when using a chemotherapeutic regimen that includes Oxaliplatin.

It is noteworthy that in a recent study by Fernandez-Rozadilla et al [63], seven SNPs (rs16857540, rs2465403, rs10876844, rs10784749, rs17626122, rs7325568, rs4243761) were found to be significantly associated with adverse drug reactions in the context of singular 5-FU or FOLFOX treatment. Given the relatively large sample size of 221 CRC patients and a validation set of 791 patients, these results hold strong statistical significance and provide potential predictive capacity for toxicity response on an individual patient basis if validated through a larger cohort.

Irinotecan (CPT-11): Irinotecan is a camptothecin analogue with well-established anti-neoplasia activity exerted though stabilization of the ordinarily transient DNA topoisomerase I-DNA complex, thus preventing the repair of temporary single stranded breaks during DNA replication and leading to cell death. [64] There are two primary pathways that have been implicated in variable response to Irinotecan treatment: drug transport into the extracellular environment, and metabolism of Irinotecan into its active (SN-38 and SN-38G) and inactive metabolites.

Hydrolysis of Irinotecan by carboxylesterases: CES1 and CES2 results in the production of its active metabolite, SN-38. This metabolite then undergoes detoxification via the process of glucuronidation, catalyzed by uridine diphosphate-glucurono-syltransferase 1A (UGT1A), to produce a metabolite called SN-38G which then interacts directly with the DNA topoisomerase I enzyme. However, Irinotecan can also be oxidized by members of the Cytochrome P450 3A subfamily (CYP3A) to produce inactivate metabolites. Each of these metabolites is transported out of the cell by the adenosine-triphosphate (ATP) binding cassette (ABC) transporter transmembrane proteins. As such, polymorphic variation in these enzymes has been associated with altered metabolism, transport and therapeutic efficacy of this drug and its metabolites. A selection of these SNPs is detailed in the Table 4.

Gene	SNP	Molecular effect	Associated treatment outcome	Reference
CES2	IVS10-88	Decreased expression	Decreased response	Bandrés et al (2007)
CYP3A	?	Decreased activity	Decreased response	Bandrés et al (2007)
UGT1A1	UGT1A1*28	Decreased activity	Increased response Increased toxicity	Bandrés et al (2007)
ABCB1	1236C"/>T	Decreased activity	Increased response Increased toxicity	Bandrés et al (2007)
ABCB1	3435C"/>T	Decreased activity	Increased response Increased toxicity	Bandrés et al (2007)
ABCC2	3792T		Increased response	Bandrés et al (2007)
ABCG2	421A	Decreased activity	Increased response	Bandrés et al (2007)

Table 4. A list of the single nucleotide polymorphism (SNP) markers associated with treatment outcome, as reported by Bandrés et al (2007), when using a chemotherapeutic regimen that includes Irinotecan (CPT-11).

Markers of treatment outcomes when treated with biological agents: In recent years there has been an emergence of a new class of antibody-based therapeutics that directly and specifically target molecules belonging to processes fundamental to cancer pathophysiology. Comprehensive reviews of the hallmarks of the cancer phenotype have been updated recently by Hanahan and Weinberg [65, 66]; in addition, comprehensive reviews of biomarkers associated with monoclonal antibody therapies that are currently in being used in the treatment of this disease have also been published recently. [56, 60]

Vascular endothelial growth factor as a target: It is well understood that tumours have angiogenic potential, i.e. they possess the ability to induce the production of new blood vessels, and thereby increase their supply of oxygen and nutrients; this characteristic provides an opportunity for therapeutic intervention, targeting the vascular endothelial growth factor (VEGF) and associated VEGF receptors (VEGFR-1, -2, and -3). In particular, overexpression of VEGF has been associated with vascularity, endothelial cell migration and invasion, poor prognosis and aggressiveness in most malignancies [67]; mAbs have thus been designed to target VEGF, thereby reducing the amount of free VEGF, reducing VEGF receptor activation, and ultimately reducing angiogenesis. [68] A recombinant humanized IgG1 monoclonal antibody, Bevacizumab, that specifically targets VEGF is currently indicated as part of combination therapy in metastatic colorectal cancer; however, a biomarker that is predictive of response to anti-VEGF therapy is yet to be discovered.

Epidermal growth factor receptor as a target: Another fundamental hallmark of the cancer phenotype is the ability for tumours to alter their response to growth factors through differential gene expression of growth factor receptors. This too presents the opportunity interrupt aberrant growth mechanisms. In colorectal cancer, it has been shown that there is an abnormal activation of epidermal growth factor receptor (EGFR). [69] As such, a humanized monoclonal antibody, Cetuximab, targeted at the extracellular domain of EGFR has been evaluated in clinical trials. This mAb blocks specific EGF-mediated signal transduction events [70], thereby inhibiting cellular proliferation and inducing apoptosis. [71] Treatment with Cetuximab also leads to increased responses to classic chemotherapeutic agents and radiotherapy, as well as inhibiting cellular proliferation, angiogenesis and metastasis. [72] Another recombinant human IgG2 monoclonal antibody, Panitumumab, which also targets EGFR is currently indicated in metastatic colorectal carcinoma where there has been resistance to fluoropyrimidine, Oxaliplatin, and Irinotecan containing regimens.

To date there have been a small but useful number of genes harboring mutations that provide insight into the outcome of anti-EGFR therapy. For example, the mutational status of the Kirsten-ras (KRAS) gene is currently being used in predicting treatment benefit in the context of anti-EGFR therapy for patients with metastatic disease. Other common genes with mutations relevant to anti-EGFR mAb therapy include BRAF and PIK3CA, as well as loss of expression of PTEN.

Conclusion: It is clear that SNP biomarkers associated with treatment outcome are generally found in genes with specific characteristics of cancer pathophysiology, or with drug metabolism and transport, and numerous low-throughput, focused, yet fruitful studies have resulted in clinically translatable SNP biomarkers being identified. This contrasts with the high-throughput transcriptomic approach to identification of biomarker gene panels that is typically initially blind to the functional significance of each individual gene. As such, these simple SNP markers present a cost-effective option to predicting the efficacy of a specific therapeutic agent, or combination thereof, prior to prescription, enabling design of individualized therapy that will result in increased efficacy and improved treatment outcomes.

5. Epigenomics and epigenetics

Molecular studies of cancer have revealed the presence of not only of genetic mutations, copy number alterations, altered gene expression, but also of aberrant epigenetic changes. Intense investigation in recent years has shown that epigenetic regulation of gene expression plays a crucial role in embryonic development, imprinting, and tissue differentiation. [73] Therefore, deregulation of such a fundamental mechanism might offer insight into the driving molecular mechanisms associated with the development, and regulation, of a carcinoma phenotype, particularly in cases where other genomic perspectives have not yet provided an answer.

In cancer studies, the field of epigenomics has encompassed investigations into aberrant DNA methylation, post-translational modification of histones that affects chromatin structure, altered expression of microRNAs and non-coding RNAs, and nucleosome positioning. [73-75] For complete reviews of this specific topic see Ballestar et al [76], Hatziapostolou et al [77], Khare et al [74], Lao et al [75], Liu et al [78], Sawan et al [79], Sharma et al [73], Ting et al [80], and van Engeland et al [81].

DNA methylation studies have focused particularly on the methylation patterns of cytosine and guanine (CpG)-rich DNA sequences. In particular, regions of the genome that have a higher than expected number of CpG nucleotides compared to the rest of the genome – so-called "CpG islands" – are of particular interest because they have been shown to overlap the promoter regions of 60-70% of genes. [75] An extension of this concept has been the discovery of CpG sites outside of promoter regions, referred to as "CpG Island shores", that are within two kilobases of the 5′ end of a CpG island. [75] Methylation of CpG islands is largely associated with transcriptional repression [75, 82] and, in general, CpG islands are protected from aberrant methylation but in cancer this does not appear to be the case. Since methylation changes can significantly alter gene expression profiles and thereby deregulate important biological pathways, a sound understanding of which genes and which associated pathways are affected in which individual patients might in the future be applied in the clinic to guide the selection of appropriate treatment regimens.

The first report of epigenetic alterations in tumours of the colon revealed an extensive loss of 5′-methylcytosine when compared to normal colon tissue. [83] However, it is only recently that this area of research has gained increased attention. Today, high-throughput methylation-specific microarray and sequencing technologies, together with a well-established array of commercially available methylation assay kits, have facilitated large-scale epigenomic investigations and contributed to an increased understanding of the methylome on a multi-gene scale.

Arguably the most important epigenetic finding to date, in the context of colorectal cancer, has been the identification of a unique molecular subtype characterized by a high frequency of gene methylation. Colorectal tumours of this variety are now referred to as having the CpG island Methylator Phenotype (CIMP). The exact panel for diagnosing CIMP varies from study to study, but the panel of genes proposed by Weisenberger et al [84] has been commonly used, i.e. *NEUROG1, SOCS1, RUNX3, IGF2,* and *CACNA1G.* In general, if a panel has more than 60% of its genes methylated, then is considered to be CIMP positive. Despite, the lack of a standardized CIMP diagnostic panel, this type of tumour is reported to be predominantly associated with right-sided colon cancer, and tends to be more common in woman. [84, 85]

Diagnosing CIMP tumours is clinically relevant because approximately 20% of colorectal tumours have this phenotype and generally share a high frequency of the BRAF c.1799T>A (p. V600E) mutation [75] that has been reported to negatively impact treatment outcomes in anti-

EGFR mAb-mediated therapy in patients with KRAS wild-type tumours and metastatic disease. [60, 86, 87] As such, classifying a patient's tumour as having the CIMP phenotype could be used in the future to guide the selection of biological therapeutics to ensure that the most efficacious treatment regimen is utilised.

The current lack of a standardized panel of genes from which to assess the status of genomic methylation highlights the fact that this is an emerging field of study. As such, the translation of these panels into the clinic as diagnostic or prognostic biomarkers is still premature. However, as the field progresses and more literature-based evidence is published in support and validation of a particular panel, the full potential of such epigenomic biomarkers may ultimately be translated into patient benefit.

While the field is currently in its infancy, there are a number of encouraging studies that represent good examples of novel discoveries of methylation markers that have highly significant associations. For example, Wang et al [88] examined the methylation status of five tumour suppressor genes in eighty-five paired colorectal tumours and normal mucosa samples from Chinese patients and showed that the methylation status of two genes, CDH13 and FLBN3, were significantly associated with stage of disease and prognosis. In particular, CDH13 was significantly associated with poor differentiation ($p=0.019$) and had a relatively strong association with advanced stage of disease ($p=0.084$). In a similar fashion, FLBN3 was significantly associated with advanced disease ($p=0.027$) and with the presence of lymph node metastasis ($p=0.029$). Furthermore, CDH13 and/or FLBN3 methylation status was found to be predictive of a poor overall survival ($p=0.001$) and conversely the presence of methylated hMHL1 indicated a better chance of survival ($p=0.046$).

In a clinical setting, samples that are obtained in a non- or minimally invasive manner are preferred and there have been a number of studies based on stool and blood plasma samples to assess aberrant methylation patterns. One example is the clinically validated methylation status of the Vimentin gene (*VIM*) - which has been found in the majority of colorectal tumours (53 – 84%; Lao et al 2011) – with assays conducted on stool samples, thus providing a non-invasive mechanism for early detection of colorectal cancer. This assay is currently commercially available in the United States as the ColoGuard assay (LabCorp), and reports a sensitivity of 83% and a specificity of 82%. [89, 90] Outside of the United States, in Europe and the Middle East there is now an additional non-invasive test for early detection of colorectal cancer by assessing the methylation status of *SEPT9*. This assay is currently commercially available as Epi *pro*Colon (Epigenomics AG).

The field of epigenomics, and epigenetics, applied to colorectal cancer is providing valuable insights into underlying mechanisms of this disease and seems to be a promising avenue of research. It is clear that assessing the status of DNA methylation alone holds prognostic and predictive value, and as such we would expect this field to gain much momentum towards translating these findings into a routine clinical setting. As this field of study can be conducted on a broad spectrum of sample types, along with commercially available kits to assess methylation, this field is likely to see an increased number of significant findings in the near future. However, as in the case of gene expression-based biomarkers, each epigenetic finding will need to be assessed in patients of diverse ethnicities. A recent study by Nieminen et al [91] highlighted this in observing that colorectal carcinomas in an Egyptian cohort had a significantly higher state of methylation, in microsatellite stable tumours, compared with sporadic colorectal cancers in a Finnish cohort.

5.1. Proteomics

The field of proteomics deals with identification of the total complement of peptides and proteins expressed in a cell, tissue or an organism and is in principle more directly related to phenotypic changes associated with disease pathogenesis. Proteomic studies are able to define: the functional state of protein activities; protein-ligand interactions; protein-protein interactions; and a host of dynamic post-translational modifications such as glycosylation, phosphorylation, ubiquitinylation, SUMOylation, proteolytic cleavage, lipoylation and acetylation of proteins. The proteome of a cell may vary from one time point to another and in different states of health and disease so proteomics techniques have been employed to identify cancer specific proteomes as a means to identify candidate biomarkers of early disease. A huge amount of data is generated from single proteomic experiments and these are typically analyzed to understand the mechanistic pathways of pathologic events in protein networks using various databases, workflows and algorithms. For proteomics analysis, complex mixtures of proteins derived from a given biological sample are typically rendered into a set of peptides via proteolysis, most commonly using the enzyme trypsin; direct liquid chromatography-tandem mass spectrometry (LC-MS/MS) based methods are then typically employed to separate, quantify and identify thousands of individual tryptic peptides in a sample [92-94], from which the identity and quantity of the parent proteins in the original biological sample can be inferred. For example, one notable recent study identified and quantified >7,000 unique proteins from FFPE tissue blocks from individual colorectal cancer patients [95], amply demonstrating the potential of the technology.

Common sources of current proteomics biomarkers for CRC include stool, blood, biopsy and urine samples. A common fecal proteomics biomarker in use today is hemoglobin [96], while carcinoembryonic antigen (CEA) is a common blood-based biomarker currently in use. [97] Tissue inhibitor of metalloproteinase 1 (TIMP-1) has also been used and has been found useful in the early detection of cancer although, paradoxically, other studies using multivariate analysis have described TIMP-1 as independent of the stage of cancer. [98] Proteasome activator complex subunit-3 (PSME-3), nicotinamide N-methyltransferase (NNMT), collapsin response mediator protein-2 (CRMP-2), MIF, M2-PK, M-CSF, HNP 1-3, CCSA-2, CCSA-3, CCSA-4, laminin, MMP-9, MMP-7, and a host of other serum proteomics biomarkers are being developed and optimized for clinical use. For example, surface enhanced laser desorption-ionisation (SELDI) mass spectrometry was used to analyze the serum of 62 CRC patients compared to 31 controls, and four proteomic markers were found in detectable levels in the serum of CRC patients: apolipoprotein C1, alpha-1-antitrypsin, C3a-desArg and transferrin. [99] A separate study carried out at the Mayo Clinic revealed elevated levels of 5 serum biomarkers in CRC: DcR3, TRAIL-2, spondin-1, MIC 1 and Reg IV [100]; usefully, this '5-biomarker panel' has been reported to exceed the performance of CEA both in specificity and sensitivity. Immunoproteomics - involving techniques such as immunoblotting, ELISA and immunocapture-mass spectrometry - has also yielded candidate biomarkers in CRC, including antibodies against inosine monophosphate dehydrogenase II [101], MUC-5A, MUC-1, MAPKAPK3, AVCR2B, HlpA, RpL7/L12, and nucleobindin- 1. [102-106]

5.2. Lipidomics

Lipidomics is a novel 'omics field which deals with complex large scale analysis of the full complement of various classes of lipids and lipid networks expressed by a cell, tissue or organism (the 'lipidome') and involves the high throughput systems-level identification and quantification of lipid metabolic pathways that may be involved in disease using chromatographic methods coupled to mass spectrometry. Generally, lipids are hydrophobic molecules that are involved in energy storage, structural components of a cell, cell signaling, endocrine actions, signal transduction, membrane trafficking, and morphogenesis. Structurally, lipids can be classified as: fatty acids; glycerolipids; glycerophospholipids; sphingolipids; sterol lipids; prenol lipids; saccharolipids; and polyketides. These 8 classes of lipids can also be further subdivided into several subclasses.

Whilst there is currently a paucity of clinically validated lipidomics biomarkers for colorectal cancer, the prospects of this field to complement proteomics and genomics in a combined 'systems biology' approach for disease detection, monitoring and treatment is worth consideration since over the past two decades, numerous publications have described the perturbation of lipid metabolism and signaling in colorectal carcinogenesis. [107-110] Lipidomics analysis of primary and metastatic colorectal cancer cell lines (SW480 and SW620) identified 600 and 694 lipids respectively in 'shotgun' study [111]; increased level of triglyceride lipid and plasmacholine were observed, while a decrease in the level of C-16 containing sphingomyelin, ceramide lipid and plasmenylethanolamine were observed in the metastatic CRC cell line compared to the primary isogenic CRC cell line, implying that lipidomic biomarkers of metastatic CRC disease might be plausible.

Empirically, polyunsaturated fatty acids have been known to be more beneficial in the prevention of colorectal diseases compared to saturated long-chain types, but the pathways related to this were largely unclear. The emergence of lipidomics techniques however has revealed that metabolic control of long chain fatty acids is an important factor in development of CRC, with short chain fatty acids from the gut microflora/ microbiome being described as onco-preventive. [112]

Elevated level of lysophosphatidic acid - a phosphoglyceride - has been described as a prospective cancer biomarker of ovarian tumours [113-115] but, paradoxically, a marked decrease in the serum level of lysophosphatidylcholine has been reported in CRC. [116] Similarly, elevated profiles of phosphatidylcholine and choline kinase activity have been demonstrated it colon cancers [117] and a high ratio of phosphatidylcholine to phosphatidylethanolamine has been used to differential metastatic colon cancers from localized ones. [118] Elevated levels of sphingomyelin have also been reported to characterize human colon cancer, based on nuclear magnetic resonance (NMR) studies [119], whilst cancer cell motility was shown to be down-regulated by the interaction between CD9 and sialoglycosphingolipid GM3 using CRC cell lines [120] and ceramides have been found to induce apoptosis in CRC cell lines

(HT-29, LOVO, and HCT-116). [121-123] Urinary phospholipids analysis using nanoflow LC-ESI MS/MS has been previously used for the analysis of breast [124, 125]) and prostate cancer [124], but there is a dearth of literature on the application of this method to colorectal cancer. Interestingly though, urinary levels of metabolites of prostaglandin E_2 have been used as a biomarker for colorectal cancer risk evaluation. [126, 127] Overall, these observations of disease-associated variation in colorectal cancer lipid profiles provide a sound precedent for the future development of reliable lipidomics biomarkers.

5.3. Metabolomics

The relatively new field of 'omics techniques that investigates the presence and abundance of low molecular weight metabolites in cells and body fluids is known as 'metabolomics'. This new branch in the 'omics world has emerged to address molecular biologic problems that have hitherto not been amenable to genomics or proteomics approaches. Common specimens compatible with metabolomics experiments include urine, serum and tissue. As is the case for genomics, proteomics and lipidomics, the 'metabolome' changes depending on physiologic and pathologic states of an individual and identification of unique metabolites provides potentially useful insight into pathogenetic mechanism of disease.

A number of analytical techniques have been used for metabolomics research, including: gas chromatography mass spectrometry (GC-MS); liquid chromatography mass spectrometry (LC-MS); capillary electrophoresis mass spectrometry (CE-MS); matrix assisted laser desorption-ionization mass spectrometry (MALDI-MS); and nuclear magnetic resonance (NMR). [128] By way of example, metabolomics studies on CRC patient serum samples, using a combination of proton-NMR and GC-MS techniques, was used to differentiate locoregional CRC from metastatic types as well as to identify CRC that metastasized to the liver. [129] Separately, in a review of eight metabolomics studies on CRC for diagnostic accuracy and distinguishing metabolites, twelve metabolites were found to be elevated. [130] In a further study using GC-MS, 34 endogenous metabolites were found significantly elevated in CRC compared with health individual, whilst the serum 3-hydroxybutyric acid level was noted to be reduced. [131] A predictive model developed in yet another study comprised of 2-hydroxybutyrate, kynurenine, cystamine and aspartic acid and was found to have specificity, sensitivity and accuracy as high as 85%, 85%, and 85% respectively. [128] Finally, Cheng et al [132] found evidence of dysregulation of several metabolic pathways through urine analysis of colorectal cancer patients, whilst Qui et al [133] also observed evidence of similar perturbations in tricarboxylic acid (TCA) and tryptophan metabolic pathways. With a solid foundation, a panel of metabolite markers may ultimately be developed for metabolomic profiling of colorectal patients as a means to improve diagnosis.

5.4. Molecular Imaging

Visualisation of precursor lesions and of malignant tissue is a major aspect of diagnosis and monitoring of therapeutic interventions in oncology. Classically this has been carried out using anatomical and functional technologies, such as Ultrasound (US), Computerised Tomography (CT), and Magnetic Resonance Imaging (MRI). While these approaches have been the mainstay of medical imaging, they are limited to information at the gross anatomical and physiological levels respectively. Recent years have however seen the emergence of molecular imaging and its addition to the repertoire of techniques to visualise disease.

In previous sections we have discussed how a range of different 'omics technologies have facilitated an in-depth view of the pathophysiology and molecular pathology of cancer. These insights provide candidate biomarkers based on the identification of differentially expressed genes and proteins between tumours and normal tissue. These biomarkers have either been associated with prognosis, stage of disease, molecular subtypes, predictors of treatment outcome, and markers of discriminating carcinoma from benign lesions at the molecular level.

In this light, molecular imaging is then the science of utilising the ever-increasing knowledge of cancer molecular pathology to: identify the appropriate molecular targets; design molecular constructs to selectively and specifically interact with them; and produce a visual signal that is measurable through an imaging technology. In order for this methodology to succeed at the molecular level, the target should be available for interaction and should be unique enough to ensure selective and specific interactions. Furthermore, once a signal has been generated from the appropriate interaction, it is important that a suitably sensitive imagining technology exists in order to visualise, and quantify, signal emission.

In the context of colorectal cancer, plasma-membrane associated proteins are generally considered good candidate targets since they are reasonably accessible and a subset of them play vital roles in signal transduction. In a similar fashion, aberrantly expressed or deregulated intracellular and secreted enzymes represent potentially useful targets for molecular imaging, based on their ability to catalyse formation of spectroscopically-measurable products. Both of these types of targets are accessible through the extensive vascularisation of the colorectum, but more importantly these targets can be accessed via the luminal surface through topical application of an appropriately designed molecular construct.

Molecular imaging provides tremendous opportunities to enhance the early detection of CRC, as well as potentially aiding the demarcation of clear margins during surgical resection, as reviewed recently by Abdullah [134], Seaman et al [135] and Akin et al [136].

By way of illustration of the potential of molecular imaging methods, colorectal cancers have been found to naturally emit a red fluorescent signal due to the accumulation of protoporphyrin IX (PpIX) in primary colorectal tumours and associated metastases located in lymph nodes. [137] These authors postulated that endogenous PpIX accumulates as a result of aberrant metabolic changes in the CRC cells; Kemmner et al [138] subsequently provided supporting evidence for this hypothesis by showing that there is a significant down-regulation of ferrochelatase (FECH) mRNA expression in gastric, colon, and rectal carcinomas, leading to accumulation of PpIX. In an effort to utilise this information Moesta et al [137] found that metastatically involved lymph nodes could be identified compared to all other palpable nodes; in the context of previously untreated patients (n=24), this observation had a sensitivity of 62% and a specificity of 78% ($p < 0.0001$). However, in a neoadjuvant setting there was a reduction in PpIX fluorescence in primary tumours, and a drastic reduction of fluorescent signal in metastases that resulted in not being able to discriminate between lymph nodes containing metastatic cells. In a follow-up study by Wan et al [139], conducted in xenografted nude mice, a novel siRNA-mediated knockdown of FECH was used to enhance the accumulation of PpIX, thereby increasing the endogenous fluorescence in tumour cells. While these results still need to be developed further, and tested in a clinical trial, they do hold promise for increasing the accuracy of early detection of primary and metastatic lesions and monitoring therapeutic response based on the size of the visualised tumour.

In different work, differential gene expression profiling, confirmed by immunohistochemistry, demonstrated that matrix-metalloproteases (MMPs) are differentially expressed in the context of colorectal adenocarcinoma by macrophage subpopulations and, at times, by the tumours themselves. MMPs are a family of zinc-dependent endopeptidases with multiple human peptidase members. For example, MMP-9 is able to degrade specific components of the extracellular matrix, including type IV collagen, after activation of the secreted zymogen [140] and as a direct consequence, malignant cells are thereby able to become mobile and achieve metastatic potential.

Of particular interest to surgical resection was the finding that colorectal adenocarcinomas express MMP-9 *via* a distinct macrophage subpopulation found at the edge of primary tumours and local lymph node metastases. [140] Fudala et al [141] have subsequently designed a dual fluorophore beacon molecule that is specifically cleaved by MMP-9, resulting in the emission of a specific fluorescent signal, suggesting that if a suitably non-invasive and anti-immunogenic method is developed to administer the beacon molecule to an anatomical structure under investigation, then accurate measurement of the tumour edge may be possible during surgical resection procedures.

As can be seen from the above examples, molecular imaging holds considerable promise for application in CRC. As this field becomes more developed and is validated through clinical trials, it should provide improved visualisation ability coupled with the ability to quantify specific molecules, enabling novel insights into diagnosis, prognosis, treatment response monitoring, and underlying tumour physiology and molecular pathology in CRC.

5.5. Cancer nanotechnology

Nanotechnology as a division of engineering concerned with the manipulation of atomic and subatomic molecules has recently found its place in the detection, staging, imaging, and management of human cancers. Various physical, chemical and biologic principles have been applied to improve the diagnosis and treatment using elements and molecules in the Nano-range ($\sim 10^{-9}$). [142]

For diagnosis of CRC, nanoparticles have been used to enhance the precision and reliability of colonoscopy and other conventional diagnostic methods, largely resulting in earlier detection and obviating variables such as operator skills and speed of examination. Quantum dots (QD) and surface-enhanced Raman scattering (SERS) are two important nano- methodologies used to improve tissue based diagnosis of cancer, avoiding the cumbersome protocols and lower reliability of multiplexed tissue staining. Both methods have the ability to detect multiple biomolecular signals in a single cancer cell. Gold and silver particles have been derivatized and stabilized with Raman active particles and silica respectively for used in generating composite organic and inorganic nanoparticles (COINs) for potential improvement of biopsy diagnosis. [143] Simultaneous Multiple Aptamers and RGD Targeting (SMART) cancer probes have also been used to detect multiple cancer biomarker signals using currently available imaging techniques. [144] Superconducting quantum interference device (SQUID) sensors and magnetic relaxometry - which are both nanotechnology based techniques - have been reported to be more accurate in the diagnosis of breast cancer than mammography and MRI respectively. KRAS mutant alleles have been detected in gastrointestinal malignancies, including colorectal carcinoma, using nanofluidic digital PCR which showed a better performance in detection of mutation KRAS in colorectal adenomas compared to conventional PCR. [145] Nanoparticles have been coupled with short cancer specific oligonucleotides (aptamers) for targeted binding to prostate specific membrane antigen positive cells in prostate cancer cell lines. [146] Finally, serum detection of colorectal cancer has been achieved with gold nanoparticles using SERS spectroscopy in a study which exemplified the use of this approach as a viable, minimally invasive screening method for colorectal cancer. [147]

Nanotechnology also has significant potential in the development of targeted therapeutics for cancer, with many studies currently at experimental- and a few at clinical validation stages. Different types of nanostructures, including mesoporous silica nanoshells, dendrimers, supramagnetic iron cores, nanosuspensions, gold nanoparticles, nanolipogels, nanoemulsions, carbon nanotubes, titanium oxide nanoparticles, liposomes, polymeric miscelles, and other lipid based nanoparticles have been used as drug delivery vehicles and facilitators of targeted cancer therapies. [148-155] Although most of the cancer nanodiagnostic and nanotherapy studies are still in their infancy, it seems clear that nanotechnology will play an important role in colorectal cancer diagnostics and therapeutics in the future.

6. Prospects of 'Omics based molecular approaches in colorectal cancer diagnosis and treatment in a developing country: A case study in Cape Town

Groote Schuur Hospital, situated in Cape Town, South Africa, is a quaternary hospital where the many colorectal cancer patients from the Western Province region are treated by combinations of radiotherapy, colonic resection and standard chemotherapeutic regimens. However, there are two complicating factors involved in treating these patients with the greatest efficacy: (1) the relatively high cost of utilising platinum- or modern monoclonal antibody-based regimens; and (2) the fact that the majority of patients present with advanced stages of disease, typically between TNM stage II and III. As mentioned earlier, these stages of disease have relatively high recurrence rates and as such timely diagnosis and efficacious treatment schedules are needed to reduce disease recurrence and improve patient prognoses.

To illustrate this point, consider the cost of the standard chemotherapeutic regimen of 5-fluorouracil (5-FU) alone versus Oxaliplatin: One cycle of Oxaliplatin costs approximately ZAR 5,000.00 (~USD 560), while one cycle of 5-FU is drastically less at a cost of ZAR 200 (~USD 22).

The response rate obtained with 5-FU alone can be improved by utilising Leucovorin (LV) in a combination therapy approach. However, it has been observed that the further addition of Oxaliplatin or Irinotecan can improve the stage II/III CRC response rates drastically to around 40 – 50%. [156, 157] The relatively recent appearance of monoclonal antibody based therapies has also offered significant gains in treatment response rates.

South Africa is a developing nation with a limited budget for treating non-communicable diseases such as cancer, not least because a large proportion of the country's healthcare budget is understandably spent on addressing the concurrent HIV/AIDS and TB epidemics (see for example the Lancet series on "Health in South Africa" published in 2009, with particular emphasis on the following publications: Abdool et al [158]; Chopra et al [159]; Coovadia et al [160]; and Mayosi et al [161]). Considering these financial constraints, two possible situations can be envisaged in which a patient treated in the public sector (i.e. subject to government healthcare budgets) could access platinum-based regimens and/or modern biological therapeutic agents:

The first opportunity for a patient to access medication with greater efficacy would be through participation in clinical trials conducted by pharmaceutical companies either wanting to assess their treatment in ethnically diverse cohorts (which could be required by local regulatory authorities) or to explore a new disease indication for an existing therapeutic agent. The second opportunity might be one afforded by the use of 'omics approaches, leveraging biomarker panels to provide predictive indications of whether or not a patient might benefit from a particular chemo- or biological therapeutic agent. Furthermore, given the heterogeneity of tumours and the unique molecular subtypes of colorectal cancer, it would be instructive to assess the relative likelihood of recurrent disease. Such a measurement could be used to motivate the aggressiveness of the treatment regimen prescribed.

In terms of possible cost effective benefits from the addition of platinum-based drugs to the standard regimen of 5-FU and LV, a trial conducted in the United Kingdom found that the relative levels of topoisomerase-1 (Topo1), assessed by routine immunohistochemistry, could be used to identify patient subpopulations who could potentially benefit from the addition of Oxaliplatin to their 5-FU/LV regimen [162]. Furthermore, Paré and colleagues [163] reported that a particular polymorphism in the excision repair cross-complementing 1 *ERCC1* gene (codon 118) can predict response and overall survival in patients treated with an Oxaliplatin/ 5-FU/LV regimen. Provided that these markers are further validated in a clinical setting, it then stands to reason that a simple immunohistochemical or real-time polymerase chain reaction assay could therefore be routinely requested to determine likely response to Oxaliplatin and therefore to motivate additional expenditure on an Oxaliplatin-supplemented regimen. This type of personalised approach has the obvious advantage of improving treatment efficacy, and reducing the risk of disease recurrence with a concomitant cost saving for the hospital authority from not having to conduct lengthy additional treatments, after possible first round treatment failure.

Similarly, assessment of the common SNPs that are predictive of benefit from the limited array of biological agents (e.g. the mutational status of the KRAS and BRAF genes) could provide an indication of whether or not the comparatively expensive anti-epidermal growth factor receptor mAb therapy should be prescribed.

As discussed above, a number of gene expression panels could also be used to predict patient prognosis and the associated likelihood of disease recurrence, with results being used to design a personalised treatment regimen in which the aggressiveness of the treatment schedule correlates with the severity of disease, the most likely prognosis and the likelihood of recurrence. In this context, Genomic Health's Onco*type* DX® Colon Cancer Assay costs ~USD 3,200 [45], which translates to approximately ZAR 28,560 in South Africa; this assay could provide a very useful clinical metric of the likelihood of recurrence, particularly in complicated TNM stage II cases and stage III cases where recurrence rates are still unfavorably high, but in reality such a test is beyond the financial means available for treatment of CRC disease at a public facility in South Africa today, not least since its cost dwarfs even that of Oxaliplatin-based treatments. The prospects for wide uptake of the Onco*type* DX® Colon Cancer Assay in South Africa therefore seem remote.

As the complexities of biopsy heterogeneity are addressed by the biomedical community, it is thus clear that local validation studies of simple and cost-effective, assays will be necessary to ensure that the prognostic and treatment outcome biomarkers reported in the literature apply to the diverse ethnicities in South Africa. Given the financial constraints imposed by the government funded healthcare system, it appears that relatively inexpensive techniques such as PCR based SNP assays would be well-suited to the public sector since, despite being a simple, low cost assay, the results could have a profound impact on treatment outcomes for the patients afflicted with this disease. Importantly, if utilised correctly such a molecular diagnostics strategy could actually result in significant cost savings mid-term for the hospitals administering care by avoiding the complexities of treatment failures.

7. Conclusion

'Omics based techniques represent novel, scientifically sound approaches to the diagnostic and therapeutic aspects of managing colorectal cancer patients, but there remain very significant challenges regarding their uptake and wide utilisation in developing world healthcare settings, primarily due to financial considerations. None-the-less, surgeons, clinicians, basic medical researchers and all other healthcare workers at the cutting edge of colorectal cancer management need to remain abreast of the prospects and potential effectiveness of integrating molecular approaches in to colorectal cancer management. The old paradigm where patients had no active choice or participation in their disease management, with treatment choices being exclusively the decision of the clinician, is under threat today since many patients now have access to information about emerging therapeutic options *via* the internet. It is therefore important that surgeons and clinicians, in spite of their invariably tight schedules, consider some form of participation in basic medical research in order to contribute clinical perspectives as well as to improve their understanding of molecular approaches to diagnosis and treatment.

Acknowledgements

HA thanks the ICGEB for a PhD scholarship; RWG thanks the National Research Foundation (NRF), South Africa, for a PhD scholarship; JB thanks the NRF for a Research Chair.

Author details

Henry Adeola[1,2], Ryan William Goosen[1], Paul Goldberg[1,3] and Jonathan Blackburn[1]

1 Institute of Infectious Disease & Molecular Medicine, Department of Clinical Laboratory Science, Faculty of Health Sciences, University of Cape Town, South Africa

2 International Centre for Genetic Engineering and Biotechnology, Cape Town, South Africa

3 Surgical Gastroenterology Unit, Department of Surgery, Groote Schuur Hospital, Cape Town, South Africa

References

[1] Cancer Genome Atlas Research Network. Comprehensive genomic characterization defines human glioblastoma genes and core pathways. Nature 2008; 455: 1061-68.

[2] Cancer Genome Atlas Research Network. Integrated genomic analyses of ovarian carcinoma. Nature 2011; 474: 609-15.

[3] Cancer Genome Atlas Network. Comprehensive molecular characterization of human colon and rectal cancer. Nature 2012; 487: 330-37.

[4] GLOBOCAN cancer fact sheets 2008 (IARC). Available at: http://globocan.iarc.fr/factsheets/cancer/colorectal.asp. Accessed June 26, 2012.

[5] Mqoqi N, Kellet P, Sitas F et al. Cancer in South Africa, 1998-1999. National Cancer Registry of South Africa, National health Laboratory Service, Johannesburg, 2004.

[6] Slaughter DP, Southwick HW, Smejkal W. "Field Cancerization" in oral stratified squamous epithelium. Cancer 1953; 6 (5): 963-968.

[7] Tabor MP, Braakhuis BJ, Van der Waal JE et al. Comparative molecular and histological grading of epithelial dysplasia of the oral cavity and the oropharynx. J Pathol 2003; 199: 354-360.

[8] Braakhuis BJ, Brakenhoff RH, Leeman CR. Second field tumors: a new opportunity for cancer prevention. The Oncologist 2005; 10: 493-500.

[9] Bernstein C, Bernstein H, Payne CM et al. Field defects in progression to gastrointestinal tract cancers. Cancer Letters 2008; 260: 1-10.

[10] McDonald SA, Greaves LC, Gutierrez- Gonzalez L et al. Mechanism of field cancerization in the human stomach: the expansion and spread of mutated gastric stem cells. Gastroenterology 2008; 134: 500-510.

[11] Jass JR. Classification of colorectal cancer based on correlation of clinical, morphological and molecular features. Histopathology 2007; 50: 113-130.

[12] Yap TA, Gerlinger M, Futreal PA et al. Intratumor heterogeneity: Seeing the wood for the trees. Sci Transl Med 2012; 4 (127): 127ps10.

[13] Michor F, Polyak K. The origin and implication of intratumor heterogeneity. Cancer Prev Res (Phila) 2010; 3(11): 1361-1364.

[14] Gerlinger M, Rowan AJ, Horswell S et al. Intratumour heterogeneity and branched evolution revealed by multiregion sequencing. N Engl J Med 2012; 366 (10): 883-93.

[15] Rocco A, Compare D, Nardone G. Cancer stem cell hypothesis and gastric carcinogenesis: experimental evidence and unsolved questions. World J Gastrointest Oncol 2012; 4 (3): 54-59.

[16] Luo W, Wu F, Atlas SR et al. Defining genetic intra-tumour heterogeneity: a chronological annotation of mutational pathways. Proceedings in Obstetrics and Gynecology 2010; 1 (1): 9.

[17] Durrett R, Foo J, Leder K et al. Intratumor heterogeneity in evolutionary models of tumor progression. Genetics 2011; 188 (2): 461-77.

[18] Iwasa Y, Michor F. Evolutionary dynamics of intratumor heterogeneity. PLoS One 2011; 6 (3): e17866.

[19] Polley AC, Mulholland F, Pin C et al. Proteomic analysis reveals field-wide changes in protein expression in the morphologically normal mucosa of patients with colorectal neoplasia. Cancer Res. 2006 Jul 1;66(13):6553-62.

[20] Chen LC, Hao CY, Chiu YS et al. Alteration of gene expression in normal-appearing colon mucosa of APC(min) mice and human cancer patients. Cancer Res. 2004 May 15;64(10):3694-700.

[21] Hao CY, Moore DH, Wong P et al. Alteration of gene expression in macroscopically normal colonic mucosa from individuals with a family history of sporadic colon cancer. Clin Cancer Res. 2005 Feb 15;11(4):1400-7.

[22] Hao CY, Moore DH, Chiu YS et al. Altered gene expression in normal colonic mucosa of individuals with polyps of the colon. Dis Colon Rectum. 2005 Dec;48(12): 2329-35.

[23] Suter CM, Martin DI, Ward RL. Hypomethylation of L1 retrotransposons in colorectal cancer and adjacent normal tissue. Int J Colorectal Dis. 2004 Mar;19(2):95-101. Epub 2003 Oct 8.

[24] Kreso A, O'Brien CA, van Galen P et al. Variable clonal repopulation dynamics influence chemotherapy response in colorectal cancer. Science 2013 Feb 1;339(6119):543-8. doi: 10.1126/science.1227670. Epub 2012 Dec 13.

[25] Fisher R, Larkin J, Swanton C. Inter and intratumour heterogeneity: a barrier to individualized medical therapy in renal cell carcinoma. Frontiers in oncology 2012; 2 (49): 1-5.

[26] Swanton C, Larkin JM, Gerlinger M et al. Predictive biomarker discovery the parallel integration of clinical trial and functional genomics datasets. Genome Med 2010; 2: 53-63.

[27] Duke CE. The classification of Cancer of the rectum. Journal of Pathologic Bacteriology 1932; 35: 323-32.

[28] Astler VB, Coller FA, The prognostic significance of direct extension of carcinoma of the colon and rectum. Am Surg 1954; 139 (6): 846- 852.

[29] Edge SB, Byrd DR, Compton CC et al. Cancer staging manual. AJCC (American joint committee on cancer). 7th ed. New York, Springer 2010.

[30] Ogino S, Goel A. Molecular Classification and Correlates in Colorectal Cancer. Journal of Molecular Diagnostics 2008; 10 (1): 13-27.

[31] Bohanes P, LaBonte MJ, Winder T et al. Predictive Molecular Classifiers in Colorectal Cancer. Seminars in Oncology 2011; 38 (4): 576-87.

[32] Vogelstein B, Kinzler KW. Cancer genes and the pathway they control. Nat Med 2004; 10 (8): 789-99.

[33] Chan SK, Griffith OL, Tai IT et al. Meta-analysis of Colorectal Cancer Gene Expression profiling studies identifies Consistently Reported Candidate Biomarkers. Cancer Epidemiol Biomarkers Prev 2008; 17: 543-52

[34] Diaz- Cano SJ. Tumour Heterogeneity: Mechanism and bases for a reliable application of molecular marker design. Int. J. Mol. Sci. 2012; 13: 1951-2011.

[35] Nirmalan NJ, Harnden P, Selby PJ et al. Mining the archival formalin-fixed paraffin-embedded tissue proteome: opportunities and challenges. Mol BioSyst 2008; 4: 712-20.

[36] Dotti I, Bonin S, Basili G et al. Effect of formalin, Methacarn, and FineFIX fixatives on RNA preservation. Diagn Mol Pathol 2010; 19 (2): 112-22.

[37] Chung JY, Braunschweig T, Williams R et al. Factors in tissue handling and processing that impact RNA obtained from formalin-fixed, paraffin-embedded tissue. J Histochem Cytochem 2008;56:1033–42.

[38] Gnanapragasam VJ. Unlocking the molecular archive: the emerging use of formalin-fixed paraffin-embedded tissue for biomarker research in urological cancer. BJU International 2009; 105: 274-78.

[39] Bakay M, Chen Y, Borups R et al. Sources of variablility and effect of experimental approaches on expression profiling data interpretation. BMC Bioinformatics 2002; 3:4.

[40] Popat S, Hubner R, Houlston RS. Systematic review of microsatellite instability and colorectal cancer prognosis. J Clin Oncol 2005; 23: 609-18.

[41] Mori S, Ogata Y, Shirouzu K et al. Biological features of sporadic colorectal carcinoma with high-frequency microsatellite instability: special reference to tumor proliferation and apoptosis. Int J Clin Oncol 2004; 9: 322-29.

[42] Soreide K, Gudlaugsson E, Skaland I et al. Metachronous cancer development in patients with sporadic colorectal adenomas- multivariate risk model with independent and combined value of hTERT and surviving. Int J Colorectal Dis 2008; 23: 389-400.

[43] Soreide K, Nedrebo BS, Knapp JC et al. Evolving molecular classification by genomic and proteomic biomarkers in colorectal cancer: potential implication for the surgical oncologist. Surgical Oncology 2009; 18: 31-50.

[44] Markowitz SD, Dawson DM, Willis J et al. (2002). Focus on colon cancer. Cancer cell; 1: 233-6.

[45] Carlson B. Putting a lid on chemotherapy costs. Biotechnol Healthc. 2011; 8(2):15-8.

[46] Libutti SK, Saltz LB, Tepper JE. Colon cancer. In: DeVita, V. T. Jr, Lawrence, T. S., Rosenberg, S. A. eds. DeVita, Hellman, and Rosenberg's cancer: principles and practice of oncology. Vol. 1. Philadelphia: Lippincott Williams & Wilkins 2008, 1232-1284.

[47] Compton C, Hawk ET, Grochow L et al. Colon cancer. In: Abeloff, M.D., Armitage J., Niederhuber J. E et al, eds. Abeloff's clinical oncology. Philadelphia: Churchill Livingstone 2008, 1477-1534.

[48] O'Connell MJ, Lavery I, Yothers G et al. Relationship between tumor gene expression and recurrence in four independent studies of patients with stage II/III colon cancer treated with surgery alone or surgery plus adjuvant fluorouracil plus leucovorin. J Clin Oncol 2010 Sep 1;28(25):3937-44. doi: 10.1200/JCO.2010.28.9538.

[49] Kerr D, Gray R, Quirke P, Watson D, Yothers G, Lavery IC, Lee M, O'Connell MJ, Shak S, Wolmark N, and Genomic Health and QUASAR Colon Teams.A quantitative multigene RT-PCR assay for prediction of recurrence in stage II colon cancer: Selection of the genes in four large studies and results of the independent, prospectively designed QUASAR validation study Journal of Clinical Oncology, 2009 ASCO Annu-

al Meeting Proceedings (Post-Meeting Edition). Vol 27, No 15S (May 20 Supplement), 2009: 4000

[50] Salazar R, Roepman P, Capella G et al. Gene expression signature to improve prognosis prediction of stage II and III colorectal cancer. J Clin Oncol. 2011 Jan 1;29(1): 17-24. doi: 10.1200/JCO.2010.30.1077.

[51] Agesen TH, Sveen A, Merok MA et al. ColoGuideEx: a robust gene classifier specific for stage II colorectal cancer prognosis. Gut. 2012; 61(11): 1560-67.

[52] Tabas-Madrid D, Nogales-Cadenas R, Pascual-Montano A: GeneCodis3: a non-redundant and modular enrichment analysis tool for functional genomics. Nucleic Acids Research 2012; doi: 10.1093/nar/gks402.

[53] Nogales-Cadenas R, Carmona-Saez P, Vazquez M et al: GeneCodis: interpreting gene lists through enrichment analysis and integration of diverse biological information. Nucleic Acids Research 2009; doi: 10.1093/nar/gkp416.

[54] Carmona-Saez P, Chagoyen M, Tirado F et al: GENECODIS: A web-based tool for finding significant concurrent annotations in gene lists. Genome Biology 2007 8(1):R3.

[55] Shi M, Beauchamp RD, Zhang B. A network-based gene expression signature informs prognosis and treatment for colorectal cancer patients. PLoS One 2012; 7(7): e41292. doi: 10.1371/journal.pone.0041292.

[56] Asghar U, Hawkes E, Cunningham D. Predictive and prognostic biomarkers for targeted therapy in metastatic colorectal cancer. Clin Colorectal Cancer. 2010 Dec;9(5): 274-81. doi: 10.3816/CCC.2010.n.040.

[57] Bandrés E, Zárate R, Ramirez N et al. Pharmacogenomics in colorectal cancer: the first step for individualized-therapy. World J Gastroenterol. 2007 Nov 28;13(44): 5888-901.

[58] Benhaim L, Labonte MJ, Lenz HJ. Pharmacogenomics and metastatic colorectal cancer: current knowledge and perspectives. Scand J Gastroenterol. 2012 Mar;47(3): 325-39. doi: 10.3109/00365521.2012.640832.

[59] Coate L, Cuffe S, Horgan A et al. Germline genetic variation, cancer outcome, and pharmacogenetics. J Clin Oncol. 2010 Sep 10;28(26):4029-37. doi: 10.1200/JCO.2009.27.2336.

[60] De Roock W, De Vriendt V, Normanno N et al. KRAS, BRAF, PIK3CA, and PTEN mutations: implications for targeted therapies in metastatic colorectal cancer. Lancet Oncol. 2011 Jun;12(6):594-603. doi: 10.1016/S1470-2045(10)70209-6.

[61] Ross JS, Torres-Mora J, Wagle N et al. Biomarker-based prediction of response to therapy for colorectal cancer: current perspective. Am J Clin Pathol. 2010 Sep;134(3): 478-90. doi: 10.1309/AJCP2Y8KTDPOAORH.

[62] Heidelberger C., Chaudhuri NK, Danneberg P et al. Fluorinated Pyrimidines, A New Class of Tumor Inhibitory Compounds. Nature 179: 663-666.

[63] Fernandez-Rozadilla C, Cazier JB, Moreno V et al.Pharmacogenomics in colorectal cancer: a genome-wide association study to predict toxicity after 5-fluorouracil or FOLFOX administration. Pharmacogenomics J. 2012. doi: 10.1038/tpj.2012.2.

[64] Hsiang YH, Liu LF, Wall ME et al. DNA topoisomerase I-mediated DNA cleavage and cytotoxicity of camptothecin analogues. Cancer Res. 1989; 49(16): 4385-9.

[65] Hanahan D, Weinberg RA. The hallmarks of cancer. Cell 2000;100(1):57-70.

[66] Hanahan D, Weinberg RA. Hallmarks of cancer: the next generation. Cell 2011; 144(5): 646-74. doi: 10.1016/j.cell.2011.02.013.

[67] Takahashi Y, Kitadai Y, Bucana CD et al. Expression of vascular endothelial growth factor and its receptor, KDR, correlates with vascularity, metastasis, and proliferation of human colon cancer. Cancer Res 1995; 55: 3964-3968.

[68] Presta LG, Chen H, O'Connor SJ et al. Humanization of an anti- vascular endothelial growth factor monoclonal antibody for the therapy of solid tumors and other disorders. Cancer Res 1997; 57: 4593-4599.

[69] Mayer A, Takimoto M, Fritz E et al. The prognostic significance of proliferating cell nuclear antigen, epidermal growth factor receptor, and mdr gene expression in colorectal cancer. Cancer 1993; 71: 2454-2460.

[70] Ciardiello F, Tortora G. A novel approach in the treatment of cancer: targeting the epidermal growth factor receptor. Clin Cancer Res 2001; 7: 2958-70.

[71] Ciardiello F, Tortora G. EGFR antagonists in cancer treatment. N Engl J Med 2008; 358: 1160–74.

[72] Baselga J. The EGFR as a target for anticancer therapy--focus on cetuximab. Eur J Cancer 2001; 37 Suppl 4: S16-S22

[73] Sharma S, Kelly TK, Jones PA. Epigenetics in cancer. Carcinogenesis 2010; 31:27–36.

[74] Khare S, Verma M. Epigenetics of colon cancer. Methods Mol Biol 2012;863:177-85. doi: 10.1007/978-1-61779-612-8_10.

[75] Lao VV, Grady WM. Epigenetics and colorectal cancer. Nat Rev Gastroenterol Hepatol. 2011 Oct 18;8(12):686-700. doi: 10.1038/nrgastro.2011.173.

[76] Ballestar E, Esteller M. Epigenetic gene regulation in cancer. Adv Genet. 2008; 61:247–267.

[77] Hatziapostolou M, Iliopoulos D. Epigenetic aberrations during oncogenesis. Cell Mol Life Sci. 2011;68(10):1681-702. doi: 10.1007/s00018-010-0624-z.

[78] Liu M, Chen H. The role of microRNAs in colorectal cancer. J Genet Genomics. 2010 Jun;37(6):347-58. doi: 10.1016/S1673-8527(09)60053-9.

[79] Sawan C, Herceg Z. Histone modifications and cancer. Adv Genet. 2010; 70:57–85.

[80] Ting AH, McGarvey KM, Baylin SB. The cancer epigenome--components and functional correlates. Genes Dev. 2006; 20:3215–3231.

[81] Van Engeland M, Derks S, Smits KM et al. Colorectal cancer epigenetics: complex simplicity. J Clin Oncol. 2011; 29:1382–1391.

[82] Bird A. DNA methylation patterns and epigenetic memory. Genes Dev. 2002; 16:6–21.

[83] Feinberg A, Vogelstein B. Hypomethylation distinguishes genes of some human cancers from their normal counterparts. 1983; 301:89, 92.

[84] Weisenberger DJ, et al. DNA methylation analysis by digital bisulfite genomic sequencing and digital MethyLight. Nucleic Acids Res. 2008; 36:4689–4698.

[85] Curtin K, Slattery ML, Samowitz WS. CpG island methylation in colorectal cancer: past, present and future. Patholog Res Int. 2011; 2011:902674.

[86] Mao C, Liao RY, Qiu LX et al. BRAF V600E mutation and resistance to anti-EGFR monoclonal antibodies in patients with metastatic colorectal cancer: a meta-analysis. Mol Biol Rep 2011 Apr;38(4):2219-23. doi: 10.1007/s11033-010-0351-4.

[87] Tol J, Dijkstra JR, Klomp M et al. Markers for EGFR pathway activation as predictor of outcome in metastatic colorectal cancer patients treated with or without cetuximab. Eur J Cancer 2010 Jul;46(11):1997-2009. doi: 10.1016/j.ejca.2010.03.036.

[88] Wang Z, Yuan X, Jiao N et al. CDH13 and FLBN3 gene methylation are associated with poor prognosis in colorectal cancer. Pathol Oncol Res. 2012 Apr;18(2):263-70. doi: 10.1007/s12253-011-9437-0.

[89] Itzkowitz SH, Jandorf L, Brand R et al. Improved fecal DNA test for colorectal cancer screening. Clin Gastroenterol Hepatol. 2007; 5:111–117.

[90] Itzkowitz S,Brand R, Jandorf L et al. A simplified, noninvasive stool DNA test for colorectal cancer detection. Am J Gastroenterol. 2008; 103:2862–2870.

[91] Nieminen TT, Shoman S, Eissa S et al. Distinct genetic and epigenetic signatures of colorectal cancers according to ethnic origin. Cancer Epidemiol Biomarkers Prev 2012 Jan;21(1):202-11. doi: 10.1158/1055-9965.EPI-11-0662.

[92] Mallick P, Kuster M. Proteomics: a pragmatic perspective. Nature Biotech 2010; 27: 695-709.

[93] Domon B, Aebersold R. Options and considerations when selecting a quantitative proteomics strategy. Nature Biotech 2010; 27: 710-721.

[94] Duncan MW, Aebersold R, Caprioli RM. The pros and cons of peptide-centric proteomics. Nature Biotech 2010; 27: 659-664.

[95] Wisniewski JR, Ostasiewicz P, Dus K et al. Extensive quantitative remodeling of the proteome between normal colon tissue and adenocarcinoma. Molecular Systems Biology 2012; 8: 611.

[96] Huang CS, Lal SK, Farraye FA. Colorectal cancer screening in average risk individuals. Cancer Causes Control 2005; 16: 171-88.

[97] Bates J. Cancer Biomarkers: adoption is driving growth. Insight Pharma Reports 2008, Needham, MA, USA.

[98] Holten-Andersen M, Christensen IJ, Nilbert M et al. Association between preoperative plasma levels of tissue inhibitor of metalloproteinases 1 and rectal cancer patient survival: a validation study. Eur J. cancer 2004; 40: 64-72.

[99] Ward DG, Suggett N, Cheng Y et al. Identification of serum biomarkers for colon cancer by proteomic analysis. Br J cancer 2006; 94: 1898-1905.

[100] diaDexus Inc (2007). Clinical application of diaDexus diagnostics in colorectal cancer. http://www.diadexus.com/products/research/oncology_diagnostics.php

[101] He YJ, Mou ZR, Li WL et al. Identification of IMPDH2 as a tumor-associated antigen in colorectal cancer using immunoproteomics analysis. Int J. Colorectal Dis. 2009; 24: 1271-79.

[102] Tjalsma H. Identification of biomarkers for colorectal cancer through proteomics-based approaches. Expert Rev. Proteomics 2010; 7 (6): 879-95.

[103] Kocer B, McKolanis J, Soran A. Humoral immune response to MUC5AC in patients with colorectal polyps and colorectal carcinoma. BMC Gastroenterol 2006; 6: 4.

[104] Chen Y, Lin P, Qui SM et al. Autoantibodies to Ca+ binding protein Calnuc is a potential marker in colon cancer detection. Int J. Oncol 2007; 30: 1137-44.

[105] Babel I, Barderas R, Diaz-Uriarte R et al. Identification of tumor-associated autoantigens for the diagnosis of colorectal cancer in serum using high density protein microarrays. Mol. Cell Proteomics 2009; 8: 2382-95.

[106] Silk AW, Schoen RE, Potter DM et al. Humoral immune response to abnormal MUC1 in subjects with colorectal adenoma and cancer. Mol Immunol 2009; 47: 52-56.

[107] Merchant TE, Kasimos JN, de Graaf PW et al. Phospholipid profile of human colon cancer using 31P magnetic resonance spectroscopy. Int J Colorectal Dis 1991; 6 (2): 121-6.

[108] Dueck DA, Chan M,Tran K et al. The modulation of choline phosphoglyceride metabolism in human colon cancers. Mol Cell Biochem 1996; 162 (2): 97-103.

[109] Schonberg SA, Lundemo AG, Fladvad T et al. Closely related colon cancer cell lines display different sensitivity to polyunsaturated fatty acids, accumulate different lipid

classes and downregulates sterol regulatory element-binding protein 1. FEBS J 2006; 273 (12): 2749-65.

[110] White- Gilbertson S, Muller T, Senkal C et al. Ceramide synthase 6 modulates TRAIL sensitivity and nuclear translocation of active caspase-3 in colon cancer cells. Oncogene 2009; 28 (8): 1132-41.

[111] Fhaner CJ, Liu S, Ji H et al. Comprehensive Lipidome Profiling of Isogenic Primary and Metastatic Colon Adenocarcinoma Cell Lines. Anal Chem. 2012; 84: 8917-26.

[112] Gassler N, Klaus C, Kaemmerer E et al. Modifier-concept of colorectal carcinogenesis: Lipidomics aa a technical too in pathway analysis, World J Gastroenterol 2010; 16 (15): 1820-27.

[113] Sutphen R, Xu Y, Wilbanks GD et al. Lysophospholipids are potential biomarkers for ovarian cancer. Cancer Epidemiol Biomarkers Prev 2004; 13: 1185-91.

[114] Pozlep B, Melch M, Kobal B et al. Use of lysophosphatidic acid in the management of benign and malignant ovarian tumors. Eur J Gynaecol Oncol 2007; 28: 394-99.

[115] Melch M, Pozlep B, Mlakar A et al. Determination of serum lysophosphatidic acid as a potential biomarker for ovarian cancer. J Chromatogr B Analyt Technol Biomed Life Sci 2007; 858: 287-91.

[116] Zhao Z, Xiao Y, Elson P et al. Plasma lysophosphatidylcholine levels: potential biomarkers for colorectal cancer. J Clin Oncol 2007; 25: 2696-701.

[117] Nakagami K, Uchida T, Ohwada S et al. Increased choline kinase activity and elevated phosphocholine levels in human colon cancer. Jpn J Cancer Res 1999; 90: 419-24.

[118] Dobrzynska I, Szachowicz-Petelska B, Sulkowski S et al. Changes in electrical charge and phospholipids composition in human colorectal cancer cells. Mol Cell Biochem 2005; 276: 113-19.

[119] Merchant TE, Diamantis PM, Lauwers G et al. Characterization of malignant colon tumors with 31P nuclear magnetic resonance phospholipid and phosphate metabolite profiles. Cancer 1995; 76 (10): 1715-23.

[120] Ono M, Handa K, Sonnino S et al. GM3 ganglioside inhibits CD9- facilitated haptotactic cell motility: coexpression of GM3 and CD9 is essential in the downregulation of tumor cell motility and malignancy. Biochemistry 2001; 40: 6414-21.

[121] Zhang XF, Li BX, Doug CY et al. Apoptosis of human colon carcinoma HT-29 cells induced by ceramide. W J Gastroenterol 2006; 12: 3581-84.

[122] Tan X, Zhang Y, Jiang B et al. Changes in ceramide level upon catechins-induced apoptosis in LoVo cells. Life Sci 2002; 70: 2023-29.

[123] Ahn EH, Schroeder JJ. Sphingoid bases and ceramide induce apoptosis in HT-29 and HCT-116 human colon cancer cells. Exp Biol Med (Maywood) 2002; 227: 345-53.

[124] Min HK, Lim S, Chung BC et al. Shotgun lipidomics for candidate biomarkers of urinary phospholipids in prostate cancer. Anal Bioanal Chem 2011; 399 (2): 823-30.

[125] Kim H, Min HK, Kong G et al. Quantitative analysis of phosphatidylcholines and phosphatidylethanolamine in urine of patients with breast cancer by nanoflow liquid chromatography/ Tandem mass spectrometry. Anal Bioanal Chem 2009; 393 (6-7): 1649-56.

[126] Johnson JC, Schmidt CR, Shrubsole MJ et al. Urine PGE-M: A metabolite of Prostaglandin E2 as a potent biomarker of Advanced Colorectal Neoplasia. Clinical Gastroenterology and Hepatology 2006; 4: 1358-1365.

[127] Cai Q, Gao Y, Chow W et al. Prospective Study of Urinary Prostaglandin E2 Metabolite and Colorectal cancer Risk. Journal of Clinical Oncology 2006; 24 (31): 5010-16.

[128] Nishiumi S, Kobayashi T, Ikeda A et al. A Novel Serum Metabolomics-Based diagnostic Approach for Colorectal Cancer. PloS ONE 2012; 7 (7): e40459.

[129] Farshidfar F, Weljie AM, Kopciuk K et al. Serum metabolomic profile as a means to distinguish stages of colorectal cancer. Genome Medicine 2012; 4: 42.

[130] Wang H, Tso VK, Slupsky CM et al. Metabolomics and detection of colorectal cancer in humans: a systematic review. Future Oncology 2010; 6 (9): 1395-1406.

[131] Ma YL, Liu WJ, Peng JY et al. Study on specific metabonomic profiling of serum from colorectal cancer patients by gas chromatography-mass spectrometry. Zhonghua Wei Chang Wai Ke Za Zhi 2009; 12 (4): 386-90.

[132] Cheng Y, Xie G, Chen T et al. Distinct Urinary Metabolic Profile of Human Colorectal Cancer. J Proteome Res 2012; 11: 1354-62.

[133] Qui Y, Cai G, Su M et al. Urinary metabonomic study on colorectal cancer. Journal of Proteome Research 2010; 9: 1627-1634.

[134] Abdullah B. Molecular imaging: spawning a new melting-pot for biomedical imaging. Biomed Imaging Interv J 2006; 2(4): e28. doi: 10.2349/biij.2.4.e28.

[135] Seaman ME, Contino G, Bardeesy N et al. Molecular imaging agents: impact on diagnosis and therapeutics in oncology. Expert Rev Mol Med. 2010 Jul 15;12:e20. doi: 10.1017/S1462399410001511.

[136] Akin O, Brennan SB, Dershaw DD et al. Advances in oncologic imaging: update on 5 common cancers. CA Cancer J Clin. 2012 Nov-Dec; 62(6): 364-93. doi: 10.3322/caac.21156.

[137] Moesta KT, Ebert B, Handke T et al. Protoporphyrin IX occurs naturally in colorectal cancers and their metastases. Cancer Res. 2001; 61(3):991-9.

[138] Kemmner W, Wan K, Rüttinger S et al. Silencing of human ferrochelatase causes abundant protoporphyrin-IX accumulation in colon cancer. FASEB J. 2008; 22(2): 500-9.

[139] Wan K, Ebert B, Voigt J, Wang Q, Dai Y, Haag R, Kemmner W. In vivo tumor imaging using a novel RNAi-based detection mechanism. Nanomedicine. 2012; 8(4): 393-8. doi: 10.1016/j.nano.2012.02.004.

[140] Illemann M, Bird N, Majeed A et al. MMP-9 is differentially expressed in primary human colorectal adenocarcinomas and their metastases. Mol Cancer Res. 2006 May; 4(5):293-302.

[141] Fudala R, Ranjan AP, Mukerjee A et al. Fluorescence detection of MMP-9. I. MMP-9 selectively cleaves Lys-Gly-Pro-Arg-Ser-Leu-Ser-Gly-Lys peptide. Curr Pharm Biotechnol. 2011; 12(5):834-8.

[142] Fortina P, Kricka LJ, Graves DJ et al. Application of nanoparticles to diagnostics and therapeutics in colorectal cancer. Trends in Biotechnology 2007; 25 (4): 145-52.

[143] Sun L, Sung K, Dentinger C et al. Composite organic-inorganic nanoparticles as Raman labels for tissue analysis. Nano Letters 2007; 7 (2): 351-56.

[144] Ko HY, Choi K, Lee CH et al. A multimodal nanoparticle-based cancer imaging probe simultaneously targeting nucleolin, intergrin $\alpha v\beta 3$ and tenascin-C proteins. Biomaterials 2011; 32: 1130-38.

[145] Azuara D, Ginesta MM, Gausach M et al. Nanofluidic digital PCR for KRAS mutation detection and quantification in gastrointestinal cancer. Clin Chem 2012; 58 (9): 1332-41.

[146] Farokhzad OC, Jon S, Khademhosseini A et al. Nanoparticle-Aptamer Biconjugates: a New Approach for Targeting Prostate cancer Cells. Cancer Res 2004; 64: 7668-72.

[147] Lin D, Feng S, Pan J et al. Colorectal cancer detection by gold nanoparticle based surface-enhanced Raman spectroscopy of blood serum and statistical analysis. Opt Express 2011; 19 (14): 13565-77.

[148] Jordan M, Navel A, Brownlow B et al. Development and evaluation of tocopherol-rich argan oil-based nanoemulsions as vehicles possessing anticancer activity. J Biomed Nanotechnol 2012; 8 (6): 944-56.

[149] Goncalves AS, Macedo AS, Souto EB. Therapeutic nanosystems for oncology nanomedicine. Clin Transl Oncol 2012. 14: 883-90.

[150] Ruggeiro A, Villa CH, Holland JP et al. Imaging and treating tumor vasculature with targeted radiolabeled carbon nanotubes. Int J Nanomedicine 2010; 5: 783-802

[151] Gianella A, Jarzyna PA, Mani V et al. Multifunctional nanoemulsion platform for imaging guided therapy evaluated in experimental cancer. ACS Nano 2011; 5 (6): 4422-33.

[152] Yao L, Zhao X, Li Q et al. In vitro and in vivo evaluation of camptothecin nanosuspension: a novel formulation with high antitumor efficacy and low toxicity. Int J Pharm 2012; 423 (2): 586-88.

[153] Komizu Y, Ueoka H, Goto K et al. Remarkable inhibitory effects of hybrid liposomes on growth of human colon cancer cells through induction of cell cycle arrest along with apoptosis. Int J Nanomedicine 2011; 6: 1913-20.

[154] Cho H, Kwon GS. Polymeric miscelle for neoadjuvant cancer therapy and tumor-primed optical imaging. ACS Nano 2011; 5 (11): 8721-29.

[155] Zhang AP, Sun YP. Photocatalytic killing effect of TiO2 nanoparticles on Ls-174-t human colon carcinoma cells. World J Gastroenterol 2004; 10 (21): 3191-93.

[156] Giacchetti S, Itzhaki M, Gruia G et al. Long-term survival of patients with unresectable colorectal cancer liver metastases following infusional chemotherapy with 5-fluorouracil, leucovorin, oxaliplatin and surgery. Ann Oncol. 1999; 10(6): 663-9.

[157] Douillard JY, Cunningham D, Roth AD et al. Irinotecan combined with fluorouracil compared with fluorouracil alone as first-line treatment for metastatic colorectal cancer: a multicentre randomised trial. Lancet 2000;355(9209):1041-47.

[158] Abdool Karim SS, Churchyard GJ, Karim QA, Lawn SD. HIV infection and tuberculosis in South Africa: an urgent need to escalate the public health response. Lancet. 2009; 374(9693): 921-33. doi: 10.1016/S0140-6736(09)60916-8.

[159] Chopra M, Daviaud E, Pattinson R et al. Saving the lives of South Africa's mothers, babies, and children: can the health system deliver? Lancet 2009; 374(9692): 835-46. doi: 10.1016/S0140-6736(09)61123-5.

[160] Coovadia H, Jewkes R, Barron P et al. The health and health system of South Africa: historical roots of current public health challenges. Lancet. 2009; 374(9692):817-34. doi: 10.1016/S0140-6736(09)60951-X.

[161] Mayosi BM, Flisher AJ, Lalloo UG et al. The burden of non-communicable diseases in South Africa. Lancet 2009; 374(9693): 934-47. doi: 10.1016/S0140-6736(09)61087-4

[162] Braun MS, Richman SD, Quirke P, Daly C, Adlard JW, Elliott F, Barrett JH, Selby P, Meade AM, Stephens RJ, Parmar MKB, Seymour MT. Predictive Biomarkers of Chemotherapy Efficacy in Colorectal Cancer: Results From the UK MRC FOCUS Trial. JCO JUNE 1, 2008 vol. 26 no. 16 2690-2698

[163] Paré L, Marcuello E, Altés A, del Río E, Sedano L, Salazar J, Cortés A, Barnadas A, Baiget M. Pharmacogenetic prediction of clinical outcome in advanced colorectal cancer patients receiving oxaliplatin/5-fluorouracil as first-line chemotherapy. Br J Cancer. 2008 Oct 7;99(7):1050-5. doi: 10.1038/sj.bjc.6604671. Epub 2008 Sep 16.

Chapter 16

COL11A1 — Genetic Biomarker Targeted in Stool Samples for Early Diagnosis of Colorectal Cancer in Patients at Risk

Andra Iulia Suceveanu, Laura Mazilu and Adrian-Paul Suceveanu

Additional information is available at the end of the chapter

http://dx.doi.org/10.5772/57327

1. Introduction

Colorectal cancer (CRC) is the third most frequently diagnosed cancer in both men and women and the second leading cause of cancer death after lung cancer. Even though CRC is considered to be 90% curable if detected in early stage, the majority of patients are diagnosed with advanced stages, III or IV [1].

Screening tests applied according to well known strategies make the early diagnosis of CRC possible and there is is strong evidence evidence that screening lowers mortality and incidence rates of cancer, if recommended at proper time in people at risk [2]. Still, the existing tests practiced on a large scale in CRC screening do not fully accomplish the goal of best specificity and sensitivity or either an optimal cost/efficiency ratio. A more effective screening test may significantly decrease disease burden.

Extensive research over the past two decades provided large information about genetic aberrations underlying CRC and revealed complex and heterogeneous mechanisms in the occurrence of the disease [3, 4]. Genetic changes occurred in normal colonic epithelium cells promoting the neoplastic transformation into benign adenomas and subsequently malignant adenocarcinomas were the essence for understanding the disease behavior and related clinical outcome, and created a perspective for future improvements in diagnosis, treatment and survival rates.

2. Colorectal cancer genesis — Gene mutations and underlying stool testing

A cancer cell develops through a collection of gene mutations. Mutations left uncorrected by cell cycle regulation before division are fixed in that cell and in its future progenitors. A cell undergoes full carcinogenic transformation once a sufficient number of genes are mutated and the cell can no longer respond to the external signals that act as brakes on cell growth. Comparing with breast cancer, in which a single gene is required for disease initiation, in CRC there are 7 to 10 genes responsible for neoplastic transformation and thereforee, the genetic-based screening for CRC is a more laborious task than screening breast cancer [5].

Although a smaller subgroup can arise as a result of inherited mutations or previous inflammatory bowel disease (Crohn's disease or ulcerative colitis), the great majority of CRC arise sporadically. This means that mutated genes are present only in precancerous and cancerous lesions in the colon and rectum, and are not present in all cells of the body. Therefore, CRC cannot be detected by a blood test, as breast cancer does [6].

Over the time, mutations of three different classes of genes have been described in colon cancer etiology: oncogenes, suppressor genes, and mismatch repair genes [7]. Knowledge of many of the specific mutations responsible for colon carcinogenesis allowed understanding the phenotypic manifestations and provided a large field for genetic testing from stool cell's DNA [8]. Although genetic testing is possible and available, it is not yet clear what battery of genetic tests are more accurate to use as an alternative diagnostic tool instead present widely accepted stool test.

Until now, the genetic changes targeted in the stool cell's DNA involved in the development of some colorectal cancers included: activating mutations of the K-RAS oncogene, inactivating mutations of the adenomatous polyposis cancer (*APC*) and *TP53* tumor suppressor genes [9] and germline or somatic mutations of mismatch repair genes (*MMR*) [10, 11].

A much less studied biomarker targeted in stool samples for early diagnosis of CRC in patients at risk is *COL11A1* gene, mutations of which have been first described in Marshall's syndrome and Stickler's syndrome [12]. The normal function of this gene is the production of collagen type XI, which participate to build the structure and the resistance of conjunctive tissues. Beside its main role in the assembly, organization and development of cartilage, *COL11A1* was found to be expressed at low level in a wide variety of normal adult human tissues, including lung, parotid gland and colorectal cells.

Few studies have found overexpression of the *COL11A1* gene in various types of cancers, such as non-small cell lung cancer (NSCLC), ovarian, oral cavity and colorectal cancers. In particular, overexpression of the *COL11A1* gene was found to be correlated with invasive and metastatic potential of these cancers [13-16].

This gene is located on chromosome 1, arm p, site 21, between the 103.055.015 and 103.286.072 pair of bases, and is composed of 231 kbase. It contains 68 exons, not yet wholly sequenced [17]. A major contribution to the *COL11A1* gene sequencing knowleddgee, especially with the purpose of detecting mutations, is *Annune S* research and results [18]. Recent extented studies demonstrated that some polymorphysms of *COL11A1* are associated with different types of adenocarcinoma [19].

3. AIM

This study was designed to analyze *COL11A1* gene mutations identified in the DNA of exfoliated epithelial cells of the colon in the stool of the patients diagnosed with CRC through screening and to demonstrate the perfect similarity between the detected mutations in tumor samples and in exfoliated stool cells, in order to prove the reliability of the method as a diagnostic tool for early CRC diagnosis.

4. Patients and method

We selected 250 patients diagnosed in the Endoscopy Department of Emergency Hospital of Constanta with adenomatous polyps and CRC using colonoscopy and biopsy and confirmed by histopathological exam, during screening programme or admitted and investigated for intestinal disturbances such as chronic diarrhea or recent exacerbated constipation, stool bleeding or association of the above symptoms in their recent history.

We collected samples biopsied from tumors during colonoscopy and stool sample from each patient.

Colonoscopy and biopsies were performed with Olympus Exera equipment.

The bowel preparation was done according to guidelines and its quality was noted.

The colonoscopist documented the presence, size, location and extension of colonic tumors.

Biopsy or surgical resection samples were examined histopathologically and genetically.

Subjects were instructed prior stool collection. No dietary or medication modifications were required. Until shipping samples to genetic lab, these were disposed in a coded container into a refrigerator, between 0 and 4°C. Specimens were required to arrive within 3 days after collection.

The minimum quantity of stool sample required was 30 g. Samples were stored at –80°C until genetic analysis.

DNA was extracted from biopsy and feaces samples for mutation analysis:

- from stool, with QIAmp stool extraction kit (QIGene, Germany);
- from biopsy sample, with IQ-DNA Extraction Kit (Promega USA).

Primers for PCR amplification were provided by TIB MOLBIOL, Germany.

The *COL11A1* gene, examined in the present study, produces a component of the colagen type XI, named pro-alpha1 chain, an important factor for connective tissue structure and resistance.

The method used for *COL11A1* mutations was polyacrylamide gel electrophoresis method for the heteroduplex analysis (HA).

Investigation of *COL11A1* gene is made sequentially by setting fragments to be analyzed. To do this, fragments that usually carry most mutations are identified. Each fragment of *COL11A1* gene that is proposed for investigation is amplified by PCR. For this, primers flanking each particular fragment are used.

PCR conditions are dependent on the characteristics of each pair of primers. Each program contains a PCR initial denaturing step, lasting for 3 minutes at 94°C, followed by 30-35 reaction cycles (depending on the length of the fragment of interest and the size and composition of the primers), each cycle comprising: denaturation, alignment, elongation (conditions are established for each pair of primers used), and the final elongation step, lasting for 5 minutes at 72°C. Obtained amplicons are subjected to additional steps of forced denaturation-renaturation (to encourage heteroduplex formation), and then migrated in a 6% polyacrylamide gel.

The heteroduplex is represented by a fragment of double-stranded DNA in which the two strands do not express perfect complementarity. When DNA is denatured, the two strands are separated. Through renaturation, complementary chains come together to form a homoduplex. If there is a mutation in one of the two strands, heteroduplex is formed (figure 1).

Heteroduplex analysis was imagined by *Ziemmermann et al* in 1993 [20] and has been used to enhance the sensitivity of denaturing gradient gel electrophoresis (DGGE) in the detection of point mutation [21-23]. DNA fragments for HA can be visualized via a variety of methods including bromide staining, labelling with radioisotopes and silver staining. The mutations detection rate of HA under ideal conditions is near 90%.

Heteroduplex differ from homoduplex by electrophoretic migration speed in polyacrylamide gel. Mutational alteration of a single base pair is sufficient to produce changes in mobility. Electrophoretic mobility of heteroduplex is lower than that of homoduplex, and it can be detected as a slower migrating band. This method can detect insertions, deletions and substitutions of even a single base pair in fragment lengths smaller than 200 bp.

The working protocol for this technique is very simple and quick and consists of a denaturation-renaturation step for which we set the following conditions: 94°C – 1 minute, 72°C – 1 minute, 65°C – 1 minute, 40°C – 1 minute and thermal shock at 4°C. Each stage is covered by one cycle. The existence of deletion mutations will result in the formation of four bands, two heteroduplex and two homoduplex (heterozygous condition) (Figure 1).

Migration occurs differently based on molecular weight. Samples from patients and healthy individuals (control samples) are migrated in the same gel, in order to analyze the difference in migration. If the investigated individual is a normal homozygous or a homozygous for analyzed mutation, a single band will be displayed in each case. The difference between these conditions is based on different migration and reported to the molecular weight marker used. If there is a substitution mutation, two bands are visualized on polyacrylamide gel: a band representing heteroduplex and a band representing homoduplex. In this case, the difference in migration is explained on the basis of different chemical composition of the four DNA

http://dx.doi.org/10.5772/57327

strands. For optimal view of amplification products, we used 6% polyacrylamide gel, containing 0.5 µg ethidium bromide, migrated 6 V/cm. The gel is observed and photographed on UV transilluminator.

In the latter stages of a PCR amplification the polymerase is limiting, so that during the final annealing and synthesis steps, a proportion of the single stranded products spontaneously reanneals without primer extension. When amplifying from individuals heterozygous for any sequence difference, the single strands do not necessarily rehybridize exactly with the complementary strand. They can alternatively form a DNA hybrid (heteroduplex) consisting of a sense strand with one sequence variant and an antisense strand with another variant.

As a consequence, the heteroduplex DNA has a region of at least one base pair mismatch. The region of mismatch can elicit a mobility shift by altering the conformation adopted by the heteroduplex DNA, probably by causing it to bend at the location of the mismatch. The mobility shifts are usually small but can be visualized after prolonged electrophoresis on native polyacrylamide gels.

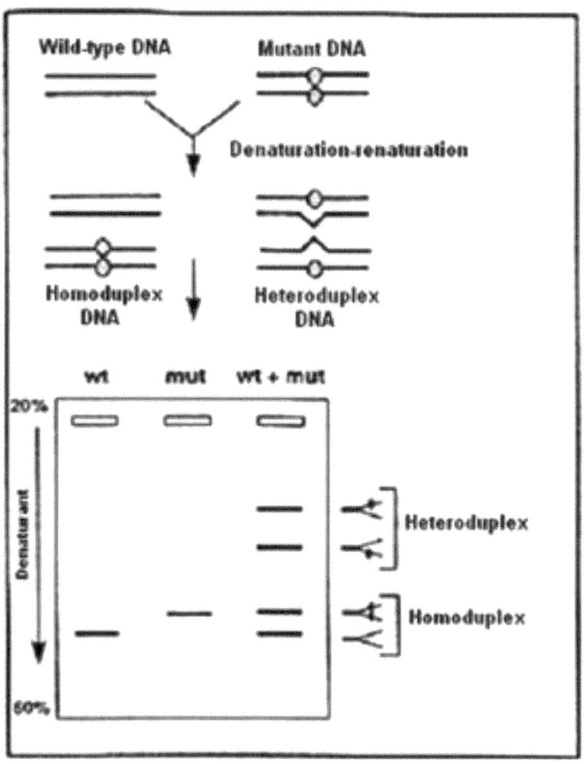

Figure 1. Denaturation and renaturation of normal and mutated DNA fragments in order to generate four types of fragments: two heteroduplex and two homoduplex. Fragments were migrated parallel on denaturating gradient gel. "Melting" heteroduplex are modified in the sense that they denaturate at a lower concentration of denaturant, allowing their visualization.

1. Detection of *COL11A1* gene mutations included the following steps:
2. Genomic DNA extraction from the analyzed samples: tumor tissue obtained through biopsy and exfoliated cells from feces;
3. Amplification of the interested gene amplicons through PCR reaction;
4. Amplification check up through electrophoresis in agarosis gel and bromide ethidium staining;
5. Mutations identification through DGGE technique and silver or ethidium bromide staining.

5. DNA extraction from proposed samples

DNA extraction from stool has been made by a specific kit for stool extraction [24, 25]. DNA tissue extraction from the colorectal biopsy has been performed using DNA IQ (TM) System kit [26]. DNA IQ (TM) System kit uses the principle of DNA extraction based on a paramagnetic resine. In addition, the kit contains a series of denaturating agents ("lysis buffer"), having the role of disintegrating the biologic product that is the DNA source.

An important advantage of this kit is that it provides extraction of an optimal DNA quantity for PCR reaction (100 ng/µl).

6. DNA extraction from stool

DNA extraction from stool was performed with a kit designed for extraction from faeces (QIAGEN GmbH, Hilden Germany). The technique included the following steps:

1. 200 mg of faeces were suspended in 2 ml of ASL buffer by vortexing for 1 minute.
2. 1.6 ml of this lysate was transferred to a new tube.
3. Suspension was boiled for 5 minutes.
4. Centrifuged at maximum speed for 1 minute.
5. Transfered 1.2 ml of supernatant into a new tube containing an InhibitEX tablet.
6. Vortexed the tube for 1 minute and incubated for 1 minute at room temperature.
7. Centrifuged the tube for 3 minutes.
8. Transfered 200 µl of supernatant into a new tube containing 15 µl of proteinase K.
9. Added 200 µl of Buffer AL and vortex.
10. Incubated at 70°C for 10 minutes.

http://dx.doi.org/10.5772/57327

11. Added 200 μl of ethanol to lysate and vortex.
12. Content was applyed in a column of centrifugation and centrifuged at 10,000 x g for 1 minute.
13. The column was washed once with 500 μl of Buffer AW1 at 10,000 x g for 1 minute and then with 500 μl of Buffer AW2 at 10,000 x g for 1 minute.
14. DNA was eluted from the column at 10,000 x g, 1 minute, with 100 μl heated buffer AE.

7. DNA tissue extraction from colorectal biopsy

DNA extraction from biological product was performed with DNA kit IQTM System, manufactured by Promega, USA. DNA IQTM System is a kit that uses a new DNA extraction principle based on the use of paramagnetic resin. In addition, the kit contains a number of denaturating agents ("lysis buffer") which are designed to disintegrate biological product that is the source of DNA.

For some biological products (hair, tissue) which are resistant to this type of disintegration, an additional pretreatment with proteinase K is used, an enzyme that produces sample lysis.

A considerable advantage of this kit is that it provides an optimal quantity of DNA extraction for PCR reaction, respectively 100 ng/μl, regardless of used biological product.

Used magnetic resin binds only a limited amount of DNA even if it is in excess. Finally, DNA is eluted from the resin with 100 μl of eluent solution yielding a final concentration of 1 ng/μl. Thus, it is no longer necessary to quantify the amount of extracted DNA.

In principle extraction kit use the following steps:

- Extraction of the sample and its lysis;
- Resin-capture DNA;
- Magnetic resin-washing;
- Elution of DNA from the resin.

8. Purification of DNA from a tissue sample

1. We place about 1 mg of tissue in a 1.5 ml tube.
2. We added 50-100 μl of incubation buffer solution/freshly prepared proteinase K and incubated at 56°C for 2 hours. Usually all tissue is digested after 2 hours, and if it doesn't occur, incubation is extended.
3. We removed the source sample incubation and added 2 volumes of lysis buffer.

4. We added 7 μl of magnetic resin. The sample was vortex 3 seconds and left at room temperature for 5 minutes.
5. Then the simple was vortex for 2 seconds and left the tube on the magnetic stand. Separation occured instantly.
6. Carefully we aspirated all the solution without disturbing the resin at the bottom of the tube.
7. We add 100 μl of prepared lysis buffer. We removed the tube from the magnetic stand and vortex 2 seconds.
8. Placed the tube again on the magnetic stand and vacuum lysis buffer.
9. Added 100 μl of Wash Buffer preparation. We removed the tube from the magnetic stand and vortex 2 seconds.
10. We replaced the tube in the magnetic stand and aspirated the solution.
11. We repeated steps 9 and 10, 2 times to make a total of three washes.
12. Tubes were allowed in the magnetic stand with the lid open for 5 minutes to dry.
13. We added 25-100 μl of elution buffer, depending on the amount of biological material used.
14. Then we closed the lid and vortexed 2 seconds. We incubated at 65°C for 5 minutes.
15. Removed the tube from the heating device, vortexed 2 seconds and immediately puted the tube on the magnetic stand.
16. Finally, we aspirated DNA containing solution and left the tube in conservation.

9. Validation of human origin of DNA extracted from stool by STR loci typing

The analysis of the nuclear DNA extracted from stools is a recent new method for CRC diagnostics.

In the preliminary phase of our study, we comparatively analyzed the DNA extracted from the biopsy samples of the patients with the DNA extracted from the stool samples of the same patients. This comparative analysis was performed by investigating a number of 9 human STR loci, frequently used in the DNA typing techniques of forensic medicine.

The STR type loci ("short tandem repeat" or "microsatellite repeats") contain 4 bases of segments that repeat 5-50 folds, depending on the loci. These STR are of a very small size (100-400 bases) and are very useful for the degraded DNA analysis. These repetitive sequences are largely spread in the human genome, being a rich source of polymorphic markers that may be detected through PCR.

For the DNA typing in our cases, we used a number of 9 STR loci. Determination of the 9 loci can be made by using kits of molecular biology, forming GenePrintSTR Systems of Multiplex type.

10. Amplification of the interested gene amplicons through PCR reaction

Primers the analysis of all the 68 exons of *COL11A1* gene are not yet available. We managed to obtain sequence for primers of two groups of amplicons containing amplified segments in exons where most frequently mutations in various cancers were found.

Amplification groups are:

- Group 1:
  - Amplicon 38;
  - Amplicon 41;
  - Amplicon 16.
- Group 2:
  - Amplicon 54;
  - Amplicon 55;
  - Amplicon 56;
  - Amplicon 57.

PCR reactions were done simultaneously for each of the two groups above. We used PCR amplification kit manufactured by Promega (USA) called "PCR Core System". It was designed to enhance any type of amplicon, by usind standard type Taq polymerase.

Materials required:

- Thermal cicler for 0.2 ml tubes;
- microcentrifuge;
- Taq DNA polymerase;
- Nucleases-free water;
- Mineral Oil;
- 0.2 ml Amplification tubes;
- 1.5 ml microcentrifuge tubes;
- Anti-aerosol pipette tips;
- Ice.

11. Thermal cycling protocol

Manufacturing company recommends several types of thermal cycling protocols and the choice depends on the thermo-cicler and optimized version that has been established. We have optimized the following protocol – protocol *COL11A1*:

- Step 1: 94°C, 1 minute;
- Step 2: 52°C, 1 minute;
- Step 3: 72°C, 1 minute;

Repeated successive steps 1, 2 and 3, in 5 cycles.

- Step 4: 94°C, 1 minute;
- Step 5: 50°C, 1 minute;
- Step 6: 72°C, 1 minute;

Repeated successive steps 4, 5 and 6, in 5 cycles.

- Step 7: 94°C, 1 minute;
- Step 8: 48°C, 1 minute;
- Step 9: 72°C, 1 minute;
- Step 10: 72°C, 3 minutes;
- Step 11 (rest): 4°C.

12. Amplification setting

To prevent contamination it is strongly recommended the use of gloves and anti-aerosol pipette tips. Maneuvers that must be cosidered are as follows:

1. Defrost kit components and pairs of primers and then put them on ice.
2. Mark each 0.2 ml amplification tube and place it in the stand.
3. Determine the number of reactions to be performed. This number must include the positive and negative control reaction, respectively. Add to this number another 1-2 reactions in addition, to compensate for pipetting errors.
4. Prepare the amplification (PCR Master Mix) solution, according to the table below (table 1). Multiply the volume per sample (μl) with the total number of reactions, to obtain the final volume.

http://dx.doi.org/10.5772/57327

PCR Master Mix Component	Volume per sample (μl)
$MgCl_2$ 25 mM sol.	1.5
10X Buffer Taq DNA Polymerase	2.5
PCR Nucleotide mix, 10 mM	0.5
"Primer Upstream", 15 μM	1.65
"Primer "Downstream", 15 μM	1.65
Taq DNA Polymerase (at 5 u/μl)	0.12
Distilled water without nucleases	17.08
Total volume	22.5

Table 1. Preparation of PCR Master Mix.

1. In order from above table lay the final volume of each reagent in a sterile tube. Shake gently (not vortex) and place the tube on ice.
2. Add 22.5 μl of PCR Master Mix to each reaction tube and place tubes on ice.
3. Pipette 2.5 μl of each DNA sample to respective tubes containing 22.5 μl of PCR Master Mix.
4. Pipette 2.5 μl (5 ng) of K562 DNA (diluted to 2 ng/μl) in a reaction tube containing 22.5 μl of PCR Master Mix, which is a positive control.
5. Pipette 2.5 μl of sterile distilled water (instead of DNA) in a reaction tube containing 22.5 μl of PCR Master Mix, which is a negative control.
6. Add 1 drop of mineral oil to each tube. Close the tubes.
7. Centrifuge tubes to bring the contents to the bottom of the tube.
8. Assemble the tubes in thermal triggers cicler and start amplification.
9. After amplification, the tubes must be kept at –20°C.

12.1. Electrophoresis of amplified samples for evidence heteroduplex

For this complex electrophoresis technique, we used a device type "DCode Universal Mutation Detection System" manufactured by Bio-Rad (Germany).

12.2. Formation reaction of heteroduplex

Protocol consists of a denaturation-renaturation step of PCR sample obtained from normal witness mixed with PCR sample from analyzed patient was established under the following conditions:

- 94°C – 1 minute;
- 72°C – 1 minute;

- 65°C – 1 minute;
- 40°C – 1 minute;
- heat shock at 4°C.

Heteroduplex are generated by adding to the same PCR reaction the mold of mutant and normal DNA, or by PCR product mixing, denaturation and ultimately their renaturation. A heteroduplex contains a mismatch base in the double chain, causing a distortion in its conformation; bands containing heteroduplex always migrates more slowly compared to bands containing homoduplex.

12.3. Preparation of reagents

Acrylamide concentration used generally depends on the sample to be analyzed, and we used a 40% stock solution containing acrylamide and bis-acrylamide.

- Acrylamide/Bis – 40% (37.5:1);
- Acrylamide – 38.9 g;
- Bis-acrylamide – 1.07 g;
- Water dist. – ad. 100 ml.

In the table below (table 2) we present the concentration of acrylamide/bis used to separate different DNA molecules:

Gel concentration	Separation of base pairs
6%	300-1000 bp
8%	200-400 bp
10%	100-300 bp

Table 2. Concentration of acrylamide/bis used to separate DNA molecules.

We worked with a solution of acrylamide/bis 6%, given the length of amplified fragments.

- Acrylamide/Bis solutions, 6% (1.25 x TAE, 6M urea);
- Acrylamide/Bis 40% 6.0 ml;
- 50X TAE buffer 1 ml;
- Urea 14.4 g;
- TEMED 40 μl;
- Ammonium persulfate 10% 400.0 μl;
- Total volume 40 ml.

We added water to 40 ml. Pour gel immediately after adding TEMED and ammonium persulphate.

- 50X TAE buffer:
  - Tris base 242.0 g;
  - glacial acetic acid 57.1 ml;
  - 0.5M EDTA, pH 8.0, 100 ml;
  - water dist. ad. 1000 ml.
- Ammonium persulfate 10%:
  - ammonium persulfate 0.1 g;
  - water dist. 1 ml;
- Staining solution DCode;
  - bromophenol blue 0.05 g;
  - xylene cyanol 0,05 g;
  - 1X TAE buffer 10 ml;
- Solution for implementing samples:
  - bromophenol blue 0.25 ml 2%;
  - xylene cyanol 0.25ml 2%;
  - glycerol 7.0 ml;
  - water dist. 2.5 ml;
- 1.25 X TAE buffer migration:
  - 50X TAE buffer 175 ml;
  - water dist. 6825 ml.

13. Sample preparation

1. It is important that PCR is optimized to decrease the formation of artifact products that may interfere with test itself. PCR products should be assessed for purity by agarose gel electrophoresis before being used for electrophoresis.
2. On gel we applied 180-300 ng of amplified DNA per well. On each gel and for each amplicon there were joined migration of the sample and normal DNA.
3. At each sample, we added a volume of 2X sample application solution.

13.1. Preheating migration buffer

1. Electrophoresis tank was filled with a quantity of 7 L of 1X TAE buffer.
2. We placed the temperature control module above the electrophoresis tank.
3. Then we adjusted the temperature to 60°C. To achieve this temperature 1-1.5 hours wereneeded. If the buffer is preheated in the oven, this time can be reduced.

13.2. Assemble gel sandwich

Casting procedure is extremely laborious and is was done by strict electrophoresis guidelines provided by equipment manufacturer. A system of 16x16cm plates was used and the prepared gel was "sandwich" type.

1. "Sandwich" gel is mounted on a clean surface. We have placed large plate first, then we have set the spacers on the short edges of this plate.
2. Lower plate was disposed over the large plate so the bottom was flush with large plate edge.
3. We loosen the black screw of the two sandwich cutters. We placed plates in these pliers so that the arrows were facing upwards.
4. We tightened the clamps so that the glass plates were well fixed.
5. Sandwich assembly was inserted into the alignment (without clips into place) so short board was facing forward. We loosen the clips and clamps easily inserted between the plates alignment plate which serves to align the spacers.
6. We aligned the plates and spacers by moving laterally and obliquely claws. We must ensure that the spacers are perfectly parallel and the lower edge of the two plates was perfectly aligned. We tightened the screw clamps for immobilizing overall assembly.
7. We removed the plate alignment between glass plates. Then we removed the sandwich from the stand and check the lower edges of the plates and spacers are aligned perfectly.

13.3. Casting the gel

1. We placed the gray foam in the space provided for pouring the gel. Pins of the base were completely relaxed. Placed plates mounted on the lower plate to the front pad. After it was placed correctly by turning the cam, pressing the lower edge of the foam boards was performed.
2. In a 50 ml tube we puted the required amount of gel solution. Ammonium persulfate and TEMED were added to a final concentration of 0.09% (v/v). Stopped the tube and mixed by inversion.
3. We inserted the comb into sandwich and positioned it so that it was slightly bent (angle) to the edge boards. This prevented the formation of air bubbles between the gel and the comb teeth.

4. Poured the gel solution into the sandwich until comb teeth were covered. Then pressed the comb in its correct position. Solution was added to the filling.

5. We allowed the gel to polymerize for 60 minutes. After polymerization we carefully removed the comb.

13.4. Migrating samples

1. Electrophoresis tank must contain 7 liters of buffer migration.

2. After the temperature was reached by the migration buffer (60°C) we disconnected temperature maintenance system.

3. Removed the temperature module from the electrophoresis tank. Gel fitting with gel electrophoresis was introduced into the tank and the temperature module was placed again into position.

4. Filled the volume of migration buffer until the level mark on the camera, and added also into the anode upper chamber.

5. Before applying the samples we left the machine running again to reach a migration temperature of 60°C.

6. Applied the samples after each well was previously rinsed with buffer. Sample application was made through a specially designed device that is provided.

7. Samples prepared as described above were applyed by automated pipetting carefully so that they do not spread outside the wells.

8. Closed the device and connected to the source. Migration was 5 hours at a voltage of 5 V/cm.

13.5. Gel staining

Electrophoresis was performed after the gel is removed from the tank, and glass plates carefully unfold. The gel sticks to the glass plate. Staining can be done by two procedures: simple procedure with Ethidium Bromide and fluorescence examination or staining procedure Argent. We opted for the second.

Protocol described below is an adaptation of that offered by the company with the Promega kit "DNA Silver Staining System".

A kit contains the following ingredients required for 10 stains:

- 500μl Bind silane;
- 20 G Silver Nitrate (10 x 2g);
- 60 Ml Formaldehyde, 37% (20 x 3 ml);
- 10 Ml Sodium thiosulfate, 10 mg/ml (10 x 1 ml);

- 600 G Sodium Carbonate (10 x 60g).

13.6. Materials required

- Fixing solution/stop:
  - 200 ml glacial acetic acid;
  - 1800 ml distilled water;
- Coloring solution:
  - silver nitrate ($AgNO_3$) 2 g;
  - 3 ml 37% formaldehyde;
  - 2000 ml distilled water;
- Developing solution:
  - 3 ml 37% formaldehyde;
  - Sodium thiosulfate 10 mg/ml, ($Na_2S_2O_3 \times 5H_2O$) 400 µl ;
  - 2000 ml distilled water;
  - sodium carbonate (Na_2CO_3) 60 g.

We prepared the solution just in time to use it, cooled at 4-10°C before use.

14. Technique used

1. Gel plates were placed on a flat surface. With a plastic "feather" glass was removed. The gel was caught on the short board.
2. The gel attached on short plate was placed in a plastic tray.
3. Argent coloring followed few steps:
   a. fixing /stop solution – 20 minutes;
   b. distilled water – 2 minutes;
   c. Repeat step "b" 2 times 2 x 2 minutes;
   d. staining solution – 30 minutes;
   e. distilled water – 10 seconds;
   f. developing solution (4-10°C) up to 5 minutes (to become visible Ladder allele);
   g. fixing/stop solution* – 5 minutes;
   h. distilled water – 2 minutes;

*Solution was added directly above solution developer to stop the developer reaction.

4. We placed the gel upright and dry overnight.

15. Mutations identification through DGGE technique and silver or ethidium bromide staining

After amplification the samples were checked to confirm successful amplification by agarose gel electrophoresis. For migration were applied two tests, one that was considered the normal type (same in all cases) and the other representing the analyzed case.

To see if amplifyed amplicons in the studied cases presented mutations, we used samples examined by agarose gel electrophoresis, for electrophoresis on polyacrylamide 6%.

16. Statistical analysis

Statistical analysis was performed using Graph Pad InState and Graph Pad State Mate.

17. Results

Demographic and clinical characteristics of patients examined during study period were as follows (table 3).

Histopathological classification and localization of tumors in patients investigated through colonoscopy and biopsy referred to genetic analysis of *COL11A1* mutations can be seen in table 4.

From the total of 250 patients genetically explored, 178 (71.20%) were diagnosed with adenocarcinoma and TNM staged after hiistopathological and imagistic examinations. Most of the patients were staged as stage II or III (18.80%, respectively 23.60%).

We analyzed 51 patients diagnosed with advanced adenomatous polyps. Polyps were classified according to hiistopathological features in: 26 polyps with high-grade dysplasia (10.40%), 17 villous adenoma (6.80%), and 8 tubular adenoma bigger than 1 cm (3.20%).

Among the 250 patients studied, 178 had adenocarcinomas, 51 had advanced adenomas, and the rest 21 had minor polypspolyps.

All samples analyzed for fecal *COL11A1* mutations were processed in a single laboratory.

The plan for *COL11A1* analyses in feces or biopsy has been described previously and is shown in figure 2.

Characteristic	No.	%
Age		
Mean (yr)	67.44 ± 8.97	20.40
40-49	51	31.60
50-59	79	34.80
60-69	87	9.20
70-79	23	4.00
≥ 80	10	
Sex		
Male	189	75.60
Female	61	24.4
Ethnicity		
Caucasians	203	81.20
Other	47	18.80
Family history		
APC (adenomatous polyposis coli)	16	6.40
CRC	49	19.60
Other cancer	37	14.80
Without family history of cancer/polyps	148	59.20

Table 3. Demographic characteristics of patients enrolled in the study.

Histopathological feature	No./%	Localisation – no./%				
		Ascendinging Colon	Transvers	Descendinging colon	Sigmoid	Rectumum
Adenocarcinoma	178/250 [71.2]	41/178 [23.03]	21/178 [11.79]	62/178 [34.83]	44/178 [24.71]	10/178 [4.00]
Stage TNM I	33 [13.20]	6 [3.37]	5 [2.80]	12 [6.74]	7 [3.93]	3 [1.68]
Stage TNM II	47 [18.80]	7 [3.93]	6 [3.37]	18 [10.11]	12 [6.74]	4 [2.24]
Stage TNM III	59 [23.60]	14 [7.86]	8 [4.49]	22 [12.35]	12 [6.74]	3 [1.68]
Stage TNM IV	39 [15.60]	14 [7.86]	2 [2.23]	10 [5.61]	13 [7.30]	0 [0.00]
Advanced adenoma	51/250 [20.40]	12/51 [23.52]	7/51 [13.72]	16/51 [31.72]	14/51 [27.45]	2/51 [3.92]
High-grade dysplasia	26 [10.40]	8 [15.6]	4 [7.84]	7 [13.72]	7 [13.72]	–
Villous adenoma	17 [6.80]	3 [5.88]	1 [1.96]	5 [9.80]	6 [11.76]	2 [3.93]
Tubular adenoma ≥ 1cm	8 [3.20]	1 [1.96]	2 [3.93]	4 [7.84]	1 [1.96]	–
Minor polyps	21/250 [8.40]	3/21 [14.28]	5/21 [23.80]	5/21 [23.80]	6/21 [28.57]	2/21 [9.52]
Tubular adenoma <1cm	9 [3.60]	1 [4.76]	2 [9.52]	2 [9.52]	3 [14.28]	–
Hiperplastic	10 [4.00]	1 [4.76]	3 [14.28]	3 [14.28]	2 [9.52]	2 [9.52]
Unspecified	2 [0.8]	1 [4.76]	–	–	1 [0.56]	–

Table 4. Hiistopathological classification and tumor localization.

http://dx.doi.org/10.5772/57327

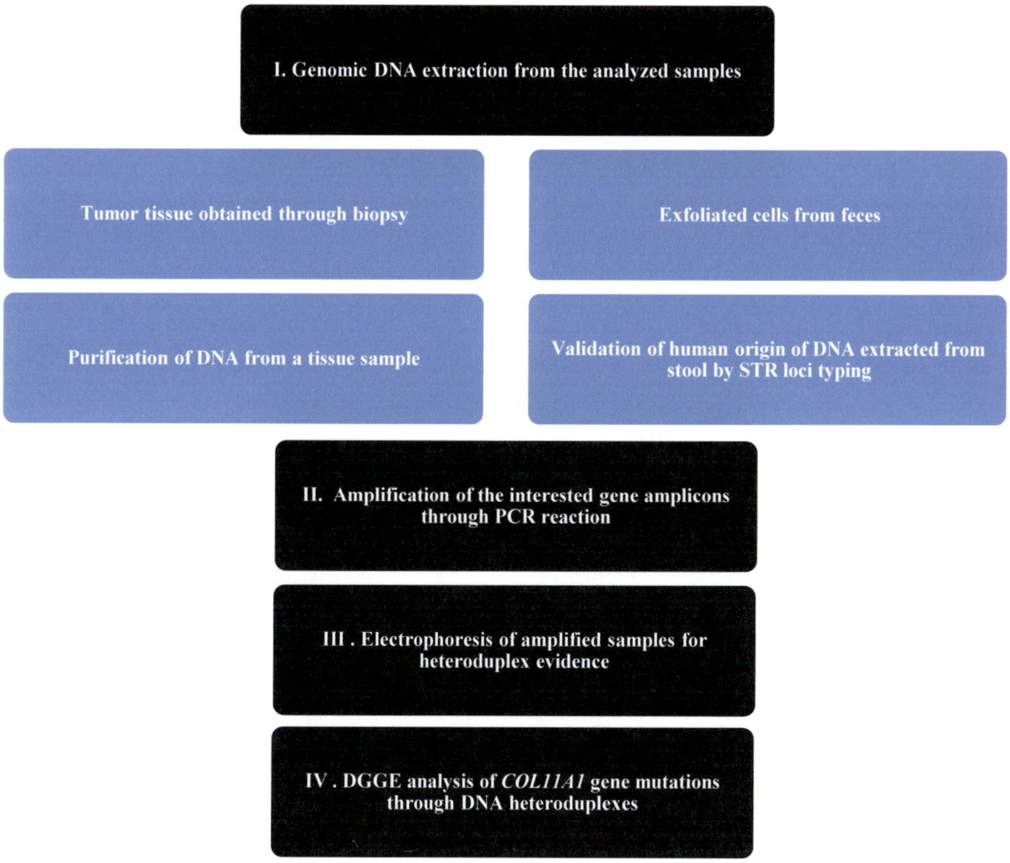

Figure 2. Approach to Extraction and Analysis of Fecal and Tumor DNA analysis.

Also laboratory handling of all samples was fully described above.

Each exon of gene *COL11A1* studied was assessed independently.

We considered a positive result any modified component of the study gene, and we noted any mutation as a positive fecal DNA test.

18. DGGE analysis of *COL11A1* gene mutations through DNA heteroduplexes

COL11A1 is located on chromosome 1p21 and consists of 232,030 bases. It contains 68 exons, yet not wholly sequenced, of which exons 38, 41, 16, 54, 55, 56 and 57 were until now studied.

HE analysis for exons 38, 41 and 16

For all 3 analyzed amplicons in all 250 studied cases, the migration speed was identical for both control and samples.

HE analysis for exons 54, 55, 56 and 57

HE analysis of exons 54 clearly demonstrated in 52 cases (20.80%) the presence of the same displaced bands pattern in the biopsy and stool extracted cells samples compared with the control. This pattern of mutation was correlated positively with male gender, TNM stage II/III tumors, vegetative pattern, descendent and sigmoid localization – table 5.

No.	Pacient no.	DNA sample	Mutations/amplicons						
			38	41	16	54	55	56	57
1	1	Biopsy	-	-	-	+	-	-	-
		Faeces	-	-	-	+	-	-	-
2	4	Biopsy	-	-	-	-	-	+	-
		Faeces	-	-	-	-	-	+	-
3	7	Biopsy	-	-	-	+	-	-	-
		Faeces	-	-	-	+	-	-	+
4	8	Biopsy	-	-	-	+	-	-	-
		Faeces	-	-	-	+	-	-	+
5	11	Biopsy	-	-	-	+	-	-	+
		Faeces	-	-	-	+	-	-	+
6	13	Biopsy	-	-	-	+	-	-	+
		Faeces	-	-	-	+	-	-	-
7	14	Biopsy	-	-	-	-	-	+	-
		Faeces	-	-	-	-	-	+	-
8	16	Biopsy	-	-	-	+	-	-	-
		Faeces	-	-	-	+	-	-	-
9	17	Biopsy	-	-	-	-	-	+	-
		Faeces	-	-	-	+	-	+	-
10	20	Biopsy	-	-	-	-	-	+	-
		Faeces	-	-	-	-	-	+	-
11	21	Biopsy	-	-	-	+	-	-	-
		Faeces	-	-	-	+	-	-	+
12	26	Biopsy	-	-	-	+	-	+	-
		Biopsy	-	-	-	+	-	+	-
13	29	Faeces	-	-	-	+	-	+	-
		Biopsy	-	-	-	+	-	+	-
14	34	Biopsy	-	-	-	+	-	+	-
		Faeces	-	-	-	+		+	-
15	38	Biopsy	-	-	-	+	-	-	-

http://dx.doi.org/10.5772/57327

No.	Pacient no.	DNA sample	Mutations/amplicons						
			38	41	16	54	55	56	57
		Biopsy	-	-	-	+	-	-	-
16	46	Faeces	-	-	-	+			-
		Biopsy	-	-	-	+	-	+	-
17	48	Biopsy	-	-	-	+	-	-	-
		Faeces	-	-	-	+			-
18	56	Biopsy	-	-	-	-	-	+	-
		Faeces	-	-	-			+	-
19	59	Biopsy	-	-	-	+	-	+	-
		Faeces	-	-	-	-	-	+	-
20	74	Biopsy	-	-	-	-	-	+	+
		Faeces	-	-	-	-	-	+	-
21	78	Biopsy	-	-	-	+	-	-	-
		Faeces	-	-	-	+			-
22	84	Biopsy	-	-	-	+	-	-	-
		Biopsy	-	-	-	+	-	-	-
23	89	Faeces	-	-	-	+			-
		Biopsy	-	-	-	+	-	-	-
24	93	Biopsy	-	-	-	+	-	-	-
		Faeces	-	-	-	+			-
25	96	Biopsy	-	-	-	+	-	+	-
		Biopsy	-	-	-	+	-	-	-
26	104	Faeces	-	-	-	+			+
		Biopsy	-	-	-	+	-	-	+
27	107	Biopsy	-	-	-	+	-	-	-
		Faeces	-	-	-	+	-	-	-
28	109	Biopsy	-	-	-	-	-	+	-
		Faeces	-	-	-	-	-	+	
29	116	Biopsy	-	-	-	+	-	-	-
		Biopsy	-	-	-	+	-	-	-
30	119	Faeces	-	-	-	+	-	-	-
		Biopsy	-	-	-	+	-	-	-
31	121	Biopsy	-	-	-	+	-	+	-
		Faeces				+	-	-	-
32	129	Biopsy	-	-	-	+	-	-	+
		Faeces	-	-	-	+	-	-	+
33	132	Biopsy	-	-	-	+	-	-	-
		Faeces	-	-	-	+	-	-	-

No.	Pacient no.	DNA sample	Mutations/amplicons						
			38	41	16	54	55	56	57
34	134	Biopsy	-	-	-	+	-	+	-
		Faeces	-	-	-	+	-	-	-
35	138	Biopsy	-	-	-	+	-	-	-
		Faeces	-	-	-	+	-	-	-
36	143	Biopsy	-	-	-	+	-	+	-
		Biopsy	-	-	-	+	-	+	-
37	146	Faeces	-	-	-	-	-	+	-
		Biopsy	-	-	-	-	-	+	-
38	147	Biopsy	-	-	-	+	-	-	-
		Faeces	-	-	-	+	-	-	-
39	159	Biopsy	-	-	-	-	-	+	-
		Biopsy	-	-	-	-	-	+	-
40	166	Faeces	-	-	-	+	-	+	-
		Biopsy	-	-	-	+	-	+	+
41	168	Biopsy	-	-	-	+	-	+	-
		Faeces	-	-	-	+	-	+	-
42	171	Biopsy	-	-	-	-	-	+	-
		Faeces	-	-	-	-	-	+	-
43	177	Biopsy	-	-	-	+	-	-	-
		Biopsy	-	-	-	+	-	-	-
44	179	Faeces	-	-	-	+	-	-	-
		Biopsy	-	-	-	+	-	-	-
45	182	Biopsy	-	-	-	+	-	-	+
		Faeces	-	-	-	+	-	-	+
46	189	Biopsy	-	-	-	+	-	-	-
		Faeces	-	-	-	+	-	-	-
47	201	Biopsy	-	-	-	+	-	-	-
		Faeces	-	-	-	+	-	-	-
48	203	Biopsy	-	-	-	+	-	-	-
		Faeces				+	-	-	-
49	208	Biopsy	-	-	-	+	-	-	-
		Faeces	-	-	-	+	-	-	-
50	211	Biopsy	-	-	-	+	-	-	-
		Biopsy	-	-	-	+	-	-	-
51	220	Faeces	-	-	-	-	-	+	+
		Biopsy	-	-	-	-	-	+	+
52	224	Biopsy	-	-	-	+	-	-	-

http://dx.doi.org/10.5772/57327

No.	Pacient no.	DNA sample	Mutations/amplicons						
			38	41	16	54	55	56	57
		Faeces	-	-	-	+	-	-	-
53	228	Biopsy	-	-	-	-	-	-	-
		Biopsy	-	-	-	-	-	-	-
54	230	Faeces	-	-	-	+			
		Biopsy	-	-	-	+	-	-	-
55	236	Biopsy	-	-	-	+	-	-	-
		Faeces	-	-	-	+	-	-	-
56	237	Biopsy	-	-	-	+	-	-	+
		Faeces	-	-	-	+	-	-	-
57	211	Biopsy	-	-	-	-	-	-	+
		Biopsy	-	-	-	-	-	-	+
58	220	Faeces				+			-
		Biopsy	-	-	-	+	-	-	-
59	224	Biopsy	-	-	-	+	-	-	+
		Faeces				+			+
60	228	Biopsy	-	-	-	+	-	-	-
		Faeces	-	-	-	+	-	-	-
61	230	Faeces	-	-	-	-	-	-	+
		Biopsy	-	-	-	-	-	-	+
62	236	Biopsy	-	-	-	+	-	-	-
		Faeces	-	-	-	+	-	-	-
63	237	Biopsy	-	-	-	+	-	-	-
		Faeces	-	-	-	+	-	-	-
64	238	Biopsy	-	-	-	+	-	-	-
		Faeces	-	-	-	+	-	-	-
65	241	Biopsy	-	-	-	-	-	-	+
		Biopsy	-	-	-	-	-	-	+
66	244	Faeces	-	-	-	+	-	-	+
		Biopsy	-	-	-	+	-	-	+
67	248	Biopsy	-	-	-	+	-	-	-
		Faeces	-	-	-	-	-	-	-
68	249	Biopsy	-	-	-	+	-	-	-
		Faeces	-	-	-	+	-	-	-
69	250	Faeces	-	-	-	+	-	-	-
		Biopsy	-	-	-	+	-	-	-

Table 5. Patients with *COL11A1* gene mutations

We also noticed the same pattern of different speed migration in case of HE analysis of exon 56 in 18 patients (7.20%) and exon 57 in 11 patients (4.40%).

Statistic analysis revealed that the last two kind of mutations were correlated with tumor stage IV, male gender and advanced age (> 70 yrs old) – table 6.

Histopathological and clinical features	*COL11A1 mutations (No./%)*
Adenocarcinoma	
Stage TNM I	2 [2.89]
Stage TNM II	18 [26.08]
Stage TNM III	27 [39.13]
Stage TNM IV	3 [4.34]
Advanced adenoma	
High-grade dysplasia	0
VillousVillous adenoma	1 [1.44]
Tubular adenoma ≥1cm	1 [1.44]
Minor polyps	
Tubular adenoma <1cm	0
HyperplasticHyperplastic	0
Unspecified	0
Age (only for exon 56, 57)	> 70 yrs (p=0.0478, 95%CI 11.781-49.552)
Gender ratio	M/F=3.72 (p=0.021, 95%CI 26.330-49.312)
EthnicityEthnicity	CaucasianCaucasian/other (p=0.0037, 95%CI 14.114-49.226)
Localisation	Descendent/Sigmoid (p=0.02, 95%CI 29.481-50.227)
TNM classification	Stage II/III (p=0.009, 95%CI 7.336-39.386)

Table 6. Correlation between hiistopathological examination and genetic analysis.

The migrating front presented two bands, out of which the slowest part generates the heteroduplexes obtained through denaturation-renaturation, and the faster one, the homoduplexes (figure 3).

The samples were different from the wild type due to the fact that they contain amplified mutant type DNA, which through electrophoresis leads to speed migration modification.

The mutation detected by us is a substitutive type one as a series of 2 bands was evident on the migration front.

There were no seen mutations for the rest of the analyzed cases for the exon 55.

All detected mutations can be observed in table no. 5

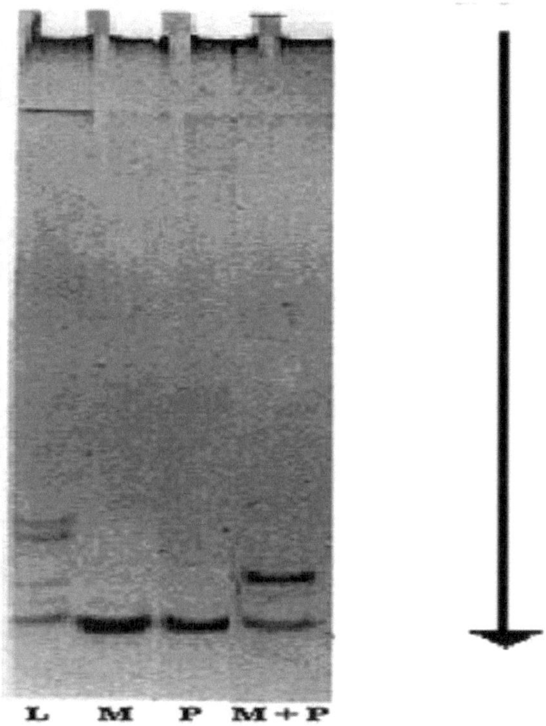

L – molecular weight ladder. M – healthy individual allele (control). P – unprocessed allele for exon 54. M+P – denatured-renatured sample.

Figure 3. Electrophoresis in 6% polyacrylamid gel of the processed samples in order to point out heteroduplexes for exon 54, using silver staining.

Among 229 patients with advanced neoplasia (tubular adenoma 1 cm in diameter or larger, villous polyp, polyps with high-grade dysplasia, or cancer), 69 patients (27.60%) presented mutations in *COL11A1* gene in at least 1 exon (table no. 5 and 6).

Regarding benign polyps, none of patients presented *COL11A1* mutations.

19. Disscusions and conclusions

COL11A1 gene overexpression has been implicated as a candidate marker of various types of cancers [26]. Previous studies have found overexpression of the *COL11A1* gene in different types of cancers, such as non-small cell lung (NSCLC), ovarian, oral cavity and colorectal cancers [13-16]. In particular, overexpression of the *COL11A1* gene was found to be correlated with invasion and metastasis of these cancers [13-16].

As we previously detected in a pilot study regarding genetic mutations related to *COL11A1* gene in exfoliated epithelial cells in the stool, we found mutations involving exon 54 [27].

Our present study confirmed the presence of *COL11A1* mutations in patients with colorectal adenomas or cancer. Polyacrylamide gel electrophoresis method for the heteroduplex analysis (HA) was a sensitive genetic method to diagnose mutations of *COL11A1*.

Mutations detected in biopsy cells were present in exfoliated cells from feaces, proving the usefulness of this genetic approach for noninvasive early diagnosis. Genetic alterations were detected at the level of exons 54, 56 and 57.

Our results are similar with the results of other studies which have previously shown that *COL11A1* is upregulated in the majority of sporadic colorectal cancer [28], emphasizing the fact that the expression of *COL11A1* could be the primary change giving rise to a tumorigenic response in epithelial cells [28].

1. Another study found a statistically significant overexpression of *COL11A1* in polyps from a patient with FAP [29]. The results from this study suggested that the expression of COL11A1 could directly contribute to tumorigenesis in fibroblasts in FAP and explain osteomas and desmoids, or indirectly to polyp-formation and tumor progression in sporadic CRC [29].
2. The study of Croner R et al [30] also showed up-regulation of *COL11A1* in CRC versus normal colonic mucosa ($p<0.001$). The same result was shown by Lascorz et al study, in which extracellular matrix receptor interaction and focal adhesion shared nine genes (*COL1A1, COL1A2, COL3A1, COL4A1, COL11A1, FN1, ITGA2, SPP1*, and *THBS2*) were upregulated in colorectal cancer [31].

Joined by other well known genetic tools already examined in the stool cell's DNA involved in the development of some colorectal cancers, *COL11A1* could be a feasible genetic biomarker targeted in stool samples for early diagnosis of colorectal cancer at risk patients.

Acknowledgements

This work was accomplished with the support of Professor Mixici Fr.

Author details

Andra Iulia Suceveanu[1], Laura Mazilu[2] and Adrian-Paul Suceveanu[3]

*Address all correspondence to: andrasuceveanu@yahoo.com

1 Gastroenterology Department, Emergency Hospital of Constanta, Faculty of Medicine, Ovidius University of Constanta, Romania

2 Oncology Department, Emergency Hospital of Constanta, Faculty of Medicine, Ovidius University of Constanta, Romania

3 Internal Medicine Department, Emergency Hospital of Constanta, Faculty of Medicine, Ovidius University of Constanta, Romania

References

[1] Jemal A, Murray T, Ward E, et al. Cancer statistics, 2005. *CA Cancer J Clin,* 2005; 55(1): 10-30.

[2] Whitlock EP, Lin J, Liles E, Beil T, Fu R, O'Connor E, Thompson RN, Cardenas T. Screening for Colorectal Cancer: An Updated Systematic Review. Evidence Synthesis No. 65, Part 1. AHRQ Publication No. 08-05124-EF-1. Rockville, Maryland, Agency for Healthcare Research and Quality, October 2008.

[3] Vogelstein B, Fearon ER, Hamilton SR, Kern SE, Preisinger AC, Leppert M, et al. Genetic alterations during colorectal-tumor development. *N Engl J Med,* 1988; 319: 525-532.

[4] Siena S, Sartore-Bianchi A, Di Nicolantonio F, Balfour J, Bardelli A. Biomarkers predicting clinical outcome of epidermal growth factor receptor-targeted therapy in metastatic colorectal cancer. *J Natl Cancer Inst,* 2009; 101: 1308-1324.

[5] Renée M. Ned, Stephanie Melillo, and Michael Marrone. Fecal DNA testing for Colorectal Cancer Screening: the ColoSure™ test PLoS Curr, 2011, March 22; 3: RRN1220.

[6] Hall MJ, Olopade OI. Disparities in genetic testing: Thinking outside the BRCA box. *J Clin Oncol,* 2006; 24: 2197-203.

[7] Calvert PM, Frucht H. The genetics of colorectal cancer. *Ann Intern Med*, 2002; 137(7): 603-12.

[8] Fearon ER, Vogelstein B. A genetic model for colorectal tumorigenesis. *Cell,* 1990; 61: 759-67.

[9] Kinzler KW, Vogelstein B. Lessons from hereditary colorectal cancer. *Cell*, 1996; 87: 159-70.

[10] Lynch HT, de la Chapelle A. Genetic susceptibility to non-polyposis colorectal cancer. *J Med Genet*, 1999; 36: 801-18.

[11] Perucho M. Cancer of the microsatellite mutator phenotype. Biol Chem, 1996; 377: 675-84.

[12] Zlotogora J, Sagi M, Schuper A, Leiba H & Merin S. Variability of Stickler syndrome. *Am J Med Genet*, 1992; 42: 337-379.

[13] Wang KK, Liu N, Radulovich N, et al. Novel candidate tumor marker genes for lung adenocarcinoma. *Oncogene*, 2002; 21: 7598-7604.

[14] Chong IW, Chang MY, Chang HC, et al. Great potential of a panel of multiple *hMTH1, SPD, ITGA11* and *COL11A1* markers for diagnosis of patients with non-small cell lung cancer. *Oncol Rep*, 2006;16: 981-988.

[15] Kim H, Watkinson J, Varadan V, Anastassiou D. Multi-cancer computational analysis reveals invasion-associated variant of desmoplastic reaction involving *INHBA, THBS2* and *COL11A1*. *BMC Med Genomics*, 2010; 3: 51.

[16] Schmalbach CE, Chepeha DB, Giordano TJ, et al. Molecular profiling and the identification of genes associated with meta-static oral cavity/pharynx squamous cell carcinoma. *Arch Otolaryngol Head Neck Surg*, 2004; 130: 295-302.

[17] Bernard M, Yoshioka H, Rodriquez E, van der Rest M, Kimura T, Ninomiya Y, Olsen BR & Ramirez F. Cloning and sequencing of pro-a1(XI) collagen cDNA demonstrates that type XI belongs to the fibrillar class of collagens and reveals that the expression of the gene is not restricted to cartilagenous tissue. *J Biol Chem*, 1988; 263: 17159-17166.

[18] Annunen, S. From rare syndrome to a common disease. Mutations in minor cartilage collagen genes cause Marshall and Stickler syndromes and intervertebral disc disease. Oulu University Library, Finland, 1999.

[19] M Erkan, N Weis, Z Pan, C Schwager et al. Organ-inflammation-and cancer specific transcriptional fingerprints of pancreatic and hepatic stellate cells. *Molecular Cancer*, 2010, 9:88.

[20] Ziemmermann PA, Carrington MN, Nutman TB. Exploiting structural differences among heteroduplex molecules to simplify genotyping the *DQA1* and *DQB1* alleles in human lymphocyte typing. *Nucleic Acids Res*, 1993; 25: 4541-4547.

[21] Mülhardt C. DNA analysis. Heteroduplex analysis. In: Molecular biology and genomics, 2006, 165.

[22] Lorkowski S, Cullen P. Analyzing gene expression. A handbook of methods and pitfalls, 2001.

[23] QIAGEN Gmbh. Midi/Maxi Handbook, 2nd ed. QIAGEN Gmbh, Hilden, Germany, 2001.

[24] Edwards A, et al. DNA typing with trimeric and tetrameric tandem repeats: polymorphic loci, detection systems, and population genetics. In: The 2nd International Symposium on Human Identification 1991, Promega Corporation, 31.

[25] Pellestor F. Methods in Molecular Biology, PRINS and In Situ PCR Protocols. *Humana Press*, 2006; 211-220.

[26] Park JH, et al. Association between collagen type XI $\alpha 1$ gene polymorphisms and papillary thyroid cancer in a Korean population. *Exp Ther Med*, 2011; 2(6): 1111-1116.

[27] Suceveanu AI, Suceveanu AP, Voinea Fl, Mazilu L, Mixici F, Adam T. Introduction of cytogenetic tests in CRC screening. *Journal of Gastrointestinal and Liver Diseases (JGLD)*, An International Journal of Gastroenterology and Hepatology, march 2009, vol. 18 (1): 33-38, Print ISSN 1841-8724, Online ISSN 1842-1121, www.jgld.ro.

[28] Fischer H, Stenling R, Rubio C, Lindblom A. Colorectal carcinogenesis is associated with stromal expression of *COL11A1* and *COL5A2*. *Carcinogenesis*, Volume 22, Issue 6, 2001; 875-878.

[29] Fischer H, Salahshor S, Stenling R, Björk J, Lindmark G, Iselius L, Rubio C, Lindblom A. *COL11A1* in FAP polyps and in sporadic colorectal tumors. *BMC Cancer*, 2001; 1: 17.

[30] Croner R, et al. Common denominator genes that distinguish colorectal carcinoma from normal mucosa. *Int Journal Colorectal Disease*, 2005; 20: 353-362.

[31] Lascorz J, Hemminki K, Fösti A. Systematic enrichment analysis of gene expression profiling studies identifies consensus pathways implicated in colorectal cancer development. *J Carcinog*, 2011; 10: 7.

Chapter 17

The Complexity of Colorectal Cancer Biology — Putting Bricks on the Path to Personalized Medicine

Emilia Balboa, Angel Carracedo and
Francisco Barros

Additional information is available at the end of the chapter

http://dx.doi.org/10.5772/57172

1. Introduction

Boveri's hypothesis about the genetic basis of cancer, a century ago, subsequently confirmed by Loeb et al. in 1974, opened the gate for genetic studies that became essential for cancer management. [1, 2]

Cancer is a disease that arises from altered cell due to multiple genetic and epigenetic alterations that confer them the properties of apoptosis evasion and growth advantage. These properties represent a competitive advantage over normal cells, leading to the expansion and colonization of other tissues by these cells, which cause patient´s death by interfering with the normal function of its organs. [3]

Introduction of chemotherapy in cancer treatments has supposed an important improvement in progression-free survival but, it is also associated to life threatening secondary effects, in the worst scenario, and an important quality life reduction in the best one. Furthermore, due to the difficulty to stratify patients in low and high risk, there are a substantial number of them that will receive the therapy but will not experience any benefit from it. These consequences, underline the importance of personalized treatment in cancer management. [4, 5]

The first chemotherapy treatments were based on a frequently observed characteristic of cancer cells, this is, a high proliferation index. Their effectiveness rates vary among cancers, but all of them are characterized by important secondary effects as consequence of their low specificity, since these chemotherapeutics also affects normal cells.

The use of this traditional chemotherapy effectively shrinks tumor mass but, observation of tumor metastases and recurrences led to the idea of the existence of cell populations unaffected by the treatment, either because they are a type of cells with different characteristics from the cells that the drug was designed to, because they have undergone genetic changes that confer them resistance or because the microenvironment protects them. Identification of the resistance cause is one of the cornerstones of cancer treatment and in this attempt, identification of cells that have tumorigenic potential to sustain cancer is fundamental. [6]

Based on this, studies of tumor organization were performed. As indicated by Shackleton et al, research on tumor organization intends to determine which cells have tumorigenic potential to sustain cancer, this is, all cells in a cancer or only a specific population of them. There are two principal models of tumor organization, not mutually exclusive, the clonal evolution model [stochastic] and the stem cell model [hierarchical], that have been subjected to deep examination owing to their implications in cancer management. [6]

The clonal evolution model was described by Nowell in 1976, and it is quite verified that it seems to be ubiquitous in all cancers. It describes cancer development by the successive acquisition of differential features in the derived cells giving rise to the formation of cell clones, this is, group of cells with common features because they originate from the same progenitor cell that can be a stem cell or not. Some of these features can be positive and provide a selective advantage to these cells over the others, with the consequent establishment of these clones. This model supports the idea that all cells in a tumor are important since the cancer can be sustained due to the possible acquisition of resistance or advantage features in the derived cells. On the other hand, this process is not random, tumors share similarities, but these similarities will be modulated by the tumor environment turning each tumor into unique entities. [3, 7]

To establish a model of tumor organization is fundamental since it should drastically change treatment cancer approach. Identification of cells that drive tumor progression will allow us to design target drugs against this cells instead of nonspecific drugs that treat all cancer cells, even normal cells. Tumors that have a hierarchical organization from stem cells to more differentiated cells are said to follow the stem cell model that have been recently proved in a few cancers, among them, the colorectal cancer. [3, 6-13] Stem cells are a very specific type of cells that possess differential capabilities such as being pluripotent, remain in a quiescent state, have a long life as well as self-renewal capacity which allows them to perpetuate themselves and repopulate different cells linages.

Nonetheless, both models are not incompatible, mutation causing clonal expansion may happen in the stem cell compartment and manifests its effects on the progenitors cells or may happen in the progenitors cells that can re-activate the auto-renewal machinery to generate stem cells. [14] As long as the disease progresses, these changes can induce alterations in the normal patterns of development of these cells, reducing their ability to differentiate and increasing their auto-renewal capacity, causing the uncontrolled increase of undifferentiated cells, as it happens in leukemia. [15] As Nowell denoted the observation of non-differentiation of tumor cells is explained by focus the cell resources in increasing cell proliferation and invasiveness. [3]

Both models describe a scenario of intratumor genetic heterogeneity that reproduces the tumor tissue heterogeneity observed in patients, and also describes the heterogeneity observed in the different stages of cancer as consequence of selection in different environments. [3, 7]

Nonetheless, cells in this tissue are not independent units, there is a communication between them and even collaboration has been proved in leukemogenic cells. [16] This communication is performed through the extracellular matrix by different signals to which cells respond and its behavior is modulated by these signals as them change over time. Hence, during cancer development, cells in a tumor, experiment different genetic alterations selected by their fitness which is determined by the tumor microenvironment and tissue characteristics where the tumor is being developed. All these characteristics explain the observed intra-tumor heterogeneity in cancer and the different subtypes identify in a specific type of cancer, which added to the modification performed by the individual genetic background makes each cancer a unique entity. [7]

To add more complexity to the system, not all the mutations within a tumor are important for its progression or survival. Due to alterations in DNA repair systems, numerous mutations are produced that do not provide any advantage nor disadvantage to cells at a given moment but, its presence and proportion in the tumor mass will depend on if they are produced in clones which have driver mutations, this is mutations that will lead tumor development and response to the environment. Differentiate which mutations are drivers from passengers it is another important and confounding factor for both, identification of tumor and pharmacogenetic markers. [7, 17, 18]

Equally importantly is to determine the global effects that mutations cause, since understanding the aims of the tumor through the modulation of the pathways that performs will help us to predict the compensatory mechanism that executes. [3] Knudson's two hits hypothesis postulates that more than one mutation is needed in cells to become malignant. [19, 20] The fine regulation that tumor cells exert, and the importance of the molecular pathways implied is exemplified by the °Just-right hypothesis° that postulates that the second mutation in the adenomatous polyposis coli [APC] gene [which is a gene where germline mutations are found to be associated to an hereditary form of colorectal cancer] produces in a tumor is dependent on the type and localization of the germline mutation in a patient in order to maintain some basal APC activity, which it is needed for cell functioning. [21]

Apart from all these convolutions, each tumor has an inherent progression; there is a pattern of genetic alterations typical of each tumor, whose establishment is a priority when designing cancer treatments. The goal is to increase drug efficiency along with its specificity in order to diminish the secondary effects. In this road, there have been two important events that have helped us to achieve this ultimate goal.

Firstly, advances in knowledge of genetics have allowed us to discover the hereditary component of cancer as well as the steps that follow in cancer development, the more important pathways trigger in them and have pointed out the key deregulated molecules against to specific drugs can be designed. The studies realized to determine the cancer characteristics have also contributed to the discovery of specific and differential patterns of each cancer. [22-25]

Secondly, drug development research has focused their efforts in the development of target drugs that act specifically on those molecules in order to avoid the important secondary effects of classical chemotherapy.

Molecular specific drugs, like tyrosine kinase inhibitors or antibody-based therapies are the next-generation cancer treatment. [4] As result of this molecular specificity, effectiveness of these selective treatments is more dependent on the biology of the target cell. Consequently, the pace of the improvements in cancer treatments is highly dependent on the knowledge of cancer cells biology.

But, as stated above, cancer cells are not islands, its behavior is modulated by the signals that its surroundings emit, as well as its surroundings control the quantity of nutrients, oxygen and chemicals that reach the tumor. Therefore, treatment efficiency is influenced by drug pharmacokinetics, that is dependent of the biology of the normal cells, as well as the secondary effects are determined by drug pharmacodynamics, that is subject to drug specificity and the inherited sensibility of normal cells to chemotherapeutic agents determined by different mechanisms, for example, detoxifying mechanisms. [3] Subsequently, when trying to personalize treatments it is important to identify both, the genetic of the tumor and the genetic of normal cells. This is one of the causes that explain the variability in response to chemotherapy observed in patients with similar tumor characteristics. [4]

Despite the efforts realized, the only pharmacogenetics markers used today in clinic are KRAS and BRAF mutations. Some of the causes of this delay in markers discovery are then. No intention of this chapter is to provide a deep review of the different subtypes but offer an outline of the principal characteristics of the diverse subtypes according to the literature, in order to expose the cause of the delay in markers discovery that was previously mentioned, and reflect that problems in pharmacogenetic studies obtained are due, in part, to the high heterogeneity in colorectal cancer which makes difficult to establish clearly differentiated groups of study and at the same time, to reflect that intense research has a positive point of view, since important advances in tumor characterization and target molecules discovery have also been done.

2. Colorectal cancer biology — Heterogeneity of colorectal cancer

Colon tissue is organized in a repetition of structural subunits called crypts. Cells in each crypt have an ordered configuration, being the stem cells at the base of the crypt and the subsequent differentiated cells upwards along the crypt. The main conductor in the colonic cell differentiation is the Wnt/β-catenin signaling pathway. [26] β-Catenin is a transcriptional co-activator of genes implicated in cell growth and differentiation. Activation of the Wnt pathway disrupts the cytoplasmatic complex that marks β-catenin for degradation allowing it to enter the nucleus were exerts its activity. [27-29] APC protein forms part of the degradation complex. Concordant to their function in the differentiation and growing pattern, there is an inverse gradient of APC/β-catenin expression along the crypt axle, being APC mostly expressed in the upper part of the crypt and β-catenin in the lower part on the crypt. [30]

Colorectal cancer is a highly heterogeneous malignancy caused by genetic and epigenetic alterations in the stem cells of the crypt of the bowel which give rise to precancerous lesion, aberrant crypt foci, that overgrow usually forming polyps that after a successful accumulation of genomic alterations become tumor cells. [11-13, 31, 32] It can arise in a sporadic form or it can have a hereditary component.

Identification of the cause that predisposes to cancer in the hereditary syndromes have given us clues, due to the similarities of the mechanisms identified, to understand what happen in the sporadic tumors, that involves the majority of the colorectal cancer cases. Germline mutations in known oncogenes or DNA repair genes have been identify as causative of a predisposition to endure colorectal cancer but the origin of the sporadic form is still unclear and it is attributed to genetic alterations caused by the environmental as chemical carcinogens, age related factors which increase DNA errors rate and nutritious factors. All these conditions will probably determine the activated cancer mechanism depending on which factor has triggered the cancer. But, environment is also an important factor that modulates colorectal cancer appearance in patients with a hereditary component since germline mutations cause a predisposition to cancer, but another mutation is needed in the cells for them to become malignant, as it is postulated in Knudson´s two hits hypothesis. [19, 20]

In recent times it has become evident the need of establish subtypes in colorectal cancer due to the differential characteristics of the proximal and distal segments of the colon as well as diverse features, at both histological and molecular level, observed in colorectal cancer.

Proximal and distal colon, proceed from a different embryological origin, midgut and hindgut respectively. Besides the embryological origin, its distinctions span from innervation and blood supply to functional differences and differential gene expression. [33, 34]

At histological level, most the polyps are adenomatous [95%], but only a small percentage of them progress to cancer and not all the colorectal cancer cases are presented with polyps. [35-37] Actually, prevalence of each type of polyp is only rough since it is population dependent, due to its genetic background and environmental dependence apart from the expertise of the pathologist to identify the polyp, which sometimes is difficult. [37, 38] Histological features of the tumors are associated to the underlying molecular pathway. So far, two main types of carcinoma have been identified, traditional and serrated carcinomas, that have several subtypes and whose development is driven by three main molecular mechanisms, chromosomal instability (CIN), microsatellite instability (MSI) and CpG island methylator phenotype (CIMP). Combinations of these mechanism and some additional genetic and epigenetics changes according to the tumor environment give raise to the large varieties of histological forms observed. [38]

On molecular basis, colorectal cancer development is mainly, but not exclusively, driven by the deregulation of one of these mechanisms (CIN, MSI or CIMP), CIN being the most prevalent. [23, 39-44] But it not clear if these mechanisms are the cause or the major alterations trigger in cancer. [2]

The predominance, of one of these mechanisms over the others, since they are not mutually exclusive, provides the tumor their differential features, which includes morphological characteristics, cancer prognosis and treatment efficiency. This heterogeneity observed in colorectal cancer is due to the diverse scenarios in which colorectal cancer develops so, characterization of the colorectal cancer in different subtypes, according to its distinctive signatures, will help us to stratify cancer progression risk and personalize treatments. [45-47]

But these subtypes are not mutually exclusive, the intra-heterogeneity observed in a patient´s polyps reflects the heterogeneity of the molecular pathways and mechanisms that can be implicated. [37]

Despite this overlap, predominant characteristics can be distinguished into the subtypes and even alterations that are, in principal, mutually exclusive have been identified, that reflect the unique signature of each tumor. [48, 49]

2.1. Molecular mechanism

2.1.1. Chromosomal instability mechanism – CIN

Chromosomal instability mechanism (CIN) is detected in the 65-70% of the colorectal cancers. It is defined by the identification of changes at chromosomal level in tumor cells that cause gene dose variations. [2] This mechanism is associated to the major hereditary syndrome, the polyposis adenomatous familiar (FAP) as well as its attenuated variant (AFAP), that accounts for 1% of the colorectal cases and it is the most frequently detected in the sporadic form [38, 50-52]. Less commonly, CIN is categorized in subtypes as CIN-high and low. [47, 52, 62]

The molecular steps that describe this mechanism were proposed by Fear and Vogelstein in the °adenoma-carcinoma sequence°, where mutations in the APC gene (chr.5q) is the first step identified in a sequence of genetic alterations on oncogenes and tumor suppressor genes that leads to its keys characteristics, the aneuploidy and loss of heterozigosity. [22, 52-54]

Germline mutations in the APC gene are associated with these hereditary syndromes, as well as mutations in this gene are detected in the 72%-85 of sporadic colorectal cancer cases and hypermethylation of its promoter in the 18%. According to the importance of the Wnt pathway in the colorectal cancer, in half of the patients where genetic alterations in APC are not detected, gain of function mutations in the β-catenin gene have been found that account for 10% of colorectal cases. [52, 55-57]

Besides its function in the repression complex of the β-catenin, APC has numerous functions, among which highlights its implication in chromosomal segregation and, according to its parallel increasing expression with cell differentiation, plays a role in different features of cell differentiation. [52, 55, 56]

Mutations in APC are followed by genetic alterations with a different frequency, in KRAS, DCC, SMAD4 and p53 that are detected in the progression of a tumor from adenoma to carcinoma. [22, 58] All these genes are key points of regulation of important pathways that control cell behavior thus, KRAS [chr.12p] is member of the Ras and PI3K pathway, which are usually dysregulated in cancer and is implicated in cell proliferation, differentiation, survival, metabolism and apoptosis. Its activation triggers both pathways. [58, 59]

SMAD4 belongs to the transforming growth factor β pathway signaling which is a tumor suppressor pathway. Its inactivation is related to tumor progression and invasion, being associated to the transition from adenoma to carcinoma. This pathway has also a function on the microenvironment regulation of cell by autocrine and paracrine factors. [58, 60]

Because of its important and numerous functions in cells, like cell cycle regulation or maintenance of genomic integrity, p53 (chr.17p) is called the guardian of the genome. Being one of the most frequently mutated genes in cancer, its inactivation is associated to metastasis. [58, 61]

Nonetheless, the establishment of the adenoma-carcinoma sequence does not implied that all mutations described are needed for the progression of cancer nor the uniques but the more frequently ones detected, with different prevalence across the stages. [22]

2.1.2. Microsatellite instability (MSI)

Microsatellite instability (MSI) is defined by the detection of alterations in the length of short repeated sequences known as microsatellite, which is indicative of defects in the DNA mismatch repair system (MMR). These alterations influence expression of the affected genes. [63] The genes that have been found associated to this altered mechanism are MLH1, PMS2, PMS1 and MSH6. This mechanism is detected in 15-20% of colorectal cancers in both sporadic and hereditary tumors. It is the main feature of another hereditary syndrome, Lynch syndrome that accounts for 2-3% of colorectal cases. [38, 64] The number of altered microsatellites, is also important, defining two subtypes as this number is high, MSI-H, or low, MSI-L. [65]

Mutations in MUTYH are associated to another hereditary syndrome, rarely found in sporadic cases, called adenomatous polyposis associated to Mutyh (MAP). This protein belongs to the DNA base-excision repair system, which is important in DNA oxidative damage repair that causes guanosine (G) to thymidine (T) transversions. [66] Molecular mechanisms are not yet totally clarified and polyps from MAP have some of the features but not all of both, CIN and MSI mechanism. [67, 68]

2.1.3. Methylator Phenotype (CIMP)

CpG island methylator phenotype (CIMP) is defined by the detection of high degree of methylation. [69] Hypermethylation of the promoter region causes silencing expression of affected genes. It is generally age-related and it is related to cell response to inflammation. [65]

This mechanism is frequent in sporadic tumor and has also been detected associated to hereditary mechanisms with a non-Darwinian patter of inheritance. [58, 70-75] There are two panels of genes studied to identify the CIMP state, which define two subtypes, CIMP-high and CIMP-low. CIMP-H is associated to neoplastic methylation meanwhile CIMP-L are age related.

2.2. Molecular pathways

2.2.1. Traditional pathway (Chromosomal instability mechanism – CIN)

The traditional pathway of colorectal cancer is the most prevalent, 60% of CCR arise by this pathway. [76] Histologically, tumors that follow the traditional pathway are tubular polyps that can be subdivided into tubular, tubulovillous and villous, being the former the most prevalent. Colorectal cancer from FAP and AFAP patients, are the canonical tumors develop by these pathway. This type of adenomas affects the epithelial layer and are originated from dysplastic aberrant crypt foci. [77]

CIN is the most prevalent molecular mechanism in the traditional pathway of colorectal cancer, which is also characterized for being microsatellite stable (MSS) and CIMP-. Tumors driven by this mechanism are more frequently detected in distal localization and have a worse prognosis than MSI tumors. They recently have showed the use of CIN as useful marker for predicting survival, being patients that harbors CIN high tumors associated with a poor survival. [62]

Adenoma – carcinoma sequence also lies beneath Lynch syndrome polyps but develops at a faster tempo. [78, 79] Lynch syndrome polyps are more frequently associated to the proximal colon, and even though it can be tubular, are more frequently associated with a mucinous or signet ring histology and villous structures. These polyps show a high grade dysplasia, poorly differentiated cells and Crohn's-like infiltration of lymphocytes which has been found associated to an increased survival. These polyps have higher risk of cancer but are less invasive, have a better prognosis and a different response to chemotherapeutics. Less frequently these polyps have KRAS or p53 mutations. [64, 65, 78-80]

Although, presence of this mechanism in tumors has been reported to be inversely related to CIMP, either CIMP-L or CIMP-H, [81, 82] there is a subgroup of CIN/MSS tumors characterized by the presence of BRAF mutation that seems to be correlated with CIMP and poor survival. [83] BRAF is implicated in MERK-ERK activation pathway by its recruitment by KRAS. Confirming previous reports of KRAS and BRAF mutations as mutually exclusive, these tumors are wild type KRAS. [84]

2.2.2. *Alternative pathway (KRAS)*

The alternative pathway is still not very well characterized. Some studies indicate the presence of KRAS as its hallmark. [85] Histologically, the presence of KRAS, p53 mutation and recently GNAS, has been associated to villous histology and a high grade dysplasia [86-88] and the presence of CIMP+ to tubule villous size, right side localization and amount of villous, [89, 90] as well as to a differential pattern of the Wnt pathway genes. [91] Villous polyps are also characterized for being microsatellite stable [MSS] and CIMP-L.

2.2.3. *Serrated pathway CpG Island [methylator phenotype (CIMP)*

The serrated pathway underlines the 20-35% of colorectal cancer cases. [37, 76] Histologically, it is characterized by hyperplastic polyps, sessile serrated polyps or traditional serrated adenomas, originated from non-dysplastic aberrant crypt foci that can either be mucinous or not mucinous. [77, 85, 92] This type of tumor is mostly localized in the proximal colon and has bad prognosis. [37]

Serrated polyps can be hyperplastic (HP) (20-30%), sessile serrated adenomas (SSA) (2-9%) and traditional serrated adenomas (TSA) (0.3%) that are subsequently divided into subtypes.

HP can distinguish polyps of microvesicular type (MVHP), Goblet cell–rich type (GCHP) or Mucin poor type (MPHP), according to their content in mucin. SSA can be with/without cytological dysplasia as well as TSA can be with/without conventional dysplasia. [37, 76]

The molecular characteristic of the majority of serrated polyps is the BRAF mutation and CIMP + mechanism. [93]

The CpG island methylator phenotype (CIMP) is detected in 15%-40% of the colorectal tumors. [94, 95] This kind of tumor is mostly related to ageing and environmental factors. One of these genes identified as susceptible of hypermethylation is MLH1, which belongs to the DNA mismatch repair system (MMR), being the causal mechanism of MSI in the serrated pathway. [37, 65, 69]

The sequential steps described in this pathway from normal mucosa to carcinoma goes from the presence of BRAF mutation in microvesicular hyperplastic polyps and posterior acquisition of CIMP phenotype in sessile serrated polyps to a co-occurrence of both genetics alteration leading to sessile serrated polyps. The acquisition of MLH1 promoter methylation is related to the carcinoma stage. [76]

Goblet cell-rich hyperplastic polyps (GCHP) and traditional serrated adenomas (TSA) are associated to KRAS mutations and while it has not been demonstrated a progression of GCHP to carcinoma, it was proved in TSA. It has also been suggested MSI-L after MGMT methylation or partial MLH1 methylation. [76]

Tumors associated to MUTYH can be since hyperplastic and sessile serrated polyps to no polyps at CRC presentation. A higher association of KRAS mutations (70%) has been found in MAP tumors that follow the serrated pathway compared to sporadic (17%), as well as an increased on G:C to T:A transversions (94% vs. 29%). The findings of mutations on APC in adenomas indicate two pathways of development of MAP tumors. [67, 96]

These data seem to confirm that are, at least, as many cancers as patients.

3. State of the art of pharmacogenetics

Personalized medicine is based on the clinical use of molecular biomarkers. A biomarker is any specific physical trait or measurable biological change in the organism related to disease or health conditions, being a very broad concept that includes many different measurements of a biologic status.

Besides being diagnostic [used for the establishment of a particular disease present in the patient sample [97]] or prognostic [used for the establishment of an association with clinical outcomes, such as overall survival or recurrence-free survival independently of the treatment [98] biomarkers can be predictive, by the assessment of the likely benefit of a specific treatment to a specific patient, [99] or pharmacodynamic, by the measurement of the drug effect in a disease [100].

The term, Pharmacogenetics, was first used by Vogel in 1959 as the science about the effects of heritability on drug response [101]. According to the definitions approved by the US Food and Drug Administration (FDA), pharmacogenetics is 'the study of variations in DNA sequence as related to drug response' [102] while the more comprehensive term Pharmacogenomics is defined as 'the study of variations of DNA and RNA characteristics as related to drug response' [103]. Sometimes used indistinctly, Pharmacogenomics is related to the study of whole genome, the gene transcripts and population variability, with the aim of predicting the right treatment in individual patients and designing new drugs.

In last years work in the field has grown almost exponentially [104], at the same pace as the expectations about the increasing of clinical benefit and reduction of the risk of adverse drug reactions (ADR), at least in outliers, i.e. people whose drug responses are not "average" [105].

Nonetheless, adoption of validated pharmacogenetic markers into routine clinical practice has been slow, mainly in the oncological field. Pharmacogenetics has mainly focused on the association between monogenic polymorphisms and in variations in drug metabolism. [102] But, limitations exist on the role of pharmacogenetics in cancer therapy, mainly because of the non-concordance at genetic level between germinal and somatic line of patients [106]. Heritability can be used to assess toxicity, but there are major concerns in their use to assess effectivity.

Today, more than a 100 drugs have pharmacogenomic biomarkers in drug labels approved by the U.S. Food and Drug Administration (FDA), being 35 oncology drugs [107]. In the opposite sense, the European Medicines Agency (EMA) has been more conservative in the implementation of pharmacogenetic markers in drug labels.

In the oncology field, hematology has been the more rewarding, due in part to the lack of some of the architectural barriers found in solid tumors. As result of the pharmacogenetic management, survival rates of some leukemias have improved drastically. Albeit the efforts realized to infer drug efficiency from germline markers, the only ones that have been consistently replicated across the studies for efficiency, are tumor markers, leaving germline markers for the identification of patients with toxicity risk and posterior evaluation of risk/benefit of the drug.

3.1. Colorectal cancer treatment efficiency

In colorectal cancer, 75% of patients with stage I to III can be treated with surgery alone or in combination with chemotherapy, with a 5-year survival rate of 93.2%, 82.5%, and 59.5%, respectively, in contrast with only 8.1% survival rate of patients harbouring stage IV disease. [108]

For patients management, the probability of distant metastasis and response to chemotherapy, are the most important clinical variables. With or without surgery, adjuvant chemotherapy is routinely employed to treat those colorectal cancer patients at high risk of developing recurrence or, those who already have metastatic disease at the time of diagnosis (up to 20 %).

The initial standard treatment with 5-fluorouracil (5-FU), with a median overall survival of 12 months or less and an overall response rate of 10%, has evolved to combinations with oxaliplatin or irinotecan that have dramatically improved survival. [109-111]. The preoperative application of radiotherapy with infusional 5-FU have significantly decreased, the rate of local recurrence [112-114]. In advanced colorectal cancer fluoropyrimidine chemotherapies are basics for treatment in combination with oxaliplatin or irinotecan [115]. The integration of biological agents with conventional cytotoxic drugs has expanded the treatment of metastatic disease, resulting in an increased response rate and survival and achieving downstaging for surgical resection and potential cure. The currently approved and widely used targeted treatments are the monoclonal antibodies bevacizumab that recognizes the vasculature endothelial growth factor (VEGF) and cetuximab and panitumumab, targeting the epidermal growth factor receptor [EGFR]. These combinations reach response rates of up to 50% with a median time of progression free survival of 10–12 months for patients with advanced CRC.

Biomarker development is now essential to aid selection of patients likely to respond to therapy, rationalizing treatments and improving outcomes. But the different approaches used in order to establish biomarkers of the response to treatments in patients with CRC are not lacking in controversial. Even though numerous biomarkers have been postulated to be used as pharmacogenetic markers, only a few of them are actually being used to manage cancer treatment [116].

3.2. Biomarkers of 5-FU response

Thymidylate synthase (TS) is the primary intracellular target of 5-FU. 5-FU acts by preventing the methylation of the deoxyuridine monophosphate to deoxythymidine monophosphate by forming a stable complex, 5-FU–TYMS, causing a thymine deficiency. [117] In CRC, the overexpression of TS has been associated with 5-FU resistance. [118] Several studies analysed genetic polymorphisms as potential predictive factors to 5-FU response [119] but the association between TS expression or TS polymorphisms and response after 5-FU adjuvant treatment is still largely unclear. Thus, although most studies report a TS expression decrease with a better response, [120] there are studies that contradict this association, regarding both the genotype and level of expression, and that link genotypes of high expression of TS with a better response [121] and even a lack of association. [116, 122] Among the several factors that can explain the variability of results, a relevant role might be played by the use of germline genetic data despite the target of 5-FU is the tumor cell. In fact, the TS genotypes from germline and tumor cells from a single patient can differ widely in rectal cancer, distorting the influence of TS on the response to 5-FU. [116]

Although MSI CRCs have a prognostic advantage, [123] mainly due to the minor metastatic potential of MSI CRCs, [124] the predictive value of MSI is still controversial. [125-127] MSI is a strong and well validated prognostic marker to be used in the decision making process in an appropriate clinical setting, for example in stage II, the favourable outcome of patients with MSI CRC suggests that adjuvant chemotherapy could be avoided. [128]

Loss of heterozygosity (LOH) or allelic imbalance (AI) is common in chromosomal instability (CIN) CRC. LOH of chromosome 18q leads to the loss of the tumor suppressor gene Deleted in Colon Cancer (DCC) and had been associated with a poor prognosis of stage II and III CRC patients in several studies [129], but these data were not confirmed. [130] In addition, their role as predictor of outcome in CCR patients following 5-FU based adjuvant therapy, is controversial too.

Near 30–50% of colorectal tumors harbour mutations in the KRAS oncogene, 90% of the mutations occurring either in codon 12 or 13. [131] However, there is no consensus about the role of KRAS as a prognostic marker [132] and KRAS mutation can hardly be expected to be a predictive marker of response to standard chemotherapy. [132, 133]

Global hypomethylation and hypermethylation of tumor, characterize epigenomic instability. Due to this context of genomic instability is difficult to know how the hypermethylated phenotype "CpG island methylator phenotype" (CIMP) affect survival rate. Despite initial results, [134] CIMP positivity in CRC seems not to be a significant independent predictor of survival benefit from 5-FU chemotherapy. [135]

3.3. Biomarkers of platinum response

Glutathione, a ubiquitous tripeptide thiol, is a vital antioxidant and has a protective role against a range of toxins including metal compounds such as cisplatin. Glutathione S-transferase P1 (GSTP1) acts directly in the detoxification of platinum compounds so it is an important factor related to resistance to platinum [136]. However, and despite initial studies [137] reporting the association between GSTP1 Ile105Val and oxaliplatin efficacy and toxicity, results of subsequent studies were inconclusive. [138, 139]

High levels of excision repair cross-complementing 1 (ERCC1), an endonuclease of the nucleotide excision repair (NER) system, are associated with an increased platinum resistance. [140, 141] The x-ray repair cross complementing group 1 (XRCC1), a member of the base excision repair (BER) pathway, links to other proteins related to the BER pathways and repair specific base damage, caused by oxaliplatin. [142] XRCC1 polymorphisms increase the risk of oxaliplatin resistance, via inadequate repair or increased damage tolerance. [143] XPD (ERCC2) has an important role in DNA repair by removing bulky DNA adducts produced by environmental toxins and xenobiotics. The XPD Lys751Gln polymorphism has been associated to clinical outcome following platinum-based chemotherapy. [136, 139, 144]

3.4. Biomarkers of monoclonal antibodies response

There is a wide consensus on the predictive value of KRAS mutations in response to treatment with anti-EGFR drugs. Interestingly, a single first study, in barely 30 patients with metastatic CRC treated with cetuximab, demonstrated the relation between KRAS mutation and non-response: KRAS mutations were found in 68% of non-responding patients but in none of the responders. [145] [145]. The fact is that KRAS is downstream in the EGFR signalling pathway and that pathway is activated by KRAS mutations irrespective of the receptor status, overriding the efficacy of anti-EGFR therapy. The Food and Drug Administration (FDA) approved, in a record time, label changes to cetuximab and panitumumab to advise against their use in patients with KRAS positive metastatic CCR [146, 147]

BRAF mutations also affects the EGFR signalling pathway and are found in CRC at lower frequency than KRAS (≤10%), in fact BRAF and KRAS mutations are mutually exclusive events in tumors. [148] The most frequent BRAF mutation (V600E) represents 50% of BRAF mutations in CCR, being more common in MSI CRC, than in microsatellite stable tumors. [128] BRAF mutation is involved in MEK-ERK pathway activation and CRC carcinogenesis. BRAF V600E is also associated with the CIMP phenotype, 70% of CIMP CRC can harbour BRAF mutations. [93] BRAF mutations have been associated with poor prognosis in patients with stage IV CRC. In agreement with the role of BRAF mutations in enhancing stimulation of downstream MEK-ERK signalling, in patients with metastatic CRC, BRAF mutations are predictive of non-response to EGFR-targeted agents. [149]

3.5. Biomarkers of toxicity

As stated previously, more than a 100 drugs have pharmacogenomic biomarkers in drug labels approved by the FDA. It is paradoxical that, while germline genetical markers should be better for the identification of patients with toxicity risk, the efforts in pharmacogenetic studies were realized to infer drug efficiency. Only six of the FDA approved oncology biomarkers are associated with toxicity. DPYD*2A for capecitabine and UGT1A1*28 irinotecan are the biomarker associated to CRC chemotherapy. [107]

With this data, the problem related to discovering biomarkers of ADRs is clear. Most studied biomarkers related to ADRs are reflected in Table 1, but they are not extensively used in clinical practice.

Gene	Treatment	Toxicity	Review
DPYD	fluoropyrimidine	myelotoxicity	Amstutz U et al. Pharmacogenomics. 2011, 12 [9]:1321-36 FDA: XELODA® [capecitabine] Label [http://www.accessdata.fda.gov/drugsatfda_docs/label/2011/020896s026lbl.pdf]
UGT1A1	irinotecan	Myelotoxicity severe diarrhea	Marques SC, Hum Genomics. 2010, 4 [4]:238-49 FDA Camptosar® Label [http://www.accessdata.fda.gov/drugsatfda_docs/label/2006/020571s030lbl.pdf]
EGFR	EGFR inhibitors	Skin rash	Galvani E, Future Oncol. 2012, 8 [8]: 1015-29
VEGF	VEGF inhibitors	hypertension	Schneider BP, J. Clin. Oncol. 2008, 26 [28]: 4672–4678
ABCB1	capecitabine	neutropenia	Gonzalez-Haba E, Pharmacogenomics. 2010, 11 [12], 1715–1723.
GSTP1 GSTM1 ERCC1 XPD [ERCC2] XRCC1	platin-based platin-based oxaliplatin oxaliplatin platin-based	Neurotoxicity neutropenia hematotoxicity hematotoxicity gastrointestinal	Cortejoso L, López-Fernández LA. Pharmacogenomics. 2012, 12 [10]:1173-1191

Table 1. Association of genes to toxicity in colorectal treatments.

3.6. Biomarkers used in clinical practice

In conclusion, currently the UICC/AJCC Tumor Node Metastasis (TNM) stage system remains the only valid prognostic marker for predicting the outcome of CRC patients. [150-155] Besides different histomorphological, immunohistochemical and molecular biomarkers have been proposed [156, 157] to improve stratification of CRC patients into prognostic subgroups. But, if no additional prognostic and predictive factors were included in the pre- and postoperative management of non-metastatic CRC until now, for metastatic CRC patients gene mutations are arising as predictive biomarker, mainly the KRAS mutational status, with the implementation of anti-EGFR therapy.

4. Establishment issue of genotype-phenotype correlations in cancer

In the last years, numerous candidate prognostic and predictive markers have been reported in hundreds of studies and failed to demonstrate clinical utility. It is difficult to review, even monthly, all described molecular markers of prognosis. Clearly a validation is necessary to establish an association between any of these markers with prognosis or with the response to therapy but the validation itself is not an explanation of why so many potential markers fail to be validated. Inconsistencies can arise between initial reports and subsequent studies because differences in assays, study design, genetic substructure of human populations, statistical power or methodologies. But the establishment of clear genotype-phenotypes correlations, mostly in solid tumors, is still a wide and difficult field of study due to several reasons:

4.1. Architecture of solid tumor

Hematologic cancers treatments have turned them, in some cases, in chronic diseases with the appropriate treatment. Even though they share a common problem with solid tumor, this is, localization and properties of the cancer stem cells, majority of leukemia cells are located in the bloodstream so once drugs reach the bloodstream do not have additional barriers to trespass but the cellular membrane. This more easily access by the drug allows reduce cancer cells load.

But in solid tumors, drugs have to overcome several barriers to access the cells. To get access to tumor drugs first have to extravasate and diffuse across the extracellular matrix to reach all the cells in a tumor, included not well irrigated zones where transportation into the cells is even more difficult due to the extracellular acidic pH. [158, 159]

Tumor mass is a not equally organized mass of cells with an equally distributed blood capillary network that supplies all cells in a tumor but a disorganized mass of different cells with unequally blood supply subject to a different interstitial fluid pressure that produce differential gradient of molecules distribution, among them, drugs. Thus, obstruction of an adequate intratumoral drug delivery in one the cause is one of the causes for cancer recurrence. [158, 159]

Indeed, modification of tumor microenvironment is one of the novel mechanisms to overcome drug resistance. [160, 161]

4.2. Tumor microenvironment

It is already established that tumor microenvironment has an important role in tumor behavior as well as physical impediment of drug delivery but its function in promoting cancer development and drug resistance by segregating molecules by stromal cells have been recently proved. [161-164]

In colorectal cancer, presence of tumor-infiltrating lymphocytes, as part of the immune system response, has been associated positively to both survival and chemotherapy response. [165, 166]

Straussman et al. showed that resistance to RAF inhibitors are not only due to gene activated mutations but mediated by the segregation of hepatocyte growth factor (HGF) by the stromal cells. Their work confirmed the microenvironment as a frequent cause of chemotherapy resistance, principally to targeted drugs [164].

4.3. Intertumor heterogeneity

Similar to other natural ecosystems, tumor growth and development is dependent on the niche conditions. In the case of a tumor, these conditions are primarily determined by the genetic background and physiological state of the patient and lately, determined by the genetic of the tumor itself. And as it happens in all ecosystems, tumor is not in a static state, as the environment changes, the tumor will be adapted to the changed conditions. The different conditions in which a tumor will be developed [a unique mixture of genomic and epigenomic features] determine its specific features, which are improbable to be parallel in another organism. [167]

Albeit colorectal cancer is governed by the general mechanisms described above, the existence of a different mutational spectrum between patients with the same type of cancer has been broadly reported. [168] The experimental confirmation of the 'just right hypothesis' [169] provided new insights into the importance of the genetic background of the patient in determining tumourigenesis and tumor progression.

Even the triggered mechanisms into the tumor cells contribute to such divergence: Bielas et al. determined the mutational rate in tumors and found that was, on average, 200 times greater than in normal cells. This finding uncovered a novel cancer mechanism called point mutation instability (PIN) [170, 171], and can have consequences over pharmacogenomic assays.

4.4. Intratumor heterogeneity

As stated before [116], intratumor heterogeneity may explain the difficulties encountered in the validation of oncology biomarkers owing to sampling bias. As consequence of the different conditions that tumor cells undergone, tumor cells have to adjust their behavior. The adaptation process to these variable circumstances is accompanied by a differential mutational process that results in a genetic heterogeneous blend of cells.

Gerlinger et al [172] demonstrated performing exome sequencing in primary renal carcinomas that 63 to 69% of all somatic mutations were not detectable in all the samples from different tumor sections. They also found biomarkers of good and poor prognosis in the analysis of different regions of the same tumor and high intratumor heterogeneity when ploidy was measured. [172] These findings indicate that intratumor heterogeneity is one of the most important obstacles in the establishment of biomarkers of both prognosis and response to treatment, what implies that the approaches that, so far, have been realized have to change.

4.5. Stem cells

Other possible pitfall can be the contribution of cancer stem cells to drug resistance. As explained before, identification of the appropriate cell to direct therapy is essential to eradicate cancer. Even though treatments can decrease tumor burden, if drugs do not target the appropriate cell, chemotherapy can, as much, become a disease in chronic but not eliminate it from the organism, as it has proved in leukemias. Stem cells are the only tumor-initiating cells within a malignancy and therefore have been shown to maintain colorectal cells population, [173] in fact, they account for about 2.5%% of cancer cells in CRC. [13] But the current chemotherapy is not specific for these cells, and possibly cancer stem cells are naturally resistant to chemotherapy through quiescence, capacity for DNA repair or expression of genes affecting transport and effective drug release into the cells as ABC-transporter. [174]

Even more, stem cells itself are related to genetic background of the tumor. Mutations in APC gene can increase the number of stem cells via Wnt signaling, promoting tumorigenesis [169].

4.6. Response to chemotherapy

Introduction of chemotherapy is a determinant selection factor of cell survival. The appearance of resistance cells to treatments due to mutations that prevent treatment efficiency either by selection of pre-existent resistant clones, either by the emergence of mutants clones induced by the drug, either by inducing the segregation of protective molecules by autocrine or paracrine mechanism or molecules that bypass the activity of the drug, adds new difficulties to both, discovery of clear biomarkers and development of drugs that cure cancer.

4.7. Difficulty of identification or characterization of specific histologic subtypes

Histological identification of different colorectal cancer subtypes can be tough due to its heterogeneity which makes it hardly dependent on the pathologist to identify the polyp. [37] This fact introduces an error in the genotype-phenotype correlations that obscures biomarkers identification.

4.8. Techniques limitations

The existence of high intratumor heterogeneity reveals the scarcity in the information that can be obtained from a tumor and the impossibility, so far, of study bigger regions of the tumor either because of the limited laboratory resources and high cost disclose high intratumor heterogeneity is a difficult obstacle to overcome.

Detection of genetic abnormalities is subject to the proper target identification and design of the methodologies used. For example, one of the difficulties to categorized CIMP is the choice of the appropriate panel of loci to study methylation. [175, 176]

4.9. Studies design

The classification of the groups is often different among studies. To analyse the statistical association of a biomarker, some studies group patients in I-II stage and III-IV of cancer, having each group a different association [positive, negative or not association with respect to the analysed trait] meanwhile others does that with II-III stages. The different criteria used to group patients, is obviously a source of contradictions, since studies compare results obtained from patients with different characteristics. The different methodologies used between studies is another source of confuse. [62, 83]

Some limitations in studies design are an obviously consequence of the resources restraints, either economic or by shortage of the sample but extrapolation of results from these studies are more hazardous.

The reality of high tumor heterogeneity and dynamic change of tumor behaviour makes easy to understand the very little information we can acquire when study only one, two or three markers in one slice of the tumor and this is even worse when study not targeted drugs since cell have more options to overcome their effect like compensatory mechanisms.

As Greaves and Maley expose °genome profiles under-estimate complexity° and continue ° It may be that only a modest number of phenotypic traits are required to negotiate all constraints and evolve to full malignant or metastatic status but the inference is that this can be achieved by an almost infinite variety of evolutionary trajectories and with multiple, different combinations of driver mutations° [7]

The limited capacity to detect low- prevalence clones are another source of a possible future selection of resistance. [7]

Another reason for inconsistencies is small study sample sizes. Typically biomarker studies are done in a subset of patients enrolled in a main study and, therefore, often not statistically adequate to answer clinical questions. Analysis is hampered further by multiple comparisons in correlative studies. Although this approach is crucial to sound statistical methodology, correction for multiple comparisons [or the failure to do so] has probably led to heterogeneity. A major statistical flaw is the potential for false-positive associations because of assessment of multiple SNPs. The opposite is a concern too; biologically important associations frequently cannot be detected after stringent correction because the selection of SNPs is too broad. Study power might also be inadequate if SNPs with excessively rare minor allele frequency are selected. Finally, racial heterogeneity within the trial is important to take into account, and proper correction or analysis of patients in subgroups by ethnic origin must be done.

Due to the need of major research projects, both in number of samples as in appropriate resources for their study, consolidate research consortia has become imperative.

The establishment of clear genotype-phenotypes correlations is still a wide and difficult field of study due to the previously exposed heterogeneity and overlapping characteristics observed in colorectal cancer in both histological and molecular level, exacerbated by the confusion in identifying some histologic subtypes of polyps and the designing problem of the studies, which often compare only a few markers and patients in different stages, and with different treatments, that as previously show have an impact in the molecular mechanism trigger. As consequence, some of the published associations are not lately replicated

5. Conclusion

The clinical application of pharmacogenetic tests is still limited to a few drugs. But, the fact that a significant number of patients obtain no advantage receiving chemotherapy encourage us to increase the efforts to get more and better biomarkers. Knowledge of the problems outlined above gives us a better understanding of the challenges of pharmacogenetics and allow us to reach a better understanding of the biological basis of cancer treatments. While that work continues, new genomic technologies now in development are enabling to bring useful biomarkers from the bench to bedside in a more rapid and effective way.

Acknowledgements

This work was supported in part by a grant from Acción Estratégica de Salud (ISCIII-Mineo) (PS09/02368)

Author details

Emilia Balboa[1], Angel Carracedo[1,2,3] and Francisco Barros[1]

1 Grupo Medicina Xenómica – CIBERER, Fundación Pública Galega de Medicina Xenómica, Santiago de Compostela, Spain

2 Grupo Medicina Xenómica – CIBERER, Universidad de Santiago de Compostela, Spain

3 Center of Excellence in Genomic Medicine Research (CEGMR), King Abdulaziz University, Jeddah, Saudi Arabia

References

[1] Loeb LA, Springgate CF, Battula N. Errors in DNA replication as a basis of malignant changes. Cancer research. 1974 Sep;34 (9):2311-21. PubMed PMID: 4136142. Epub 1974/09/01. eng.

[2] Holland AJ, Cleveland DW. Boveri revisited: chromosomal instability, aneuploidy and tumorigenesis. Nat Rev Mol Cell Biol. 2009 Jul;10 (7):478-87. PubMed PMID: 19546858. Pubmed Central PMCID: PMC3154738. Epub 2009/06/24. eng.

[3] Nowell PC. The clonal evolution of tumor cell populations. Science. 1976 Oct 1;194 (4260):23-8. PubMed PMID: 959840.

[4] Catenacci DV, Kozloff M, Kindler HL, Polite B. Personalized colon cancer care in 2010. Semin Oncol. 2011 Apr;38 (2):284-308. PubMed PMID: 21421118. Pubmed Central PMCID: 3065981.

[5] Ansfield FJ. A Less Toxic Fluorouracil Dosage Schedule. JAMA : the journal of the American Medical Association. 1964 Nov 16;190:686-8. PubMed PMID: 14217470.

[6] Shackleton M, Quintana E, Fearon ER, Morrison SJ. Heterogeneity in cancer: cancer stem cells versus clonal evolution. Cell. 2009 Sep 4;138 (5):822-9. PubMed PMID: 19737509. Epub 2009/09/10. eng.

[7] Greaves M, Maley CC. Clonal evolution in cancer. Nature. 2012 Jan 19;481 (7381): 306-13. PubMed PMID: 22258609. Pubmed Central PMCID: 3367003.

[8] Driessens G, Beck B, Caauwe A, Simons BD, Blanpain C. Defining the mode of tumour growth by clonal analysis. Nature. 2012 Aug 23;488 (7412):527-30. PubMed PMID: 22854777. Epub 2012/08/03. eng.

[9] Chen J, Li Y, Yu TS, McKay RM, Burns DK, Kernie SG, et al. A restricted cell population propagates glioblastoma growth after chemotherapy. Nature. 2012 Aug 23;488 (7412):522-6. PubMed PMID: 22854781. Pubmed Central PMCID: PMC3427400. Epub 2012/08/03. eng.

[10] La Porta CA, Zapperi S, Sethna JP. Senescent cells in growing tumors: population dynamics and cancer stem cells. PLoS Comput Biol. 2012 Jan;8 (1):e1002316. PubMed PMID: 22275856. Pubmed Central PMCID: PMC3261911. Epub 2012/01/26. eng.

[11] Dalerba P, Dylla SJ, Park IK, Liu R, Wang X, Cho RW, et al. Phenotypic characterization of human colorectal cancer stem cells. Proceedings of the National Academy of Sciences of the United States of America. 2007 Jun 12;104 (24):10158-63. PubMed PMID: 17548814. Pubmed Central PMCID: 1891215.

[12] O'Brien CA, Pollett A, Gallinger S, Dick JE. A human colon cancer cell capable of initiating tumour growth in immunodeficient mice. Nature. 2007 Jan 4;445 (7123): 106-10. PubMed PMID: 17122772.

[13] Ricci-Vitiani L, Lombardi DG, Pilozzi E, Biffoni M, Todaro M, Peschle C, et al. Identification and expansion of human colon-cancer-initiating cells. Nature. 2007 Jan 4;445 (7123):111-5. PubMed PMID: 17122771.

[14] Wang JC, Dick JE. Cancer stem cells: lessons from leukemia. Trends Cell Biol. 2005 Sep;15 (9):494-501. PubMed PMID: 16084092.

[15] Vermeulen L, Sprick MR, Kemper K, Stassi G, Medema JP. Cancer stem cells--old concepts, new insights. Cell Death Differ. 2008 Jun;15 (6):947-58. PubMed PMID: 18259194.

[16] Liu J, Joha S, Idziorek T, Corm S, Hetuin D, Philippe N, et al. BCR-ABL mutants spread resistance to non-mutated cells through a paracrine mechanism. Leukemia : official journal of the Leukemia Society of America, Leukemia Research Fund, UK. 2008 Apr;22 (4):791-9. PubMed PMID: 18216868. Epub 2008/01/25. eng.

[17] Stratton MR, Campbell PJ, Futreal PA. The cancer genome. Nature. 2009 Apr 9;458 (7239):719-24. PubMed PMID: 19360079. Pubmed Central PMCID: 2821689.

[18] Bozic I, Antal T, Ohtsuki H, Carter H, Kim D, Chen S, et al. Accumulation of driver and passenger mutations during tumor progression. Proceedings of the National Academy of Sciences of the United States of America. 2010 Oct 26;107 (43):18545-50. PubMed PMID: 20876136. Pubmed Central PMCID: 2972991.

[19] Knudson AG, Jr. Mutation and cancer: statistical study of retinoblastoma. Proceedings of the National Academy of Sciences of the United States of America. 1971 Apr; 68 (4):820-3. PubMed PMID: 5279523. Pubmed Central PMCID: 389051.

[20] Knudson AG. Two genetic hits (more or less) to cancer. Nature reviews Cancer. 2001 Nov;1 (2):157-62. PubMed PMID: 11905807.

[21] Albuquerque C, Breukel C, van der Luijt R, Fidalgo P, Lage P, Slors FJ, et al. The 'just-right' signaling model: APC somatic mutations are selected based on a specific level of activation of the beta-catenin signaling cascade. Human molecular genetics. 2002 Jun 15;11 (13):1549-60. PubMed PMID: 12045208. Epub 2002/06/05. eng.

[22] Fearon ER, Vogelstein B. A genetic model for colorectal tumorigenesis. Cell. 1990 Jun 1;61 (5):759-67. PubMed PMID: 2188735.

[23] Sjoblom T, Jones S, Wood LD, Parsons DW, Lin J, Barber TD, et al. The consensus coding sequences of human breast and colorectal cancers. Science. 2006 Oct 13;314 (5797):268-74. PubMed PMID: 16959974.

[24] Wood LD, Parsons DW, Jones S, Lin J, Sjoblom T, Leary RJ, et al. The genomic landscapes of human breast and colorectal cancers. Science. 2007 Nov 16;318 (5853): 1108-13. PubMed PMID: 17932254. Epub 2007/10/13. eng.

[25] Lin J, Gan CM, Zhang X, Jones S, Sjoblom T, Wood LD, et al. A multidimensional analysis of genes mutated in breast and colorectal cancers. Genome Res. 2007 Sep;17 (9):1304-18. PubMed PMID: 17693572. Pubmed Central PMCID: 1950899.

[26] Peifer M. Developmental biology: colon construction. Nature. 2002 Nov 21;420 (6913):274-5, 7. PubMed PMID: 12447423.

[27] Mosimann C, Hausmann G, Basler K. Beta-catenin hits chromatin: regulation of Wnt target gene activation. Nat Rev Mol Cell Biol. 2009 Apr;10 (4):276-86. PubMed PMID: 19305417.

[28] Su LK, Vogelstein B, Kinzler KW. Association of the APC tumor suppressor protein with catenins. Science. 1993 Dec 10;262 (5140):1734-7. PubMed PMID: 8259519.

[29] Rubinfeld B, Souza B, Albert I, Muller O, Chamberlain SH, Masiarz FR, et al. Association of the APC gene product with beta-catenin. Science. 1993 Dec 10;262 (5140): 1731-4. PubMed PMID: 8259518.

[30] Fodde R, Smits R, Clevers H. APC, signal transduction and genetic instability in colorectal cancer. Nature reviews Cancer. 2001 Oct;1 (1):55-67. PubMed PMID: 11900252.

[31] Siegmund KD, Marjoram P, Woo YJ, Tavare S, Shibata D. Inferring clonal expansion and cancer stem cell dynamics from DNA methylation patterns in colorectal cancers. Proceedings of the National Academy of Sciences of the United States of America. 2009 Mar 24;106 (12):4828-33. PubMed PMID: 19261858. Pubmed Central PMCID: 2651202.

[32] Barker N, Ridgway RA, van Es JH, van de Wetering M, Begthel H, van den Born M, et al. Crypt stem cells as the cells-of-origin of intestinal cancer. Nature. 2009 Jan 29;457 (7229):608-11. PubMed PMID: 19092804. Epub 2008/12/19. eng.

[33] Hull UMSaTL. Colonic Physiology. In: al. DEBe, editor. The ASCRS Textbook of Colon and Rectal Surgery: Second Edition: Springer Science+Business Media; 2011.

[34] Glebov OK, Rodriguez LM, Nakahara K, Jenkins J, Cliatt J, Humbyrd CJ, et al. Distinguishing right from left colon by the pattern of gene expression. Cancer epidemiology, biomarkers & prevention : a publication of the American Association for Cancer Research, cosponsored by the American Society of Preventive Oncology. 2003 Aug;12 (8):755-62. PubMed PMID: 12917207.

[35] Nielsen M, Joerink-van de Beld MC, Jones N, Vogt S, Tops CM, Vasen HF, et al. Analysis of MUTYH genotypes and colorectal phenotypes in patients With MUTYH-associated polyposis. Gastroenterology. 2009 Feb;136 (2):471-6. PubMed PMID: 19032956.

[36] Nielsen M, Morreau H, Vasen HF, Hes FJ. MUTYH-associated polyposis (MAP). Crit Rev Oncol Hematol. 2011 Jul;79 (1):1-16. PubMed PMID: 20663686.

[37] Makkar R, Pai RK, Burke CA. Sessile serrated polyps: Cancer risk and appropriate surveillance. Cleve Clin J Med. 2012 Dec;79 (12):865-71. PubMed PMID: 23208991.

[38] Haggar FA, Boushey RP. Colorectal cancer epidemiology: incidence, mortality, survival, and risk factors. Clinics in colon and rectal surgery. 2009 Nov;22 (4):191-7. PubMed PMID: 21037809. Pubmed Central PMCID: 2796096.

[39] Thibodeau SN, Bren G, Schaid D. Microsatellite instability in cancer of the proximal colon. Science. 1993 May 7;260 (5109):816-9. PubMed PMID: 8484122. Epub 1993/05/07. eng.

[40] Liu B, Nicolaides NC, Markowitz S, Willson JK, Parsons RE, Jen J, et al. Mismatch repair gene defects in sporadic colorectal cancers with microsatellite instability. Nature genetics. 1995 Jan;9 (1):48-55. PubMed PMID: 7704024.

[41] Issa JP, Ottaviano YL, Celano P, Hamilton SR, Davidson NE, Baylin SB. Methylation of the oestrogen receptor CpG island links ageing and neoplasia in human colon. Nature genetics. 1994 Aug;7 (4):536-40. PubMed PMID: 7951326.

[42] Gardner EJ, Rogers SW, Woodward S. Numerical and structural chromosome aberrations in cultured lymphocytes and cutaneous fibroblasts of patients with multiple adenomas of the colorectum. Cancer. 1982 Apr 1;49 (7):1413-9. PubMed PMID: 7059954. Epub 1982/04/01. eng.

[43] Ionov Y, Peinado MA, Malkhosyan S, Shibata D, Perucho M. Ubiquitous somatic mutations in simple repeated sequences reveal a new mechanism for colonic carcinogenesis. Nature. 1993 Jun 10;363 (6429):558-61. PubMed PMID: 8505985.

[44] Aaltonen LA, Peltomaki P, Leach FS, Sistonen P, Pylkkanen L, Mecklin JP, et al. Clues to the pathogenesis of familial colorectal cancer. Science. 1993 May 7;260 (5109):812-6. PubMed PMID: 8484121. Epub 1993/05/07. eng.

[45] Li FY, Lai MD. Colorectal cancer, one entity or three. J Zhejiang Univ Sci B. 2009 Mar; 10 (3):219-29. PubMed PMID: 19283877. Pubmed Central PMCID: 2650032.

[46] Lindblom A. Different mechanisms in the tumorigenesis of proximal and distal colon cancers. Curr Opin Oncol. 2001 Jan;13 (1):63-9. PubMed PMID: 11148689.

[47] Cheng YW, Pincas H, Bacolod MD, Schemmann G, Giardina SF, Huang J, et al. CpG island methylator phenotype associates with low-degree chromosomal abnormalities in colorectal cancer. Clinical cancer research : an official journal of the American Association for Cancer Research. 2008 Oct 1;14 (19):6005-13. PubMed PMID: 18829479. Pubmed Central PMCID: 3268558.

[48] Chan TL, Zhao W, Leung SY, Yuen ST, Cancer Genome P. BRAF and KRAS mutations in colorectal hyperplastic polyps and serrated adenomas. Cancer research. 2003 Aug 15;63 (16):4878-81. PubMed PMID: 12941809.

[49] Singh H, Nugent Z, Demers AA, Kliewer EV, Mahmud SM, Bernstein CN. The reduction in colorectal cancer mortality after colonoscopy varies by site of the cancer. Gastroenterology. 2010 Oct;139 (4):1128-37. PubMed PMID: 20600026.

[50] Groden J, Thliveris A, Samowitz W, Carlson M, Gelbert L, Albertsen H, et al. Identification and characterization of the familial adenomatous polyposis coli gene. Cell. 1991 Aug 9;66 (3):589-600. PubMed PMID: 1651174.

[51] Nishisho I, Nakamura Y, Miyoshi Y, Miki Y, Ando H, Horii A, et al. Mutations of chromosome 5q21 genes in FAP and colorectal cancer patients. Science. 1991 Aug 9;253 (5020):665-9. PubMed PMID: 1651563.

[52] Pino MS, Chung DC. The chromosomal instability pathway in colon cancer. Gastroenterology. 2010 Jun;138 (6):2059-72. PubMed PMID: 20420946.

[53] Powell SM, Zilz N, Beazer-Barclay Y, Bryan TM, Hamilton SR, Thibodeau SN, et al. APC mutations occur early during colorectal tumorigenesis. Nature. 1992 Sep 17;359 (6392):235-7. PubMed PMID: 1528264.

[54] Smith AJ, Stern HS, Penner M, Hay K, Mitri A, Bapat BV, et al. Somatic APC and K-ras codon 12 mutations in aberrant crypt foci from human colons. Cancer research. 1994 Nov 1;54 (21):5527-30. PubMed PMID: 7923190.

[55] Kaplan KB, Burds AA, Swedlow JR, Bekir SS, Sorger PK, Nathke IS. A role for the Adenomatous Polyposis Coli protein in chromosome segregation. Nat Cell Biol. 2001 Apr;3 (4):429-32. PubMed PMID: 11283619.

[56] Fodde R, Kuipers J, Rosenberg C, Smits R, Kielman M, Gaspar C, et al. Mutations in the APC tumour suppressor gene cause chromosomal instability. Nat Cell Biol. 2001 Apr;3 (4):433-8. PubMed PMID: 11283620.

[57] Medema JP, Vermeulen L. Microenvironmental regulation of stem cells in intestinal homeostasis and cancer. Nature. 2011 Jun 16;474 (7351):318-26. PubMed PMID: 21677748.

[58] Markowitz SD, Bertagnolli MM. Molecular origins of cancer: Molecular basis of colorectal cancer. The New England journal of medicine. 2009 Dec 17;361 (25):2449-60. PubMed PMID: 20018966. Pubmed Central PMCID: 2843693.

[59] Zhang J, Roberts TM, Shivdasani RA. Targeting PI3K signaling as a therapeutic approach for colorectal cancer. Gastroenterology. 2011 Jul;141 (1):50-61. PubMed PMID: 21723986. Epub 2011/07/05. eng.

[60] Derynck R, Akhurst RJ, Balmain A. TGF-beta signaling in tumor suppression and cancer progression. Nature genetics. 2001 Oct;29 (2):117-29. PubMed PMID: 11586292.

[61] Vogelstein B, Sur, S. & Prives, C. p53 : The Most Frequently Altered Gene in Human Nature Education 2010;3 (9):6.

[62] Watanabe T, Kobunai T, Yamamoto Y, Matsuda K, Ishihara S, Nozawa K, et al. Chromosomal instability (CIN) phenotype, CIN high or CIN low, predicts survival for colorectal cancer. J Clin Oncol. 2012 Jun 20;30 (18):2256-64. PubMed PMID: 22547595.

[63] Perucho M. Microsatellite instability: the mutator that mutates the other mutator. Nature medicine. 1996 Jun;2 (6):630-1. PubMed PMID: 8640546. Epub 1996/06/01. eng.

[64] Vilar E, Gruber SB. Microsatellite instability in colorectal cancer-the stable evidence. Nat Rev Clin Oncol. 2010 Mar;7 (3):153-62. PubMed PMID: 20142816. Pubmed Central PMCID: 3427139.

[65] Boland CR, Goel A. Microsatellite instability in colorectal cancer. Gastroenterology. 2010 Jun;138 (6):2073-87 e3. PubMed PMID: 20420947. Pubmed Central PMCID: 3037515.

[66] David SS, O'Shea VL, Kundu S. Base-excision repair of oxidative DNA damage. Nature. 2007 Jun 21;447 (7147):941-50. PubMed PMID: 17581577. Pubmed Central PMCID: 2896554.

[67] Venesio T, Balsamo A, D'Agostino VG, Ranzani GN. MUTYH-associated polyposis (MAP), the syndrome implicating base excision repair in inherited predisposition to colorectal tumors. Frontiers in oncology. 2012;2:83. PubMed PMID: 22876359. Pubmed Central PMCID: 3410368.

[68] Lipton L, Halford SE, Johnson V, Novelli MR, Jones A, Cummings C, et al. Carcinogenesis in MYH-associated polyposis follows a distinct genetic pathway. Cancer research. 2003 Nov 15;63 (22):7595-9. PubMed PMID: 14633673.

[69] Toyota M, Ahuja N, Ohe-Toyota M, Herman JG, Baylin SB, Issa JP. CpG island methylator phenotype in colorectal cancer. Proceedings of the National Academy of Sciences of the United States of America. 1999 Jul 20;96 (15):8681-6. PubMed PMID: 10411935. Pubmed Central PMCID: 17576.

[70] Gazzoli I, Loda M, Garber J, Syngal S, Kolodner RD. A hereditary nonpolyposis colorectal carcinoma case associated with hypermethylation of the MLH1 gene in normal tissue and loss of heterozygosity of the unmethylated allele in the resulting microsatellite instability-high tumor. Cancer research. 2002 Jul 15;62 (14):3925-8. PubMed PMID: 12124320.

[71] Suter CM, Martin DI, Ward RL. Germline epimutation of MLH1 in individuals with multiple cancers. Nature genetics. 2004 May;36 (5):497-501. PubMed PMID: 15064764.

[72] Chan TL, Yuen ST, Kong CK, Chan YW, Chan AS, Ng WF, et al. Heritable germline epimutation of MSH2 in a family with hereditary nonpolyposis colorectal cancer. Nature genetics. 2006 Oct;38 (10):1178-83. PubMed PMID: 16951683.

[73] Pineda M, Mur P, Iniesta MD, Borras E, Campos O, Vargas G, et al. MLH1 methylation screening is effective in identifying epimutation carriers. Eur J Hum Genet. 2012 Dec;20 (12):1256-64. PubMed PMID: 22763379. Pubmed Central PMCID: PMC3499751. Epub 2012/07/06. eng.

[74] Ward RL, Dobbins T, Lindor NM, Rapkins RW, Hitchins MP. Identification of constitutional MLH1 epimutations and promoter variants in colorectal cancer patients from the Colon Cancer Family Registry. Genet Med. 2013 Jan;15 (1):25-35. PubMed PMID: 22878509.

[75] Ohm JE, McGarvey KM, Yu X, Cheng L, Schuebel KE, Cope L, et al. A stem cell-like chromatin pattern may predispose tumor suppressor genes to DNA hypermethylation and heritable silencing. Nature genetics. 2007 Feb;39 (2):237-42. PubMed PMID: 17211412. Pubmed Central PMCID: PMC2744394. Epub 2007/01/11. eng.

[76] Snover DC. Update on the serrated pathway to colorectal carcinoma. Human pathology. 2011 Jan;42 (1):1-10. PubMed PMID: 20869746.

[77] Worthley DL, Leggett BA. Colorectal cancer: molecular features and clinical opportunities. The Clinical biochemist Reviews / Australian Association of Clinical Biochemists. 2010 May;31 (2):31-8. PubMed PMID: 20498827. Pubmed Central PMCID: 2874430.

[78] Oxentenko AS, Smyrk TC. Interval colon cancer in a Lynch syndrome patient under annual colonoscopic surveillance: a case for advanced imaging techniques? BMC Gastroenterol. 2012;12:50. PubMed PMID: 22624972. Pubmed Central PMCID: 3493301.

[79] Vasen HF. Review article: The Lynch syndrome (hereditary nonpolyposis colorectal cancer). Alimentary pharmacology & therapeutics. 2007 Dec;26 Suppl 2:113-26. PubMed PMID: 18081655.

[80] Duval A, Collura A, Berthenet K, Lagrange A, Garrido C. Microsatellite instability in colorectal cancer: time to stop hiding! Oncotarget. 2011 Nov;2 (11):826-7. PubMed PMID: 22084152. Pubmed Central PMCID: 3259994.

[81] Goel A, Nagasaka T, Arnold CN, Inoue T, Hamilton C, Niedzwiecki D, et al. The CpG island methylator phenotype and chromosomal instability are inversely correlated in sporadic colorectal cancer. Gastroenterology. 2007 Jan;132 (1):127-38. PubMed PMID: 17087942. Epub 2006/11/08. eng.

[82] Ogino S, Kawasaki T, Kirkner GJ, Ohnishi M, Fuchs CS. 18q loss of heterozygosity in microsatellite stable colorectal cancer is correlated with CpG island methylator phenotype-negative (CIMP-0) and inversely with CIMP-low and CIMP-high. BMC cancer. 2007;7:72. PubMed PMID: 17474983. Pubmed Central PMCID: PMC1876238. Epub 2007/05/04. eng.

[83] Bond CE, Umapathy A, Buttenshaw RL, Wockner L, Leggett BA, Whitehall VL. Chromosomal instability in BRAF mutant, microsatellite stable colorectal cancers. PloS one. 2012;7 (10):e47483. PubMed PMID: 23110075. Pubmed Central PMCID: 3478278.

[84] Yokota T. Are KRAS/BRAF mutations potent prognostic and/or predictive biomarkers in colorectal cancers? Anti-cancer agents in medicinal chemistry. 2012 Feb;12 (2): 163-71. PubMed PMID: 22043994. Pubmed Central PMCID: PMC3343383. Epub 2011/11/03. eng.

[85] Leggett B, Whitehall V. Role of the serrated pathway in colorectal cancer pathogenesis. Gastroenterology. 2010 Jun;138 (6):2088-100. PubMed PMID: 20420948.

[86] Maltzman T, Knoll K, Martinez ME, Byers T, Stevens BR, Marshall JR, et al. Ki-ras proto-oncogene mutations in sporadic colorectal adenomas: relationship to histologic and clinical characteristics. Gastroenterology. 2001 Aug;121 (2):302-9. PubMed PMID: 11487539.

[87] Barry EL, Baron JA, Grau MV, Wallace K, Haile RW. K-ras mutations in incident sporadic colorectal adenomas. Cancer. 2006 Mar 1;106 (5):1036-40. PubMed PMID: 16456810.

[88] Yamada M, Sekine S, Ogawa R, Taniguchi H, Kushima R, Tsuda H, et al. Frequent activating GNAS mutations in villous adenoma of the colorectum. The Journal of pathology. 2012 Sep;228 (1):113-8. PubMed PMID: 22374786.

[89] Kakar S, Deng G, Cun L, Sahai V, Kim YS. CpG island methylation is frequently present in tubulovillous and villous adenomas and correlates with size, site, and villous component. Human pathology. 2008 Jan;39 (1):30-6. PubMed PMID: 17950780. Epub 2007/10/24. eng.

[90] Rashid A, Shen L, Morris JS, Issa JP, Hamilton SR. CpG island methylation in colorectal adenomas. Am J Pathol. 2001 Sep;159 (3):1129-35. PubMed PMID: 11549606. Pubmed Central PMCID: 1850474.

[91] Nguyen AV, Albers CG, Holcombe RF. Differentiation of tubular and villous adenomas based on Wnt pathway-related gene expression profiles. Int J Mol Med. 2010 Jul; 26 (1):121-5. PubMed PMID: 20514431. Epub 2010/06/02. eng.

[92] Tanaka H, Deng G, Matsuzaki K, Kakar S, Kim GE, Miura S, et al. BRAF mutation, CpG island methylator phenotype and microsatellite instability occur more frequently and concordantly in mucinous than non-mucinous colorectal cancer. International journal of cancer Journal international du cancer. 2006 Jun 1;118 (11):2765-71. PubMed PMID: 16381005. Epub 2005/12/29. eng.

[93] Weisenberger DJ, Siegmund KD, Campan M, Young J, Long TI, Faasse MA, et al. CpG island methylator phenotype underlies sporadic microsatellite instability and is tightly associated with BRAF mutation in colorectal cancer. Nature genetics. 2006 Jul; 38 (7):787-93. PubMed PMID: 16804544. Epub 2006/06/29. eng.

[94] van Rijnsoever M, Grieu F, Elsaleh H, Joseph D, Iacopetta B. Characterisation of colorectal cancers showing hypermethylation at multiple CpG islands. Gut. 2002 Dec;51 (6):797-802. PubMed PMID: 12427779. Pubmed Central PMCID: PMC1773491. Epub 2002/11/13. eng.

[95] Hawkins N, Norrie M, Cheong K, Mokany E, Ku SL, Meagher A, et al. CpG island methylation in sporadic colorectal cancers and its relationship to microsatellite insta-

bility. Gastroenterology. 2002 May;122 (5):1376-87. PubMed PMID: 11984524. Epub 2002/05/02. eng.

[96] Boparai KS, Dekker E, Van Eeden S, Polak MM, Bartelsman JF, Mathus-Vliegen EM, et al. Hyperplastic polyps and sessile serrated adenomas as a phenotypic expression of MYH-associated polyposis. Gastroenterology. 2008 Dec;135 (6):2014-8. PubMed PMID: 19013464. Epub 2008/11/18. eng.

[97] Ong FS, Das K, Wang J, Vakil H, Kuo JZ, Blackwell WL, et al. Personalized medicine and pharmacogenetic biomarkers: progress in molecular oncology testing. Expert review of molecular diagnostics. 2012 Jul;12 (6):593-602. PubMed PMID: 22845480. Pubmed Central PMCID: 3495985.

[98] McShane LM, Altman DG, Sauerbrei W, Taube SE, Gion M, Clark GM, et al. Reporting recommendations for tumor marker prognostic studies. J Clin Oncol. 2005 Dec 20;23 (36):9067-72. PubMed PMID: 16172462.

[99] Buyse M, Michiels S, Sargent DJ, Grothey A, Matheson A, de Gramont A. Integrating biomarkers in clinical trials. Expert review of molecular diagnostics. 2011 Mar;11 (2): 171-82. PubMed PMID: 21405968.

[100] Sarker D, Workman P. Pharmacodynamic biomarkers for molecular cancer therapeutics. Adv Cancer Res. 2007;96:213-68. PubMed PMID: 17161682.

[101] Vogel F. Moderne problem der humangenetik. Ergeb Inn Med U Kinderheilk 1959;12:52-125.

[102] Wang L, McLeod HL, Weinshilboum RM. Genomics and drug response. The New England journal of medicine. 2011 Mar 24;364 (12):1144-53. PubMed PMID: 21428770. Pubmed Central PMCID: PMC3184612. Epub 2011/03/25. eng.

[103] Trent RJ. Pathology practice and pharmacogenomics. Pharmacogenomics. 2010 Jan; 11 (1):105-11. PubMed PMID: 20017676.

[104] Meyer UA. Pharmacogenetics - five decades of therapeutic lessons from genetic diversity. Nature reviews Genetics. 2004 Sep;5 (9):669-76. PubMed PMID: 15372089.

[105] Woodcock J, Lesko LJ. Pharmacogenetics--tailoring treatment for the outliers. The New England journal of medicine. 2009 Feb 19;360 (8):811-3. PubMed PMID: 19228625.

[106] Balboa E, et al. Role of Tumor Tissue Analysis in Rectal Cancer Pharmacogenetics, Rectal Cancer - in A Multidisciplinary Approach to Management. In: G.A. Santoro, editor. Rectal Cancer - A Multidisciplinary Approach to Management: InTech.; 2011.

[107] Bertotti A, Migliardi G, Galimi F, Sassi F, Torti D, Isella C, et al. A molecularly annotated platform of patient-derived xenografts ("xenopatients") identifies HER2 as an effective therapeutic target in cetuximab-resistant colorectal cancer. Cancer discovery. 2011 Nov;1 (6):508-23. PubMed PMID: 22586653.

[108] O'Connell JB, Maggard MA, Ko CY. Colon cancer survival rates with the new American Joint Committee on Cancer sixth edition staging. Journal of the National Cancer Institute. 2004 Oct 6;96 (19):1420-5. PubMed PMID: 15467030.

[109] Tournigand C, Andre T, Achille E, Lledo G, Flesh M, Mery-Mignard D, et al. FOLFIRI followed by FOLFOX6 or the reverse sequence in advanced colorectal cancer: a randomized GERCOR study. J Clin Oncol. 2004 Jan 15;22 (2):229-37. PubMed PMID: 14657227.

[110] Colucci G, Gebbia V, Paoletti G, Giuliani F, Caruso M, Gebbia N, et al. Phase III randomized trial of FOLFIRI versus FOLFOX4 in the treatment of advanced colorectal cancer: a multicenter study of the Gruppo Oncologico Dell'Italia Meridionale. J Clin Oncol. 2005 Aug 1;23 (22):4866-75. PubMed PMID: 15939922. Epub 2005/06/09. eng.

[111] de Gramont A, Figer A, Seymour M, Homerin M, Hmissi A, Cassidy J, et al. Leucovorin and fluorouracil with or without oxaliplatin as first-line treatment in advanced colorectal cancer. J Clin Oncol. 2000 Aug;18 (16):2938-47. PubMed PMID: 10944126. Epub 2000/08/16. eng.

[112] Kapiteijn E, Marijnen CA, Nagtegaal ID, Putter H, Steup WH, Wiggers T, et al. Preoperative radiotherapy combined with total mesorectal excision for resectable rectal cancer. The New England journal of medicine. 2001 Aug 30;345 (9):638-46. PubMed PMID: 11547717.

[113] Sauer R, Becker H, Hohenberger W, Rodel C, Wittekind C, Fietkau R, et al. Preoperative versus postoperative chemoradiotherapy for rectal cancer. The New England journal of medicine. 2004 Oct 21;351 (17):1731-40. PubMed PMID: 15496622.

[114] Cunningham D, Atkin W, Lenz HJ, Lynch HT, Minsky B, Nordlinger B, et al. Colorectal cancer. Lancet. 2010 Mar 20;375 (9719):1030-47. PubMed PMID: 20304247.

[115] National Comprehensive Cancer Network Guidelines Version 2. 2011 Colon Cancer. NCCN Home Page. Available from: http://www.nccn.org/professionals/physician_gls/pdf/colon.pdf (15 February 2011).

[116] Balboa E, Duran G, Lamas MJ, Gomez-Caamano A, Celeiro-Munoz C, Lopez R, et al. Pharmacogenetic analysis in neoadjuvant chemoradiation for rectal cancer: high incidence of somatic mutations and their relation with response. Pharmacogenomics. 2010 Jun;11 (6):747-61. PubMed PMID: 20504250. Epub 2010/05/28. eng.

[117] Zhang N, Yin Y, Xu SJ, Chen WS. 5-Fluorouracil: mechanisms of resistance and reversal strategies. Molecules. 2008;13 (8):1551-69. PubMed PMID: 18794772.

[118] Etienne MC, Ilc K, Formento JL, Laurent-Puig P, Formento P, Cheradame S, et al. Thymidylate synthase and methylenetetrahydrofolate reductase gene polymorphisms: relationships with 5-fluorouracil sensitivity. Br J Cancer. 2004 Jan 26;90 (2): 526-34. PubMed PMID: 14735204. Pubmed Central PMCID: 2409555.

[119] Afzal S, Gusella M, Jensen SA, Vainer B, Vogel U, Andersen JT, et al. The association of polymorphisms in 5-fluorouracil metabolism genes with outcome in adjuvant treatment of colorectal cancer. Pharmacogenomics. 2011 Sep;12 (9):1257-67. PubMed PMID: 21919605.

[120] Villafranca E, Okruzhnov Y, Dominguez MA, Garcia-Foncillas J, Azinovic I, Martinez E, et al. Polymorphisms of the repeated sequences in the enhancer region of the thymidylate synthase gene promoter may predict downstaging after preoperative chemoradiation in rectal cancer. J Clin Oncol. 2001 Mar 15;19 (6):1779-86. PubMed PMID: 11251009. Epub 2001/03/17. eng.

[121] Edler D, Glimelius B, Hallstrom M, Jakobsen A, Johnston PG, Magnusson I, et al. Thymidylate synthase expression in colorectal cancer: a prognostic and predictive marker of benefit from adjuvant fluorouracil-based chemotherapy. J Clin Oncol. 2002 Apr 1;20 (7):1721-8. PubMed PMID: 11919227.

[122] Gusella M, Frigo AC, Bolzonella C, Marinelli R, Barile C, Bononi A, et al. Predictors of survival and toxicity in patients on adjuvant therapy with 5-fluorouracil for colorectal cancer. Br J Cancer. 2009 May 19;100 (10):1549-57. PubMed PMID: 19384296. Pubmed Central PMCID: 2696766.

[123] Walther A, Houlston R, Tomlinson I. Association between chromosomal instability and prognosis in colorectal cancer: a meta-analysis. Gut. 2008 Jul;57 (7):941-50. PubMed PMID: 18364437.

[124] Malesci A, Laghi L, Bianchi P, Delconte G, Randolph A, Torri V, et al. Reduced likelihood of metastases in patients with microsatellite-unstable colorectal cancer. Clinical cancer research : an official journal of the American Association for Cancer Research. 2007 Jul 1;13 (13):3831-9. PubMed PMID: 17606714.

[125] Elsaleh H, Iacopetta B. Microsatellite instability is a predictive marker for survival benefit from adjuvant chemotherapy in a population-based series of stage III colorectal carcinoma. Clinical colorectal cancer. 2001 Aug;1 (2):104-9. PubMed PMID: 12445368.

[126] Jover R, Zapater P, Castells A, Llor X, Andreu M, Cubiella J, et al. The efficacy of adjuvant chemotherapy with 5-fluorouracil in colorectal cancer depends on the mismatch repair status. European journal of cancer. 2009 Feb;45 (3):365-73. PubMed PMID: 18722765.

[127] Sargent DJ, Marsoni S, Monges G, Thibodeau SN, Labianca R, Hamilton SR, et al. Defective mismatch repair as a predictive marker for lack of efficacy of fluorouracil-based adjuvant therapy in colon cancer. Journal of clinical oncology : official journal of the American Society of Clinical Oncology. 2010 Jul 10;28 (20):3219-26. PubMed PMID: 20498393. Pubmed Central PMCID: 2903323.

[128] French AJ, Sargent DJ, Burgart LJ, Foster NR, Kabat BF, Goldberg R, et al. Prognostic significance of defective mismatch repair and BRAF V600E in patients with colon

cancer. Clinical cancer research : an official journal of the American Association for Cancer Research. 2008 Jun 1;14 (11):3408-15. PubMed PMID: 18519771. Pubmed Central PMCID: 2674786.

[129] Popat S, Houlston RS. A systematic review and meta-analysis of the relationship between chromosome 18q genotype, DCC status and colorectal cancer prognosis. European journal of cancer. 2005 Sep;41 (14):2060-70. PubMed PMID: 16125380.

[130] Popat S, Zhao D, Chen Z, Pan H, Shao Y, Chandler I, et al. Relationship between chromosome 18q status and colorectal cancer prognosis: a prospective, blinded analysis of 280 patients. Anticancer research. 2007 Jan-Feb;27 (1B):627-33. PubMed PMID: 17348452.

[131] Gnanasampanthan G, Elsaleh H, McCaul K, Iacopetta B. Ki-ras mutation type and the survival benefit from adjuvant chemotherapy in Dukes' C colorectal cancer. The Journal of pathology. 2001 Dec;195 (5):543-8. PubMed PMID: 11745689.

[132] Arrington AK, Heinrich EL, Lee W, Duldulao M, Patel S, Sanchez J, et al. Prognostic and Predictive Roles of KRAS Mutation in Colorectal Cancer. International journal of molecular sciences. 2012;13 (10):12153-68. PubMed PMID: 23202889. Pubmed Central PMCID: 3497263.

[133] Bianchi P, Laghi L, Delconte G, Malesci A. Prognostic Value of Colorectal Cancer Biomarkers. Cancers. 2011;3:2080-105.

[134] Van Rijnsoever M, Elsaleh H, Joseph D, McCaul K, Iacopetta B. CpG island methylator phenotype is an independent predictor of survival benefit from 5-fluorouracil in stage III colorectal cancer. Clinical cancer research : an official journal of the American Association for Cancer Research. 2003 Aug 1;9 (8):2898-903. PubMed PMID: 12912934.

[135] Jover R, Nguyen TP, Perez-Carbonell L, Zapater P, Paya A, Alenda C, et al. 5-Fluorouracil adjuvant chemotherapy does not increase survival in patients with CpG island methylator phenotype colorectal cancer. Gastroenterology. 2011 Apr;140 (4): 1174-81. PubMed PMID: 21185836. Pubmed Central PMCID: 3073650.

[136] Le Morvan V, Smith D, Laurand A, Brouste V, Bellott R, Soubeyran I, et al. Determination of ERCC2 Lys751Gln and GSTP1 Ile105Val gene polymorphisms in colorectal cancer patients: relationships with treatment outcome. Pharmacogenomics. 2007 Dec; 8 (12):1693-703. PubMed PMID: 18085999.

[137] Stoehlmacher J, Park DJ, Zhang W, Yang D, Groshen S, Zahedy S, et al. A multivariate analysis of genomic polymorphisms: prediction of clinical outcome to 5-FU/oxaliplatin combination chemotherapy in refractory colorectal cancer. British journal of cancer. 2004 Jul 19;91 (2):344-54. PubMed PMID: 15213713. Pubmed Central PMCID: 2409815.

[138] Ruzzo A, Graziano F, Loupakis F, Rulli E, Canestrari E, Santini D, et al. Pharmacogenetic profiling in patients with advanced colorectal cancer treated with first-line

FOLFOX-4 chemotherapy. Journal of clinical oncology : official journal of the American Society of Clinical Oncology. 2007 Apr 1;25 (10):1247-54. PubMed PMID: 17401013.

[139] Lamas MJ, Duran G, Balboa E, Bernardez B, Touris M, Vidal Y, et al. Use of a comprehensive panel of biomarkers to predict response to a fluorouracil-oxaliplatin regimen in patients with metastatic colorectal cancer. Pharmacogenomics. 2011 Mar;12 (3):433-42. PubMed PMID: 21449681.

[140] Reed E. ERCC1 and clinical resistance to platinum-based therapy. Clinical cancer research : an official journal of the American Association for Cancer Research. 2005 Sep 1;11 (17):6100-2. PubMed PMID: 16144907.

[141] Viguier J, Boige V, Miquel C, Pocard M, Giraudeau B, Sabourin JC, et al. ERCC1 codon 118 polymorphism is a predictive factor for the tumor response to oxaliplatin/5-fluorouracil combination chemotherapy in patients with advanced colorectal cancer. Clinical cancer research : an official journal of the American Association for Cancer Research. 2005 Sep 1;11 (17):6212-7. PubMed PMID: 16144923.

[142] Moreno V, Gemignani F, Landi S, Gioia-Patricola L, Chabrier A, Blanco I, et al. Polymorphisms in genes of nucleotide and base excision repair: risk and prognosis of colorectal cancer. Clinical cancer research : an official journal of the American Association for Cancer Research. 2006 Apr 1;12 (7 Pt 1):2101-8. PubMed PMID: 16609022.

[143] Stoehlmacher J, Ghaderi V, Iobal S, Groshen S, Tsao-Wei D, Park D, et al. A polymorphism of the XRCC1 gene predicts for response to platinum based treatment in advanced colorectal cancer. Anticancer research. 2001 Jul-Aug;21 (4B):3075-9. PubMed PMID: 11712813.

[144] Park DJ, Stoehlmacher J, Zhang W, Tsao-Wei DD, Groshen S, Lenz HJ. A Xeroderma pigmentosum group D gene polymorphism predicts clinical outcome to platinum-based chemotherapy in patients with advanced colorectal cancer. Cancer research. 2001 Dec 15;61 (24):8654-8. PubMed PMID: 11751380.

[145] Lievre A, Bachet JB, Le Corre D, Boige V, Landi B, Emile JF, et al. KRAS mutation status is predictive of response to cetuximab therapy in colorectal cancer. Cancer research. 2006 Apr 15;66 (8):3992-5. PubMed PMID: 16618717.

[146] FDA US. ERBITUX® (cetuximab).

[147] FDA US. Vectibix® (panitumumab).

[148] Yuen ST, Davies H, Chan TL, Ho JW, Bignell GR, Cox C, et al. Similarity of the phenotypic patterns associated with BRAF and KRAS mutations in colorectal neoplasia. Cancer research. 2002 Nov 15;62 (22):6451-5. PubMed PMID: 12438234.

[149] Tol J, Nagtegaal ID, Punt CJ. BRAF mutation in metastatic colorectal cancer. The New England journal of medicine. 2009 Jul 2;361 (1):98-9. PubMed PMID: 19571295.

[150] Andre T, Boni C, Navarro M, Tabernero J, Hickish T, Topham C, et al. Improved overall survival with oxaliplatin, fluorouracil, and leucovorin as adjuvant treatment in stage II or III colon cancer in the MOSAIC trial. J Clin Oncol. 2009 Jul 1;27 (19): 3109-16. PubMed PMID: 19451431. Epub 2009/05/20. eng.

[151] Andre T, Quinaux E, Louvet C, Colin P, Gamelin E, Bouche O, et al. Phase III study comparing a semimonthly with a monthly regimen of fluorouracil and leucovorin as adjuvant treatment for stage II and III colon cancer patients: final results of GERCOR C96.1. J Clin Oncol. 2007 Aug 20;25 (24):3732-8. PubMed PMID: 17704423. Epub 2007/08/21. eng.

[152] Le Voyer TE, Sigurdson ER, Hanlon AL, Mayer RJ, Macdonald JS, Catalano PJ, et al. Colon cancer survival is associated with increasing number of lymph nodes analyzed: a secondary survey of intergroup trial INT-0089. J Clin Oncol. 2003 Aug 1;21 (15):2912-9. PubMed PMID: 12885809. Epub 2003/07/30. eng.

[153] Mamounas E, Wieand S, Wolmark N, Bear HD, Atkins JN, Song K, et al. Comparative efficacy of adjuvant chemotherapy in patients with Dukes' B versus Dukes' C colon cancer: results from four National Surgical Adjuvant Breast and Bowel Project adjuvant studies (C-01, C-02, C-03, and C-04). J Clin Oncol. 1999 May;17 (5):1349-55. PubMed PMID: 10334518.

[154] Saltz LB, Niedzwiecki D, Hollis D, Goldberg RM, Hantel A, Thomas JP, et al. Irinotecan fluorouracil plus leucovorin is not superior to fluorouracil plus leucovorin alone as adjuvant treatment for stage III colon cancer: results of CALGB 89803. J Clin Oncol. 2007 Aug 10;25 (23):3456-61. PubMed PMID: 17687149. Epub 2007/08/10. eng.

[155] Van Cutsem E, Labianca R, Bodoky G, Barone C, Aranda E, Nordlinger B, et al. Randomized phase III trial comparing biweekly infusional fluorouracil/leucovorin alone or with irinotecan in the adjuvant treatment of stage III colon cancer: PETACC-3. J Clin Oncol. 2009 Jul 1;27 (19):3117-25. PubMed PMID: 19451425.

[156] Deschoolmeester V, Baay M, Specenier P, Lardon F, Vermorken JB. A review of the most promising biomarkers in colorectal cancer: one step closer to targeted therapy. The oncologist. 2010;15 (7):699-731. PubMed PMID: 20584808. Pubmed Central PMCID: 3228001.

[157] Jass JR. Classification of colorectal cancer based on correlation of clinical, morphological and molecular features. Histopathology. 2007 Jan;50 (1):113-30. PubMed PMID: 17204026.

[158] Iessi E MM, Lozupone F, Fais St, De Milito A. Tumor acidity and malignancy: novel aspects in the design of anti-tumor therapy. Cancer Therapy 2008;6:55-66.

[159] Tredan O, Galmarini CM, Patel K, Tannock IF. Drug resistance and the solid tumor microenvironment. Journal of the National Cancer Institute. 2007 Oct 3;99 (19): 1441-54. PubMed PMID: 17895480.

[160] Provenzano PP, Cuevas C, Chang AE, Goel VK, Von Hoff DD, Hingorani SR. Enzymatic targeting of the stroma ablates physical barriers to treatment of pancreatic ductal adenocarcinoma. Cancer cell. 2012 Mar 20;21 (3):418-29. PubMed PMID: 22439937. Pubmed Central PMCID: 3371414.

[161] Meads MB, Gatenby RA, Dalton WS. Environment-mediated drug resistance: a major contributor to minimal residual disease. Nature reviews Cancer. 2009 Sep;9 (9): 665-74. PubMed PMID: 19693095.

[162] Sun Y, Campisi J, Higano C, Beer TM, Porter P, Coleman I, et al. Treatment-induced damage to the tumor microenvironment promotes prostate cancer therapy resistance through WNT16B. Nature medicine. 2012 Sep;18 (9):1359-68. PubMed PMID: 22863786. Epub 2012/08/07. eng.

[163] Roodhart JM, Daenen LG, Stigter EC, Prins HJ, Gerrits J, Houthuijzen JM, et al. Mesenchymal stem cells induce resistance to chemotherapy through the release of platinum-induced fatty acids. Cancer cell. 2011 Sep 13;20 (3):370-83. PubMed PMID: 21907927. Epub 2011/09/13. eng.

[164] Straussman R, Morikawa T, Shee K, Barzily-Rokni M, Qian ZR, Du J, et al. Tumour micro-environment elicits innate resistance to RAF inhibitors through HGF secretion. Nature. 2012 Jul 26;487 (7408):500-4. PubMed PMID: 22763439. Epub 2012/07/06. eng.

[165] Nosho K, Baba Y, Tanaka N, Shima K, Hayashi M, Meyerhardt JA, et al. Tumour-infiltrating T-cell subsets, molecular changes in colorectal cancer, and prognosis: cohort study and literature review. The Journal of pathology. 2010 Dec;222 (4):350-66. PubMed PMID: 20927778. Pubmed Central PMCID: 3033700.

[166] Halama N, Michel S, Kloor M, Zoernig I, Benner A, Spille A, et al. Localization and density of immune cells in the invasive margin of human colorectal cancer liver metastases are prognostic for response to chemotherapy. Cancer research. 2011 Sep 1;71 (17):5670-7. PubMed PMID: 21846824.

[167] Ogino S, Goel A. Molecular classification and correlates in colorectal cancer. The Journal of molecular diagnostics : JMD. 2008 Jan;10 (1):13-27. PubMed PMID: 18165277. Pubmed Central PMCID: 2175539.

[168] Ogino S, Fuchs CS, Giovannucci E. How many molecular subtypes? Implications of the unique tumor principle in personalized medicine. Expert review of molecular diagnostics. 2012 Jul;12 (6):621-8. PubMed PMID: 22845482. Pubmed Central PMCID: PMC3492839. Epub 2012/08/01. eng.

[169] Lewis A, Segditsas S, Deheragoda M, Pollard P, Jeffery R, Nye E, et al. Severe polyposis in Apc (1322T) mice is associated with submaximal Wnt signalling and increased expression of the stem cell marker Lgr5. Gut. 2010 Dec;59 (12):1680-6. PubMed PMID: 20926645. Pubmed Central PMCID: PMC3002835. Epub 2010/10/12. eng.

[170] Bielas JH, Loeb KR, Rubin BP, True LD, Loeb LA. Human cancers express a mutator phenotype. Proceedings of the National Academy of Sciences of the United States of America. 2006 Nov 28;103 (48):18238-42. PubMed PMID: 17108085. Pubmed Central PMCID: 1636340.

[171] Loeb LA. Human cancers express mutator phenotypes: origin, consequences and targeting. Nature reviews Cancer. 2011 Jun;11 (6):450-7. PubMed PMID: 21593786.

[172] Gerlinger M, Rowan AJ, Horswell S, Larkin J, Endesfelder D, Gronroos E, et al. Intratumor heterogeneity and branched evolution revealed by multiregion sequencing. The New England journal of medicine. 2012 Mar 8;366 (10):883-92. PubMed PMID: 22397650.

[173] Crea F, Duhagon MA, Farrar WL, Danesi R. Pharmacogenomics and cancer stem cells: a changing landscape? Trends in pharmacological sciences. 2011 Aug;32 (8): 487-94. PubMed PMID: 21529973. Pubmed Central PMCID: 3448442.

[174] Dean M, Fojo T, Bates S. Tumour stem cells and drug resistance. Nature reviews Cancer. 2005 Apr;5 (4):275-84. PubMed PMID: 15803154.

[175] Issa JP. Colon cancer: it's CIN or CIMP. Clinical cancer research : an official journal of the American Association for Cancer Research. 2008 Oct 1;14 (19):5939-40. PubMed PMID: 18829469.

[176] Wu C, Bekaii-Saab T. CpG Island Methylation, Microsatellite Instability, and BRAF Mutations and Their Clinical Application in the Treatment of Colon Cancer. Chemotherapy research and practice. 2012;2012:359041. PubMed PMID: 22792460. Pubmed Central PMCID: PMC3389642. Epub 2012/07/14. eng.

Chapter 18

The Role, Significance and Applicability of Aberrant Crypt Foci in Clinical Practice

Martina Perše and Anton Cerar

Additional information is available at the end of the chapter

http://dx.doi.org/10.5772/57474

1. Introduction

Colorectal cancer (CRC) is one of the leading causes of cancer-related mortalities in the Western world, with over 1.2 million new cases and over 0.6 million deaths being recorded in 2008 [1].

Major risk factors of CRC are personal history of precursor lesion, inflammatory bowel disease, age (about 90% of cases occur after age 50) and family history of CRC or a genetic susceptibility to the development of CRC resulting from DNA mutations. It is estimated that approximately 15% of CRC cases develop as a result of inherited factors and 5-10% of them result from known genetic syndroms, e.g., familial adenomatous polyposis (FAP) and hereditary non-polyposis colorectal carcinoma (HNPCC), while most cases of CRC occurs sporadically (70-80%) [2]. In patiens with inherited genetic factors CRC occurs early in life, usualy before 40 years of their age, while in sporadic cases cancer develops after 40 years of age with the highest incidence between 60 and 70 years of age. CRC remains asymptomatic for years. Symptoms develop insidiously and are frequently present for months, sometimes years, before being diagnosed. If colon tumors are not identified and removed at the precancerous or adenoma stage, the disease gradually progresses into carcinoma stage where cancer cells invade the wall of the intestine and distant organs [1].

There are different approaches and strategies concerning how to reduce the mortality due to CRC. The surgical and chemotherapeutic treatment of CRC is usually costly, painful and the prognosis is not promisig. Therefore, in clinical practice efforts have been directed toward identification and removal of precancerous lesions. Screening programs, which are based upon detection and removal of visible polypoid adenomas, have been implemented in a number of countries on nationwide scale.

Global cancer statistics shows that CRC-related mortality has been decreasing in Western countries due to improved treatment and early detection, which indicates that screening program is one of the important steps in reducing the mortality due to CRC [1]. However, although screening programs are promising and represent one of the important steps in reducing the mortality due to CRC, reports demonstrate that there is still 25% of false-negative results due to flat or depressed precancerous lesions, which are commonly missed during conventional colonoscopy [3].

Recently, another promising approach has been demonstrated. It is directed toward identification of aberrant crypt foci (ACF), intermediate biomarkers predictive for CRC. The association of ACF with CRC is supported by shared histological and molecular features of ACF with colonic polyps and adenomas [4-7].

The aim of the present chapter is to summarize experimental and clinical results regarding morphological, histological and molecular characteristics of ACF with emphasis on current progress in the knowledge of CRC development. The role, significance and applicability of ACF in clinical practice is also presented and discussed.

2. Aberrant crypt foci (ACF)

ACF are the first lesions in multistep development of CRC, which can be seen on the colon surface with aid of magnification and/or dye.

ACF were first identified in 1987 by Bird on whole unembedded colon of carcinogen treated mouse [8]. Colon was fixed, stained with methylene blue and observed under low-magnification (10-40x M) stereomicroscope [9; 10]. This simple and rapid methodological approach enabled visualization of all crypts on the surface of the colon mucosa. Since their first identification numerous studies investigating morphology, distribution, histology and molecular characteristics of ACF have been performed. In 1991 reports on identification of ACF in the human colon were published. ACF were identified under a dissecting microscope after methylene blue staining on the mucosal surface of both formalin-fixed human colon resections and fresh (unfixed) colon resections [11-13].

Based on morphological appearance of crypts on the colon surface crypts can be regarded as normal or aberrant. Aberrant crypts can be observed as single altered crypt or as a cluster of altered crypts that form a focus termed ACF [8; 14; 15].

It is important to keep in mind that ACF is a term that denotes topographic or endoscopic observation. ACF can be identified as clusters of altered crypts in unembedded colon mucosa (fixed or fresh) under magnification after visualization by different dyes. In studies using animal models ACF are usually observed under stereomicroscope on whole colon mucosa that is fixed flat (to prevent excessive unevenness while viewing) and stained with methylene blue [9; 10]. In clinical practice ACF can be observed *in vivo* endoscopically with aid of dye spray (methylene blue or indigo carmine) using high magnification colonoscopy [6; 7; 16].

ACF is not a histological diagnosis. Structural and cytological features of ACF can be recognized or confirmed only after histological examination. However, at the same time it is noteworthy to mention that lesions seen in histologic sections of colon without prior topographic identification on colon surface can not be termed ACF.

http://dx.doi.org/10.5772/57474

To better understand the histological background of ACF as well as molecular alterations recognized and described at this stage of colon carcinogenesis, the next section is brief overview of histological criteria and classification of ACF, histologically denoted as colorectal intraepithelial lesions [17; 18].

3. Histological characteristics of ACF

Histologically, ACF are heterogeneous group of intraepithelial lesions that exhibit variable features, ranging from almost normal or mild atypia to severe dysplasia. Based on their histological characteristics they can be divided into three main categories [7; 14]:

1. ACF that are almost histologically normal,
2. ACF with hyperplastic crypts and
3. ACF with dysplastic crypts.

According to World Health Organization ACF are histologically classified into two groups, i.e. ACF with hyperplastic crypts and ACF with dysplastic crypts [19].

It has been demonstrated that the majority of observed ACF, including ACF identified in patients with sporadic CRC, are classified as almost histologically normal (Figure 1). These ACF are composed of crypts with almost normal histological appearance. The major histologic difference that distinguishes this type of ACF from normal crypts is slightly enlarged crypt diameter. The crypt diameter in this type of ACF measures up to 1.5 times the diameter of a normal crypt. They show no other histological or molecular alterations and they even spontaneously regress. Accordingly, it was found that this type of ACF has no clinical diagnostic value [7; 14].

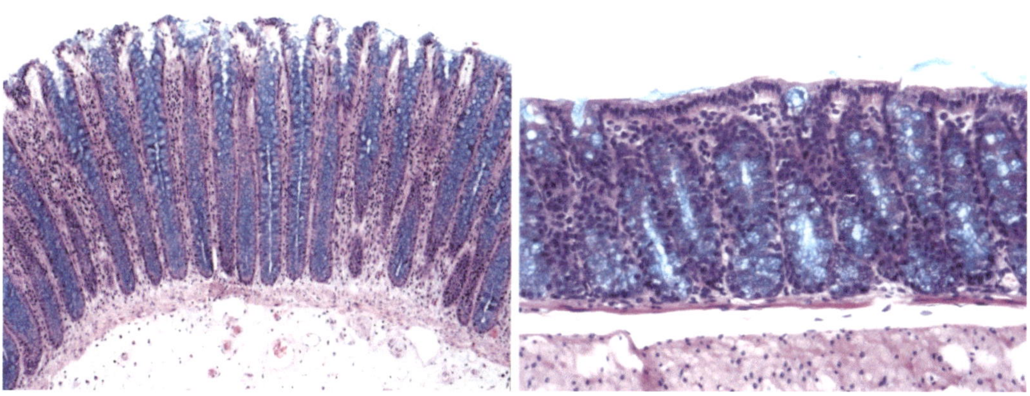

Figure 1. A normal human (left) and rat (right) colorectal mucosa. Crypts are parallel. The mucin is stained blue (Kreyberg trichrom stain).

On the other hand, other two groups of ACF have been found to have potential clinical value as biomarker predictive for CRC risk [7; 14].

4. ACF with hyperplastic crypts (hyperplastic intraepithelial lesions)

Hyperplastic epithelial lesions are composed of mixture of goblet and absorptive cells with enlarged or sometimes crowded nuclei without stratification (Figure 2).

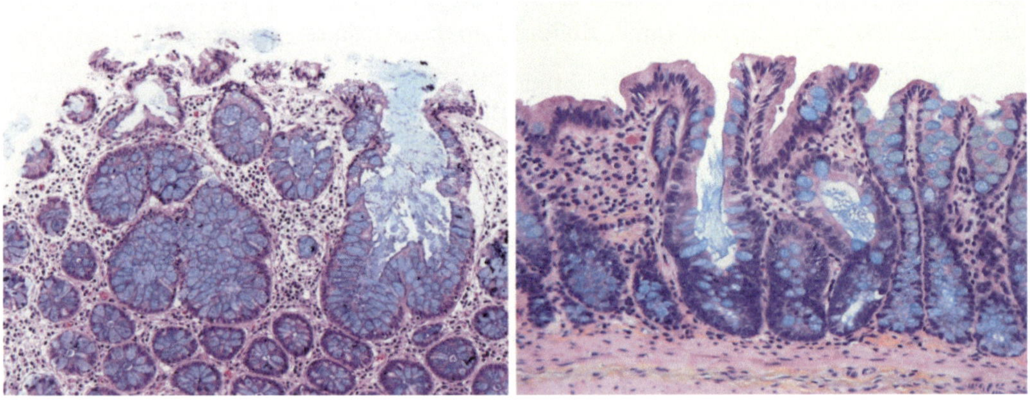

Figure 2. Hyperplastic aberrant crypts of human (left) colorectal mucosa accompanying resected sporadic colorectal adenoma. The focus is composed of 3 hyperplastic crypts that are much wider then surrounding normal crypts. The epithelial cells of the hyperplastic crypts are higher and composed of one layer. On the right there are hyperplastic aberrant crypts of rat colorectal mucosa, induced by carcinogen. The focus is composed of 3 crypts with slight mucin depletion. The level of focus is higher then of the surrounding mucosa. The epithelial cells of the hyperplastic crypts are higher and composed of one layer (Kreyberg trichrom stain).

Mitotic figures are limited to the lower two-thirds of the crypts and are never observed on the surface of crypts. Nuclei are basally located, ovoid or round, with occasional visible nucleoli and usually uniformly dark. The luminal opening of crypts is slightly elevated from the surrounding normal mucosa and the crypts are elongated and occasionally branching with partial mucin depletion [17]. The role of hyperplastic aberrant crypts in the process of colon carcinogenesis is not clear and is a matter of debate and further investigations [15].

5. ACF with dysplastic crypts (intraepithelial neoplasia/dysplasia)

Presence of dysplasia is regarded as early histopathological changes in the precursor lesions of colon cancer. The word dysplasia is histological term that describes structural and cytological alterations in the epithelium that predispose an organ to cancer development. Inraepithelial neoplasia (IEN) is a histological term for dysplastic lesions in the epithelial layer of colon mucosa that can be identified only after careful histological examination (Figure 3). IEN is

http://dx.doi.org/10.5772/57474

synonymous with terms atypical hyperplasia, microadenoma, carcinoma *in situ* and dysplasia. Depending on cytological and architectural features IEN is classified as low-grade or high grade. The differential histological criteria involve hypercellularity with enlarged, hyperchromatic nuclei, varying degrees of nuclear stratification, loss of polarity, high nuclear/cytoplasmic ratio, nuclear crowding, increased mitotic index and decreased mucin excretion [17; 20].

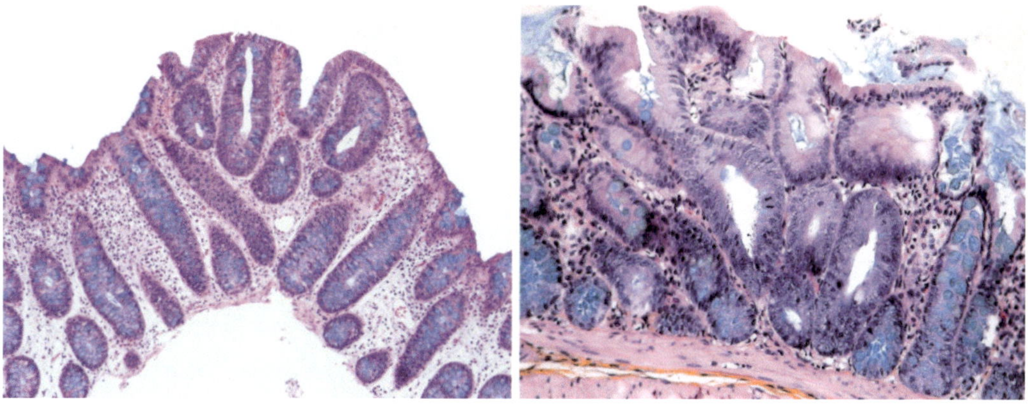

Figure 3. Dysplastic aberrant crypts of human colorectal mucosa accompanying FAP (left). The focus is composed of 4 crypts. The level of focus is higher then that of the surrounding mucosa. The epithelial cells covering the aberrant crypts are classified as mild dysplasia. On the right there are dysplastic aberrant crypts of rat colorectal mucosa induced by carcinogen. The focus is composed of 3 crypts that show severe mucin depletion. Numerous mitoses, stratification of nuclei, atypical epithelial cells, and architectural atypia are the components of dysplasia (Kreyberg trichrom stain).

6. Molecular characteristics of ACF

Evidence from experimental and clinical studies demonstrates that ACF share similar histological and molecular features as colonic tumors (i.e. adenomas and adenocarcinomas) [15; 21; 22]. Today, high-magnification chromoscopic colonoscopy allows detection and biopsy of ACF *in vivo* in man. It also provides opportunity to investigate and characterize the earliest genetic and molecular alterations in CRC development in man. ACF exhibit many of the molecular and genetic abnormalities that form the basis for the adenoma-carcinoma sequence in CRC.

It has been found that ACF exhibit many of the molecular and genetic abnormalities that form the basis for the adenoma-carcinoma sequence in CRC. Genetic alterations found in human ACF include mutations in tumor suppressor genes, microsatellite instability, aberrant methylation as well as aberrant expression of proteins (summarized in Figure 4). Up to date, three molecular pathways of CRC development have been identified and described, i.e. chromosomal instability, microsatellite instability and CpG island methylator phenotype. All three types of molecular alterations have also been found in ACF [22; 23].

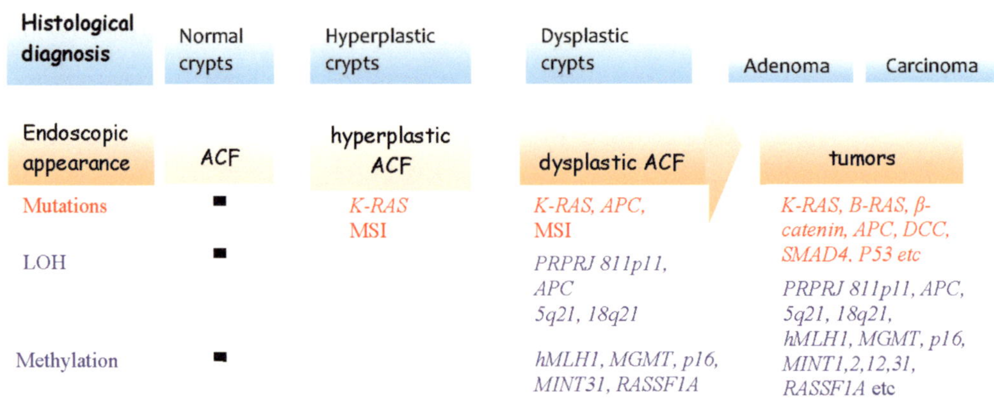

Figure 4. Phenotypic, genetic and epigenetic alteration involved in multistep development of colon carcinogenesis.

7. The chromosomal instability (CIN)

CIN is the most common in sporadic CRC and shows chromosomal abnormalities such as chromosome breaks, duplication, rearrangements, loss of heterozygosity (LOH) and sequential inactivation of tumor suppressor genes such as APC (5q), P53 (17p) and SMAD4 (18q), which are frequently found in sporadic carcinomas. It is known that germ line mutations in APC lead to the hereditary syndrome of FAP [22; 23].

Loss of heterozygosity (LOH) was observed in ACF at 18q (locus that maps close to the DCC and DPC4 genes) [24], in 67% LOH was found at locus 11p11, the location of the gene for protein tyrosine phosphatase receptor type J (PTPRJ; tumor suppressor gene), at locus 5q21 and 18q21 [25]. LOH was identified near the APC tumor suppressor gene (at the D5S346 marker) [26].

APC mutation was found in ACF with dysplastic crypts but not in ACF with hyperplastic crypts. This was frequently observed in ACF obtained from patients with FAP, while in ACF obtained from patients with sporadic CRC APC mutation was rarely observed [7; 27; 28].

β-catenin mutation, which is found in 12% of adenomas and 16% of carcinomas, was not found in ACF, regardless of the histologic type of ACF [5; 29]. Only increased expression of β-catenin was found in the cytosol of ACF with dysplastic crypts (54%) [30; 31].

K-RAS mutation was found in 13%-95% of ACF and was much more frequent in ACF with hyperplastic crypts (80%-100%) that in ACF with dysplastic crypts (0%-57%) [7; 27; 28; 32-35].

8. The microsatellite instability (MSI)

MSI is a hallmark of defective DNA mismatch repair (MMR) genes such as *hMLH1* or *hMSH2* and leads to the accumulation of a high frequency of somatic mutations [24]. It is frequent in patients with HNPCC (90%) but also found in sporadic CRC (15%).

MSI was identified in 30% ACF from patients of elevated risk (family or personal history) and 13% lesions from average risk patients (subjects without family or personal history) [24-26].

9. The CpG island methylator phenotype (CIMP)

CIMP is epigenetic mechanism characterized by hypermethylation of cytosine residue within CpG islands in the promoter regions of certain genes (which are particularly rich in CpG nucleotides such as tumor suppressor and MMR genes) and results in their inactivation (loss of gene expression). Genes that have been shown to be silenced by promoter hypermethylation in human CRC are *p16, hMLH1, MGMT, MINT1,2,12,* and *31 [22; 23].*

Methylation of CpG islands was found in 34% ACF obtained from patients with both FAP and sporadic CRC, but was more frequent in sporadic ACF (53%), especially dysplastic ACF (75%) and less hyperplastic ACF (7%) [32].

In ACF hypermethylation of the MMR genes such as *hHLM1* and *MGMT* (in hyperplastic ACF) [26] and tumor suppressor genes such as *p16, MINT31* [32], *RASSF1A* were found [26].

10. ACF revealing new insight into CRC development

As high-magnification chromoscopic colonoscopy now allow detection and biopsy of ACF in the mucosa of large bowel, ACF might serve as a research tool for revealing new insights and knowledge into first alterations and risk factors in CRC development.

Evidence shows that ACF in FAP patients differ from ACF in subjects with sporadic CRC. Differences can be observed regarding endoscopic, histological and molecular characteristics. Patients with FAP have significantly increased number of ACF than patients with sporadic CRC. Most of the ACF in FAP patients is histologically diagnosed as dysplastic (89%), while patients with sporadic CRC have mostly ACF with hyperplastic crypts (82%). *K-RAS* mutation was found very rarely in dysplastic ACF of FAP patients, but frequently in ACF obtained from patients with sporadic CRC (82%) [7].

Conversely, *APC* mutations were very rarely found in dysplastic ACF from patients with sporadic CRC, while in ACF from FAP patients were almost always present. Methylation of CpG islands was found in sporadic ACF but not in ACF from FAP patients [32].

Differences in the endoscopic appearance and genetic features were observed also in ACF obtained from patients with ulcerative colitis (UC). In ACF from patients with UC *K-RAS* mutation was rarely observed and *APC* mutation was not found. However, in dysplastic ACF frequent methylation of promoter region of *p16* (73%) and *P53* mutation (60%) was found [36].

All these data show that ACF provide opportunity to get closer insight into first molecular events that are responsible for initiation and formation of CRC.

11. Endoscopic characteristics of ACF

As already mentioned ACF are the first lesions that can be found on the surface of the fixed or fresh colorectal mucosa. ACF are invisible to standard endoscopic instruments but can now be visualized *in vivo* endoscopically by using specialized magnifying colonoscopes in conjunction with dye sprays (methylene blue, indigo carmine), the technique termed high-magnification chromoscopic colonoscopy [6].

Staining of the colonic mucosa at colonoscopy improves the visibility of the morphological characteristics of the crypts in the mucosa, such as shape, size or luminal openings of the crypts. Most prominent feature of aberrant crypts is that they stain more darkly than do normal surrounding crypts. However, there are also other morphological features important for identification of ACF. By definition, ACF are colon crypts that are larger than normal surrounding crypts, have increased pericryptal space that separates them from the normal crypts, they have a thicker layer of epithelial cells that often stains darker, their luminal openings are not circular but rather oval or even compressed. They are usually not in the same level as the surrounding normal crypts but they are either slightly elevated above the mucosa or may be even depressed. ACF may be composed of one to few hundreds of aberrant crypts per focus (1 to 412) [10; 14; 15].

As explained, ACF are heterogeneous group of lesions that exhibit variability in histological and molecular characteristics as well as variability in morphological characteristics.

Based on the surface morphologic features of ACF, researchers are able to distinguish three types of ACF and predict histologic characteristics of ACF [6].

Aberrant crypts that stain more darkly and are larger, have a thicker epithelial lining and a larger pericryptal zone than normal crypts and exhibit large oval (smooth, dilated) lumens have been histologically diagnosed as almost normal. Such ACF have slight enlargement, irregularity, and elongation of the ducts but show no signs of hyperplasia or dysplasia [6].

Aberrant crypts that have all above-mentioned characteristics and exhibit asteroid or slit shape of lumens have been histologically diagnosed as hyperplastic with serrated luminal pattern. Aberrant crypts that have ticker epithelial lining than both above mentioned types and exhibit compressed or undistinguishable lumen are classified in the third group of ACF, histologically diagnosed as dysplastic. Such ACF show loss of polarity, hyperchromatism and stratification of the nuclei in the crypt epithelium [6; 12; 14].

12. Prevalence and density of ACF

First data about density (average number of ACF per cm^2 of mucosa) and anatomical location of ACF in colonic mucosa are based on investigations of colorectal resections. Results have shown that patients with increased risk (personal or family history) have higher average number of ACF per cm^2 than persons with average risk (subjects without personal or family history). It was found that FAP patients have significantly higher density of ACF in colon mucosa than patients with sporadic CRC or benign bowel disease. Higher frequencies of ACF were observed in left than in right colon. Results have shown that density of ACF increases from proximal to distal part of the colon, being the highest in the rectosigmoidal region, which corresponds to anatomical location of CRC development [11-14; 34].

13. Endoscopic detection of ACF

Similar findings regarding prevalence and distribution of ACF in colorectal mucosa have been observed in humans *in vivo* by using magnifying (40x) endoscopy after endoscopic staining of colon mucosa (methylene blue). Takayama et al. [6] examined 370 subjects (147 normal subjects, 130 patients with adenoma, and 48 patients with carcinoma) and found that ACF were present in almost all patients with adenoma or carcinoma. ACF were most frequently observed in the left colon, where polyps are often found. Additionally, it was found that patients with adenoma or carcinoma had significantly higher estimated relative risks for ACF with dysplastic crypts than normal subjects [6].

In normal subjects, both the prevalence and the number of ACF in subjects under 40 years of age were very low (10%) but increased with age, particularly after the age of 40 (54% - 66%). Conversely, patients with cancer had a consistently high prevalence (100%) and large number of ACF regardless of age. In patients with adenoma, the age-associated increment in the prevalence and number of ACF was intermediate [6].

Takayama et al. [6] investigated number, density, and dysplastic features of distal colorectal ACF in patients with exophytic adenomas and carcinomas, while Hurlstone et al. [16] assessed the prevalence and features of ACF in patients with flat and depressed colorectal neoplastic lesions, which account for around one third of all colorectal lesions. High magnification chromoscopic colonoscopy was performed on 574 healthy subjects, 281 patients with flat adenomas and 14 patients with flat carcinomas in which 602 (3% of them dysplastic), 2796 (18% dysplastic) and 594 (61 % dysplastic) ACF were identified, respectively. Similarly as in patients with exophytic colorectal lesions, the number of ACF increased in a stepwise fashion from normal subjects to patients with flat or depressed adenoma and then to patients with flat or depressed carcinoma [16].

In another study 103 patients with average age of 61 (range of 28-87) were examined by using magnification (60x) chromoscopic colonoscopy. 788 ACF were found in the distal 20 cm of colon/rectum. Patients with a family history of CRC had a significantly higher mean number of ACF than the average risk subjects (7.6% dysplastic and 46% hyperplastic) [5].

Rudolph et al. [37] have demonstrated that the number of ACF is significantly increased in patients with personal history of adenoma in comparison to subjects without personal or family history. They also observed that number of ACF is higher in older persons than in younger subjects [37].

14. Clinical application

Clinical application of ACF as an intermediate biomarker for CRC in humans is under development and is thus less conclusive [4; 38].

Recently, few studies investigated relationship of human colorectal ACF and formation of colorectal polyps on repeat colonoscopy. It was found that the number of ACF in the colorectum was associated with substantial risk for future advanced neoplasia [39-42].

Ohkubo et al. [39] investigated natural history of human ACF and correlation with risk factors for CRC. They examined 82 subjects who underwent total colonoscopy and whose ACF number was examined at least 2 times. They retrospectively evaluated the changes in the ACF number at four different surveillance periods (6 months, 1 year, 2 years, 3 years) and in groups with and without colorectal neoplasms. The subjects were classified into an increased ACF group and a no change/decreased ACF group, and investigated the relationship between the changes in the ACF number and known risk factors for CRC. No significant differences were observed in the ACF number between the first and second observations in any surveillance period groups, and in the groups classified according to the presence or absence of colorectal neoplasms. There were no significant differences between the increased and no change/decreased ACF groups in terms of gender, smoking habit, current alcohol consumption, age, BMI, HbA1c or serum triglyceride level, whereas a significant difference between the groups was observed in the serum total cholesterol level [39].

All these data strongly implicate that detection and quantification of ACF in the distal colon may be useful in predicting CRC risk and may be considered as a useful marker in chemopreventive trials. Furthermore, it is expected that one of the most important clinical applications of ACF observation with magnifying endoscopy will be its use as a target lesion for chemoprevention. Because ACF are small lesions, they are suggested to be eradicated during a short time by administration of chemopreventive agents [43]. Takayama et al. [43] performed an open chemopreventive trial of sulindac and found that the number of ACF was reduced markedly in 2 months. Patients receiving sulindac for more than one year had no ACF in colon mucosa. After 8 to 12 months of follow-up, the number of ACF in colorectal mucosa significantly decreased or even completely disappeared. In the untreated control subjects the number of ACF was either unchanged or slightly increased [6]. Another short-term chemoprevention trial of metformin for colorectal ACF showed suppressive effect of the drug on the formation of ACF [44]. Other chemopreventive a double blind randomized controlled trial targeting ACF are under investigations [43-45].

15. Difficulties or pitfalls in detection of ACF

All these data strongly suggest that ACF in the distal colon may be useful and reliable surrogate marker in predicting CRC risk. However, there are also limitations and difficulties. The main limitation is the fact that chromoendoscopy and magnifying endoscopes are largely research tools and not the equipment in gastrointestinal practice. Difficulties were reported in some studies in which endoscopic criteria failed to predict histologic confirmation of ACF or correlation between the number of ACF and CRC risk [46; 47]. It was also found that there was considerable variability among endoscopists regarding accuracy to correctly identify ACF. It was found that in spite of training, accuracy to correctly identify ACF did not improve [46].

Current knowledge about rodents ACF, which share many similarities with human pathology, might be helpful to understand tricks and traps when using ACF. In rodents, ACF are widely accepted as intermediate biomarkers of CRC risk assessment. They have been used as an endpoint in identifying and assessing preventive or promotional role of natural and pharmacological compounds, as well as dietary and environmental factors in the process of colon carcinogenesis [48; 49]. However, limitations to the use of ACF as a biomarker to identify cancer preventive agents exist. Increasing number of studies has demonstrated that ACF in both animals and humans are heterogeneous group of lesions that contain multiple genetic, epigenetic and phenotypic alterations [15; 22; 50]. In rodents, total number of ACF may be considered as a valid biomarker only at very early stage of carcinogenesis, while in subsequent weeks ACF with higher crypt multiplicities (more than 4 crypts) are considered more specific biomarker than total number of ACF. In more advanced stages of colon carcinogenesis ACF may not be reliable intermediate biomarker of colon carcinogenesis (explained in detail in [9] and [51]). It is also important to mention that ACF are not equally distributed among the proximal, middle or distal colon. The majority of ACF develop in the middle and distal colon [52-54], which need to be taken into consideration when using ACF as biomarkers (comprehensively discussed in [9; 10] and [51]. Nevertheless, when considering all above mentioned facts ACF are useful biomarkers for the screening of compounds for their chemopreventive activities [49; 51].

16. Conclusion

Based on experimental and clinical studies evidence demonstrates that ACF share similar histological and molecular features as colonic tumors (i.e. adenomas and adenocarcinomas). ACF exhibit many of the molecular and genetic abnormalities that form the basis for the adenoma-carcinoma sequence in CRC. Today, high-magnification chromoscopic colonoscopy allows detection and biopsy of ACF *in vivo* in man. It also provides opportunity to investigate and characterize the earliest genetic and molecular alterations in CRC development in man.

However, it has been shown that ACF are heterogeneous group of lesions that exhibit variable endoscopic, histological and molecular features. This fact has been shown to cause some difficulties in accuracy of detection and quantification of ACF among endoscopists. However, chromoendoscopy and magnifying endoscopes are largely research tools and future research on that field will bring new information about reliability and applicability of ACF as biomarker of CRC risk in clinical practice.

Acknowledgements

This work was funded by the Slovenian Ministry of Higher Education, Science and Technology (grant number P3-0054).

Author details

Martina Perše* and Anton Cerar

*Address all correspondence to: martina.perse@mf.uni-lj.si

Institute of Pathology, Medical Experimental Centre, Faculty of Medicine, University of Ljubljana, Slovenia

References

[1] Jemal, A., Bray, F., Center, M. M., Ferlay, J., Ward, E., and Forman, D., "Global cancer statistics," *CA Cancer J.Clin.*, Vol. 61, No. 2, 2011, pp. 69-90.

[2] Souglakos, J., "Genetic alterations in sporadic and hereditary colorectal cancer: implementations for screening and follow-up," *Dig.Dis.*, Vol. 25, No. 1, 2007, pp. 9-19.

[3] Orlando, F. A., Tan, D., Baltodano, J. D., Khoury, T., Gibbs, J. F., Hassid, V. J., Ahmed, B. H., and Alrawi, S. J., "Aberrant crypt foci as precursors in colorectal cancer progression," *J.Surg.Oncol.*, Vol. 98, No. 3, 2008, pp. 207-213.

[4] Stevens, R. G., Swede, H., and Rosenberg, D. W., "Epidemiology of colonic aberrant crypt foci: review and analysis of existing studies," *Cancer Lett.*, Vol. 252, No. 2, 2007, pp. 171-183.

[5] Stevens, R. G., Swede, H., Heinen, C. D., Jablonski, M., Grupka, M., Ross, B., Parente, M., Tirnauer, J. S., Giardina, C., Rajan, T. V., Rosenberg, D. W., and Levine, J., "Aberrant crypt foci in patients with a positive family history of sporadic colorectal cancer," *Cancer Lett.*, Vol. 248, No. 2, 2007, pp. 262-268.

[6] Takayama, T., Katsuki, S., Takahashi, Y., Ohi, M., Nojiri, S., Sakamaki, S., Kato, J., Kogawa, K., Miyake, H., and Niitsu, Y., "Aberrant crypt foci of the colon as precursors of adenoma and cancer," *N.Engl.J.Med.*, Vol. 339, No. 18, 1998, pp. 1277-1284.

[7] Takayama, T., Ohi, M., Hayashi, T., Miyanishi, K., Nobuoka, A., Nakajima, T., Satoh, T., Takimoto, R., Kato, J., Sakamaki, S., and Niitsu, Y., "Analysis of K-ras, APC, and beta-catenin in aberrant crypt foci in sporadic adenoma, cancer, and familial adenomatous polyposis," *Gastroenterology*, Vol. 121, No. 3, 2001, pp. 599-611.

[8] Bird, R. P., "Observation and quantification of aberrant crypts in the murine colon treated with a colon carcinogen: preliminary findings," *Cancer Lett.*, Vol. 37, No. 2, 1987, pp. 147-151.

[9] Bird, R. P. and Good, C. K., "The significance of aberrant crypt foci in understanding the pathogenesis of colon cancer," *Toxicol.Lett.*, Vol. 112-113, 2000, pp. 395-402.

[10] Bird, R. P., "Role of aberrant crypt foci in understanding the pathogenesis of colon cancer," *Cancer Lett.*, Vol. 93, No. 1, 1995, pp. 55-71.

[11] Pretlow, T. P., Barrow, B. J., Ashton, W. S., O'Riordan, M. A., Pretlow, T. G., Jurcisek, J. A., and Stellato, T. A., "Aberrant crypts: putative preneoplastic foci in human colonic mucosa," *Cancer Res.*, Vol. 51, No. 5, 1991, pp. 1564-1567.

[12] Roncucci, L., Medline, A., and Bruce, W. R., "Classification of aberrant crypt foci and microadenomas in human colon," *Cancer Epidemiol.Biomarkers Prev.*, Vol. 1, No. 1, 1991, pp. 57-60.

[13] Roncucci, L., Stamp, D., Medline, A., Cullen, J. B., and Bruce, W. R., "Identification and quantification of aberrant crypt foci and microadenomas in the human colon," *Hum.Pathol.*, Vol. 22, No. 3, 1991, pp. 287-294.

[14] Fenoglio-Preiser, C. M. and Noffsinger, A., "Aberrant crypt foci: A review," *Toxicol.Pathol.*, Vol. 27, No. 6, 1999, pp. 632-642.

[15] Pretlow, T. P. and Pretlow, T. G., "Mutant KRAS in aberrant crypt foci (ACF): initiation of colorectal cancer?," *Biochim.Biophys.Acta*, Vol. 1756, No. 2, 2005, pp. 83-96.

[16] Hurlstone, D. P., Karajeh, M., Sanders, D. S., Drew, S. K., and Cross, S. S., "Rectal aberrant crypt foci identified using high-magnification-chromoscopic colonoscopy: biomarkers for flat and depressed neoplasia," *Am.J.Gastroenterol.*, Vol. 100, No. 6, 2005, pp. 1283-1289.

[17] Boivin, G. P., Washington, K., Yang, K., Ward, J. M., Pretlow, T. P., Russell, R., Besselsen, D. G., Godfrey, V. L., Doetschman, T., Dove, W. F., Pitot, H. C., Halberg, R. B., Itzkowitz, S. H., Groden, J., and Coffey, R. J., "Pathology of mouse models of intestinal cancer: consensus report and recommendations," *Gastroenterology*, Vol. 124, No. 3, 2003, pp. 762-777.

[18] Tanaka, T., "Colorectal carcinogenesis: Review of human and experimental animal studies," *J.Carcinog.*, Vol. 8, 2009, pp. 5.

[19] Hamilton, S. R., Vogelstein, B., Kudo, S., Riboli, E., Nakamura, S., Hainaut, P., Rubio, C. A., Sobin, L. H., Fogt, F., Winawer, S. J., Goldar, D. E., and Jass, J. R., "Tumours of

the colon and rectum," *Pathology and Genetics of Tumours of the Digestive System*, edited by S. R. Hamilton and L. A. Aaltonen IARC Press, Lyon, 2000, pp. 103.

[20] "The Paris endoscopic classification of superficial neoplastic lesions: esophagus, stomach, and colon: November 30 to December 1, 2002," *Gastrointest.Endosc.*, Vol. 58, No. 6 Suppl, 2003, pp. S3-43.

[21] Perse, M. and Cerar, A., "Morphological and molecular alterations in 1,2 dimethylhydrazine and azoxymethane induced colon carcinogenesis in rats," *J.Biomed.Biotechnol.*, Vol. 2011, 2011, pp. 473964.

[22] Cheng, L. and Lai, M. D., "Aberrant crypt foci as microscopic precursors of colorectal cancer," *World J.Gastroenterol.*, Vol. 9, No. 12, 2003, pp. 2642-2649.

[23] Orlando, F. A., Tan, D., Baltodano, J. D., Khoury, T., Gibbs, J. F., Hassid, V. J., Ahmed, B. H., and Alrawi, S. J., "Aberrant crypt foci as precursors in colorectal cancer progression," *J.Surg.Oncol.*, Vol. 98, No. 3, 2008, pp. 207-213.

[24] Heinen, C. D., Shivapurkar, N., Tang, Z., Groden, J., and Alabaster, O., "Microsatellite instability in aberrant crypt foci from human colons," *Cancer Res.*, Vol. 56, No. 23, 1996, pp. 5339-5341.

[25] Luo, L., Shen, G. Q., Stiffler, K. A., Wang, Q. K., Pretlow, T. G., and Pretlow, T. P., "Loss of heterozygosity in human aberrant crypt foci (ACF), a putative precursor of colon cancer," *Carcinogenesis*, Vol. 27, No. 6, 2006, pp. 1153-1159.

[26] Greenspan, E. J., Cyr, J. L., Pleau, D. C., Levine, J., Rajan, T. V., Rosenberg, D. W., and Heinen, C. D., "Microsatellite instability in aberrant crypt foci from patients without concurrent colon cancer," *Carcinogenesis*, Vol. 28, No. 4, 2007, pp. 769-776.

[27] Jen, J., Powell, S. M., Papadopoulos, N., Smith, K. J., Hamilton, S. R., Vogelstein, B., and Kinzler, K. W., "Molecular determinants of dysplasia in colorectal lesions," *Cancer Res.*, Vol. 54, No. 21, 1994, pp. 5523-5526.

[28] Smith, A. J., Stern, H. S., Penner, M., Hay, K., Mitri, A., Bapat, B. V., and Gallinger, S., "Somatic APC and K-ras codon 12 mutations in aberrant crypt foci from human colons," *Cancer Res.*, Vol. 54, No. 21, 1994, pp. 5527-5530.

[29] Sparks, A. B., Morin, P. J., Vogelstein, B., and Kinzler, K. W., "Mutational analysis of the APC/beta-catenin/Tcf pathway in colorectal cancer," *Cancer Res.*, Vol. 58, No. 6, 1998, pp. 1130-1134.

[30] Hao, X., Frayling, I. M., Willcocks, T. C., Han, W., Tomlinson, I. P., Pignatelli, M. N., Pretlow, T. P., and Talbot, I. C., "Beta-catenin expression and allelic loss at APC in sporadic colorectal carcinogenesis," *Virchows Arch.*, Vol. 440, No. 4, 2002, pp. 362-366.

[31] Hao, X. P., Pretlow, T. G., Rao, J. S., and Pretlow, T. P., "Beta-catenin expression is altered in human colonic aberrant crypt foci," *Cancer Res.*, Vol. 61, No. 22, 2001, pp. 8085-8088.

[32] Chan, A. O., Broaddus, R. R., Houlihan, P. S., Issa, J. P., Hamilton, S. R., and Rashid, A., "CpG island methylation in aberrant crypt foci of the colorectum," *Am.J.Pathol.*, Vol. 160, No. 5, 2002, pp. 1823-1830.

[33] Losi, L., Roncucci, L., Di, G. C., de Leon, M. P., and Benhattar, J., "K-ras and p53 mutations in human colorectal aberrant crypt foci," *J.Pathol.*, Vol. 178, No. 3, 1996, pp. 259-263.

[34] Pretlow, T. P., Brasitus, T. A., Fulton, N. C., Cheyer, C., and Kaplan, E. L., "K-ras mutations in putative preneoplastic lesions in human colon," *J.Natl.Cancer Inst.*, Vol. 85, No. 24, 1993, pp. 2004-2007.

[35] Shivapurkar, N., Huang, L., Ruggeri, B., Swalsky, P. A., Bakker, A., Finkelstein, S., Frost, A., and Silverberg, S., "K-ras and p53 mutations in aberrant crypt foci and colonic tumors from colon cancer patients," *Cancer Lett.*, Vol. 115, No. 1, 1997, pp. 39-46.

[36] Kukitsu, T., Takayama, T., Miyanishi, K., Nobuoka, A., Katsuki, S., Sato, Y., Takimoto, R., Matsunaga, T., Kato, J., Sonoda, T., Sakamaki, S., and Niitsu, Y., "Aberrant crypt foci as precursors of the dysplasia-carcinoma sequence in patients with ulcerative colitis," *Clin.Cancer Res.*, Vol. 14, No. 1, 2008, pp. 48-54.

[37] Rudolph, R. E., Dominitz, J. A., Lampe, J. W., Levy, L., Qu, P., Li, S. S., Lampe, P. D., Bronner, M. P., and Potter, J. D., "Risk factors for colorectal cancer in relation to number and size of aberrant crypt foci in humans," *Cancer Epidemiol.Biomarkers Prev.*, Vol. 14, No. 3, 2005, pp. 605-608.

[38] Sakai, E., Takahashi, H., Kato, S., Uchiyama, T., Hosono, K., Endo, H., Maeda, S., Yoneda, M., Taguri, M., and Nakajima, A., "Investigation of the prevalence and number of aberrant crypt foci associated with human colorectal neoplasm," *Cancer Epidemiol.Biomarkers Prev.*, Vol. 20, No. 9, 2011, pp. 1918-1924.

[39] Ohkubo, H., Takahashi, H., Yamada, E., Sakai, E., Higurashi, T., Uchiyama, T., Hosono, K., Endo, H., Taguri, M., and Nakajima, A., "Natural history of human aberrant crypt foci and correlation with risk factors for colorectal cancer," *Oncol.Rep.*, Vol. 27, No. 5, 2012, pp. 1475-1480.

[40] Takahashi, H., Yamada, E., Ohkubo, H., Sakai, E., Higurashi, T., Uchiyama, T., Hosono, K., Endo, H., and Nakajima, A., "Relationship of human rectal aberrant crypt foci and formation of colorectal polyp: One-year following up after polypectomy," *World J.Gastrointest.Endosc.*, Vol. 4, No. 12, 2012, pp. 561-564.

[41] Uchiyama, T., Takahashi, H., Endo, H., Kato, S., Sakai, E., Hosono, K., Yoneda, M., Inamori, M., Hippo, Y., Nakagama, H., and Nakajima, A., "Number of aberrant crypt foci in the rectum is a useful surrogate marker of colorectal adenoma recurrence," *Dig.Endosc.*, Vol. 24, No. 5, 2012, pp. 353-357.

[42] Anderson, J. C., Swede, H., Rustagi, T., Protiva, P., Pleau, D., Brenner, B. M., Rajan, T. V., Heinen, C. D., Levine, J. B., and Rosenberg, D. W., "Aberrant crypt foci as predic-

tors of colorectal neoplasia on repeat colonoscopy," *Cancer Causes Control*, Vol. 23, No. 2, 2012, pp. 355-361.

[43] Takayama, T., Miyanishi, K., Hayashi, T., Kukitsu, T., Takanashi, K., Ishiwatari, H., Kogawa, T., Abe, T., and Niitsu, Y., "Aberrant crypt foci: detection, gene abnormalities, and clinical usefulness," *Clin.Gastroenterol.Hepatol.*, Vol. 3, No. 7 Suppl 1, 2005, pp. S42-S45.

[44] Higurashi, T., Takahashi, H., Endo, H., Hosono, K., Yamada, E., Ohkubo, H., Sakai, E., Uchiyama, T., Hata, Y., Fujisawa, N., Uchiyama, S., Ezuka, A., Nagase, H., Kessoku, T., Matsuhashi, N., Yamanaka, S., Inayama, Y., Morita, S., and Nakajima, A., "Metformin efficacy and safety for colorectal polyps: a double-blind randomized controlled trial," *BMC.Cancer*, Vol. 12, 2012, pp. 118.

[45] Higurashi, T., Hosono, K., Endo, H., Takahashi, H., Iida, H., Uchiyama, T., Ezuka, A., Uchiyama, S., Yamada, E., Ohkubo, H., Sakai, E., Maeda, S., Morita, S., Natsumeda, Y., Nagase, H., and Nakajima, A., "Eicosapentaenoic acid (EPA) efficacy for colorectal aberrant crypt foci (ACF): a double-blind randomized controlled trial," *BMC.Cancer*, Vol. 12, 2012, pp. 413.

[46] Gupta, A. K., Pinsky, P., Rall, C., Mutch, M., Dry, S., Seligson, D., and Schoen, R. E., "Reliability and accuracy of the endoscopic appearance in the identification of aberrant crypt foci," *Gastrointest.Endosc.*, Vol. 70, No. 2, 2009, pp. 322-330.

[47] Mutch, M. G., Schoen, R. E., Fleshman, J. W., Rall, C. J., Dry, S., Seligson, D., Charabaty, A., Chia, D., Umar, A., Viner, J., Hawk, E., and Pinsky, P. F., "A multicenter study of prevalence and risk factors for aberrant crypt foci," *Clin.Gastroenterol.Hepatol.*, Vol. 7, No. 5, 2009, pp. 568-574.

[48] Corpet, D. E. and Pierre, F., "How good are rodent models of carcinogenesis in predicting efficacy in humans? A systematic review and meta-analysis of colon chemoprevention in rats, mice and men," *Eur.J.Cancer*, Vol. 41, No. 13, 2005, pp. 1911-1922.

[49] Wargovich, M. J., Jimenez, A., McKee, K., Steele, V. E., Velasco, M., Woods, J., Price, R., Gray, K., and Kelloff, G. J., "Efficacy of potential chemopreventive agents on rat colon aberrant crypt formation and progression," *Carcinogenesis*, Vol. 21, No. 6, 2000, pp. 1149-1155.

[50] Pretlow, T. P., O'Riordan, M. A., Spancake, K. M., and Pretlow, T. G., "Two types of putative preneoplastic lesions identified by hexosaminidase activity in whole-mounts of colons from F344 rats treated with carcinogen," *Am.J.Pathol.*, Vol. 142, No. 6, 1993, pp. 1695-1700.

[51] Raju, J., "Azoxymethane-induced rat aberrant crypt foci: relevance in studying chemoprevention of colon cancer," *World J.Gastroenterol.*, Vol. 14, No. 43, 2008, pp. 6632-6635.

[52] Park, H. S., Goodlad, R. A., and Wright, N. A., "The incidence of aberrant crypt foci and colonic carcinoma in dimethylhydrazine-treated rats varies in a site-specific

manner and depends on tumor histology," *Cancer Res.*, Vol. 57, No. 20, 1997, pp. 4507-4510.

[53] Rodrigues, M. A., Silva, L. A., Salvadori, D. M., de Camargo, J. L., and Montenegro, M. R., "Aberrant crypt foci and colon cancer: comparison between a short- and medium-term bioassay for colon carcinogenesis using dimethylhydrazine in Wistar rats," *Braz.J.Med.Biol.Res.*, Vol. 35, No. 3, 2002, pp. 351-355.

[54] Ghirardi, M., Nascimbeni, R., Villanacci, V., Fontana, M. G., Di, B. E., and Salerni, B., "Azoxymethane-induced aberrant crypt foci and colorectal tumors in F344 rats: sequential analysis of growth," *Eur.Surg.Res.*, Vol. 31, No. 3, 1999, pp. 272-280.

Section 6

Post operative care

Chapter 19

ERAS (Enhanced Recovery after Surgery) in Colorectal Surgery

Raúl Sánchez-Jiménez, Alberto Blanco Álvarez,
Jacobo Trebol López, Antonio Sánchez Jiménez,
Fernando Gutiérrez Conde and
José Antonio Carmona Sáez

Additional information is available at the end of the chapter

http://dx.doi.org/10.5772/57136

1. Introduction

Evidence-based medicine has led to an extensive investigation and development of new therapies and programs to improve the care of the surgical patient, both in the postoperative and in the pre-operative period, known as enhanced recovery after surgery (ERAS) programs, "fast-track" programs or multimodal rehabilitation programs.

1.1. Definition

ERAS programs are evidenced-based protocols designed to standardize and optimize perioperative medical care in order to reduce surgical trauma, perioperative physiological stress and organ dysfunction related to elective procedures [1]. In addition, improved outcomes, decreased hospital length of stay and faster patient recovery to normal life are expected to be obtained. Other advantages of this philosophy are the reduction of clinical complications and the health costs together with and increase of patient satisfaction. A diagram with all the core principles of an ERAS program can be seen on Figure 1.

This approach could not be understood and implemented without the participation and commitment of a multidisciplinary team including surgeons, anesthesiologists, nursing staff and hospital administration. Moreover, it is important to make the patient and their families a partner in their care and give them join responsibility for the recovery.

These kinds of programs are not exclusive of a type of surgery or surgical procedure since they can be applied to different specialties (digestive, vascular, thoracic, etc.), different procedures (colon resection, pancreatic procedures, etc.) or different approaches (laparoscopic or open procedures).

In this chapter we will focus on ERAS protocols applied to colorectal surgery.

1.3. Background

Patients undergoing major open colorectal surgery traditionally undergo prolonged rehabilitation and complication rates even as high as 30% have been reported after this procedure [2].

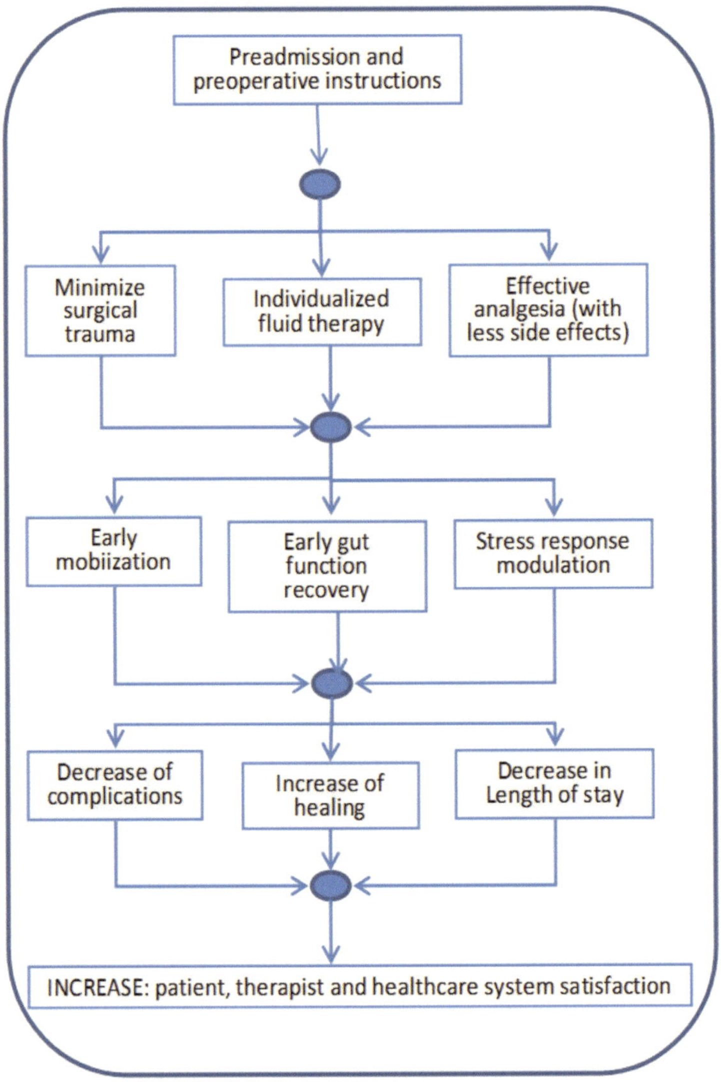

Figure 1. Core principles of an ERAS program applied to digestive tract surgery.

http://dx.doi.org/10.5772/57136

Surgeons learned over the years that surgery was an aggression and that the bigger the procedure was, the bigger the aggression emerged. For example, surgeons understood that patients undergoing major open colorectal surgery suffered prolonged rehabilitation with profound changes in endocrine, metabolic, neural and pulmonary function during the postoperative period. However, the scientific interest was not focused on how to control these changes.

In digestive surgery there were some inviolable principles that were transferred between generation of surgeons over a long period of time. Senior clinicians had strong principles and they were assumed as a dogma. We will highlight some of them:

- Preoperative prolonged fasting is necessary to empty the bowel, prevent intraoperative contamination and the early passage of bowel content through an anastomosis.
- Mechanical bowel preparation is imperative in colorectal surgery to prevent intraoperative contamination and the passage of faeces through a suture line while it is healing. This passage could increase leaking and dehiscence risk or infections.
- Systematic use of nasogastric tubes is imperative to empty stomach and prevent its content to come into the bowel protecting sutures.
- Drains usage is essential in all kind of digestive procedures.
- Extended periods of bed rest are recommended to facilitate abdominal wall healing.
- Postoperative period is a "resting time" in which surgeons are expecting spontaneous patient recovery.

The majority of these paradigms were only based on clinical experience instead of the scientific evidence and, subsequently, they were passed down from masters to disciples, who preserved them as a non-questionable tradition. However, stepwise, published studies have dispelled these and other "truths" and the evidence has taught us that some of them may be unnecessary and maybe they can contribute to postoperative functional deterioration. For example, the return of bowel function is essential for postoperative recovery and this is influenced negatively by several perioperative factors such as preoperative fasting and bowel mechanical preparation, opioid analgesic, fluid overload, immobilization and postoperative prolonged fasting. Thus, several reviews and meta-analyses have focused in the absence of benefits in routinely mechanical bowel preparation, routine nasogastric decompression or prolonged postoperative fasting [3].

In 1990's, several revolutionary changes were seen: in the field of anesthesia the development of regional anesthetic techniques and new drugs to control pain and sedation; and in the field of surgery the widespread use of minimally invasive (laparoscopic) techniques. As a result, a great improvement in postoperative recovery and earlier return of patients to normal function were achieved. Moreover, it was thought that a minimally invasive approach, with reduced operative trauma, conducted to an earlier return of bowel function and allowed for early oral tolerance. The next step was the thinking that some of the improvements seen were simply due to overall changes in perioperative care attitudes.

In the late 1990´s, based on those findings, the "fast track" concept to major abdominal surgery was pioneered by Professor Henrik Kehlet and a solid doctrine concerning perioperative care was born. He was a researcher surgeon interested in perioperative medicine, from the Hvidovre University Hospital in Denmark. Kehlet and colleages were investigating in combined pain relief, early feeding and mobilization since 1995 [4], observing that no more complications were seen and that patients even could be discharged earlier [3]. The concept of a "multimodal" approach was first published in 1997 [4] and subsequently prospective studies appeared [5]. The aims of Kehlet´s study were to reduce postoperative morbidity and mortality and to promote a faster recovery through a multimodal approach, thus minimizing the impact of the factors that lead to surgical stress. On the other hand, in the study of Basse *et al* the multimodal rehabilitation program significantly reduced the postoperative hospital stay in high-risk patients undergoing colonic resection (two days compared to more than 10 days in some historical series) and it might also reduce postoperative ileus and cardiopulmonary complications [5].

During the following decade published studies in this issue grew exponentially. Subsequently, cohort studies, controlled trials and several reviews and meta-analyses were published. It is important to highlight those from Wind [6], Goubas [7], and the meta-analyses directed by Cochrane Collaborative Group in 2011 that will be analyzed in the following chapter´s sections [8]. Moreover, an ERAS Society was officially founded in 2010 as a natural evolution of the ERAS Study Group. This group started its works in 2001 trying to change from tradition to best-practice because there was a great discrepancy between the existing practices and those which were already known to be best practice based on the existing literature. More information is provided in the official website http://www.erassociety.org/.

To summarize, we can conclude that published results and their meta-analyses have shown the benefits of this package of measures, so that evidence-based medicine supports the ERAS concept. Nevertheless, recent surveys have demonstrated slow adaptation and implementation of the fast-track methodology. In this setting, it has been shown by Kehlet *et al* in an international multicenter study based on 1,082 patients who had undergone elective colonic operations that strategies that could contribute to improved recovery and reduce complications were not been applied and that major improvements in outcomes and reduction of costs could be obtained applying ERAS methodology [9].

Little by little, ERAS implementation and application in the clinical setting continued growing in the following years until the present. Nowadays ERAS protocols, with little modifications to adapt them to each center´s functioning, are been applied in a great number of colorectal units worldwide. The information communicated in different conventions and published makes us think that ERAS has changed from a promising "published" issue to a real application in the clinical practice.

1.4. The stress response to surgery

Surgeons have shown interest in metabolic and endocrine response to the surgical trauma long time ago. Such interest has increased by the recognition that to modulate this response to the surgical aggression might reduce the postoperative morbidity and mortality.

The overall metabolic changes in the stress response involve protein and fat catabolism to provide energy. Protein from skeletal muscle and glycerol from fat breakdown are utilised in glucogenogenesis in the liver. In addition surgery induces hormonal, haematological and inmunological changes and activate the sympathetic nervous system (stimulated by hypotension, hypoxaemia or metabolic acidosis, pain, anxiety and distress, autonomic and afferent nerves and directly hypothalamus) [10]. The initial stimulus for this response comes from cytokines, especially IL-6 and TNF, release by leucocytes and endotelial cells present at the site of injury and they are the principal mediators of the response in the acute-phase. Postoperative levels of these cytokines are correlated with the magnitude of the surgery and the presence of complications. On the other hand, leucocytes are key effector cells in the response to surgery, they mobilize quickly to devitalizated or injured tissue to begin repair and prevent secondary microbial invasion. A few minutes after the start of surgery an ACTH, vasopresine, cortisol, catecholamines, aldosterone and glucagon release occur pretending to provide to the disabled organism energy, to retain liquid and salt, and supporting the cardiovascular homeostasis [11].

A randomized controlled trial has shown that Multimodal Rehabilitation programs attenuate the response to the surgical stress as it demonstrates a significant descent of IL-1, IL-6, TNF-α and INF-gamma levels in the postoperative period.

Summarizing, the stress response to surgery increase the levels of ACTH, cortisol, GH, IGF1, ADH and glucagon, reduce the insulin, mobilizes glycogen (by glycogenolysis and skeletal muscle breakdown) and promotes formation of acute phase proteins and lipolysis.

This response also generates adverse effects; some of the most important are:

- Increased myocardial oxygen demand.
- Hypoxaemia.
- Splanchnic vasoconstriction wich may impact intestinal anastomoses healing.
- Exhaustion of energy supplies and loss of lean muscle mass, leading to weakness of both peripheral and respiratory muscle if it is severe.
- Impaired wound healing and increased risk of infections.
- Hypercoagulability (risk of Deep Vein Thrombosis).
- Sodium and water retention.

The response to the surgical trauma is protective since his final target is the survival of the disabled organism. It depends on a delicate balance between pro-inflammatory and anti-inflammatory mechanisms; nevertheless, it is known that it can be harmful when this balance is altered. Thus, if the pro-inflammatory component predominates, a Systemic Inflammatory Response Syndrome (SIRS) could be induced; on the other hand patients can suffer the effects derived from the inmunosupresion as infections or tumor progression if predominates anti-inflammatory components.

2. Aim and concerns

The aims of ERAS programs are:

- To standardize and optimize perioperative medical care.
- To atenuate the stress response to surgery: metabolic, endocrine and inflamatory response as well as reduce protein cathabolism.
- To decrease hospital length stay and a faster patient recovery to normal life.
- Regarding hospital discharge, factors such as pain, lack of gastrointestinal function and immobility complications are the main delaying patient discharge after colorectal surgery. So ERAS objectives will be to promote pain control, to improve gastrointestinal function and to avoid immobility.
- Despite the discharge criteria with ERAS programs are similar than in traditional care, patients usually reach these criteria sooner.

3. ERAS protocol components

ERAS programs are composed of preoperative, intra-operative and postoperative strategies combined to form a multimodal pathway:

3.1. Preoperative

3.1.1. Pre-admission

Pre-operative optimization: it is focused on targeting areas to optimize patient comorbidities (previous or related to the presenting complaint) such as anemia, diabetic and blood pressure control, optimizing cardiovascular disease treatments, respiratory functioning,.... It is also imperative avoid smoking and alcohol consumption. Patient´s individualized Risk stratification is also important to make good patient information and treatment decision.

Information: It is shown that this information reduces the patient's anxiety and facilitates the compliance of the program [12].

Patients and their families should be very knowledgeable about the process. It is very important to make them a partner in the process and give them the responsibility for their recovery and they should be clearly informated about the perioperative care, normal course of the protocol, discharge criteria, possible complications and the outpatient follow-up after discharge. Targets like postoperative oral intake or early mobilization are given in this stage to the patient.

Patient education: including ostomy management and its appropiate localization for it.

Pre-operative nutritional management: drinks and any new medication and nutritional supplements should be given at this time.

3.1.2. Pre-operative care

Admission on the day of surgery: because the patient has been prepared for surgery in the pre-admission period.

Pre-operative fasting and carbohydrate loading:

- Fasting is required to reduce the risk of aspiration during a general anesthesia The duration of preoperative fasting should be two hours for liquids and six hours for solids (grade A recommendation) [13].
- Major surgery is associated with postoperative insulin-resistance. Non-diabetic patients should receive carbohydrate (CHO) loading pre-operatively because they increase glycerol deposits, reduce thirst, hunger and postoperative insulin resistance [14], reducing protein catabolism, postoperative ileus and loss of lean muscle mass. CHO has to be taken in the evening before surgery and 2 hours before anaesthetic induction [15].

Avoid mechanical bowel preparation:

Mechanical bowel preparation can cause dehydration and fluid and electrolyte abnormalities, particularly in elderly patients, increasing morbidity and post-operative ileus [16].

Medication:

- Medication causing long-term sedation from midnight prior to surgery must not been used, in order to conserve the sleep pattern (grade A recommendation).
- Prophylaxis against thromboembolism with low-dose unfraccionated heparin or low-molecular-weight heparin (grade A recommendation) and the use of elastic stockings or pneumatic compression are recommended.
- Antibiotic prophylaxis with single-dose antibiotic prophylaxis against both anaerobes and aerobes about one hour before surgery is recommended (grade A recommendation).

3.2. Intraoperative

Normothermia:

Changes in body temperature can lead to coagulopathy, adverse cardiac events, and decreased resistance to surgical wound infections. An upper-body forced-air heating cover should be used routinely (grade A recommendation).

Prevention of post-operative ileus:

Mid-thoracic epidural analgesia and avoidance of fluid overload are recommended to prevent post-operative ileus (grade A recommendation) [16], [17].

Approach:

The use of minimally invasive techniques, where possible is advisable. Laparoscopic approach is recommended if locally validated (grade A recommendation) [18]. It has been shown to reduce the length of hospital stay, initial wound complications and time to return of gastro-intestinal tract function in colorectal surgery. If an open procedure is required, transverse incisions should be made preferentially to reduce postoperative pain.

Peri-operative fluid management:

Perioperative fluid management for fast-track protocols must be balanced between avoiding hypovolemia and excessive fluid administration. Overhydration has previously been common in the perioperative period, and comparisons of liberal and restrictive fluid regimes suggest that this may be detrimental.

Perioperative fluid overload can cause fluid retention and increase body weight; this is related with generalized edema (which can cause a descense in tissue oxygenation [19]), visceral edema (related with postoperative ileus), can impaire wound and anastomosis healing, can increase cardiorespiratory complications [20,21] and also thrombotic risk.

Intra-operative and post-operative fluid restriction in major colonic surgery with avoidance of hypovolaemia is safe (grade A recommendation) and reduce the time for return of gastro-intestinal tract function, improves healing, reduce length of hospital admission and avoid pulmonary dysfunction [21] and reduce overall postoperative complications by up to two thirds [22]. Early commencement of oral intake also allows reducing intravenous fluids sooner. Postoperative serious hypotension may best treated with vasopressors rather than large quantities of intravenous fluids.

No clear consensus exists regarding the optimal fluid (crystalloid or colloid), the fluid amount (liberal, restricted or supplemental) and the fluid administration (goal-directed fluid therapy by oesophageal Doppler-derived variables –such as stroke volume, the blood volume pumped with each beat- versus conventional haemodynamic variables) for fluid management after and during colectomy.

Fluid management can be then optimized using transesophageal monitoring of the cardiac stroke volume with goal-directed administration of fluid boluses. This methodology can improve outcome (patients recovered gut function significantly faster and suffered significantly less gastrointestinal and overall morbidity) in patients with significant medical comorbidities allowing an earlier hospital discharge [23]. These results have been confirmed with posterior literature review that showed a reduced hospital stay, fewer complications and ICU admissions, less requirement for inotropes and faster return of normal gastro-intestinal function [24].

In the last years literature reviews and metaanalyses have been published trying to give light to these doubts: which fluid, how many and how to control the administration. We want to highlight the one from Rahbari *et al* [25]. Authors included nine randomized controlled trials, finding that restrictive fluid amount (OR 0.41 with 95% CI 0.22 to 0.77; P = 0.005) and goal-directed fluid therapy by means of oesophageal Doppler-derived variables (OR 0.43 with 955

CI 0.26 to 0.71; P = 0.001) significantly reduced overall morbidity after colorectal resection compared with standard fluid amount and fluid therapy guided by conventional haemodynamic variables respectively. No significant differences were founded in mortality, cardiopulmonary morbidity, wound infection, anastomotic failure, recovery of bowel function and hospital stay.

Nasogastric tubes:

They should be inserted only if ileus develops. They are associated with discomfort and a delay in oral intake. Nasogastric tubes should not be used routinely in the elective situations in postoperative period (grade A recommendation) [26],[27].

Surgical drains:

Drains are avoided, as there is no evidence of beneficial effect in reducing postoperative morbidity, mortality, or reduce the effect of anastomotic leakage [28],[29]. Short-term (24-hour) use of drains after low anterior resections may be advisable. They are not indicated following routine colonic resection above the peritoneal reflection.

Epidural analgesia:

The aim of their use is to reduce the dose of general anesthetic needed and the stress response to surgery. In order to reduce the release of stress hormones and post-operative insuline resistance it is very important start with the epidural analgesia before the surgery. (Grade A recommendation).

3.3. Postoperative

Hydration:

Maintenance of hydration, avoiding overcharge and encouraging the discontinuation of intravenous fluid therapy as soon as possible and early commencement of oral intake, including carbohydrate drinks.

Analgesia:

Patients should receive continuous epidural mid-thoracic low-dose local anesthetic and opioid combinations (grade A recommendation) for approximately 48 hours following elective colonic surgery and approximately 96 hours following pelvic surgery. This provides postoperative analgesia and reduces postoperative ileus by blockade of the sympathetic nervous system. Low concentration local anesthetic mixtures reduce motor block and improve early mobilization. Intravenous analgesia is used with paracetamol and non-esteroid anti-inflammatory drugs [30]. Intravenous opioids are avoided because of increase sedation, ileus and respiratory complications.

Nausea and vomiting:

It is very important a risk stratification of patients during surgery using the Apfel scoring system with prophylaxis given for moderate or high risk patients. Risk factors are: female sex, non-smokers, administration of opioids postoperatively, motion sickness or previous postoperative nause and vomitig [31]. Patients with two ore more risk factors should be treated. Dexamethasone or 5HT3 receptor antagonist, droperidol or metoclopramide near the end of surgery are recomended. It is preferred those medication that have a minimal post-operative hang-over and effects on gastrointesinal motility. Also short-acting anesthetic and analgesic agents should be used, avoiding long-lasting opiates where possible [32].

Nutrition support:

Early commencement of an oral intake (frequently in theater recovery) after surgery should be encouraged (grade A recommendation). Oral nutritional supplements should be prescribed (approximately 200 mL, energy dense, 2-3 times daily) from the day of surgery until normal food intake is achieved. These supplements can be continued beyond the return of normal intake if pre-operative nutritional status is poor. Early resumption of oral intake is associated with fewer wound infections and shorter hospital admissions as well.

Early mobilization:

Early mobilization should occur in accordance with pre-operative plan and is a key element of ERAS in colorectal surgery [10]. For patients to be out of bed for two hours on the day of surgery and six hours thereafter is recommended. The aim is to reduce muscle loss and improve respiratory function, reducing the risk of pneumonia, and maximizing oxygen delivery to tissues. This is also essential to reducing the risk of venous thromboembolism. The breathing exercises should be done, especially in patients with previous lung pathology and these exercises must be trained before surgery.

Urinary catheter and drains:

Urinary catheters and peritoneal drains should bre removed as soon as possible in order to reduce the incidence of urinary tract infection and because of early mobilization respectively

Early discharge:

At the end, early discharge, when the discharge criteria have been reached, is the goal of fast-track along with the early recovery and return to normal activity.

A summary of all of these commented components of the perioperative management can be seen on Figure 2.

4. From theory to practice — How to organize an ERAS program

- A well-educated multidisciplinary team will be needed composed by: surgeons, anesthesiologists and pain care specialists, nursing staff, physiotherapysts and occupational therapists and social workers
- ERAS programs involve a selected number of individual interventions. It is necessary to implement all together, because only in this way they demonstrate a greater impact on outcomes than when we implement them as individual interventions [1],[33].

http://dx.doi.org/10.5772/57136

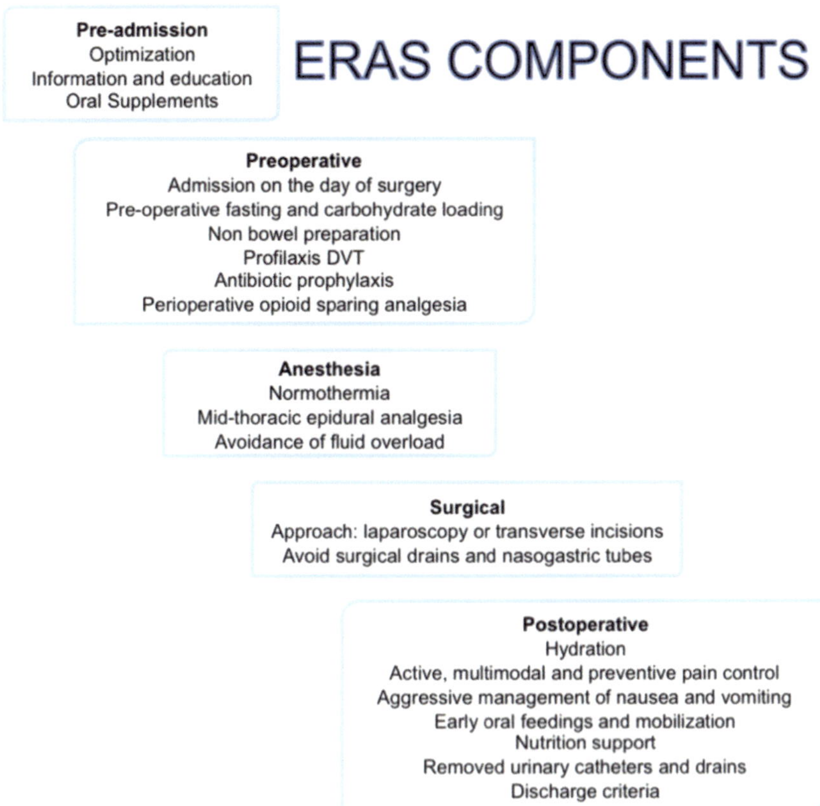

Figure 2. Components of the ERAS protocols

- It is necessary a review of the literature and a carefully study of the hospital resources where the ERAS program will be implemented.
- The program should be designed in agreement with consensus documents.
- A systematic audit should be performed including length of stay, morbidity, mortality and hospital readmissions to allow direct comparison with other institutions and provide motivation for staff and patients.

An example of an ERAS protocol in colorectal surgery can be seen on Table 1.

PREOPERATIVE	
Pre-admission	Indication for surgery, information and signed consent
	Optimization of the patient and education (including stoma)
	Preoperative studies (anesthetist and other if is required)
	Hyperproteic supplement 3 times every day during the week before surgery
Pre-operative	Day before surgery

	Ostomy location Enemas (10 am- 10 pm) if laparoscopic approach is validated No mecanical bowel preparation, except if ileostomy or intraoperative colonoscopy is expected Neomycin and Erythromycin 1g po at 1 pm- 2 pm- 9 pm Liquids on demand and carbohydrate loading during the evening (800 mL) Prophylaxis for DVT at 6 pm (dose depends on the risk) Gabapentin 300 mg and ranitidine 150 mg at 10 pm Day of surgery Carbohydrate loading 2 hours before surgery (400 mL) Antiseptic shower, shaved and elastic stockings Preoperative medication - Dexamethasone 4 mg and ranitidine 150 mg 30 minutes before surgery - Augmentin 2 g immediately before anesthesia
INTRAOPERATIVE	
Anesthetist	Normothermia: upper-body forced-air heating cover and liquid heater (37ºC) Mid-thoracic (T10) epidural analgesia with levobupivacaine Maintenance Oxygen/air FiO2 0.6 – 0.8 Avoid fluids overload maintaining 5cc/kg/h (Hartmann). Hb > 8.0 g/dL Vasoconstrictive drugs if hypotension Ondansetron 4 mg or droperidol 1.25 mg 30 minutes before the end Adittional dose of Augmentine 2 g if surgery takes more than 4h Remove nasogastric tube at the end of surgery
Surgeons	Laparoscopy or transverse incisions Avoid surgical drains except short-term (24-hour) drains after low anterior resection Local anesthesia with levobupivacaine
POSTOPERATIVE	
Day of surgery (Recovery room)	Mask with 4 l/m oxygen flow for 2h independent of saturation, after that nasal cannulae for SpO2 > 95% Epidural analgesia according with protocol of anesthesia
Day of surgery	In seat for at least 2h in the evening Fluids: 1.5 L Ringer lactate solution + 0.5 expander fluids x 24 hours Paracetamol 1 g/6h+/- metamizol 2g/8h Epidural analgesia according to protocol of anesthesia Metroclopramide 10 mg/8h and ondansetron 4 mg/8h Nasal cannulae for SpO2 > 95% Liquid diet 2 hours after surgery including 400 mL of Hyperproteic supplement
Postoperative day 1	Mobilization 6 h a day Suspend fluid e.v. if tolerated diet, maintaining heparine injection Paracetamol 1g/6h +/- metamizol 2g/8h Epidural analgesia according to protocol of anesthesia

http://dx.doi.org/10.5772/57136

	Liquid diet at least 2 L, including 600 mL of high protein/high calories Laxative /12h with MgO (2g / 24h) Heparine in order to protocol Ranitidine t.d.s
Postoperative day 2	See day 1 recommendations Mobilisation on demand Remove epidural catheter Bland/normal diet including 600 mL of high protein/high calorie Verify if Discharge criteria have been reached by the patient
Postoperative day 3	See day 2 recommendations Normal diet including 600 mL of high protein/high calorie Verify if Discharge criteria have been reached by the patiente
Follow-up	Telephone monitoring for 48 h Out-patient visit after 10-14 daysRanitidine v.o. /8 h

Table 1. An ERAS protocol example in colorectal resections.

5. Discharge criteria

The goal of ERAS programs is an accelerated recovery and return to normal activity but it is not the only focus of the protocol [34]. Discharge criteria and time-based discharge depends on the community support and possibility to follow-up.

Patients and their families should feel comfortable with the discharge. In this setting they should know that they will be followed as outpatient and they could return to hospital if required.

Discharge criteria must be previously established (see Table 2):

Discharge criteria
Good mobilization
Adequate oral intake for liquids and solids
Gastrointestinal transit for gas
Normal urinary function
No wound problems
Pain control
No fever
Patient know about possible complications and their detection
Patient feel comfortable with discharge

Table 2. Discharge criteria most usually used in colorectal surgery ERAS programs.

6. Outcomes

The expanding evidence-based medicine shows that ERAS program benefits not only all patients (including the elderly or potentially malnourished patients) but also the health service [35].

Patients accomplish surgery in the best condition. They have better management during and after operation and the best post-operative recovery.

Randomized trials and meta-analysis identified a significantly shorter length of stay and lower in-hospital postoperative complications (maybe secondary to the shorter length of hospital stay) [6].These advantages are mainly attributed to fluid restriction and epidural analgesia.

Other outcome improvements attributed to ERAS programs are shorter duration of postoperative ileus [6], better oral intake, better pain control, less cardiopulmonary morbidity, better preservation of body mass and exercise performance [36], an improvement in grip strength (all of them suggesting an overall improvement in muscular function), earlier resumption of normal activities and a reduced need for daytime sleep [37].

Early discharge is the goal of Fast-Track protocols, and should not be offset by a higher rate of hospital readmission. However, the overall rate of readmission for patients managed with early discharge is comparable to patients with a longer median length of hospital stay [34].Regarding the economical issues, it must be pointed out that the increased cost in laparoscopic approach must be balanced with savings from a shorter length of hospital stay, lower morbidity and no differences in readmission rates.

7. The research initiatives

The confirmation of the initial results should prompt the ERAS methodology embracing in other kind of major surgical procedures as gastric or pancreatic procedures.

The possibility of applying some components of fast-track programs in patients undergoing emergency colorectal surgery must be also evaluated, especially in order to reduce preoperative stress.

New drugs like Ketamina, Lidocaina, Alvimopan could have an important role in the future because of their properties in analgesia and in gastrointestinal resumption.

8. Summary and recommendations

ERAS programs for colorectal surgery were developed to reduce inpatient hospital costs through improvements in preoperative, intra-operative and postoperative strategies.

http://dx.doi.org/10.5772/57136

The success of this program depends on pre-operative setting of expectations including the concept of patients being partners in their care and taking part-ownership of post-operative rehabilitation.

Best results are achieved when the whole multidisciplinary team believe and take part in the program and individual interventions are implemented all together.

The keys of ERAS are: patient information, preservation of gastrointestinal function, minimize organ dysfunction, active pain control and to promote the patient´s autonomy.

Early discharge is the goal of ERAS protocols and patients usually reach the discharge criteria sooner than in traditional care.

Although most of the studies tend to find a lower morbidity, there are no clear advantage in mortality and we think that more studies are needed to confirm the results and focalized in mortality and long-term results of ERAs methodology. We can conclude that at least there are no significant differences in mortality and morbidity with traditional care (ERAs methodology is not dangerous for patients and probably represents a big benefice) and ERAS are more cost-effectiveness than traditional care.

Author details

Raúl Sánchez-Jiménez[1*], Alberto Blanco Álvarez[2], Jacobo Trebol López[1], Antonio Sánchez Jiménez[3], Fernando Gutiérrez Conde[4] and José Antonio Carmona Sáez[1]

*Address all correspondence to: raulsj34@gmail.com

1 Department of General Surgery, Nuestra Señora de Sonsoles Hospital, Ávila, Spain

2 Department of General Surgery, Santos Reyes Hospital, Burgos, Spain

3 Physiotherapist, Cadiz University, Cádiz, Spain

4 Department of General Surgery, University Hospital of Salamanca, Salamanca, Spain

References

[1] Kehlet H, Wilmore DW. Fast-track surgery. Br.J.Surg. 2005;92:3-4.

[2] Kehlet H, Mogensen T. Hospital stay of 2 days after open sigmoidectomy with a multimodal rehabilitation programme. Br.J.Surg. 1999;86:227-230.

[3] Kehlet H. Multimodal approach to control postoperative pathophysiology and rehabilitation. Br.J.Anaesth. 1997;78:606-617.

[4] Basse L, Hjort JD, Billesbolle P, Werner M, Kehlet H. A clinical pathway to accelerate recovery after colonic resection. Ann.Surg. 2000;232:51-57.

[5] Wind J, Polle SW, Fung Kon Jin PH et al. Systematic review of enhanced recovery programmes in colonic surgery. Br.J.Surg. 2006;93:800-809.

[6] Gouvas N, Tan E, Windsor A, Xynos E, Tekkis PP. Fast-track vs standard care in colorectal surgery: a meta-analysis update. Int.J.Colorectal Dis. 2009;24:1119-1131.

[7] Spanjersberg WR, Reurings J, Keus F, van Laarhoven CJ. Fast track surgery versus conventional recovery strategies for colorectal surgery. Cochrane.Database.Syst.Rev. 2011CD007635.

[8] Kehlet H, Buchler MW, Beart RW, Jr., Billingham RP, Williamson R. Care after colonic operation--is it evidence-based? Results from a multinational survey in Europe and the United States. J.Am.Coll.Surg. 2006;202:45-54.

[9] Zutshi M, Delaney CP, Senagore AJ, Fazio VW. Shorter hospital stay associated with fastrack postoperative care pathways and laparoscopic intestinal resection are not associated with increased physical activity. Colorectal Dis. 2004;6:477-480.

[10] Desborough JP. The stress response to trauma and surgery. Br.J.Anaesth. 2000;85:109-117.

[11] Carli F, Charlebois P, Baldini G, Cachero O, Stein B. An integrated multidisciplinary approach to implementation of a fast-track program for laparoscopic colorectal surgery. Can.J.Anaesth. 2009;56:837-842.

[12] Practice guidelines for preoperative fasting and the use of pharmacologic agents to reduce the risk of pulmonary aspiration: application to healthy patients undergoing elective procedures: an updated report by the American Society of Anesthesiologists Committee on Standards and Practice Parameters. Anesthesiology 2011;114:495-511.

[13] Soop M, Carlson GL, Hopkinson J et al. Randomized clinical trial of the effects of immediate enteral nutrition on metabolic responses to major colorectal surgery in an enhanced recovery protocol. Br.J.Surg. 2004;91:1138-1145.

[14] Mathur S, Plank LD, McCall JL et al. Randomized controlled trial of preoperative oral carbohydrate treatment in major abdominal surgery. Br.J.Surg. 2010;97:485-494.

[15] Guenaga KK, Matos D, Wille-Jorgensen P. Mechanical bowel preparation for elective colorectal surgery. Cochrane.Database.Syst.Rev. 2009CD001544.

[16] Kehlet H. Postoperative ileus--an update on preventive techniques. Nat.Clin.Pract.Gastroenterol.Hepatol. 2008;5:552-558.

[17] Vlug MS, Wind J, Hollmann MW et al. Laparoscopy in combination with fast track multimodal management is the best perioperative strategy in patients undergoing colonic surgery: a randomized clinical trial (LAFA-study). Ann.Surg. 2011;254:868-875.

[18] Lobo DN, Bostock KA, Neal KR et al. Effect of salt and water balance on recovery of gastrointestinal function after elective colonic resection: a randomised controlled trial. Lancet 2002;359:1812-1818.

[19] Cheatham ML, Chapman WC, Key SP, Sawyers JL. A meta-analysis of selective versus routine nasogastric decompression after elective laparotomy. Ann.Surg. 1995;221:469-476.

[20] Petrowsky H, Demartines N, Rousson V, Clavien PA. Evidence-based value of prophylactic drainage in gastrointestinal surgery: a systematic review and meta-analyses. Ann.Surg. 2004;240:1074-1084.

[21] Urbach DR, Kennedy ED, Cohen MM. Colon and rectal anastomoses do not require routine drainage: a systematic review and meta-analysis. Ann.Surg. 1999;229:174-180.

[22] Francom M. Stop drug price increases. Am.Pharm. 1991;NS31:6, 8.

[23] Tiippana EM, Hamunen K, Kontinen VK, Kalso E. Do surgical patients benefit from perioperative gabapentin/pregabalin? A systematic review of efficacy and safety. Anesth.Analg. 2007;104:1545-56, table.

[24] Kehlet H, Holte K. Review of postoperative ileus. Am.J.Surg. 2001;182:3S-10S.

[25] Leslie JB, Viscusi ER, Pergolizzi JV, Jr., Panchal SJ. Anesthetic Routines: The Anesthesiologist's Role in GI Recovery and Postoperative Ileus. Adv.Prev.Med. 2011;2011:976904.

[26] Wilmore DW, Kehlet H. Management of patients in fast track surgery. BMJ 2001;322:473-476.

[27] Hendren S, Morris AM, Zhang W, Dimick J. Early discharge and hospital readmission after colectomy for cancer. Dis.Colon Rectum 2011;54:1362-1367.

[28] Adamina M, Kehlet H, Tomlinson GA, Senagore AJ, Delaney CP. Enhanced recovery pathways optimize health outcomes and resource utilization: a meta-analysis of randomized controlled trials in colorectal surgery. Surgery 2011;149:830-840.

[29] Basse L, Madsen JL, Kehlet H. Normal gastrointestinal transit after colonic resection using epidural analgesia, enforced oral nutrition and laxative. Br.J.Surg. 2001;88:1498-1500.

[30] Jakobsen DH, Sonne E, Andreasen J, Kehlet H. Convalescence after colonic surgery with fast-track vs conventional care. Colorectal Dis. 2006;8:683-687.

Chapter 20

Psychosocial Care for Patients with Colorectal Cancer

Hitoshi Okamura

Additional information is available at the end of the chapter

http://dx.doi.org/10.5772/57140

1. Introduction

As medical care based on information disclosure has been promoted, the concept of informed consent has also come to be understood in cancer care, and its faithful practice is now required. However, reactions ranging from ordinary psychological reactions (such as discouragement and feelings of isolation, alienation, despair, etc.) to psychological changes requiring the attention of a specialist (i.e., depression) are sometimes seen when information is disclosed, especially after conveying bad news, and healthcare providers must constantly keep the psychological states of their patients in mind. In this chapter, I will first describe the usual psychological reactions that cancer patients exhibit after the disclosure of cancer-related information. Additionally, I will discuss general matters to keep in mind when delivering bad news to cancer patients. Then, I will summarize the diagnosis and management of psychological distress requiring psychiatric attention that healthcare providers in cancer care settings should know.

In addition, healthcare providers are expected to strive for good communication with the patient and the patient's family during the process of conveying bad news about a patient's condition and obtaining informed consent. In reality, however, training in communication skills and support skills is only rarely available, and as a result, many healthcare providers experience stress as a result of having been unable to acquire such skills adequately. With this background in mind, I will describe the need for communication skills in cancer care and review recent literature regarding the effectiveness of training designed to improve such skills.

2. Typical psychological reactions to information disclosure (especially bad news) (Table 1)

Bad news must be conveyed more often than good news when disclosing information during the clinical course of cancer. Here, the typical psychological reactions displayed by patients after being informed of such bad news will be explained by providing examples of reactions after having been informed of a diagnosis of cancer. First, the initial few days are characterized by not being ready to believe or by temporarily denying what they have been told, saying,: "That can't be...," or by a sense of despair, saying,: "Oh, I've got cancer...." Later, a time is reached when they sometimes say,: "My mind went blank, and it was as though it hadn't happened to me," or "I don't clearly remember what happened after I was told I had cancer. I don't remember how I got home." Thus, it is important for attending physicians to recognize that patients may not clearly remember any subsequent explanations after they have been told that they have cancer, and that even if they describe tests and treatment in great detail, the patients may not understand the explanations adequately.

A. First phase: period of early reaction / within a few days Patients do not believe the information or temporarily deny the facts. Some patients retrospectively describe this period as, 'My mind ceased to function as if these things were not happening to me'. Others experience despair, i.e. 'I was told what I feared'.
B. Second phase: period of distress / after 1–2 weeks Patients repeatedly develop symptoms such as anxiety, depression, insomnia, appetite loss or decreased concentration. Owing to marked anxiety and decreased concentration, patients repeatedly ask the same questions.
C. Third phase: period of adaptation / after 2 weeks–1 month, sometimes 3 months Patients face reality and begin to or try to adapt to the new situation.

Table 1. Psychological reactions to being given a bad news

Then, after a little while, a time comes when symptoms such as a sinking feeling, anxiety, feelings of isolation from their surroundings, difficulty sleeping, or a loss of appetite might occur repeatedly. Symptoms in the form of getting excited or upset over petty matters are also sometimes seen. There are also times when the patient's behavior may take the form of repeatedly asking the same question because patients are very anxious and their ability to concentrate has declined. As a result of these conditions, patients sometimes experience a certain degree of interference with their daily lives, because the things that they were usually able to do have become troublesome or take longer to complete.

After 2 weeks have gone by, however, patients gradually begin to face their real problems and become able to adapt to their new reality. More specifically, they begin to gather information, saying, "There's nothing I can do about having been diagnosed with cancer. From here on, I'm going to think about how best to make things better," or they become capable of an optimistic outlook, saying, "My cancer may get better." Moreover, because they always have the feeling

http://dx.doi.org/10.5772/57140

that, "I have to go about my daily life living with my cancer," although it may be difficult to go about their lives with the same feeling as when they were completely healthy, it does not create a very severe obstacle to their everyday lives, and they are able to return to a living pattern that is almost the same as before.

It is important to have a good understanding of the "typical" psychological reactions described above that cancer patients exhibit.

3. General matters to keep in mind when delivering bad news to cancer patients

1. Basic principles

a. The bad news should first be discussed with the patients themselves whenever possible.

b. The same physician should take charge of the patient from the initial contact until the definitive treatment whenever possible. This allows for true informed consent, during which the patient can calmly decide among several choices of treatment modalities. If a situation arises where a change in the physician-in-charge is necessary, care should be taken not to destroy patient rapport.

c. The location for discussing the bad news must be carefully chosen, providing an environment of privacy where the patients can fully express their feelings, as necessary. On no account should the bad news be communicated via the telephone or while passing in a corridor or in any public place. It was reported that 55% of patients who were told the news by telephone expressed negative feelings [2]. Patients and their families who are given bad news in an inconsiderate manner may never forget the thoughtlessness of the physician.

d. From the initial interview, physicians should try to tell the truth consistently and should provide as much information as they have available at the time. Bad news based on unconfirmed information should not be delivered.

e. Although an accurate explanation is necessary, the patient should not be bombarded with facts with no consideration given to the patient's state. Physicians should be prepared to explain facts as clearly and as simply as necessary. Patients should not be expected to cope with everything by themselves.

f. Patients are sometimes told, "You have advanced cancer and there is nothing I can do. There is no effective treatment in your case." Such cruel attitudes presented by the physician causes a loss of hope, anger, resignation and a sense of alienation in patients. Physicians should recognize that they can generate either hope or despair in patients by their verbal expressions or attitude. Physicians should present other positive features, including supportive care, instead of abandoning a patient with such a statement.

g. Breaking bad news is commonly performed in an outpatient clinic. An adequate amount of time to provide an explanation and subsequent consideration is necessary. When patients are very anxious, the physician-in-charge should provide a consultation with a psychiatrist. Options such as talking to patients on another occasion after completing all their duties at the outpatient clinic or offering encouragement by talking again on the telephone on the day that the bad news has been divulged can sometimes be very effective.

h. Patients may show reservation towards physicians and sometimes fear them. Therefore, some patients cannot express their feelings when they are given bad news or cannot ask physicians questions, believing that they should do what the physician has told them. However, some patients are able to be more frank when talking to nurses and may ask them questions about the news. Therefore, it is important for physicians to hear the patient's true feelings and complaints through nurses. Cooperation between physicians and nurses is very important in this situation.

i. The physician should not hurry to explain all the details on one occasion. Several interviews with each patient are recommended to discuss the bad news in a step-by-step manner.

j. The physician should put himself or herself in the patient's place and should not judge the patient's reactions prematurely.

2. Approaches to speaking with family members

a. In principle, family members should not be told the bad news before the patient has been told. Families who want the patient to be ignorant of the news may be worried that "... the patient may commit suicide because of fears or shock." However, such a risk is much lower than generally believed [3], though this risk should always be taken into consideration.

b. When a patient is referred to our hospital and only the family has been told the bad news at another hospital and the family strongly opposes telling the patient the truth, the family should be repeatedly encouraged to change their minds, taking as much time as necessary. In such cases, it is important not to blame the initial physicians for their old-fashioned approach, since the rapport between the patient and the physicians may be impaired.

c. Families play a very important role in cancer treatment. When the bad news is told definitively, the explanation should ideally be given to the patient and family together. Although the patient takes priority over the family, it is very important to inform the family of the patient's state as accurately as possible.

d. Families sometimes become more agitated than patients and cannot remember or understand the explanation accurately Therefore, physicians should not take it for granted that "...families will be alright when receiving bad news, because they are not patients." When necessary, families should also be supported. It is often helpful for the physician-in-charge to ask a psychiatrist for advice.

3. Psychological distress requiring psychiatric attention

Derogatis et al. [4] conducted interviews with 215 inpatients and outpatients at three leading cancer centers in the eastern United States, and investigated the prevalence of psychological problems based on the DSM-III (The DSM-III is a set of comprehensive diagnostic criteria for all mental disorders that was drawn up by the American Psychiatric Association in 1980 and is widely used throughout the world in prevalence surveys, etc. The revised DSM-III-R was published in 1987, the DSM-IV in 1994, and the DSM-IV-TR in 2000). They reported that 32% of the 215 subjects met the diagnostic criteria for adjustment disorders, 6% for depression, and 4% for delirium. These 3 psychological manifestations appear to be characteristic of the psychological distress experienced by cancer patients who require psychiatric attention. Moreover, because all these psychological manifestations reduce patients' quality of life (QOL), their proper diagnosis and treatment is needed.

The incidence of adjustment disorders, depression, or delirium has not been previously assessed in colorectal cancer patients. However, some reports have described the prevalence of psychological distress using various symptom rating scales. These reports are summarized in Table 2 [5-13]. The reports suggest that the prevalence of psychological distress in colorectal cancer patients is 7% - 44%. Zabora et al. [14] assessed the prevalence of psychological distress among a large sample of cancer patients and variations in distress among 14 cancer diagnoses; the overall prevalence of distress in this sample was 35.1% (colorectal cancer: 31.6%), and a greater patient burden was associated with similar rates of distress.

Author, Journal (year) [Reference No.]	**Subjects**	**Outcome variables**	**Major results**
Dunn et al, *Psychooncology* (2012) [5]	1966 colorectal cancer survivors	Psychological distress: Brief Symptom Inventory-18 (BSI-18) at six time points from 5 months to 5 years post-diagnosis	Over the 5-year trajectory, the prevalence of high overall distress ranged between 44% and 32%.
Graa Pereira et al, *Eur J Oncol Nurs* (2012) [6]	114 colorectal cancer patients who received treatments	Anxiety and depression: Hospital Anxiety and Depression Scale (HADS) Traumatic stress: Impact of Events Scale Revised (IES-R) during the period of 12 months after treatment	Patients who received only surgery, as treatment, had lower levels of depression, anxiety and traumatic stress symptoms when compared with patients who received surgery and chemotherapy or surgery plus radiotherapy.
Daudt et al, *Support* Care Cancer (2012) [7]	252 colorectal cancer patients referred to an outpatient clinic	Anxiety and depression: Psychosocial Screen for Cancer (PSSCAN) at the first visit to a clinic	The prevalence of anxiety and depression were determined to be 10% and 7%, respectively.
Hyphantis et al, *J Psychosom Res* (2011) [8]	144 early non-metastatic colorectal cancer patients	Psychological distress: Symptom Distress Checklist (SCL-90-R) at baseline and one year after the initial assessment	Paranoid ideation, psychoticism, interpersonal sensitivity, anxiety and depressive symptoms increased significantly over the one-year period of the study.

Author, Journal (year) [Reference No.]	Subjects	Outcome variables	Major results
Patel et al, *J Affect Disord* (2011) [9]	99 colorectal cancer patients	Clinical interview: Composite International Diagnostic Interview (CIDI) Psychological distress: Distress Thermometer (DT) Anxiety and depression: Hospital Anxiety and Depression Scale (HADS) within 9 weeks of receiving diagnosis	Seventeen patients (17%) were diagnosed with a current mood or anxiety disorder, 11 (11%) met criteria for a depressive disorder and 7 (7%) with a primary anxiety disorder, and one patient had a secondary diagnosis of generalized anxiety disorder.
Medeiros et al, *J Gastrointest Cancer* (2010) [10]	37 colorectal cancer patients	Anxiety and depression: Questionnaires of Depression and Anxiety After surgical resection; at the beginning and at the end of the treatment in the chemotherapy group (CHG) and at the first and after 6 months of follow-up in the control group (CG)	Mild or moderate depression was diagnosed in 31.6% of the CHG patients in the first evaluation and in 38.6% at the second one. There was a higher number of patients with moderate state or trait anxiety in the CHG when compared to the CG in both evaluations.
Alacacioglu et al, *Support Care Cancer* (2012) [11]	110 colorectal cancer patients undergoing chemotherapy	Depression: Beck Depression Inventory (BDI) Anxiety: State-Trait Anxiety Inventory (STAI) during chemotherapy	The mean Beck depression scores were 11.2±9.0 (range 0–44) and the mean STAI scores were 41.9±8.8 (range 22–71). 23.6% were determined as depressive.
Lynch et al, *Cancer* (2008) [12]	1822 colorectal cancer patients	Psychological distress: Brief Symptom Inventory-18 (BSI-18) at baseline (after diagnosis), approximately 6 (Time 1) and 12 months (Time 2) postdiagnosis	The prevalence of global psychological distress was low: 8.3% and 6.7% at 6 and 12 months postdiagnosis, respectively. Of the143 participants who met caseness for distress at Time 1, 38% remained highly distressed at Time 2.
Pugliese et al, *Health Qual Life Outcomes* (2006) [13]	98 advanced colorectal cancer patients during chemotherapy	Descriptive diagnosis: DSM III-R criteria before initiating treatment	According to the clinical interview, 20 (20%) met criteria for adjustment disorders, 3 (3%) for phobia, and 3 (3%) for generalized anxiety disorder.

Table 2. A summary of psychological distress in colorectal cancer patients

Below, the special features of each of these psychological manifestations are summarized.

http://dx.doi.org/10.5772/57140

1. Adjustment disorders

Adjustment disorders are the most common psychological manifestation exhibited by cancer patients, but few studies or reports have examined adjustment disorders alone. Problems with the diagnostic criteria for adjustment disorders themselves are likely to be one of the reasons for the lack of studies on this topic. The diagnostic criteria in the DSM-IV-TR state that adjustment disorders are "reactions such as anxiety and depression or behavior disorders that occur in association with psychosocial stress." The diagnosis of adjustment disorders is made when the degree of the reaction is stronger than expected or when symptoms interfere with social functions from everyday life to social activities, and such disorders are said to be a continuous condition, without any strict division from normal reactions. Thus, the criteria are vague, and the term "adjustment disorders" is used as a "wastebasket diagnosis" when there is a mood disorder but other diagnoses, including depression, do not apply. Nevertheless, the term has the advantage of being able to include a variety of psychological manifestations that would be difficult to accept as specific mental disorders.

Inadequate pain control can be listed as a primary cause of adjustment disorders. According to a study by Derogatis et al. [1], a higher percentage of cancer patients who met the diagnostic criteria for adjustment disorders had severe pain, compared with cancer patients who did not meet the criteria. Anxiety, depression, and agitation are known to readily develop when pain of unknown cause persists [15]. Clearly, understanding patients' pain, which is a typical symptom that requires symptomatic relief, and adequately controlling such pain seems to be also useful for relieving psychological distress. Moreover, feelings of difficulty breathing [16] or malaise [17], which (similar to pain) often occur in colorectal cancer patients, can have an impact on patient QOL and can be difficult to treat, and their presence appears to be a cause of anxiety or depression.

These adjustment disorders should be evaluated and properly managed, but few patients are actually diagnosed correctly and treated properly [18]. One reason for this situation appears to be that healthcare providers often miss psychological manifestations. Although the issue of physicians and nurses who are not specialists in psychiatric care overlooking mild depression and anxiety symptoms occurring during the course of cancer is, to some extent, unavoidable, there seems to be a need for education regarding the diagnosis and treatment of adjustment disorders, which are the most common psychological manifestations of cancer patients.

Psychotropic drugs, such as anxiolytic agents, hypnotics, and, depending on the circumstances, antidepressants, are often used for treatment, but it is important to make an effort to identify the cause of the adjustment disorders described above by sufficiently listening to what the patient has to say, and then eliminating the cause. To accomplish this task, supportive psychiatric care in which caregivers encourage patients to express how they are really feeling at the present time (especially feelings of fear and anxiety), that supports and empathizes with the patients, and that does not provide unrealistic information but provides assurance within the realm of reality is said to be effective. In other words, supportive psychiatric care can become a valid treatment only when the patients feel that their present suffering is understood by the healthcare provider.

2. Depression

Table 3 shows the diagnostic criteria for depression based on the DSM-IV-TR. A diagnosis of depression is made when either a depressed mood or a loss of interest or pleasure or both occurs, and a total of 5 or more other symptoms are present for at least 2 weeks. However, because some of the physical symptoms included among the listed symptoms of depression, such as sleep disturbance, anorexia and weight loss, a decreased ability to concentrate, and malaise, are common symptoms, especially in palliative care settings, these symptoms are often not regarded as unusual even when present, and there is a strong tendency for depression to be underestimated among cancer patients. Why is the accurate evaluation and treatment of depression important? To answer this question, a specific case is presented below.

1. Depressed mood most of the day.
2. Diminished interest or pleasure in all or most activities.
3. Significant unintentional weight loss or gain.
4. Insomnia or sleeping too much.
5. Agitation or psychomotor retardation noticed by others.
6. Fatigue or loss of energy.
7. Feelings of worthlessness or excessive guilt.
8. Diminished ability to think or concentrate, or indecisiveness.
9. Recurrent thoughts of death.
Depressed mood and/or loss of interest or pleasure in life activities for at least 2 weeks and at least five of the above symptoms that cause clinically significant impairment in social, work, or other important areas of functioning almost every day.

Table 3. Diagnostic criteria of depression

[Case]

The patient was a 65-year-old man who was being followed up for advanced colorectal cancer and had entered the terminal stage. Predominantly palliative care was being performed, and symptom control was fairly good. However, he gradually began to experience insomnia, and this symptom persisted. A short while later he was heard to say, "There's no point in living anymore. I want to die," and he exhibited minimal facial expressions. A hypnotic was prescribed, but the treatment was ineffective. Because the condition described above persisted, he was referred to a psychiatrist. Based on an examination, the psychiatrist concluded that the cause was depression, and when the patient was treated with a low dose of an antidepressant, he no longer made the above complaints, and his facial expression became peaceful.

It is not rare for cancer patients, particularly terminal patients, to speak of suicidal ideation (a feeling that they want to die or that there is no point in living), similar to the case described above, and more than half of such patients are reportedly in a depressed state [19]. However, since depression can be alleviated suicidal ideation can be stopped with proper treatment,

http://dx.doi.org/10.5772/57140

whenever a patient desires an early death, it is essential to always keep depression in mind and to evaluate the patient's decision-making ability.

A younger age, a past history of mood disorder, a history of alcohol dependence, low social support, a poor physical condition, and inadequate pain control have been implicated as risk factors for depression in cancer patients [20].

In addition, caution is also necessary with regard to the fact that depression is sometimes induced as a side effect of drugs that are used to treat physical illnesses [21]. Associations with depression have also been pointed out for some β-adrenergic antagonists and benzodiazepines as well as some anticancer drugs, including vincristine and asparaginase. Steroids are widely used to treat brain edema caused by brain metastasis and for malaise and nausea, but they are known to be possible causes of depression.

A variety of questionnaires and rating scales have become available as ways to conveniently screen for depression, and these tools have a high utility value as indicators of the presence of depression in cancer patients. However, prior to the use of these tools, healthcare providers must first take an interest in their patients' psychological distress and discuss the matter with their patients. When Chochinov et al. [22] used a 13-item short version of the depression screening scale and inquired about only a depressed mood in a study of 197 terminal-stage cancer patients, they reported that asking, "How are you feeling? Aren't you feeling depressed?" was the most useful way of screening for depression. When healthcare providers are standing in front of a patient, after inquiring "How are you?" the healthcare provider can easily ask an additional question, "How are you feeling?" without imposing any great burden on everyday clinical practice, and this additional question seems to be a convenient and effective way of not overlooking depression that healthcare providers can implement immediately.

As a general rule, depression is treated with drug therapy, primarily with antidepressants, and although it takes 1-2 weeks for them to take effect, these drugs are very effective in many cases. In the past, thirst and constipation were frequent side effects, but antidepressants with fewer side effects have been recently developed, and it seems possible to utilize them effectively. Nevertheless, the fact that some antidepressants inhibit the metabolism of anticancer drugs and affect their blood concentrations needs to be kept in mind when using them concomitantly. However, as stated above, the most important point is to evaluate accurately whether the patient is in a depressed state.

3. Delirium

Delirium is an organic mental disorder that is often seen during the early stage of cancer therapy or from an advanced to terminal stage, and it is a "consciousness" disorder that is accompanied by cognitive disorders such as psychomotor excitation manifesting as a mild clouding of consciousness, delusions, and hallucinations. Because cognition is impaired, a wide variety of accompanying psychological symptoms may develop. Classical cases of delirium are characterized by an abrupt onset of symptoms and diurnal fluctuations in symptoms (especially symptoms becoming worse during the night), as well as difficulty in focusing and maintaining attention. Sometimes, psychiatric departments are frequently consulted, and the nature of the requests is a failure to cooperate with treatment, negativity, and suspicion of dementia. The prevalence of delirium increases as the patients' physical conditions deteriorate and they reach a stage [23], and an overall prevalence of 4%-27% has been reported for all stages.

Several hypotheses, including impaired neurotransmitter metabolism in the brain and an impaired sleep-wakefulness mechanism, have been proposed with regard to the pathogenetic mechanism of delirium, but nothing definite is known. The causes of delirium in cancer patients consist of direct causes, such as cancer metastasis to the brain, and indirect causes caused by electrolyte abnormalities (caution is particularly necessary in regard to hypercalcemia secondary to bone metastasis), the side effects of drugs (drug-induced delirium is relatively common and is seen with narcotic analgesics, such as morphine, and drugs that have an anticholinergic action) or irradiation, and in association with multi-organ failure, infection, changes in nutritional status, etc., the incidences of which increase as a terminal stage is reached;, however, indirect causes are by far more common. Drug-induced delirium is relatively frequent and is seen with narcotic analgesics, such as morphine, and drugs that have an anticholinergic action.

An examination of the causes of delirium according to disease stage showed that single factors based on treatment (surgery, chemotherapy, etc.) are more common during stages when the patients' conditions are relatively good and that multiple factors tend to be involved in the terminal stage. Bruera et al. [23] conducted a study of the causes of delirium in terminal-stage cancer patients using peripheral blood biochemistry tests, CT examinations of the brain, and arterial blood gas analyses and reported that the cause was unknown in 56% of the cases. The factors identified were, listed in order starting with the most frequent,: drugs, sepsis, brain metastasis, hepatic or renal failure, hypercalcemia, and hyponatremia. They reported that the results showed that two thirds of the patients with a cognitive disorder died later without recovering and that the other third recovered before they died. A variety of factors in the etiology of delirium have often accumulated in terminal patients, making it difficult to identify a cause and to treat the condition.

The basic approach to treatment is to determine the cause of the delirium, and then to eliminate the cause. However, it is important to distinguish between whether recovery in response to treatment is possible or would be difficult and to decide upon an appropriate care goal (Table 4). A variety of factors in the etiology of delirium have often accumulated in terminal patients, and the identification of a cause and subsequent treatment are often difficult. When intense excitement is present or when the delirium interferes with everyday living as a result of hallucinations, delusions, etc., symptomatic drug therapy, including treatment with antipsychotic drugs, is often performed. In principle, drug therapy is the same as for the usual treatment of delirium: (1) benzodiazepine monotherapy is not used, (2) antiparkinsonian drugs are not used in combination, and (3) multiple drug combinations are not used. Table 5 contains points that should be kept in mind with regard to adverse events when using psychotropic drugs to treat cancer patients. Moreover, modifications of the patient's environment, family support, and the support and education of the staff of the hospital unit are also needed, in addition to the above.

http://dx.doi.org/10.5772/57140

	Possible to recover	Difficult to recover
Typical cause	Electrolyte imbalance	Organ failure
Goal of care	Drug	Brain metastasis
Drug therapy	Anemia	Relief of delirium symptoms
Content of care	Inflammatory reaction	Antipsychotic drug,
	Recovery from delirium	Benzodiazepine is used in combination, as
	Antipsychotic drug,	appropriate.
	Benzodiazepine is used at a minimum.	Relief of restlessness or agitation
	Recovery from delirium	Maintenance of sleep
	Correction of daily living rhythms	Care of families
	Care of families	

Table 4. Delirium causes for which recovery in response to treatment is possible or difficult

	Points to be paid attention to
Extrapyramidal symptom	Antiemetic with dopamine receptor antagonistic action (e.g., metoclopramide) is
Anticholinergic effect	often administered antecedently.
Hepatic dysfunction	Adverse effects of morphine (dry mouth, constipation, dysuria, sleepiness) are
Malignant syndrome	aggravated.
	In case of under administration of anticancer agents or liver metastasis.
	In case of the poor general conditions.

Table 5. Points regarding adverse events during the use of psychotropic drugs to treat cancer patients

4. Communication skills

Nothing is more important to the process of conveying bad news and obtaining informed consent than that healthcare providers strive for good communication with the patient and the patient's family. Good communication is said to have a favorable impact on physical and mental health, such as helping patients to cope with their disease, improving compliance, and bringing about the control of blood pressure and blood glucose levels, as well as pain control, and as a result of achieving a strong trusting relationship with their healthcare provider, patients are willing to engage actively in their treatment, increasing its therapeutic effect. [24]. Moreover, forging good relationships with patients also reportedly decreases the risk of burn out by healthcare providers [25]. However, in reality, training in communication skills and support skills is seldom provided, and as a result, many healthcare providers are thought to experience stress because they have not acquired adequate skills.

Against this background, a training program designed to improve communication skills was conducted in the United Kingdom with 178 highly experienced oncologists as the subjects [26]. When the physicians were the subjects of the evaluation, the results reportedly showed that the physicians were able to gain self-confidence with regard to communication, and had become able to engage in patient-centered communication, including directing their attention to patients' psychosocial aspects. This study was the first of its kind, and it was followed by the start of a succession of studies regarding the effectiveness of communication skills training (CST). The effects of CST interventions for health care professionals have been compiled and analyzed in several systematic reviews across recent decades [27-30]. These reviews have consistently concluded that CST leads to better communication behaviors among clinicians [28, 30]. A recent meta-analysis of 13 studies reported a moderate effect size of 0.54 (Cohen's d) for the impact of CST on the communication behaviors of oncology clinicians [30]. However, on the other hand, Kissane et al. [31] pointed out in the most recent review article that outcomes impacting patient satisfaction, improved adaptation, and enhanced quality of life are still lacking, and that patient benefits, such as increased treatment adherence and enhanced adaption, need to be demonstrated from CST.

Thus, evaluations of training in communication skills have not yet led to any definite conclusions, but an education system and a curriculum designed to improve communication skills is definitely needed in the near future. Bad news must often be conveyed, particularly in cancer care settings, and the acquisition of such skills by healthcare providers seems to be absolutely essential.

5. Conclusion

Based on the characteristics of colorectal cancer patients, the forms of psychological distress that are said to often be encountered in cancer care settings and to require evaluation and management from the standpoint of a psychiatrist have been summarized. The necessary communication skills, which are one of the skill sets that must be acquired to engage in cancer care, have also been described. However, the people who are closely involved with such psychosocial aspects and need such skills to deal with patients in actual clinical settings are typically the attending physicians, who are oncologists, and allied healthcare professionals, rather than psychiatrists. Thus, it is paramount that all healthcare providers involved in the care of cancer patients become proficient in communication skills so that they may interact with patients and their families and so that they may always aim to provide medical care with patients' psychological aspects in mind.

Author details

Hitoshi Okamura*

Address all correspondence to: hokamura@hiroshima-u.ac.jp

Institute of Biomedical & Health Sciences, Hiroshima University, Japan

References

[1] Holland JC, Rowland JH. Handbook of Psychooncology. New York: Oxford Univ Press; 1990, p273-282

[2] Lind SE, Good MD, Seidel S, Csordas T, Good BJ. Telling the diagnosis of cancer. J Clin Oncol 1989; 7: 583-9.

[3] Oken D. What to tell cancer patients. A study of medical attitudes. JAMA 1961; 175: 1120-8.

[4] Derogatis LR. The prevalence of psychiatric disorders among cancer patients. JAMA 1983; 249: 751-7.

[5] Dunn J, Ng SK, Holland J, Aitken J, Youl P, Baade PD, Chambers SK. Trajectories of psychological distress after colorectal cancer. Psychooncology. 2012; doi: 10.1002/pon.3210.

[6] Graça Pereira M, Figueiredo AP, Fincham FD. Anxiety, depression, traumatic stress and quality of life in colorectal cancer after different treatments: A study with Portuguese patients and their partners. Eur J Oncol Nurs 2012; 16: 227-32.

[7] Daudt HM, Cosby C, Dennis DL, Payeur N, Nurullah R. Nutritional and psychosocial status of colorectal cancer patients referred to an outpatient oncology clinic. Support Care Cancer 2012; 20: 1417-23.

[8] Hyphantis T, Paika V, Almyroudi A, Kampletsas EO, Pavlidis N. Personality variables as predictors of early non-metastatic colorectal cancer patients' psychological distress and health-related quality of life: a one-year prospective study. J Psychosom Res 2011; 70: 411-21.

[9] Patel D, Sharpe L, Thewes B, Bell ML, Clarke S. Using the Distress Thermometer and Hospital Anxiety and Depression Scale to screen for psychosocial morbidity in patients diagnosed with colorectal cancer. J Affect Disord 2011; 131: 412-6.

[10] Medeiros M, Oshima CT, Forones NM. Depression and anxiety in colorectal cancer patients. J Gastrointest Cancer 2010; 41: 179-84.

[11] Alacacioglu A, Binicier O, Gungor O, Oztop I, Dirioz M, Yilmaz U. Quality of life, anxiety, and depression in Turkish colorectal cancer patients. Support Care Cancer 2010; 18: 417-21.

[12] Lynch BM, Steginga SK, Hawkes AL, Pakenham KI, Dunn J. Describing and predicting psychological distress after colorectal cancer. Cancer 2008; 112: 1363-70.

[13] Pugliese P, Perrone M, Nisi E, Garufi C, Giannarelli D, Bottomley A, Terzoli E. An integrated psychological strategy for advanced colorectal cancer patients Health Qual Life Outcomes 2006; 4: 9.

[14] Zabora J, BrintzenhofeSzoc K, Curbow B, Hooker C, Piantadosi S. The prevalence of psychological distress by cancer site. Psychooncology 2001; 10: 19-28.

[15] Foley KM. The treatment of cancer pain. N Engl J Med 1985; 313: 84-95.

[16] Tanaka K, Akechi T, Okuyama T, Nishiwaki Y, Uchitomi Y. Factors correlated with dyspnea in advanced lung cancer patients: organic causes and what else? J Pain Symptom Manage 2002; 23: 490-500.

[17] Okuyama T, Tanaka K, Akechi T, Kugaya A, Okamura H, Nishiwaki Y, Hosaka T, Uchitomi Y. Fatigue in ambulatory patients with advanced lung cancer: prevalence, correlated factors, and screening. J Pain Symptom Manage 2001; 22: 554-64.

[18] Minagawa H, Uchitomi Y, Yamawaki S, Ishitani K. Psychiatric morbidity in terminally ill cancer patients. A prospective study. Cancer 1996; 78: 1131-7.

[19] Chochinov HM, Wilson KG, Enns M, Mowchun N, Lander S, Levitt M, Clinch JJ. Desire for death in the terminally ill. Am J Psychiatry 1995; 152: 1185-91.

[20] Harrison J, Maguire P: Predictors of psychiatric morbidity in cancer patients. Br J Psychiatry 165: 593-598, 1994

[21] Massie MJ, Popkin MK. Depressive disorders. In: Holland JC. (ed.) Psycho-Oncology. New York: Oxford University Press; 1998, p518-540.

[22] Chochinov HM, Wilson KG, Enns M, Lander S. "Are you depressed?" Screening for depression in the terminally ill. Am J Psychiatry 1997; 154: 674-6.

[23] Bruera E, Miller L, McCallion J, Macmillan K, Krefting L, Hanson J. Cognitive failure in patients with terminal cancer: a prospective study. J Pain Symptom Manage 1992; 7: 192-5.

[24] Epstein R, Street RL Jr. Patient-Centered Communication in Cancer Care: Promoting Healing and Reducing Suffering. http://outcomes.cancer.gov/areas/pcc/communication/pcc_monograph.pdf. (accessed 1 December 2012).

[25] Ramirez AJ, Graham J, Richards MA, Cull A, Gregory WM, Leaning MS, Snashall DC, Timothy AR. Burnout and psychiatric disorder among cancer clinicians. Br J Cancer 1995; 71: 1263-9.

[26] Fallowfield L, Lipkin M, Hall A. Teaching senior oncologists communication skills: results from phase I of a comprehensive longitudinal program in the United Kingdom. J Clin Oncol 1998; 16: 1961-8.

[27] Cegala DJ, Lenzmeier Broz S. Physician communication skills training: a review of theoretical backgrounds, objectives and skills. Med Educ 2002; 36: 1004-16.

[28] Rao JK, Anderson LA, Inui TS, Frankel RM. Communication interventions make a difference in conversations between physicians and patients: a systematic review of the evidence. Med Care 2007; 45: 340-9.

[29] Uitterhoeve RJ, Bensing JM, Grol RP, Demulder PH, VAN Achterberg T. The effect of communication skills training on patient outcomes in cancer care: a systematic review of the literature. Eur J Cancer Care (Engl) 2010; 19: 442-57.

[30] Barth J, Lannen P. Efficacy of communication skills training courses in oncology: a systematic review and meta-analysis. Ann Oncol 2011; 22: 1030-40.

[31] Kissane DW, Bylund CL, Banerjee SC, Bialer PA, Levin TT, Maloney EK, D'Agostino TA. Communication skills training for oncology professionals. J Clin Oncol 2012; 30: 1242-7